Management in Laboratory Medicine

Third Edition

Management in Laboratory Medicine

Third Edition

Edited by

John R. Snyder, PhD
Professor and Dean
Louisiana State University Medical Center
School of Allied Health Professions
New Orleans, Louisiana

David S. Wilkinson, MD, PhD
Professor of Pathology and Health
  Administration
Medical College of Virginia
Chairman, Department of Pathology
Richmond, Virginia

with 36 contributors

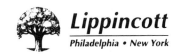

Lippincott
Philadelphia • New York

Acquisitions Editor: Lawrence McGrew
Assistant Editor: Holly Chapman
Project Editor: Sandra Cherrey Scheinin
Production Manager: Helen Ewan
Production Coordinator: Nannette Winsky and Michael Carcel
Design Coordinator: Nicholas Rook

Third Edition

9 8 7 6 5 4 3 2 1

Library of Congress Cataloging-in-Publications Data

Management in laboratory medicine / edited by John R. Snyder, David S.
  Wilkinson ; with 36 contributors. —3rd ed.
        p.   cm.
    Includes bibliographical references and index.
    ISBN 0-397-55149-5 (alk. paper)
      1. Medical laboratories—Management. I. Snyder, John R.
  II. Wilkinson, David S.   III. Title: Administration and supervision
  in laboratory medicine
  RB36.3.F55M36   1998
  616.07′56′068—dc21   97-36108
                                                            CIP

Care has been taken to confirm the accuracy of the information presented and to describe generally accepted practices. However, the authors, editors, and publisher are not responsible for errors or omissions or for any consequences from application of the information in this book and make no warranty, express or implied, with respect to the contents of the publication.

The authors, editors and publisher have exerted every effort to ensure that drug selection and dosage set forth in this text are in accordance with current recommendations and practice at the time of publication. However, in view of ongoing research, changes in government regulations, and the constant flow of information relating to drug therapy and drug reactions, the reader is urged to check the package insert for each drug for any change in indications and dosage and for added warnings and precautions. This is particularly important when the recommended agent is a new or infrequently employed drug.

Some drugs and medical devices presented in this publication have Food and Drug Administration (FDA) clearance for limited use in restricted research settings. It is the responsibility of the health care provider to ascertain the FDA status of each drug or device planned for use in their clinical practice.

⊗ This Paper Meets the Requirements of ANSI/NISO Z39.48-1992
(Permanence of Paper).

This book is dedicated, on behalf of all contributing authors:

first, to our teachers, under whose initial guidance we sought to become administrators, supervisors, consultants, and proponents of quality laboratory medicine;

second, to our students, whose questions prompted serious investigation of the management literature in search of practical application to the clinical laboratory; and

finally, to our spouses and families, without whose support and understanding this writing would not have reached completion.

In addition, this third edition is specially dedicated to three earlier contributors who in passing from this world left a legacy of leadership in laboratory medicine:

Arthur L. Larsen, MD, co-editor of the first edition and delegation chapter author; M. Robert Hicks, BS, MT(ASCP), safety chapter author; and Bettina G. Martin, MS, MBA, staffing and scheduling chapter author.

Contributing Authors

Lucia M. Berte, MA, MT(ASCP)SBB, DLM, CQA(ASQ)
Quality Systems Consultant
Elmhurst, Illinois

Rohn J. Butterfield, MBA
Administrator
University Operations and Ambulatory Services
University Hospital
Cincinnati, Ohio

Gary B. Clark, MD, MPA
Clinical Professor of Pathology
The George Washington University School of
    Medicine
Washington, DC

Janie Brown Crane, BS, MT(ASCP)
Kalaheo, Hawaii

John S. Davis, MBA, MT(ASCP)SC, DLM
Assistant Professor/Program Director
Department of Medical Technology
School of Allied Health Professions
Louisiana State University Medical Center
Shreveport, Louisiana

Justin Doheny, MHA
President
Wayne General Hospital
Wayne, New Jersey

David J. Fine, MHA
Vice Chancellor
Tulane University Medical Center
Columbia/HCA
New Orleans, Louisiana

David W. Glenn, BA, MT(ASCP)
Laboratory Consultant
Pathology Services, P.C.
North Platte, Nebraska

Sharon S. Gutterman, PhD
President, Alley Oop Group
The Ohio State University College of Medicine
Columbus, Ohio

Carolyn C. Hart, MS, MT(ASCP)
Administrative Site Director
Community Health Plan of Ohio
Knox Community Hospital
Mount Vernon, Ohio

Bonnie R. Hendrix, MS, MT(ASCP)
Laboratory Director
Northside Hospital
St. Petersburg, Florida

Edward A. Johnson, PhD
Professor of Management
University of North Florida
Jacksonville, Florida

Anthony S. Kurec, MS, H(ASCP)DLM
Associate Technical Director of Laboratory Services
University Hospital
State University of New York
Health Science Center
Syracuse, New York

Daniel I. Labowitz, AB, JD, MFS, EMT-P
Emergency Medical Services Administrator
Monroe County, New York

John A. Lott, PhD
Professor of Pathology
The Ohio State University
Director of Clinical Chemistry
The Ohio State University Medical Center
Columbus, Ohio

Peggy Printz Luebbert, MS, MT(ASCP), CIC
Risk Management Specialist
Alegent Health
Bergan Mercy Medical Center
Omaha, Nebraska

Diana Mass, MA, MT(ASCP), CLS (NCA)
Clinical Professor and Director
Clinical Laboratory Sciences Program
Department of Microbiology
College of Liberal Arts and Sciences
Arizona State University
Tempe, Arizona

Richard L. Moore III, EdD
Vice Chancellor for Development and University
    Relations
University of North Carolina at Greensboro
Greensboro, North Carolina

Pennell C. Painter, PhD
Director, Clinical Chemistry
University of Tennessee Memorial Hospital
Pathology Department
Knoxville, Tennessee

Barbara L. Parsons, PhD
Assistant Professor of Management
Division of Commerce
Fairmont State College
Fairmont, West Virginia

Richard B. Passey, MT (ASCP) PhD
Professor and Director
Clinical Chemistry and Microbiology
University of Oklahoma
Health Sciences Center
Oklahoma City, Oklahoma

Susan E. Perkins, MHS, CLS, (NCA)
Coordinator, Point of Care Testing
Baystate Medical Center
Springfield, Massachusetts

Barbara C. Salmon
Columbia/HCA
New Orleans, Louisiana

Dietrich L. Schaupp, DBA
Professor of Management
College of Business and Economics
West Virginia University
Morgantown, West Virginia

James Sharp, MD
Pathologist
Arlington Heights, Illinois

Walton H. Sharp
Labor and Industrial Relations
Denton, Texas

Jack W. Smith, Jr., MD, PhD
Director of Medical Informatics
Associate Professor of Pathology and Computer and
    Information Sciences
The Ohio State University
Columbus, Ohio

John R. Snyder, PhD, MT(ASCP)SH
Dean and Professor
School of Allied Health Professions
Louisiana State University Medical Center
New Orleans, Louisiana

Thomas M. Sodeman, MD, FCAP
Medical Director
Alliance Laboratory Services
Cincinnati, Ohio

Carl Speicher, MD
Director, Clinical Services
Professor and Vice-Chair, Department of Pathology
The Ohio State University
Columbus, Ohio

John R. Svirbley, MD
Department of Pathology
McCullough-Hyde Memorial Hospital
Oxford, Ohio

Diana W. Voorhees, MA, CLS, MT, SH
Principal
DV and Associates
Salt Lake City, Utah

David S. Wilkinson, MD, PhD
Professor of Pathology and Health Administration
Chairman, Department of Pathology
Medical College of Virginia
Virginia Community University
Richmond, Virginia

Stephen L. Wilson, PhD
Director and Associate Professor
School of Allied Medical Professions
The Ohio State University
Columbus, Ohio

Jana Wilson Wolfgang, MS, MT(ASCP)
Wolfgang Associates
Portland, Oregon

Kenneth Wolfgang, MS, MT(ASCP)
Wolfgang Associates
Portland, Oregon

Preface

The success of any organization in meeting its goals and objectives depends largely on the quality of management within the organization. Management of medical laboratory services is no exception. The provision of quality laboratory analyses and efficient reporting of data rely heavily on the application of sound principles of administration and supervision.

The field of laboratory medicine has been slower than some other health services in acknowledging the need for administrative personnel with managerial preparation. While appropriate degrees and professional certification are a fairly reliable index of the laboratorian's technical competence, these alone do not ensure that the individual has the ability to manage. Quite often the challenges to stay abreast of our rapidly changing technology has received a higher priority than the development of managerial skills. This dilemma is compounded because few authors have applied solid principles of management to administration of the clinical laboratory. The purpose of this text, therefore, is to bridge the gap between the theory of management and its application in the clinical laboratory setting.

Nearly a decade has elapsed since publication of the second edition of *Administration and Supervision in Laboratory Medicine*. During this time, the health-care industry has experienced dramatic changes in philosophy, size, structure, and payment mechanisms for health-service providers. Organizational hierarchies in the laboratory have also changed, prompting a broader involvement of laboratorians in day-to-day operations and management. Hence, we've titled the work, *Management in Laboratory Medicine*. At a time when medical knowledge and diagnostic technology are at an all-time high, clinical laboratory managers face tremendous challenges to meet both demands of consumers of laboratory services and expectations of technical staff in a cost-containment environment.

This third edition of the text retains most of the distinguishing features of the earlier editions. These include an emphasis on the centrality of the laboratory manager's role in achieving organizational goals and objectives; the importance of understanding the responsibility of the manager for maximizing the human, physical, and financial resources entrusted to his care; and the frequent use of examples and case studies to demonstrate the practical utility of management theory. In light of the many changes in healthcare and laboratory services delivery during the past decade, this third edition features new chapters on laboratory regulations, certification, and accreditation; making the transition to laboratory management; clinical laboratory design and refurbishment; quality management; managing point-of-care testing; consulting to physician office laboratories; assessing laboratory operating performance using the Laboratory Management Index Program (LMIP); and laboratory billing and reimbursement management. In addition, most chapters have been updated to reflect state-of-the-art laboratory management theory and practice. The net result is, we believe, a text that is interesting, readable, and relevant.

The text is directed to the basic-through-intermediate levels of management. It is written primarily for upper-division undergraduate students and postbaccalaureate medical technology students, graduate students in the clinical laboratory sciences and pathology, and pathology residents preparing for managerial roles in the medical laboratory. Because many laboratorians achieve management positions without the benefit of formal education in organizational theory and practice, this book will also be useful as a reference to practicing laboratory managers and pathologists. Its major function is to provide a resource that explores basic principles and develops them into viable managerial processes within the context of the clinical laboratory.

The first two chapters describe changes occurring in health care delivery, including the Clinical Laboratory Improvement Amendments of 1988 regulations.

The text is presented in five parts:

Part One consists of five chapters, which together address the fundamentals of managerial practice in the laboratory setting. The managerial functions of planning, organizing, and controlling are introduced, as well as decision making and problem solving. This is followed by a chapter assigned to help a laboratorian make the transition to management.

Part Two includes six chapters that focus on the concepts of managerial leardership—the human side of the directing function of laboratory administrators and supervisors. Separate chapters address managerial assumptions and their effects on motivation, communications within the laboratory organization, leadership styles and group effectiveness, employee-involvement work groups, effective meeting techniques, and the management of conflict and change.

Part Three, which focuses on processes in personnel administration, dicusses the practical procedures useful in the labor-intensive clinical laboratory setting. Considerations of interviewing techniques and employee selection are followed by a discussion of job descriptions and methods for staffing and scheduling. The focus then shifts to performance appraisal in the clinical setting and the preservice, inservice, and continuing education responsibilities of laboratory managers and supervisors. Because the context of personnel administration changes somewhat in the laboratory under union contract, a separate chapter is devoted to this subject.

Part Four includes twelve chapters dealing with essential managerial activities for effective laboratory operation. Several chapters address the physical resources and related processes entrusted to the manager: laboratory design and refurbishment, computers and laboratory information systems, and preventive maintenance for laboratory instrumentation. A separate chapter covers the basics of clinical laboratory safety and OSHA guidelines. Other chapters deal with managing quality in laboratory services and process control and method evaluation. In recognition of laboratory medicine's extension beyond the physical confines of the laboratory, separate chapters address managing point-of-care testing, consulting to physician office laboratories, and marketing of clinical laboratory services. Finally, external and internal control and evaluation of laboratory operations are described in terms of laboratory regulation, certification, and accreditation; assessing operating performance using the LMIP; quality management; and medicolegal concerns in laboratory medicine.

Part Five consists of seven chapters concerned with the principles of laboratory finance. The financial operation of the clinical laboratory is introduced, followed by a discussion of budgeting practices, cost accounting, billing and reimbursement management, wage and salary administration, and financial ratios for decision making as management tools. The last chapter deals with cost containment through inventory control techniques.

The text reflects the special expertise of 36 different contributors. We have been fortunate to work with such talented colleagues. We have not eliminated all redundancy or repetition among chapters; rather this has been encouraged when the effectiveness of a given topic was enhanced by such duplication of concepts.

Because managerial titles and responsibilities vary in laboratory medicine, the terms *director, administrator,* and *supervisor* are often used interchangeably to refer to the individuals with managerial responsibility, regardless of institutional title. The terms *subordinates* and *staff* refer to the group of individuals for whom the manager is responsible. The reader should also recognize that throughout the text ''his'' also means ''hers'' and ''he'' also means ''she.''

Special thanks are due Larry McGrew, Holly Chapman, and Sandra Cherrey Scheinin of the Lippincott-Raven organization for their editorial guidance and assistance, encouragement, and understanding. Cherry Lua-Undag, Debbie Justrabo, Lajuana Finigan, and Corie Rogers also deserve special appreciation for assistance in preparing the manuscript.

John R. Snyder, PhD
David S. Wilkinson, MD, PhD

Contents

Chapter 35

Inventory Management and Cost Containment   549

John R. Snyder

Management in Laboratory Medicine

Third Edition

Fundamentals of Laboratory Management

1

The Nature of Management in Laboratory Medicine

John R. Snyder • David S. Wilkinson

The American health-care system is large, complex, and diverse.[25] In 1981, expenditures totaled $287 billion, comprising 9.8% of the nation's gross national product.[41] According to the Health Care Financing Administration (HCFA), total expenditures in 1995 reached an estimated $1 trillion, 14.2% of the gross domestic product and 7.4% above 1994 levels. Complexity in the system is reflected by a diversity of physician and non-physician providers, organized in a variety of ways—private, group practice, health maintenance organizations—and functioning in a variety of settings--different sizes of hospitals, clinics, nursing homes, outpatient facilities, and other agencies. In reaction to this growth and complexity, health-care delivery today is undergoing profound change.

The most significant change in health care has resulted from the widely held notion that health-care costs are out of control. Thus, the expansionary climate of the 1970s abruptly gave way to universal concerns about cost containment, and indeed, cost abatement

of health-care spending.[35] These concerns have been reflected by the cascade of federal legislation, including the Tax Equity and Fiscal Responsibility Act in 1982; the introduction of prospective payment systems (PPSs), including diagnosis-related groups (DRGs), in 1983; and the Medicare provisions in the Budget Reduction Act of 1984. In 1985, the Comprehensive Omnibus Budget Reconciliation Act and the 1986 Omnibus Budget Reconciliation Act placed even greater fiscal constraints on hospitals.[34] The 1990s brought about resource-based relative value units, a complex reimbursement program for physicians that is based on overall work effort, including the correlation of multiple disciplines of medicine.[40] Not only has the public sector been concerned with cost containment, American industry, which spent an average of $3,821 per employee in health benefits costs in 1995, also has lent its support to cost-containment measures. For more than 10 years, health-care providers have found themselves in a seri-

1

ous adversarial position with government *and* industry and with third-party insurers.[30]

It is estimated that the overall size of the laboratory medicine industry is $30 to $35 billion.[31] The clinical laboratory industry consists of three major types of laboratories:

Hospital laboratories: $15 billion to $17.5 billion in revenue contribution (50% of total)
Physician office laboratories: $7 billion to $8.5 billion in revenue contribution (24% of total)
Independent laboratories: $8 billion to $9.5 billion in revenue contribution (26% of total)

Under the Clinical Laboratory Improvement Amendments of 1988 (CLIA '88), laboratories must hold a certificate for operation. This CLIA database provides important demographic information about the U.S. laboratory industry. In 1995, about 152,000 HCFA certificates were current, representing approximately 160,000 testing sites. Self-reported data from the HCFA registration process in 1992 enabled the Centers for Disease Control and Prevention (CDC) to estimate that approximately 4.2 billion tests were performed in that year. Clearly, laboratory medicine is a major component of health-care costs and a complex industry in its own right.

Perhaps the most significant change affecting hospital laboratory management today began with the advent of PPSs. Under PPS regulation, a lump sum payment is made to most hospitals for Medicare admissions that is based not on the actual cost of the services provided, but rather on the discharge diagnosis. Under this system, all discharges are classified or grouped under DRGs, with payment based on a predetermined amount for each DRG. Before the introduction of this system, clinical laboratories were considered revenue-generating centers in the hospital budget, because at least a portion of the costs to perform tests was reimbursable. Under PPS, each test performed becomes a cost charged against the lump sum payment for the DRG; hence, the laboratory is now a *cost center* for the hospital. With the full implementation of the PPS, well-managed laboratories that were profit centers and primarily concerned with high levels of service and quality have become loss leaders to the hospitals. *Cost containment* and *competition* have become the watchwords of laboratory medicine in the 1980s and 1990s.

This new climate of socioeconomic and regulatory restraint has put significant stresses on laboratory management. Cost-effective delivery of laboratory services rests more firmly than ever on the sound practice of administration and supervision, as described by McLendon and Reich:[24]

The efficient operation of a clinical laboratory and the effective delivery of medical laboratory services

to clinicians and their patients require a complex interdigitation of expertise in medical, scientific, and technical areas. . . . Although the medical, scientific, and technical expertise . . . are essential prerequisite(s) for the provision of medical laboratory services, success in applying these techniques to benefit patient care is vitally dependent on the management and communication skills of laboratory directors, supervisors, and technologists.

This concept may be criticized by those who contend that administration is an ancillary activity and that quality laboratory services result directly from the performance of competent laboratory scientists; however, the key element of a successful operation lies in the delivery of such services, a highly complex management activity. Laboratory management's task is to integrate and coordinate organizational resources (eg, personnel, equipment, money, time, and space) so that quality laboratory services can be provided as effectively and efficiently as possible. The successful administration of today's clinical laboratory, like any other organization or institution, requires a vast array of skills founded on sound principles of management science.

STRATEGIC VISION: A PARADIGM SHIFT AND RESULTING TRENDS

The challenge to exercise management science skills in laboratory medicine today is prompted by the major transformation occurring in health-care delivery. Health-care delivery is undergoing a re-engineering unlike any change in history. Industry in the United States experienced a similar re-engineering when competition from Japan and other nations threatened market share. For health care overall and clinical laboratories in particular, re-engineering has been embraced for the same reason—a basic strategy for organizational survival.[37]

Strategic Vision

Laboratories are stewards of the future of laboratory medicine. As such, both managers and practitioners must have a sense of threats and opportunities posed by the future and a strategic vision of laboratory medicine in the 21st century.[3] Key to developing a strategic vision is an understanding of both the external and internal environment (Fig. 1-1). Threats of and opportunities for change occurring in a transforming external environment need to be identified; strengths and weaknesses within an organization need to be detailed. The strategic direction of the laboratory needs to be care-

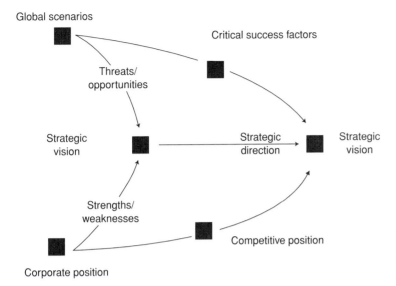

Global scenarios

Critical success factors

Threats/
opportunities

Strategic
vision

Strategic
direction

Strategic
vision

Strengths/
weaknesses

Competitive position

Corporate position

FIGURE 1-1. The role of strategic vision. (Bezold C: The future of healthcare: Implications in the allied health professions. J Allied Health 18:438, 1989)

fully planned to take advantage of critical success factors and secure the organization's competitive position.

Box 1-1 shows the results of a Delphi study conducted in collaboration with the CDC. It defines the major forces of change (both external and internal) impacting laboratory medicine in the next 5 years and changes likely to occur in research and quality assurance.

These statements about the future should help to create a vision. Figure 1-1 incorporates the essential elements of strategic planning (see Chapter 3). A *vision* is a description of the laboratory's preferred future state. It describes the ideal future, a blueprint of sorts, of the laboratory organization you will build or change and the results that will be achieved. A vision embraces the laboratory's mission and stakeholders, is as a long-term planning target, and is a measure of progress. Following is some sage advice from the many authors who have noted the importance of strategic vision: "There is one universal rule of planning: you will never be greater than the vision that guides you." To be an effective laboratory manager, one must have the ability to create a vision.

Tensions and Trends in the Changing Health-Care System

The reengineering of health care has been described by many observers. One version of the tensions shaping the system is shown in Table 1-1 as detailed by the Health Professions Commission of the Pew Foundation.[26] These are "broad brush strokes" in the dynamic environment. Some authors would label the left column "the old paradigm" and the column at the other end of

the arrow "new." In fact, these are not entirely unidirectional; there is a clear "tension" between these entities. The resulting organizational trends have particular importance for those who manage the delivery of health-care services, such as laboratory medicine.

The change from specialized care to primary care has signaled a new era for the gatekeepers of health services. Less specialization, increased use of generalists in laboratory practice, core laboratories, and other strategies are consistent with the *restructuring* and *reengineering* trends occurring in clinical laboratories.[38]

For decades, health-care value has been technology driven. The shift to care that is more client focused has in part spawned *patient-focused care* and point-of-care testing.[39] There is an increased emphasis within the health-care community to be sensitive to *client satisfaction*. For the laboratory manager, this prompts a definition of who our clients or customers are: patients, visitors, families, physicians, employees, third-party payers, referral groups, vendors, trustees, volunteers, community groups, and other departments using laboratory services. Although the most important group will always be the patients, the laboratory as a *service organization* must understand the needs and expectations of all its customers.

The shift to being cost accountable calls for an *economic alignment* of the value of laboratory services with the funds available. This typically means being aware of what constitutes costs and searching for cost-reduction measures, such as centralizing services, eliminating unnecessary testing, providing faster turnaround time, reducing personnel costs through increased flexi-

Box 1•1

Vision of the Future of Laboratory Practice: A Delphi Study

Which forces of change will have the greatest impact on the nature and quality of clinical laboratory medicine in the next 5 years?

1. Cost containment
2. Medical informatics in health care
3. Shift to managed care
4. Laboratory automation and robotics
5. Industry consolidation
6. Changes in the work force

How will clinical laboratory testing and delivery of service change in the next 5 years?

1. There will be fewer laboratories, fewer skilled positions, and more automation.
2. "Mega" laboratories will provide the majority of services and take advantage of economies of scale.
3. Networks will be the norm.
4. Point-of-care testing will replace traditional laboratory systems.
5. The standard will be lowest cost at the fastest turnaround time.
6. Clinical utility will displace current standards of acceptable accuracy.

What will be the impact of these changes on research in laboratory medicine?

1. Increased requirement for outcomes to prove medical efficacy
2. More directed, less basic research
3. Research and development that is industry based and focused on automation and molecular diagnosis
4. Profit-oriented test development

What will be the nature of clinical laboratory quality assurance?

1. Interdepartmental
2. Include clinical pathways
3. Outcomes based and patient based
4. Expert/smart systems based
5. Include real time monitors
6. Integrated and seen as a process issue
7. Standardized through benchmarking with other laboratories

bility and enhanced productivity, changing work flow by increasing automation, and standardizing tests ordered, testing techniques, and reporting.

The shift away from institution-focused care to ambulatory or community care has prompted *decentralized services* and *integration* of disparate delivery systems. Vertical integration is accomplished when services for a patient are coordinated within a given episode of illness or across episodes of illness. Horizontal integration occurs when services for a group of patients are coordinated across operating units. This shift also has led to geographic coverage (ie, access to care throughout a city or region).

Decisions about health care, once the sole domain of professionals, have recently shifted to more managerial governance in the form of managed care. This is an example of a tension that appears to be moving back toward the "old paradigm" but with new attributes like *benchmarking*[16] and *performance indicators* as newly adopted managerial tools.

An observation of what type of care should be rendered has led to the shifts toward chronic care, a population perspective on the appropriateness of care, and disease prevention/health promotion. *Cost containment* is a pervasive trend for each of these shifts, which have led to new emphasis on *clinical outcomes assessment,*[4,12,43] *patient care plans,* and *wellness and total care.*

Health-care work has shifted from content mastery to process mastery, from individual provider to team provider, and regulation of skills has led to trends of *systems thinking*[11] and *learning organizations,*[11] *self-directed teams,* and *multiskilled providers.*[2,5,9]

The once highly competitive delivery environment has shifted to cooperation between former rivals, resulting in *consolidations, mergers, partnerships* and *acquisitions.*

These trends, now in place, will most likely shape the future. The modern laboratory manager will need to accommodate or adapt to these trends in varying combinations to help the institution successfully survive.[29] Figure 1-2 illustrates a view of the plausible futures. Successful managers will temper their strategic vision to look beyond the current trends and project various scenarios that could alter the future of laboratory medicine. For example, with continued shrinkage of reimbursement dollars, will the institution likely opt for outsourcing more clinical testing? Is a likely scenario one in which managed care becomes convinced of the value of screening procedures (hence encouraging more and reimbursing more), prompting an increase in volume? An understanding of the environment and trends is crucial for effective laboratory management.

Table 1-1
Tensions and Trends in the Changing Health-Care System

Tensions Shaping the System*			Resulting Organizational Trends
Specialized care	⟵⟶	Primary care	Health services gatekeepers, restructuring, re-engineering
Technologically driven	⟵⟶	Humanely balanced	Patient-focused care, client satisfaction
Cost unaware	⟵⟶	Cost accountable	Economic alignment
Institution focused	⟵⟶	Ambulatory/community focused	Integrated delivery systems, decentralized services
Professionally governed	⟵⟶	Managerially governed	Benchmarking, performance indicators
Acute care	⟵⟶	Chronic care	Cost containment
Individual patient	⟵⟶	Population perspective	Clinical outcomes assessment, patient care plans
Curative care	⟵⟶	Preventive orientation	Wellness and total care
Content master	⟵⟶	Process mastery	Systems thinking, learning organizations
Individual provider	⟵⟶	Team provider	Self-directed teams
Competition	⟵⟶	Cooperation	Consolidations, mergers, partnerships, acquisitions
Current regulation	⟵⟶	Re-regulation	Multiskilled providers

* Source: Pew Health Professions Commission

ADMINISTRATION—ART OR SCIENCE?

Laboratory professionals are often reluctant to consider management as a science. Our educational background, laden with courses in the exacting sciences of chemistry, physics, and biology, tends to bias our acceptance of the disciplines we allow to be classified as a science. Our laboratory activities, incumbent on Gaussian statistics and predictive diagnostic value, create a mindset limiting the parameters by which we judge the "true" sciences.

Administration can, however, qualify as a science comparable to economics, psychology, and sociology, in that there exists an organized body of knowledge

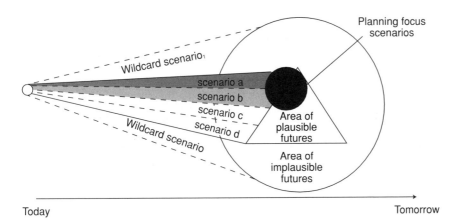

FIGURE 1-2. Focus on plausible futures. (US House of Representatives. Committee on Energy and Commerce: *Foresight in the Private Sector: How Can Government Use It?* Report of the Foresight Task Force, January 1983)

unique to the domain. Koontz and O'Donnel proposed more than 50 truths or principles to define the science of administration.[18] The search for professionalism in management led to the excesses of the secular-rationalist approach to management in the 1960s,[27] which attempted to discard the human element from management science, because "human behavior complicates immensely the task of explaining and predicting phenomena."[32]

Administration is indeed a science that, like its sister disciplines psychology and sociology, is inexact *because* it must deal to a large extent with the human element. Thus, any proposed principles of administration will be characterized by some softness and variability due to human behavior in the organization. The new wave of management theory, expressed by Peters and Waterman,[27] recognizes the variability and change that human relations bring to the science of administration.

Any proposed principles for the study of administration will be characterized by variables and change. All science is dynamic. We are more accepting of the fact that laboratory medicine as a science is constantly changing as research continues to push back the frontier of the unknown. Likewise, the science of administration continues to change as the variables inherent in the management process stimulate research and modification of generalizations into new knowledge.

Still other laboratory professionals perceive administration as an art, requiring only native ability or common sense. Art by definition is creative adaptation, and a component of the management process does require native ability. In the practice of laboratory medicine, decisions are often contingent on the specific situation. The art inherent in laboratory medicine is the application of knowledge based on perceived contingencies. In management, it is the skill that comes with experience, observation, and study of the situation.

Administration, therefore, can be considered both a science and an art. The management process requires the art of creativity based on and conditioned by an understanding of the principles of management science.

DEFINITION OF ADMINISTRATION

In this book, the terms *administration* and *management* are used interchangeably. Administration of the clinical laboratory is generally viewed as an all-inclusive concept covering the managerial skills necessary for personnel from the laboratory director to the bench supervisor. At all levels, management involves the coordination and integration of resources to accomplish spe-cific results. Management has been viewed differently by many authorities, and their various perceptions, schools of managerial thought, and experiences have resulted in nearly as many definitions as there are people who have attempted to define the term. Included are definitions such as the following:

"The process by which individual and group effort is coordinated toward superordinate goals"
"A social process comprising a series of actions that lead to the accomplishment of objectives"
"Getting from where we are to where we want to be with the least expenditure of time, money, and effort"
"The universal process of efficiently getting activities completed with and through other people"[1,18,32,33]

The most universally accepted definition bantered about has been simply "getting things done through other people." This is a fine rule for the practicing manager but leaves something to be desired from the academician's point of view. When a joint meeting was called with the primary purpose of defining *management* in terms on which the educators and executives could both agree, the following definition resulted:[1]

Management is the guiding of human and physical resources into dynamic organization units that attain their objectives to the satisfaction of those served and with a high degree of morale and sense of attainment on the part of those rendering the service.

Box 1·2

Elements of Management

Toward objectives—goals and purposes consistent with efficient delivery of laboratory services for quality health care

Through people—guiding people (leading and directing) in such a manner that these professional laboratorians feel a sense of responsibility and attainment (achievement)

Using techniques—physical resources, such as laboratory equipment, computers, and space

In an organization—into dynamic organizational units implying division of labor, specialization, protocols and procedures, and functional processing units

This definition is perhaps a bit flowery, but it is a place to begin and a measuring stick for evaluation. The definition contains four basic elements identified by Kast and Rosenzweig:[14]   (1) "toward objectives," (2) "through people," (3) "using techniques," and (4) "in an organization." The definition proposed by the educators and executives in Box 1-2 is the most comprehensive and perhaps the best working model for the clinical laboratory.

It must be pointed out that management is an activity. It is not letting each day take care of itself; rather, it is making things happen. Too often laboratory managers fall into the trap of "fighting fires" on a daily basis. For administration to be effective, it must be in control, planning ahead the steps that will ensure efficient operation of the laboratory.

MANAGEMENT: A SYSTEMS PERSPECTIVE

Given the amount of change occurring in health-care delivery, it is important for managers to adopt a systems view or "systems thinking" approach. *Systems thinking* is seeing all the interrelated effects of actions and their consequences on other components or in the future. The goal is to understand dynamic complexity and cause and effect of actions and decisions.[11]

A *system* can be defined as a set of interrelated and interdependent parts designed to achieve specific goals. Figure 1-3 is a systems conceptual model showing interrelationships among inputs, conversion processes, and outputs or outcomes.

Figure 1-4 graphically illustrates a definition of administration using a systems model.[32] Laboratory managers are entrusted with three categories of resources

(input): *financial*—operating and capital budget; *physical*—space, equipment, and supplies; and *human*—technical and support staff. As a result of the managerial role and fulfilling certain functions (ie, planning, organizing, leading, and evaluating), three categories of output are expected: *satisfactory performance*—accurate and timely testing in a cost-effective manner; *products*—legible and interpretable laboratory reports to the physician when needed; and *self-serving behavior*—a sense of accomplishment among the staff doing the work. Note also that many external and organizational forces influence the administrative process in any institution.

A systems perspective should be used to look at the function of the clinical laboratory, that is, provision of laboratory information (Fig. 1-5). On the input side, the attending physician makes *a priori* clinical diagnoses based on the patient's history and physical examination. The *a priori* diagnosis is subject to error, and laboratory information is requested to make a more accurate (higher probability) *a posteriori* diagnosis (output). If the laboratory manager views only the steps included in the laboratory under the "process" component, there is diminished value to the laboratory's function. Questions to be considered include the following: Was the right test ordered to provide maximum information? Was the correct sample acquired? Was there sufficient clinical information on the requisition to enable the laboratory to provide information rather than just data? Did the report contribute to the physician's decision making? Was the report understandable and correctly interpreted? Did the laboratory information contribute to the *a posteriori* diagnosis? Ultimately, what role did the laboratory information play in the patient's outcome?[43]

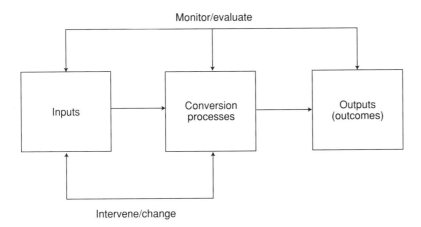

FIGURE 1-3. Basic systems model.

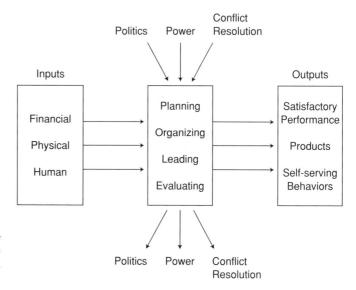

FIGURE 1-4. Advanced descriptive administrative model. (From Robbins SP: The Administrative Process, p 57. Englewood Cliffs, Prentice Hall, 1976; reprinted by permission of publisher)

Aspects of management beyond the global view shown in Figure 1-4 can also be viewed from a systems perspective. Figure 1-6 illustrates the interconnected elements of the human resource system. Poor performance at the time of a performance appraisal, for example, could necessitate retraining that might have been avoided if either different selection criteria were in place or a more comprehensive orientation provided.

One final example of a systems view is shown in Figure 1-7. This figure shows the economic relationships between tests ordered and costs to produce laboratory testing.[15]

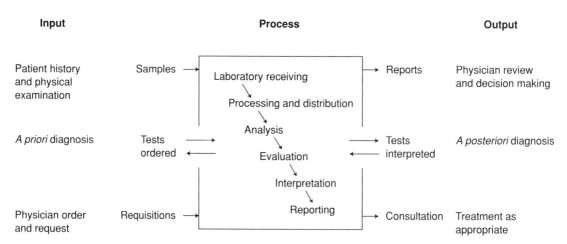

FIGURE 1-5. Laboratory information in clinical decision-making system.

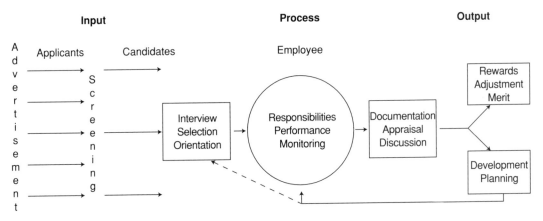

FIGURE 1-6. A systems view of the human resource cycle. (Adapted from Levy S, Loomba NP: Health Care Administration: A Managerial Perspective, 2nd ed. Philadelphia, J.B. Lippincott, 1984)

MANAGERIAL DUTIES AND RESPONSIBILITIES

The terms *director, administrator, manager,* and *supervisor* are sometimes used interchangeably. Comte and Lee have delineated each in the following manner:[6]

A *director* directs the affairs of an organization by establishing goals and priorities that determine the direction the organization will take. The director might not directly supervise or manage in a technical sense, because his role is primarily one of broad policy making.

An *administrator* administers or runs an organization within the framework of the various directives and policies given to him. Strictly speaking, he is not the person who establishes the larger goals, but a technician who knows how to make the organization move efficiently to achieve its purpose.

Input	Process	Output
Utilization	Operations	Finances
Test numbers $\longrightarrow$	Output $\longrightarrow$	Revenues
Test mix $\longrightarrow$	Input $\longrightarrow$	Expenses
	• Labor	Profits
	• Materials	
	• Equipment	

FIGURE 1-7. A systems view of economic relationships.

A *manager* takes charge of the management or oversees the functioning of an activity to achieve a set goal or purpose. His strength is in his ability to use all of these resources to get things done properly.

A *supervisor* oversees the activities of others to help them to accomplish specific tasks or to perform scheduled activities most efficiently.

There is considerable overlap in terms of duties and responsibilities among these members of the management team.[23] In the clinical laboratory, the administrative skills needed for each of these positions are largely the same. The differences rest in the amount of expertise that each member of the management team must possess. For example, the laboratory director will probably possess the greatest expertise in the overall function of the laboratory in the delivery of quality medical care; the manager, in inspection and accreditation; and the supervisor, in the technology, scheduling, and staffing of a given laboratory section.

There are several key concepts that enable distinction of three levels in the management team of the laboratory. *Laboratory directors* and *administrators* retain ultimate responsibility for seeing that the organization moves toward achievement of its goals. Changes in technology, capital investments, and services rendered are finalized by this level of laboratory management. *Laboratory managers,* sometimes termed *administrative* or *chief technologists,* create and maintain an environment designed so that other laboratory professionals can function efficiently. Laboratory managers plan, organize, direct, and control jobs. *Laboratory supervisors,* conversely, are managers whose major activities focus on people and operational provision of laboratory services. All levels of management have supervisory functions, but the first-line laboratory supervisor's major function is working with and through staff (bench-level) technologists and technicians to meet the needs of these employees and the objectives of the department.

It is noteworthy to comment on the key concept of *leader* versus *boss*. The clinical laboratory is staffed by individuals with a wide variety of backgrounds and educational preparation, from unit clerk through doctorate-level clinical associate. The cohesion of this group as a health-care team is essential for effective management. The clinical laboratory administrator is a manager of professionals. For this reason, the concept of supervisor as boss is inappropriate. Today's laboratory supervisor is a leader who promotes a climate of cooperation and respect so that the staff laboratorian will want to be led and possibly lead and direct himself.[17] One manages *things* but leads *people*.

Another important title distinction that some authors assert is the difference between a leader and a manager. Leaders are able to influence the attitudes and opinions of others in an organization; managers are able to influence actions and decisions. In this distinction, leadership is a higher order of capability.

THE ADMINISTRATIVE PROCESS

Laboratory management's task is to integrate and coordinate resources toward accomplishment of a goal. The task is thus a process composed of a series of actions, which some authors like to call the five functions of a manager. The effective use of input resources to achieve output through administrative functions is shown in Figure 1-8. Regardless of the title given the activities, the administrative process includes *planning, organizing, directing,* and *controlling*. These terms are introduced here as part of the process and are further discussed in later chapters.

Planning

A key function of managers at all levels is the planning of activities under their direction. In the medical laboratory, both long- and short-range plans are created. A laboratory director will probably be responsible for long-range planning concerned with growth potential or degree of expansion. For example, the director may want to bring in house a battery of analyses previously sent to a reference laboratory. His planning steps would include identifying sufficient equipment, space, and personnel; creating a series of written protocols and procedures; determining cost-per-test analysis; and so

forth. The laboratory director will no doubt involve the appropriate chief technologist and supervisor in some short-range planning. Short-range planning includes setting specific objectives to aid in reaching long-range goals. In this example, the supervisor may be responsible for planning a variety of steps to establish protocols and procedures (eg, method comparison research and development within the department, ordering of supplies and reagents, scheduling personnel based on the frequency with which the test is to be performed). All levels of laboratory management should be involved in various phases of both long- and short-range planning—a crucial activity in the administration process. Most management failure is due to a failure in communication.

Organizing

The organizing function involves developing a structure to facilitate the coordination of resources to achieve completion of long- and short-range plans. A division of labor is created in which various units or departments are responsible for particular activities or phases of operation. A spectrum of working relationships must then be delineated to include such things as lines of authority or responsibility and work flow for the optimal functioning of the interrelated units.

Directing

The directing function is best described as managerial leadership. Managers in the clinical laboratory, as in any organization, must be concerned with the human element. Successful managerial leadership creates a climate in which both the needs of the individual and the goals of the organization can be met. This most crucial managerial function and the parameters that increase or decrease its effectiveness are discussed more fully in Part 2 of this book.

Controlling

The wrap-up function in the administrative process is controlling, which ensures that the end-product of organized and directed events conforms to plans. Supervisors of the clinical laboratory are always aware of the importance of good quality control. In the administrative process, controlling is equally important and includes many of the same activities: defining standards and criteria for acceptable performance, developing a reporting system, and taking corrective action when and where needed.

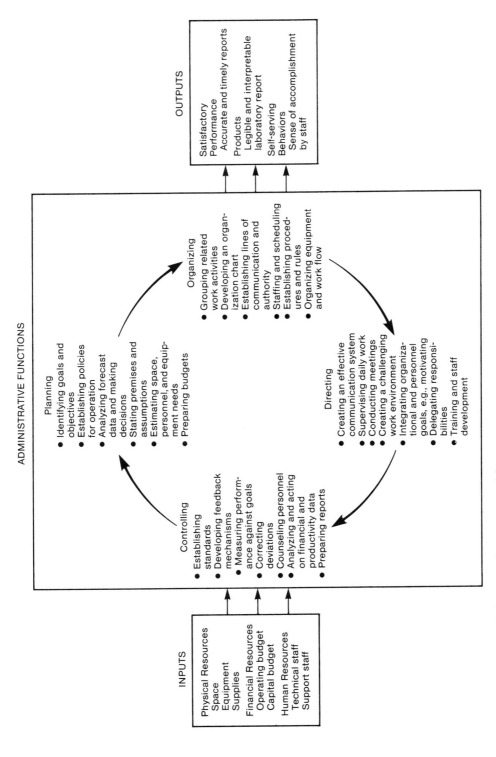

FIGURE 1–8. Clinical laboratory administration model.

Decision Making

An activity that is inherent in all other administrative process activities is decision making. This is the part of the process that ties everything together. Decisions must be made as part of planning, organizing, directing, and controlling. Because of its importance in all other process functions, we have devoted an entire chapter (Chapter 4) to the consideration of the decision-making process. Although many steps and concerns must be considered, the process itself generally includes problem analysis, development and analysis of alternative courses of action, and decision implementation and control.

The advent of prospective payment for reimbursement of laboratory services provided by hospitals has prompted top-level administration to scrutinize closely cost-effective management of clinical laboratories. As profit centers under cost reimbursement, clinical laboratories were allowed considerable latitude in their operations, and many laboratory administrators survived through the "cost be damned" attitude. Today, as a *cost* center, laboratory administrators must lead and manage. New skills under each of the traditional functions are now needed. As part of planning, for example, laboratory managers are called on to forecast accurately cost/benefit ratios, analyze new opportunities, and market to new entities, such as health maintenance organizations. When considering the laboratory's organization, managers must modify the structure for efficiency and redesign jobs, perhaps creating career ladders for technical staff. To increase productivity under the directing function, managers need to create a work environment characterized by responsibility and participative management. Under the controlling function, laboratory managers must implement cost-containment measures through reduction in overuse of testing, inventory control, and financial ratio analysis, a form of "economic grand rounds" in the laboratory.

THE TRANSITION TO LABORATORY MANAGEMENT

One of the most difficult hurdles for the new manager or supervisor is the transition from staff responsibilities to administrative responsibilities. This transition includes a shift in the focus from direct service responsibility to new relationships, new responsibilities of managing versus doing (delegation), and a new realm of influence (leadership; see Chapters 5 and 6).

Dual Hierarchy in Hospitals

Typical organizational hierarchies are bureaucratic pyramids (see Chapter 3) with specific lines of communication and authority. However, as hospitals developed over the last century, a unique governance structure evolved with them. The medical staff of the hospital (consisting of physicians with admitting privileges), who were the "users" of hospital services, including the laboratory, formed into a separate organization with an independent, but also an interdependent, relationship to the administrative structure of the hospital, thus creating a dual hierarchical structure. While the hospital administration was perceived to be primarily concerned with providing safe and efficient care for *all* of its patients, the major role of the medical staff was seen as ensuring the quality of care for the *individual* patient by controlling admission to the medical staff (credentialing) and the scope of privileges granted to a staff physician practicing within the hospital. The governance of the medical staff in its role of monitoring standards of medical practice within the institution was thought to be independent of the hospital administration and the governing board. The standards of performance of this dual hierarchy were mandated and monitored by outside accrediting agencies, such as the Joint Commission on Accreditation of Healthcare Organizations (JCAHO).

During the last decade and due to radical changes in the legal and economic environment in which hospitals and their medical staffs operate, there has been a significant and major increase in the roles and responsibilities of the governing board for the governance of the hospital. That body is now directly responsible for "establishing policy, maintaining the quality of patient care and providing for institutional management and planning." Under the pressures of these increased responsibilities, the governing boards of hospitals have moved vigorously to force both arms of the dual administrative hierarchy to become more responsive to the board itself. Thus, the hospital administrator and the chief of the medical staff both report directly, but separately, to the governing board, and board members sit on many hospital and medical staff committees. In turn, members of the executive committee of the medical staff are assigned to key subcommittees of the governing body (Fig. 1-9).

Under the new administrative pattern, the medical directors of the professional service departments (radiology, anesthesiology, and pathology [laboratory medicine]) are responsible to the governing board through the executive committee of the medical staff for all professional (medical care) activities. At the same time, they are also responsible to the hospital administrative hierarchy, which may be more concerned with the management and fiscal issues of their departments, such as the laboratory, than with direct care to the individual patient (see Fig. 1-9). This may place the medical director in a conflict situation, attempting to be responsive to the needs of the medical staff, which is primarily

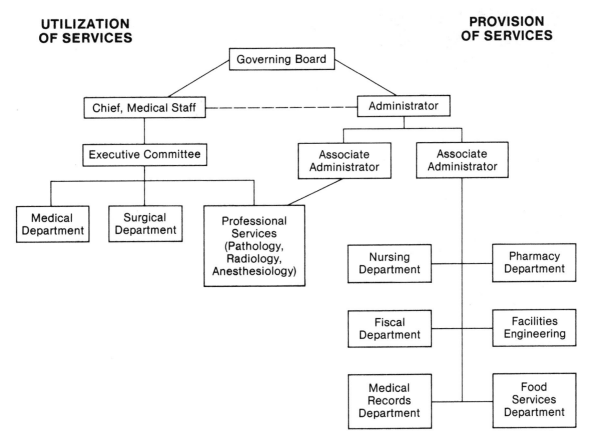

UTILIZATION OF SERVICES

PROVISION OF SERVICES

FIGURE 1-9. The dual hierarchy in health care.

concerned with quality of patient care and outcomes, and to management demands of hospital administration.

In some institutions, especially the larger hospitals, this conflict situation may be minimized by the creation of two director/manager positions—a medical director for physician and patient affairs (usually a pathologist) and a laboratory manager for laboratory administration and technical services (usually a medical technologist with additional education and experience in management). In such an arrangement, matters of professional services and quality assurance are left to the pathologist/medical director, while the laboratory manager handles the day-to-day administrative affairs of the laboratory, reporting to hospital administration. Obviously, the potential for conflict still exists under this arrangement but may be better resolved between two laboratorians who share the mutual goal of maintaining excellence in the clinical laboratory.

The increasing demand for accountability of the governing body of the hospital for matters of cost containment, utilization review, and quality assurance by the courts, governmental agencies, and accrediting bodies, such as the JCAHO, will require continuing modification of the hierarchical structures discussed previously. It is almost certain that the governing body will become more influential in the management of hospitals and other health-care organizations.

New Relationships

To be effective, the laboratory director/manager must understand individual and professional outlooks and balance his respective interests while interacting with both sides of the dual hierarchy.[12] Table 1-2 shows differences in professional "cultures" among health-care professional groups. Contrast, for example, the dif-

Table 1-2
Differences in Professional Cultures Among Health-Care Profession Groups

Attribute	Health Services Management	Clinical Laboratory Technical Staff	Physicians and Pathologists
Basis of knowledge	Social and management sciences	Combination of biomedical and social sciences	Primarily biomedical sciences
Patient focus	All patients in the larger community	Patients represented by specimen samples clustered by type of laboratory analyses requested	Individual patients categorized by type of disease
Exposure to clients while in training	Clients primarily nurses and physicians; relatively little exposure to them during graduate school training	Clients attending physicians and nurses, to whom limited exposure is possible	Great deal of exposure but not necessarily what they will see in practice
Timeframe of action	Medium to long range; gather information, analyze data; engage in long-range strategic planning	Short range with emphasis on timely results and quick turnaround of data	Generally short range; cause–effect relationships, although varies by specialty
View of resources	Limited; main challenge one of allocating scarce resources	Recognize some limitations but more narrowly than the administrator	Resources essentially unlimited; should be available to maximize the quality of patient care
Professional identity	Less cohesive	Somewhat cohesive	Most cohesive

(Adapted with permission from Shortell SM: Theory Z: Implications and relevance for health care management. Health Care Management Review, Fall 1982)

ferences in viewing resources: Hospital administrators (health services management) focus on allocating scarce resources, whereas the attending physician perceives that all required resources should be available to maximize the quality of patient care.

SUMMARY

This introductory chapter has attempted to lay the foundation for understanding the nature of management in laboratory medicine. The provision of clinical laboratory services is a large and complex enterprise operating in an environment buffeted by profound change. Understanding changes occurring in the environment is crucial for management. This chapter has offered a brief introduction to managerial functions. The next chapter deals with the most sweeping legislation to impact the laboratory industry in the last decade, CLIA '88. With these two chapters as background, the reader will be prepared to study specific aspects of management described in subsequent chapters.

REFERENCES

1. Appley LA: The nature of management, film one in a series. In Supervisory Management Course—Part One. New York, American Management Association, 1968
2. Beck SJ: Assessing the educational preparation of clinical laboratory scientists. Clin Lab Sci 7:293–299, 1994
3. Bezold C: The future of health care: Implications for the allied health professions. J Allied Health 18:437–457, 1989
4. Bissell MG: Viewpoint: Whither outcome? Clin Lab Management Rev 9:252–251, 1995
5. Castillo JB, Lien J, Steiner JW: Integrated regional laboratory systems: Implications for staffing and skill mix requirements. Clin Lab Management Rev 11:6–14, 1997
6. Comte RF, Lee LW: Management Procedures, p 16. Indianapolis, Bobbs-Merrill, 1975
7. Hammond HC: Applying the value-of-information paradigm to laboratory management. Clin Lab Management Rev 10: 98–106, 1996
8. Hickman S, Gifford C: Supervisors' perceptions of entry-level management topics appropriate for medical technology programs: A needs assessment approach. Lab Med 19:826–829, 1988
9. Hunter LL, Loscinto L: Employers' expectations of career-entry competencies: A natural survey. Lab Med 24:420–424, 1993
10. Johnson L: Computer skills deemed necessary for entry-level medical technologists. Lab Med 23:44–46, 1992
11. Johnson E: Reengineering the laboratory: Strategic process and systems innovations to improve performance. Clin Lab Management Rev 9:370–380, 1995
12. Jones H: A method for developing outcome measures in the clinical laboratory. Clin Lab Management Rev 10: 115–119, 1996

13. Karni K, Seanger D: Management skills needed by entry-level practitioners. Clin Lab Sci 1:296–300, 1988

14. Kast FE, Rosenzweig JE: Organization and Management: A Systems Approach, 2nd ed, p 6. New York, McGraw-Hill, 1974

15. Keith DM, Garza D: Utilization management in hospital clinical laboratories. Clin Lab Management Rev 10:124–133, 1996

16. Kenney M: Benchmarking: The three approaches. Qual Letter Healthcare Leaders 6(9):2–10, 1994

17. King EC: A design for laboratory managers to encourage staff motivation. Laboratory Management 16(3):45–28, 1978

18. Koontz H, O'Donnel C: Principles of Management, 5th ed. New York, McGraw-Hill, 1972

19. Lang JA: Laboratory restructuring: A move to self-directed teams. Clin Lab Management Rev 423–429, 1995

20. Lombardi DN: The healthcare manager's guide to managing change in challenging times. Clin Lab Management Rev 10:18–24, 1996

21. Matuscak R: The changing health-care market and its implications for clinical laboratory scientists. Clin Lab Sci 1:32–35, 1988

22. Matuscak R, Ducanis A: Preparing clinical laboratory scientists to meet the demands of a changing health care market: Projections for the future. Lab Med 19:661–666, 1988

23. McBride K: Task analysis of medical technology administration and supervision. Am J Med Technol 44:688–695, 1978

24. McLendon WW, Reich MD: Organization and management of the clinical laboratory. In Henry JB (ed): Clinical Diagnosis and Management by Laboratory Methods, p 1977. Philadelphia, WB Saunders, 1979

25. Miller JR: Strategic management in health care. Lab Med 16:46–48, 1985

26. O'Neil EH, Seifer SD: Healthcare reform and medical education: Forces toward generalism. Acad Med 70(Suppl.):37–48, 1995

27. Peters TJ, Waterman RH Jr: In Search of Excellence. New York, Harper & Row, 1982

28. Peterson LJ: Trends in new laboratory arrangements. MLO 18(2):27–30, 1986

29. Price GD: Clinical laboratory educators: Creating the future. Clin Lab Sci 9:134–136, 1996

30. Relman AS: Cost control, doctors' ethics and patient care. Issues in Science and Technology Winter:103–111, 1995

31. Rice AJ: Laboratory Corporation of America (LabCorp)—Company Report. Boston, CS First Boston, June 6, 1995

32. Robbins SP: The Administrative Process. Englewood Cliffs, Prentice-Hall, 1976

33. Scanlon BK: Management 18: A Short Course for Managers, pp 3–4. New York, John Wiley & Sons, 1974

34. Schwartz WB, Aron HJ: Health Care Costs: The Social Tradeoffs. Issues in Science and Technology, Winter: 39–44, 1985

35. Senhauser DA: Medical technology—the challenge to evolve. Laboratory Management 28:48–51, 1985

36. Shortell SM: Theory Z: Implications and relevance for health care management. Health Care Management Review Fall, 1982

37. Stampf SA: Strategic management skills: What are they and why are they needed? Clin Lab Management Rev 10:231–243, 1996

38. Steiner JW, Root JM, Waft DK: Roadmaps for Laboratory Restructuring: Practical Approaches and Effective Solutions, Part 2. Washington, DC, Washington G-2 Reports, 1996

39. Travers EM, Wolke JC, Johnson R, et al: Changing the way lab medicare is practical at the point of care. MLO 26(7):33–40, 1994

40. Travers EM, McClatchey KD: Laboratory management. In McClatchey KD (ed): Clinical Laboratory Medicine, pp 3–53. Baltimore, Williams and Wilkins, 1994

41. U.S. Department of Health and Human Services, Health Care Financing Administration: Health Care Financing Review. Washington, DC, U.S. Government Printing Office, September 1982

42. Watt DK, Sullivan SS: Effects of managed care on the laboratory: The Rochester, New York experience. Clin Lab Management Rev 9:161–175, 1995

43. Winkelman JW, Mennemeyer ST: Using patient outcomes to screen for clinical laboratory errors. Clin Lab Management Rev 10:134–142, 1996

44. Winsten D: The state of the lab. Healthcare Information 13(8):62–78, 1996

2

The Clinical Laboratory Improvement Amendments (CLIA)

Richard B. Passey

BACKGROUND

Clinical laboratories doing interstate business came under federal law and regulations with the Clinical Laboratory Improvement Act of 1967 (CLIA '67). The federal department of Health and Human Services (HHS) gave the Health Care Financing Administration (HCFA) the oversight responsibilities for implementing this law. Then congress passed and the president signed (October 31, 1988) a new law (Public Law 100-578—simply entitled "An Act") commonly called the Clinical Laboratory Improvement Amendments (CLIA '88). This latter law replaced CLIA '67, so it is now common to use CLIA when referring to CLIA '88.

In the United States, federal law is usually interpreted and implemented through an administrative rule-making process. This process typically involves the proposal of rules by a federal administrative division. The proposed rules (regulations) usually include a short public comment period. HCFA published the regulations implementing CLIA '67 on March 14, 1990. These rules were very difficult and intrusive into laboratory operation. On May 21, 1990, HCFA published proposed rules implementing CLIA '88 that were very similar. The public comments were so great (more than 60,000 letters) that HCFA amended the rules. The final rules were published in the *Federal Register* (vol 57, February 28, 1992, pp 7001–7288; in ordinary type, this is equivalent to 1,200 pages). These rules include the 11 sections shown in Box 2–1, along with other parts of the CLIA rules (fees, penalties, and instrument complexity assignment). HCFA has since published additional information and technical corrections in the *Federal Register* through 1994. The last edition of CLIA rules has been delayed.

The rules are written for legal regulation (to be codified in the Code of Federal Regulations), so they are redundant and somewhat convoluted for laboratory purposes. These rules are published in Part §493 of the Code. Each part of CLIA is started with a section indicator (§) followed by the part number (493), followed by a period and a specific paragraph number (eg, §493.1201 starts the quality control rules).

Who Must Comply?

The CLIA regulations apply to every facility that does clinical laboratory work on live human beings for any medical purpose. Laboratory work done on humans cannot be given away free to escape the rules. Exceptions to CLIA's coverage include work done for legal or employment eligibility purposes, such as a breath alcohol determination or a pre-employment drug screen. Research testing is exempt only if the test result is not used for patient care. Additional federal law has exempted the Veterans Administration, Armed Forces, and Substance Abuse and Mental Health Services Administration (previously called NIDA laboratories). Washington is the first state to achieve exempt status, so it evaluates its own laboratories; other states and jurisdictions (New York and Puerto Rico) are applying for this exempt status. The definition that HCFA uses for a laboratory is inclusive (§493.2).

17

Box 2•1

Summary of CLIA Parts*

Summary, highlights, and response to public comments, pp 7001–7137
   CLIA'88 laboratory rules
Part 493—Laboratory requirements or rules (pp 7137–7186)
Subpart A—General provisions (pp 7139–71142; ß493.1–493.25)
Subpart B—Certificate of waiver (pp 7142–7143; ß493.35–493.39)
Subpart C—Certificate of registration (pp 7143–7144; ß493.43–493.51)
Subpart D—Certificate of accreditation (pp 714–7146; ß493.55–493.63)
Subpart H—Participation in proficiency testing (pp 7146–7151; ß493.801–493.865)
Subpart I—Proficiency testing programs (pp 7151–7162; ß493.901–493.959)
Subpart J—Patient test management (pp 7162–7163; ß493.1101–493.111)
Subpart K—Quality control (pp 7163–72; ß493.1201–493.1285)
Subpart M—Personnel (pp 7172–7183; ß493.1401–493.1495)
Subpart P—Quality assurance (pp 7183–7184; ß493.1701–493.1721)
Subpart Q—Inspection (pp 7184–7185; ß493.1775–493.1780)
Fees (pp 7187–7218; ß493.602–649)
Penalties (pp 7218–7243; ß493.1800–493.1850)
Instrument and method complexity (pp 7245–7288)

Other CLIA Publications in the *Federal Register*

Rules for deeming authority, July 31, 1992, pp 33992–34022
Corrected sanctions, Aug. 11, 1992, pp 35760–35761
Adding back deleted sections, Jan. 19, 1993, pp 5212–5215
Technical corrections to CLIA'88 rules, Jan. 19, 1993, pp 5215–5237
Technical corrections—second installment, July 22, 1993, pp 39154–39156
Complete instrument and method complexity listing, July 26, 1993, pp 39860–39973

Additional Information

Survey procedures and interpretive guidelines for laboratories and laboratory services order document
   #PB92146174 from The National Technical Information Services at 1-800-553-6847 or 1-800-336-4700

Published in the *Federal Register* February 28, 1992.

Box 2•2

Types of CLIA Certificates

Registration—Issued until HCFA determines if the laboratory is qualified
Waiver—Permits testing of only tests in the waived category
Physician-performed microscopic tests—Permits testing of only limited microscopic tests performed by a
   physician and waived tests
Moderate complexity—Permits performance of waived and moderately complex testing
High complexity—Required for any test of high complexity and allows performance of any test
Accreditation—Certificate issued by an organization deemed by HCFA as able to act in the place of HCFA
   in providing laboratory evaluation

HCFA, Health Care Financing Administration.

Laboratory means a facility for the biological, microbiological, serological, chemical, immunohematological, hematological, biophysical, cytological, pathological, or other examination of materials derived from the human body for the purpose of providing information for the diagnosis, prevention, or treatment of any disease or impairment of, or the assessment of the health of, human beings. These examinations also include procedures to determine, measure, or otherwise describe the presence or absence of various substances or organisms in the body. Facilities only collecting or preparing specimens (or both) or only serving as a mailing service and not performing testing are not considered laboratories.

For a laboratory to operate legally in the United States, it must have a certificate, as stated in section §493.3.

A laboratory will be cited as out of compliance with Section 353 of the Public Health Services Act unless it has a current, unrevoked or unsuspended certificate.

The types of certificates that are available are found in Box 2–2, and the tests included in the certificates of waiver and physician-performed microscopic tests are found in Box 2–3. A certificate is issued to a laboratory, not to an individual.

A registration certificate is obtained by sending HCFA its form 116, "Clinical Laboratory Application," to HCFA CLIA Program, PO Box 26679, Baltimore, MD, 21207, or calling the CLIA Hotline at (410) 290-5850 or -5700 to obtain information about sending a certificate. In addition to allowing legal laboratory testing, the certificate obligates the laboratory to the list defined in Box 2–4 for any certificate type.

The complexity level of a laboratory's certificate dictates the required personnel (Table 2–1), quality control, proficiency testing, and inspection intensity. If the laboratory is lacking in personnel (director, technical consultant or supervisor, or testing personnel) qualified and trained as required for high-complexity testing, the laboratory cannot legally do high-complexity testing. In HCFA's regulations, large laboratories are organized in specialties (eg, microbiology, chemistry, hematology) and subspecialties (eg, virology, endocrinology).

Summary

As required by CLIA, each laboratory must operate under a correct active certificate with documentation that each employee is qualified, trained, and competent. The laboratory's test menu (every test) for the com-

---

Box 2·3

Waived and Physician-Performed Microscopic Tests (as of December 1994)

1. Dipstick or tablet reagent urinalysis tests for the following:
   Bilirubin
   Glucose
   Hemoglobin
   Ketone
   Leukocytes
   Nitrite
   pH
   Protein
   Specific gravity
   Urobilinogen
2. Fecal occult blood
3. Ovulation tests—visual color comparison tests for human luteinizing hormone
4. Urine pregnancy tests—visual color comparison tests
5. Erythrocyte sedimentation rate—nonautomated
6. Hemoglobin/copper sulfate—nonautomated
7. Blood glucose by glucose monitoring devices cleared by the FDA specifically for home use
8. Spun hematocrit
9. Hemoglobin by specified single-use instruments (currently HemoCue)
10. Plus others when added

Physician-Performed Microscopic Tests

1. Wet mounts:
   Vaginal
   Cervical
   Skin
2. KOH preparation
3. Pin worm preparations
4. Fern test
5. Postcoital direct qualitative examination of mucous
6. Urine sediment

---

plexity that HCFA has assigned (see Box 2–1) must be reviewed to determine if it meets the laboratory's certificate complexity. Every employee must have written duty assignments that include each CLIA required duty. The laboratory must have policies that cover each requirement. Box 2–5 is a list of many of the CLIA required policies. These policies are executed through detailed procedures (see Box 2–5). Policies must

Box 2•4

Laboratory Obligations Obtained Through the Clinical Laboratory Application

1. Pay the appropriate fee.
2. Comply with the rules for the certificate.
3. Permit inspections—either announced or unannounced (even for certificates of waiver or accreditation).
4. Notify HCFA within 30 days of changes in ownership, name, location, director, or supervisors (supervisors—high-complexity only).
5. Treat proficiency testing specimens in the same manner as patient's specimens (except waived and physician-performed microscopic tests where no proficiency testing is required).
6. Be subject to penalties specified for noncompliance.
7. Make all records available to HCFA during inspections.
8. Laboratory must notify HCFA within 6 months of adding a specialty or subspecialty, or adding to or changing test methodology.
9. All laboratories must have a director and testing personnel.
10. Follow the manufacturer's instruction or operate the test as required by the rules.

HCFA, Health Care Financing Administration.

include how the laboratory ensures that the entire testing process (preanalytical, analytical, and postanalytical phases) is done accurately and reliably.

Each laboratory must enroll in an HHS-approved proficiency testing program that monitors each test using at least five separate unknown specimens sent three times a year. For tests without proficiency testing specimens, the laboratory must have a process to ensure the accuracy of the test results. Proficiency testing for about 150 analytes have CLIA-required performance windows.

A quality control program that ensures accurate and precise test results is required by CLIA. Each testing system must perform within the laboratory's performance specifications for each test. Every laboratory must have a quality assurance system that actively looks for and solves problems affecting test results. The quality assurance program must be comprehensive and doc-

umented. The documentation must show what actions were taken and that appropriate policies and procedures were modified to ensure continued quality.

The HCFA calls laboratory inspectors "surveyors." Laboratory personnel must welcome the surveyors into the laboratory, because they have a legal right to inspect any portion of the laboratory, interview any employee, and look at any documentation. The laboratory must produce the required documents within a reasonable time. Failure to perform within these guidelines can bring penalties that HCFA calls sanctions. Sanctions are generally divided into principle sanctions, intermediate sanctions, and civil actions. Some of these sanctions can be very painful. In general, HCFA's attitude has matured from punishment to helpfulness.

PROFICIENCY TESTING

Every laboratory doing any tests (except six waived tests) is required by CLIA to participate in three proficiency testing events per year. Proficiency testing is the prime factor in the federal government's determination of which laboratories stay in business. The laboratory must now successfully participate in two out of every three events for each test. More than 150 tests have specified performance windows that define acceptable performance. Each proficiency testing service will specify how the target value is determined. Then the performance of the laboratory's testing system must meet this target value within the CLIA window. If a test value falls outside the specified limits for more than one out of five specimens (80% rule) in a proficiency testing challenge, it has failed to perform satisfactorily in that challenge. Immunohematology and cytology have different testing and grading criteria. Microbiology gets negative points for identifying organisms that are not present in the proficiency testing material. Two failures out of three events means that the laboratory has unsuccessfully participated in proficiency testing. Penalties for proficiency testing failure range from being required to make a corrective plan, denial of Medicare/Medicaid payments, removing approval to perform this test for any human patient, or more seriously, revocation of the laboratory's CLIA certificate. If serious problems continue, the laboratory may suffer monetary or even criminal punishments. The laboratory director must also certify that proficiency testing was done in the same manner (same process and testing method) used for any patient's specimen. Laboratories may not communicate with any other laboratory about the test values of the proficiency testing material before the reporting deadline specified by the proficiency testing provider. Also, no laboratory can analyze another laboratory's materials. If there is no proficiency testing program for a par-

(text continues on p. 25)

Table 2-1
CLIA Personnel Qualifications §493.1401–1495

Laboratory Complexity	Title	Education	Board Certified	Experience
Moderate	Director	(§493.1405)		Licensed as a laboratory director if required
		MD/DO AP or CP		State licensed or equivalent to practice medicine, if required
		MD/DO		State licensed to practice medicine, and 1 y directing or supervising nonwaived testing, or by Aug. 2, 1993, have 20 h continuing education for laboratory directors consistent with §493.1407, or residency training equivalent to the 20 h specified above or
		PhD(1)	Recognized Boards, or	1 y training or experience or both directing or supervising nonwaived testing, or
		PhD(1)		1 y training or experience or both and 1 y experience as a supervisor, or
		MS(2)		2 y training or experience or both and 2 y as supervisor, or
		BS(2)		Previously qualified under §493.1415 (Federal Register March 14, 1990) before Feb. 28, 1992, or before Feb. 28, 1992, qualified under State law to direct a laboratory in the State
Moderate	Technical consultant (§493.1331)			Possess a current state license if required for this position, and
		MD/DO	AP or CP or equivalent	State licensed to practice medicine, or
		MD/DO		State licensed 1 y training or experience or both in the designated specialty or subspecialty, or
		PhD(2) MS(2)		1 y training or experience or both in the designated specialty or subspecialty, or
		BS(2)		2 y training or experience or both in the designated specialty or subspecialty of service
Moderate	Clinical consultant (§493.1417)			Qualified as a director as MD/DO/PhD (see above), or
		MD/DO		State licensed to practice medicine

(continued)

Table 2-1
continued

Laboratory Complexity	Title	Education	Board Certified	Experience
Moderate	Testing personnel (§493.1423)			State licensed if required, and
		MD/DO		State licensed to practice medicine, or
		PhD/MS/BS(2), or Associates Degree(3), or High School graduate or equivalent(4),		Successfully completed a military laboratory procedures course of at least 50 wk and have held an enlisted occupational specialty of medical laboratory specialist, or
		High School graduate or equivalent(4), and		Documented training in eight specified areas
High	Director (§493.1443)			State licensed as a laboratory director, and
		MD/DO AP or CP		State licensed or equivalent to practice medicine, or
		MD/DO		State licensed to practice medicine, and 1 y laboratory training during residency, or 2 y experience directing or supervising high complexity testing, or
		PhD(1)	HHS-recognized boards, or	
		PhD(1)		Until Sept. 1, 1994, 2 y training or experience or both, 2 y experience directing or supervising high-complexity testing, and by Sept. 1, 1994, national boards, or
				Be serving as laboratory director and previously qualified or could have qualified as director under 42 CFR 493.1415 published in the *Federal Register* March 14, 1990, on or before Feb. 28, 1992, or
				On or before Feb. 28, 1992, be qualified under State law as a laboratory director in the State

(continued)

Laboratory Complexity	Title	Education	Board Certified	Experience
High	Technical supervisor (§493.1449)			Hold a current state license if required, and qualified by education and training or experience in the specialty or subspecialty of service. The director of a high-complexity laboratory may function as the technical supervisor if qualified by this section. Special qualifications apply for anatomic pathology.
		MD/DO	AP and CP or equivalent	State licensed as a laboratory director, or
		MD/DO	CP	State licensed or
		MD/DO		1 y training or experience or both in high-complexity testing within the specialty and required subspecialty training, or
		PhD(1)		1 y training or experience in high-complexity testing within the specialty and required subspecialty training, or
		MS(2)		2 y training or experience in high-complexity testing within the specialty and required subspecialty training, or
		BS(2)		4 y training or experience in high-complexity testing within the specialty and required subspecialty training

The laboratory can perform laboratory tests for the following specialties/subspecialties if the technical supervisor is qualified in and has 1 y training in the specialty and subspecialty training as listed below:

Microbiology,* virology,* bacteriology,* diagnostic immunology,† mycobacteriology,* chemistry,† mycology,* hematology,* parasitology,* radiobioassay.†

* = 6 mo subspecialty training

** = 1 y subspecialty training for PhD, 2 y for MS and 4 y for BS. Note special requirements for other specialties listed below.

Special qualifications are required in §493.1449 for cytology, histopathology, dermatopathology, ophthalmic pathology, oral pathology, histocompatibility, cytogenetics, and immunology.

Laboratory Complexity	Title	Education	Board Certified	Experience
High	Clinical consultant (§493.1455)	(See above)		Qualified as a director above as MD/DO/PhD
		MD/DO		With HHS-approved national boards or state licensed to practice medicine
	General supervisor (§493.1461) and (§493.1469)			Possess a current state license if required, and qualified as a laboratory director to technical supervisor for high-complexity testing, or

(continued)

Table 2-1
continued

Laboratory Complexity	Title	Education	Board Certified	Experience
		MD/DO		State license to practice medicine, or
		PhD(2) or MD(2) or MS(2) and BS(2) and Associates Degree(5) and		1 y training or experience or both in high-complexity testing, or
				2 y training or experience or both in high-complexity testing, or
				Could have previously qualified under 42 CFR 493.1427 (Mar 14, 1992), or
				For blood gases, be qualified as a laboratory director or technical supervisor, or
		BS respiratory therapy, and Associates Degree related to pulmonary function, and		1 y laboratory training or experience or both in blood gas analysis, or
				2 y training or experience or both in blood gas analysis
				The requirements for a general supervisor for histopathology, oral pathology, dermatopathology, and opthalmic pathology are met because the test is done by a director or technical supervisor.
High	Testing personnel (§493.1489)			Possess a state license if required, and
		MD/DO		State licensed to practice medicine, or
		PhD/MS/BS(2), Associates Degree(5), or high school diploma(4)		
			or	Previously qualified or could have qualified as a technologist under 42 CFR 493.1433 (March 14, 1990)
				Blood gas analysis: Qualified as testing personnel above or hold a BS degree in respiratory therapy from an accredited institution, or associated degree related to pulmonary therapy
High	Histopathologist:	MD/DO	AP	Tissue examined by a qualified technical supervisor (MD/DO with clinical and anatomic boards)

(continued)

Table 2-1
continued

Laboratory Complexity	Title	Education	Board Certified	Experience
High	Cytotechnologist (§493.1483)			Possess a current state license if required, and meet one of the following:
				Graduated from an accredited school of cytotechnology, or be certified by an HHS-approved agency, or before Sept. 1, 1992; have successfully completed 2 y from an accredited college with 12 semester h of science, including 8 h of biology, and had 12 mo of training in a school of cytotechnology approved by HHS, or
				Have received 6 mo formal training in a school of cytotechnology approved by HHS, and had 6 mo of full-time experience in cytotechnology acceptable to the pathologist who directed the training, or
				Qualified by an HHS-approved cytotechnologist examination, or before Sept. 1, 1992, have full-time experience of at least 2 y or equivalent within the preceding 5 y examining slide preparations under the supervision of a physician qualified as a technical supervisor in cytology, and before Jan. 1, 1969, must have
				Graduated from high school, completed 6 mo of training in cytology directed by a physician, and completed 2 y of full-time supervised experience in cytotechnology, or
				On or before Sept. 1, 1993, have full-time experience of at least 2 y or equivalent examining cytology slide preparations within the previous 5 y in the United States under the supervision of a physician qualified as a technical supervisor, and before Sept. 1, 1994, have graduated from an approved school of cytotechnology or be certified by an HHS-approved agency

Footnotes to Personnel Qualifications:
(1) Degree in a chemical, physical, biologic, or clinical laboratory science from an accredited institution.
(2) Degree in a chemical, physical, biologic, clinical laboratory science, or medical technology from an accredited institution. "Training or experience, or both in each specialty or subspecialty may be acquired concurrently in more than one of the specialties or subspecialties... excluding waived tests."
(3) Chemical, physical, or biologic science or medical laboratory technology from an accredited institution.
(4) Technical school diploma is not equivalent. Note: CLIA says that for the next 5 years, a high school graduate may perform tests of high complexity. However, as of September, 1997 he or she must be qualified with at least an associate degree. This requirement has been modified by a letter from the Department of Health and Human Services secretary Louis Sullivan on Sept. 1, 1992, to allow people who as of Sept. 1, 1992, were doing tests of high complexity and are qualified with a high school degree and training to continue until further notice.
(5) Degree in a laboratory science or medical laboratory technology from an accredited institution.
Note: All degrees must be earned and granted by an HHS-approved institution.
AP, Recognized Anatomical Pathology Boards; CP, Recognized Clinical Pathology Boards.

ticular test, the laboratory must devise a method (§493.801 [a][2][ii]) to determine the accuracy and reliability (in accordance with §493.1709) of the test.

All problems identified during proficiency testing must be addressed, and the proposed solution must be evaluated for effectiveness, with documentation of the results. Successful participation depends on three elements: policies and procedures for proficiency testing performance; analytical performance criteria; and the strategy followed to identify and solve the problems causing a failure or problem. Policies describing the laboratory's proficiency testing program can be crafted to allow testing personnel to perform proficiency testing to its advantage. For example, policies can describe

when tests can or should be repeated or must be evaluated by laboratory supervisors or directors. The policy can specify when additional calibrations can be performed, how and when methods are validated, or what methods can be used and when. Proficiency testing specimens must be treated in the same manner that is used for patient's specimens, so these policies must be used for patients' tests and for proficiency testing. In summary, proficiency testing is performed using a primary routine method, with personnel who routinely test patients' specimens, and at the frequency used for patients' specimens. Policies should then be crafted carefully to allow maximum flexibility and optimize procedures to avoid analytical problems. A laboratory

Box 2•5

CLIA-Required Policies and Procedures

1. General record-keeping policies (§493.1777):
   a. All records, at least 2 years (§493.1107)
   b. Immunohematology of blood bank, 5 years (§493.1107)
   c. Pathology, 10 years (§493.1777)
   d. All records in a readily accessible form (§493.1777)
   e. Records include instrument printouts and test requisition unless all the information from these sources automatically stored in computer file (§493.1109)
2. Proficiency testing policies (§493.801–§493.959):
   a. Handling proficiency testing specimens (§493.801)
   b. Plan of action taken when notified of a failure (§493.803 & §493.1707)
   c. Reviewing of proficiency testing results, including any failures (§493.807 & §493.1707)
3. Patient test management policies (§493.1101–§493.1111):
   a. Patient preparation and identification, specimen collection, transport, submission, processing, and patient identification (§493.1101 and §493.1103)
   b. Test requisition (§493.1105)
   c. Test records (§493.1107)
   d. Test report (§493.1109)
   e. Referral of specimens (§493.1111)
4. Quality control policies (§493.1201–§493.1269):
   a. High and moderate testing laboratories, written quality control policies (§493.1202 & §493.1203)
   b. Facilities (space and utilities) available and appropriate laboratory environment (§493.1204)
   c. Test methods, equipment, instrumentation, reagents, materials, and supplies (§493.1205)
   d. Procedure manual (§493.1211)
   e. Establishment and verification of method performance specifications (§493.1213)
   f. Demonstrating reliability of semiquantitative and qualitative tests (§493.1218)
   g. Quality control records listing each method with performance specifications (accuracy, precision, analytical sensitivity, analytical specificity or freedom from interferences, reportable range, and reference range)
   h. Equipment maintenance (§493.1215)
   i. Calibration and calibration verification procedures (§493.1217)
   j. Control procedures (§493.1218)
   k. Remedial actions (§493.1219)
   l. Quality control records (§493.1221)
   m. Specialty and subspecialty specific requirements (§493.1223–§493.1269)
5. Personnel records (§493.1401 and §493.1495)
   a. Employee application
   b. Job description
   c. Assigned duties
   d. Education (high school and above)
   e. Specifics of training
   f. Experience, including bench and supervisory duties
   g. Authorization to do specific tests or specifying supervisory duties
6. Quality assurance policies (§493.1707–§493.1721):
   a. Patient test management assessment (§493.1703)
   b. Quality control assessment (§493.1705)
   c. Proficiency testing assessment (§493.1707)
   d. Comparison of test results (§493.1709)
   e. Relationship of patient information to patient test results (§493.1711)
   f. Personnel assessment (§493.1713)
   g. Communication (§493.1715)
   h. Complaint investigations (§493.1717)
   i. Quality assurance review with staff (§493.1719)
   j. Quality assurance records (§493.1721)
7. Inspection readiness (§493.1775–§493.1780)
   a. How to handle the inspection (survey) process
   b. Self-inspection checklist of policies and procedures, including a review of readiness—following the testing system from start to finish
   c. Recording of storage, readiness, and availability
   d. Completeness of all corrective actions

may enroll in more than one proficiency testing program but must designate only one as the regulatory program.

An excellent article by Ehrmeyer and Laessig[1] gives guidance in setting the performance required to pass proficiency testing. In general, each test's imprecision should be one third of the error allowed by CLIA and the accuracy or bias less than 20%. Test performance must be evaluated to ensure that it is operating within these performance criteria. If a test performance exceeds the precision or bias that will allow the laboratory to pass proficiency testing, the laboratory will have to evaluate and perhaps change procedures for the testing. Both accuracy (bias) and precision are required to pass proficiency testing. The article "How to prepare for a proficiency testing event (and survive a failure)"[6] gives eight specific recommendations on how to prepare for a proficiency testing challenge and six items to help overcome a failed proficiency testing challenge. Preparation is the best strategy to increase chances of passing proficiency testing. Especially critical are the proper selection of methodologies, the training of personnel, well thought out policies and procedures, and appropriately handled proficiency testing materials.

PATIENT TEST MANAGEMENT

Each laboratory is required to have written procedures for handling patients' specimens from the physician's request through testing and reporting the results (preanalytical through the postanalytical phases of testing). These rules in CLIA are included under Patient Test Management.

§493.1103 Standard; Procedures for Specimen Submission and Handling

(a) The laboratory must have available and follow written policies and procedures for each of the following, if applicable: Methods used for the preparation of the patient; specimen collection; specimen labeling; specimen preservation; and conditions for specimen transportation. Such policies and procedures must assure positive identification and optimum integrity of the patient specimens from the time the specimen(s) are collected until testing has been completed and the results reported.

Several common laboratory practices may cause problems with these rules. Only an "authorized person" (authorized by state law) can order or receive laboratory information. Some states do not have laws establishing the authorized person, so the laboratory's policies must stipulate who can order laboratory tests and receive results. Laboratory requests must be in writing (which can be the patient's chart) or in electronic form (computer). The laboratory must make an effort to obtain written confirmation of oral requests for tests. The laboratory must guarantee the confidentiality of all reports. The test request form must contain specified information that includes (§493.1105): the patient's name or unique identifier, the name and address or identifier of the authorized person requesting the test, and if appropriate the individual responsible for using the test result. The test name and date of specimen collection must be clearly listed. The test request form should be designed so that the exact tests are identified. All information relevant and necessary to ensure accurate and timely testing (meets the laboratory's turn-around time) and reporting of results must be included on the request. Further, all specimens must have positive identification. The laboratory must demonstrate the link between the laboratory result and the patient from which the specimen was taken; this includes identification of the testing personnel who completed and verified the test result. Policies should stipulate how a result that represents a life-threatening condition is handled. Policies must specify how patients are prepared and specimens are labeled, transported, and stored. Patients may be given oral instructions to supplement the written information. Laboratory policies must stipulate what constitutes an unacceptable specimen (ie, hemolyzed) for each test.

The report must have the name and address of the laboratory where the test was performed (an old Medicare requirement). The original report form or an exact duplicate (duplicate information) must be available for the standard record storage time. This report must include the test's reference range and any unusual specimen problems. In the absence of manufacturer's data for reference ranges, the procedure should have accepted literature references and show that test results are in appropriate agreement. To show that reports meet the reference range, a list should be retained of a few randomly selected patients who have normal results; these data should show agreement with the laboratory's ranges.

Specimens should be referred only to outside laboratories that hold a current and unsuspended CLIA certificate of the appropriate complexity. Results or interpretations of results provided by the referral laboratory should not be changed. The referral laboratories may mail the results directly to the authorized person who ordered the test. The referral laboratory must keep an exact duplicate of the test results (information duplicate). The authorized person who received the results must be notified of the name and address of the referral laboratory where the test was done.

QUALITY CONTROL

Quality control under CLIA is a process of identification and documentation of analytical problems as they occur. The rules include a requirement to run two controls each day that testing is done. All failed quality control results (outside performance specifications) must be handled according to written policy. CLIA requires specific actions in method validation, performance specifications (accuracy, precision, analytical sensitivity, analytical specificity, reportable range, and reference range). Methods must be calibrated at least every 6 months, and calibration verification must be done under specified conditions. Each laboratory must also have written policies for instrument maintenance. The quality control rules require laboratories to have facilities, instruments, reagents, and supplies that contribute to quality laboratory results. CLIA requires that all phases (preanalytical, analytical, and postanalytical) of testing be evaluated for contribution to quality. The requirement is that quality is built in from patient preparation through reporting of test results and that this quality is part of the laboratory's procedure manual. Modified procedures or instruments require evaluation of the validity of the modification showing that the accuracy, precision, and medical usefulness of the modified method is not compromised. All problems must be documented. The following is the key quote from the CLIA rules.

Condition: General Quality Control; Moderate or High Complexity Testing or Both (§493.1201)

The laboratory must establish and follow written quality control procedures for monitoring and evaluating the quality of the analytical testing process of each method to assure the accuracy and reliability of patient test results and reports.

Each laboratory is required to look after the quality of the testing systems so that reagents, solutions, culture media, control materials, calibration materials, and other supplies are labeled to identify the material and strength or concentration. All special storage conditions and expiration dates must be documented and followed to maintain quality. Components of reagents from different lot numbers may not be interchanged unless the manufacturer allows it (§493.1205[d][e], p. 7164).

The laboratory must have a written procedure manual for the performance of all tests used by the laboratory. This manual must be approved and signed by the current laboratory director, and all changes must be witnessed by the director's signature. The manual must be readily available and followed by laboratory personnel. Textbooks or manufacturer's literature may be used as supplements to these written descriptions but may not be used in lieu of the laboratory's written procedures for testing or examining specimens. The procedure manual must follow a 16-item specific format (Box 2–6). Remedial action must be taken (according to written policy) to solve any quality control failures. These actions must be documented (§493.1219).

Each batch or shipment of reagents, discs, stains, antisera, or identification systems must be checked with controls (positive and negative). Bacterial media produced under National Committee for Clinical Laboratory Standards Publication M22A[14] can be used without doing formal quality control.

PERSONNEL

The HCFA solved the personnel shortage for clinical laboratories across the United States. A high school graduate can now do specific testing for laboratories doing tests of moderate complexity. A high school graduate can do tests of high complexity until 1995 or, according to a letter from the secretary of HHS on August 31, 1992, he or she can continue doing high complexity testing if he or she was doing those specific tests before September 1, 1992. A person who holds a bachelor's degree (specifically in biologic, chemical, physical, or medical laboratory science) can be a director of a laboratory that does only tests of moderate complexity or waived tests. A person with an associate degree can be the general supervisor of a laboratory doing high complexity testing. Historic laboratory titles are not honored by the CLIA rules except for director and cytotechnologist. Medical technologist and technician are now testing personnel. Supervisors and section directors are now either a general supervisor or a technical consultant or technical supervisor. New to the laboratory is a clinical consultant required by every laboratory with a certificate for either moderate or high complexity testing. There is no mention of manager, coordinator, clinical microbiologist, clinical chemist, laboratory assistant, or many other titles. Pathologists are only mentioned in conjunction with anatomic pathology or immunohematology. The laboratory director is responsible for all aspects of laboratory operation (Appendix 2–1 shows the 22 specific duties). Especially explicit are the requirements for establishing and monitoring the training and experience of testing personnel. HCFA's complexity model forms the basis for the personnel requirements. Laboratories holding a certificate authorizing moderate complexity testing require less rigorous education and experience for directors, consultants, and supervisors.

Box 2·6

Items Included in Procedure Manual (§493.1211)

"(b) The procedure manual must include, when applicable to the test procedure:

(1) Requirements for specimen collection and processing, and criteria for specimen rejection;

(2) Procedures for microscopic examinations, including the detection of inadequately prepared slides;

(3) Step-by-step performance of the procedure, including test calculations and interpretation of results;

(4) Preparation of slides, solutions, calibrators, controls, reagents, stains and other materials used in testing;

(5) Calibration and calibration verification procedures;

(6) The reportable range for patient test results as established or verified in §493.1213;

(7) Control procedures;

(8) Remedial action to be taken when calibration or control results fail to meet the laboratory's criteria for acceptability;

(9) Limitations in methodologies, including interfering substances;

(10) Reference range (normal values);

(11) Imminent life-threatening laboratory results or panic values;

(12) Pertinent literature references;

(13) Appropriate criteria for specimen storage and preservation to ensure specimen integrity until testing is completed;

(14) The laboratory's system for reporting patient results including, when appropriate, the protocol for reporting panic values;

(15) Description of the course of action to be taken in the event that a test system becomes inoperable; and

(16) Criteria for the referral of specimens including procedures for specimen submission and handling as described in §493.1103."

The technical supervisor has 11 named duties (see Appendix 2–1). The supervisor must set the personnel quality standards, establish training needs, evaluate procedures used for employment, provide ongoing and remedial training, and document personnel competence.

Education from high school and beyond, along with all experience and training, must be documented in each employee's personnel file. Included in this file are all tests the employee is authorized to perform. The laboratory's training system should ensure that training covers all preanalytical, analytical, and postanalytical phases of testing for each procedure. In other words, training should cover all phases from patient preparation to delivering the final report. Each employee's training and competency can be documented by a checklist. Both the testing personnel trained and the technical supervisor or consultant should sign the checklist showing the specific training and the date it was done and confirmed. Records must show that twice a year for the first year and once a year thereafter, each employee is shown to be competent to perform each test he or she is authorized to perform. The competency demonstration must be visually witnessed by the technical supervisor (see Appendix 2–1). Modification of a method starts the cycle again. The documentation must be done before any patient testing is done. This written authorization extends to all duties of supervisors, consultants, and testing personnel.

A director can direct no more than five laboratories (listed as director on five certificates). The director can delegate many duties, but none of the director's responsibilities. Delegation of duties must be done in writing and their performance documented. The director and technical supervisors or consultants must be available on site, by an electronic system, or by telephone.

Cytology is the only laboratory specialty that has workload limits set by CLIA's rules. Each cytotechnologist must have his or her work evaluated, and the technical supervisor must individually set the number of slides that can be accurately and reliably examined during each 24 hours. This limit cannot exceed 100 gynecologic or nongynecologic slides by nonautomated microscopic examination (§493.1257[b]).

The counterbalance to using less qualified (by historical standards) personnel is that the laboratory must pass proficiency testing and document all problems and corrective actions. To avoid continuously documenting problems and answering unsatisfactory proficiency testing challenges, the best employees available should be hired.

QUALITY ASSURANCE

A laboratory's personnel must use its written policies and procedures to achieve the highest quality possible. Quality assurance is the process that evaluates these policies and procedures and the resulting laboratory test results for continuing error-free operation. Quality is the responsibility of the laboratory director and technical supervisor (consultant) who ensure that all personnel carry out their responsibilities.

Condition: Quality Assurance; Moderate or High Complexity Testing or both (§493.1701)

Each laboratory performing moderate or high complexity testing, or both, must establish and follow written policies and procedures for a comprehensive quality assurance program which is designed to monitor and evaluate the ongoing and overall quality of the total testing process (preanalytical, analytical, postanalytical).

Documentation is required to show that quality is a reality through the preanalytical, analytical, and postanalytical phases of testing. CLIA allows each laboratory to establish its own policies and procedures, as long as the results meet the CLIA requirements and produce quality testing results.

Quality assurance is more than showing that each task is done; it is evaluating each task to see if it contributes any error. The quality assurance program requires that all employees are evaluated, trained, and authorized to do each test (each test listed separately). All problems must be investigated and solved with documentation. Further, there must be evidence that changes are incorporated into the laboratory's routine operations.

The elements of the laboratory's quality assurance policies include requirements for evaluation of policies and practices for patient test management (§493.1703), quality control (§493.1705), proficiency testing (§493.1707), comparison of test results (§493.1709), relationship of test results to patient condition (§493.1711), personnel assessment (§493.1713), and complaint evaluation (§493.1717). All changes in policies must be communicated to the laboratory employees and fully documented.

Additional items that should be incorporated into the quality assurance program include establishing criteria and evaluating specimen collection, including labeling, preservation, and transportation. The test requisition must be evaluated for completeness and appropriateness (Box 2–7).

Each laboratory must have effective criteria for specimen rejection. Policies must ensure that the reporting of test results is complete, useful, and accurate. They must also include how a delayed test result is handled and include policies for notification of the authorized person who ordered or will use the test results.

The laboratory's quality control activities must be included in a quality assurance report. They must include policies for corrective and remedial actions and documentation for problems identified through the evaluation of quality control data. All "out of control" conditions and unacceptable proficiency testing results must show remedial actions. The review must also include looking for errors in calibration and calibration verification policies. It must also show how known errors in reported results were corrected.

Twice a year, any method that does not have proficiency testing evaluation requires verification of its accuracy and reliability. A most difficult requirement of CLIA is to evaluate patients' test results against patient demographics and other test results. This includes evaluation of the relationship of a patient's test results with the patient's sex, diagnosis, clinical data (if provided), or relationship with other test parameters available in the laboratory. This can be done by reviewing patient charts representing a small sample of completed laboratory reports. Also included in the review are any complaints centering on test results. The selected patient's test results should be evaluated against medical condi-

---

Box 2·7

Items Included in the Test Requisition (§493.1105)

"(a) The patient's name or other unique identifier;

(b) The patient's name and address or other suitable identifiers of the authorized person requesting the test and, if appropriate, the individual responsible for utilizing the test results or the name and address of the laboratory submitting the specimen, including, as applicable, a contact person to enable the reporting of imminent life threatening laboratory results or panic values;

(c) The test(s) to be performed;

(d) The date of specimen collection;

(e) For Pap smears, the patient's last menstrual period, age or date of birth, and indication of whether the patient had a previous abnormal report, treatment or biopsy; and

(f) Any additional information relevant and necessary to a specific test to assure accurate and timely testing and reporting of results."

tion. Policies should specify appropriate actions for situations in which inappropriate test results are found. All policy and procedure changes must be communicated to all appropriate laboratory personnel. CLIA also requires documentation of the solutions for any breakdown in communication, including complaints between the laboratory and the authorized person who orders or uses results.

INSPECTIONS

The key to ensuring that each laboratory complies with HCFA's rules is the inspection process. These inspections or surveys are conducted every 2 years. Additional surveys can result from complaints to ensure that deficiencies are resolved and as a 5% reinspection of those surveys conducted by deemed organizations. HCFA's guide for these inspections is a publication entitled "Survey Procedures and Interpretative Guidelines for Laboratories and Laboratory Services." These instructions to surveyors are found in the State Operations Manual HCFA Publication 7 in Appendix C. Ordering information is found in Box 2–1. This publication sets out the inspection process in detail and provides the surveyor with guidelines and probes (questions) for most sections of the CLIA rules. This publication lists hundreds of D-tags, which is an abbreviation for deficiency tags. This is a shorthand way for surveyors to record deficiencies found during an inspection.

Inspections can now be announced a few days prior to the actual arrival of the survey team, or they may be unannounced. The laboratory's inspection policy should include instructions to welcome the survey team and provide them with access to all parts of the laboratory, all records, and all personnel. The process is composed of 11 tasks, summarized in Box 2–8.

The inspection team (one or more inspectors) will focus on the 58 condition level rules in CLIA. The difference in condition and standard level rules is that the condition level rules are the more general and carry more penalty for violation than standard level (more specific) rules.

Surveyors will focus on the following: specimen integrity and the accuracy, reliability, and timeliness of test results, including quality control and calibration data, test performance, and patient-specific information. They will also focus on the skills of testing and supervisory personnel (eg, training, delegation of responsibilities, evaluation of test results, resolution of problems). Finally, they will evaluate the general adequacy of the facilities, equipment, and supplies. The inspection will become very detailed when problems are apparent.

A key element that shows a laboratory is functioning

Box 2·8

The HCFA Survey (Inspection Process)

Task 1: Presurvey preparation

Task 2: Entrance interview

Task 3: Tour and assessment of facilities

Task 4: Sample selection for observation, personnel interview, and record review

Task 5: Assessment of specimen integrity, observations of skills and abilities of testing and supervisory staff, and evaluation of equipment and testing supplies

Task 6: Assessment of test performance and reporting of test results

Task 7: Verification of personnel qualifications

Task 8: Verification of proficiency testing enrollment and review of results

Task 9: Analysis and evaluation of findings

Task 10: Exit conference

Task 11: Formation of the statement of deficiencies

---

properly is the proficiency testing data. The survey team is supplied with this data by the laboratory's proficiency testing provider. The seriousness of deficiencies cited by the surveyors depend on the pervasiveness, frequency, and impact on the laboratory's services to patients. Small deficiencies may not be cited and may therefore be left to the laboratory to correct without follow-up.

Situations that pose an "immediate jeopardy" to a patient's or the public's health and welfare is a serious decision and will greatly affect how penalties are applied to the laboratory.

. . . a situation in which immediate corrective action is necessary because the laboratory's noncompliance with one or more condition level requirements has already caused, is causing or is likely to cause at any time serious injury or harm or death to individuals served by the laboratory or to the health or safety of the general public. This term is synonymous with imminent and serious risk to human health and significant hazard. This situation requires the application of termination procedures which are addressed specifically in the adverse action section of these instructions.

An exit conference can be an excellent opportunity to find out how the surveyors viewed the laboratory's operations. The laboratory can request an exit conference in which it presents additional information and asks about deficiencies cited by the surveyors. The survey team will formulate a written statement of deficiencies so that a "reasonably knowledgeable person" can understand the requirements. The inspectors are not to speculate why the laboratory's policies failed, only to identify deficiencies. This statement must be carefully followed by the laboratory to show resolution of all deficiencies within the time allowed by the survey team. A self-inspection can greatly increase success with the survey process.

PENALTIES

The HCFA takes its responsibilities over CLIA very seriously, and to prove it, it has developed an increasingly serious sequence of penalties for laboratories that violate the rules. Penalties are mostly imposed by the survey system, usually from infractions found during an inspection of the laboratory. If a violation is believed to pose a serious hazard to public health, the laboratory may be shut down immediately (as soon as it takes to get a court injunction). Any cited noncompliance or sanctions must be taken seriously. There are three levels of noncompliance: condition level deficiencies with immediate jeopardy, condition level deficiencies with no immediate jeopardy, and deficiencies below condition level without immediate jeopardy. Penalties can be principle sanctions, intermediate sanctions, and civil actions. CLIA's penalty section states the following:

> **SUMMARY:** These regulations set forth the rules for sanctions that HCFA may impose on laboratories that are found not to meet Federal requirements. These include the principal sanctions of suspending, limiting, or revoking the laboratory's certificate issued under the Clinical Laboratory Improvement Amendments of 1988 (CLIA), and canceling the laboratory's approval to receive Medicare payment for its services, and the alternative sanctions that may be imposed instead of or before the principal sanctions.

If the laboratory is organized so that problems can be quickly solved, policies changed, personnel trained, and data gathered to show that changes are effective, the laboratory may then be able to react quickly enough to avoid penalties. These penalties can exact a very heavy financial burden on the laboratory. In addition to stopping Medicare/Medicaid reimbursement, the laboratory can lose the privilege of doing any clinical testing, even if given away. Civil fines can range from $50 to $10,000 per incident (§493.1834), and willful endangerment of the public can result in imprisonment. Additional alternate sanctions typically include a plan of correction, publicly listing the laboratory by name along with others who have been cited, or "on-site monitor-

ing" of the laboratory's operation by an HCFA employee. The laboratory can be ordered to provide training of employees if proficiency testing is unsuccessful (§493.1838). The laboratory can voluntarily withdraw from testing, but the reinstatement process will be difficult. Each laboratory has appeal rights spelled out in the *Federal Register*, February 28, 1992 (§493.1844).

MASTER PLAN

Following an orderly master plan will help the laboratory implement and be successful under these most detailed and difficult rules. Plans should be made carefully, and all elements required by the CLIA regulations should be included. Personnel assignments are made carefully, establishing accountability and tracking progress to be prepared for the biennial HCFA survey. In the process, the laboratory will be better organized and quality instilled more deeply in the laboratory's system.

REFERENCES

1. Ehrmeyer S, Laessig R, et al: 1990 Medicare CLIA Final Rules for Proficiency Testing: Minimum Intralaboratory Performance Characteristics (CV and Bias) Needed to Pass. Clinical Chemistry 36:1736–1740, 1990
2. Passey RB: How to obtain a CLIA certificate without getting stuck in the details. Medical Laboratory Observer August: 26–31, 1992
3. Passey RB: How to meet the new personnel requirements while continuing to operate your laboratory. MLO September:47–51, 1992
4. Passey RB: How to read the *Federal Register* and other CLIA-related documents. MLO October:47–52, 1992
5. Passey RB: A master plan for implementing CLIA. MLO November:36–41, 1992
6. Passey RB: How to prepare for a proficiency testing event (and survive a failure). MLO December:32–38, 1992
7. Passey RB: How to follow the rules for patient test management. MLO January:55–57, 1993
8. Passey RB: Walking the straight and narrow on quality control. MLO February:39–43, 1993
9. Passey RB: How to prepare for and survive a CLIA inspection. MLO March:31–35, 1993
10. Passey RB: CLIA's quality assurance: A study in total devotion. MLO May:45–48, 1993
11. Passey RB: CLIA '88 penalties and how to avoid them. MLO June:31–38, 1993
12. Passey RB: Proving performance under CLIA '88. MLO July: 55–59, 1993
13. Passey RB: Coping With CLIA (a Compilation of 11 Articles), pp 1–62. Montvale, NJ, Medical Laboratory Observer, Medical Economics Publishing, 1993
14. Quality Assurance for Commercially Prepared Microbiological culture media; Approved Standard—M22A (1990). National Committee for Clinical Laboratory Standards 10(14):1–24, 1990

APPENDIX 2–1 DUTIES OF LABORATORY DIRECTORS AND TECHNICAL CONSULTANTS/SUPERVISORS

Laboratory Director Duties for Moderate and High Complexity (§493.1407 and §493.1445)

1. The laboratory director is responsible for the overall operation and administration of the laboratory, including the employment of personnel who are competent to perform test procedures; record and report test results promptly, accurately, and proficiently; and assume compliance with the applicable regulations.
2. If qualified, may perform the duties of all other personnel
3. May delegate duties but not responsibilities
4. Must be accessible to the laboratory to provide on-site, telephone, or electronic consultation as needed
5. May direct no more than five laboratories
6. The laboratory director must ensure the following:
   a. The testing systems provide quality laboratory services for all aspects of test performance, which includes the preanalytical, analytical, and postanalytical phases of testing.
   b. The physical plant and environmental conditions of the laboratory are appropriate for the testing performed and provide a safe environment in which employees are protected from physical, chemical, and biologic hazards.
   c. The test methodologies selected have the capability of providing the quality of results required for patient care.
   d. The verification procedures used are adequate to determine the accuracy, precision, and other pertinent performance characteristics of the method.
   e. The laboratory personnel are performing the test methods as required for accurate and reliable results
   f. The laboratory is enrolled in an HHS-approved proficiency testing program for the testing performed and that
      (i) The proficiency testing samples are tested as required under subpart H of this part.
      (ii) The results are returned within the timeframes established by the proficiency testing program.
      (iii) All proficiency testing reports received are reviewed by the appropriate staff to evaluate the laboratory's performance and to identify any problems that require corrective action.
      (iv) An approved corrective action plan is followed when any proficiency testing result is found to be unacceptable or unsatisfactory.
   g. The quality control and quality assurance programs are established and maintained to ensure the quality of laboratory services provided and to identify failures in quality as they occur.
   h. Acceptable levels of analytical performance for each test system are established and maintained.
   i. All necessary remedial actions are taken and documented whenever significant deviations from the laboratory's established performance characteristics are identified, and patient test results are reported only when the system is functioning properly.
   j. Reports of test results include pertinent information required for interpretation.
   k. Consultation is available to the laboratory's clients on matters related to the quality of the test results reported and their interpretation concerning specific patient conditions.
   l. A general supervisor provides on-site supervision of high-complexity test performance by testing personnel qualified under §493.1489 (b)(4). (This requirement is only for directors of high-complexity laboratories.)
   m. The laboratory employs a sufficient number of laboratory personnel with appropriate education and either experience or training to provide appropriate consultation, proper supervision and accurate performance tests and reporting of test results in accordance with the personnel responsibilities described in this subpart.
   n. Prior to testing patients' specimens, all personnel have the appropriate education and experience, receive the appropriate training for the type and complexity of the services offered, and have demonstrated that they can perform all testing operations reliably to provide and report accurate results.
   o. Policies and procedures are established for monitoring individuals who conduct preanalytical, analytical, and postanalytical phases of testing to ensure that they are competent and maintain their competency to process specimens, perform test procedures, and report test results promptly and proficiently, and whenever necessary, identify needs for remedial training or continuing education to improve skills.
   p. An approved procedure manual is available to all personnel responsible for any aspect of the testing process.

q. Specify in writing, the responsibilities and duties of each employee engaged in the performance of the preanalytical, analytical, and postanalytical phases of testing. This must identify which examinations and procedures each individual is authorized to perform; whether supervision is required for specimen processing, test performance, or result reporting, and whether supervisory or direct review is required prior to reporting patient test results.

Technical Consultant or Supervisor for Moderately and Highly Complex Laboratories (§493.1413 and §493.1451)

1. Technical supervisors/consultants are responsible for the technical and scientific oversight of the laboratory. They do not have to be onsite at all times but must be available to the laboratory as needed to provide on-site, telephone, or electronic consultation.

2. The technical supervisor/consultant is responsible for the following:
   a. Selection of test methodology appropriate for the clinical use of the test results
   b. Verification of the test procedures performed and establishment of the laboratory's test performance characteristics, including the precision and accuracy of each test and test system
   c. Enrollment and participation in an HHS-approved proficiency testing program commensurate with the services offered
   d. Establishing a quality control program appropriate for the testing performed and establishing the parameters for acceptable levels of analytical performance and ensuring that these levels are maintained throughout the entire testing process from the initial receipt of the specimen through sample analysis and reporting of test results
   e. Resolving technical problems and ensuring that remedial actions are taken whenever test systems deviate from the laboratory's established performance specifications
   f. Ensuring that patient test results are not reported until all corrective actions have been taken and the test system is functioning properly
   g. Identifying training needs and ensuring that each individual performing tests receives regular in-service training and education appropriate for the type and complexity of the laboratory services performed
   h. Evaluating the competency of all testing personnel and ensuring that the staff maintain their competency to perform test procedures and report test results promptly, accurately, and proficiently. The procedures for evaluation of the competency of the staff must include, but are not limited to, the following:
      (i) Direct observations of routine patient test performance, including patient preparation, if applicable, specimen handling, processing, and testing
      (ii) Monitoring the recording and reporting of test results
      (iii) Review of intermediate test results or worksheets, quality control records, proficiency testing results, and preventive maintenance records
      (iv) Direct observation of performance of instrument maintenance and function checks
      (v) Assessment of test performance through testing previously analyzed specimens, internal blind testing samples, or external proficiency testing samples
      (vi) Assessment of problem-solving skills
   i. Evaluating and documenting the performance of individuals responsible for high- or moderate-complexity testing at least semiannually during the first year the individual tests patient specimens. Thereafter, evaluations must be performed at least annually unless test methodology or instrumentation changes, in which case, prior to reporting patient test results, the individual's performance must be reevaluated to include the use of the new test methodology or instrumentation

3. In cytology, the technical supervisor of the individual qualified under §493.1449(k)(2)
   a. May perform the duties of the cytology general supervisor and the cytotechnologist, as specified in §§493.1471 and 493.1485, respectively
   b. Must establish the workload limit for each individual examining slides
   c. Must reassess the workload limit for each individual examining slides at least every 6 months
   d. Must perform the functions specified in §493.1257(c)
   e. Must ensure that each individual examining gynecologic preparations participates in an HHS-approved cytology proficiency testing program, as specified in §493.945, and achieves a passing score, as specified in §493.855
   f. If responsible for screening cytology slide preparations, must document the number of cytology slides screened in 24 hours and the number of hours devoted during each 24-hour period to screening cytology slides

3

Management Functions in the Clinical Laboratory

John R. Snyder • David S. Wilkinson

As described in Chapter 1, laboratory management is a complex process in which the manager is entrusted with certain physical, financial, and human resources (input) with the expectation that specific outcomes (quality results in a timely and efficient manner) will be forthcoming. Management must be viewed as a *process*. For the purpose of study, laboratory management is often described in terms of four basic functions: planning, organization, direction, and control. In practice, the boundaries between these functions are often obscure because of an interdependence of each function on the other for effective management. This chapter provides a broad, integrative framework for the functions of planning, organization, and control with some specific managerial tools for each.

The key to the management process is goal formulation. The process begins with a specification of the goals of the laboratory and ends with an evaluation of whether they were reached. To carry out the management process, laboratory supervisors and directors determine objectives as part of the planning process, construct an organization able to do the work needed to fulfill the objectives, direct the activities of staff toward meeting the objectives, and compare actual results to measure success or failure in the achievement of the goals.

STRATEGIC MANAGEMENT AND PLANNING

Recent public and government pressure aimed at controlling health-care costs has prompted significant changes in management practices for service providers in the industry. One of the most notable changes is an emphasis on strategic management and planning with a focus on goal formulation and design of specific strategies to be competitive.

Strategic management is defined as the development and implementation of the laboratory's "grand design," or overall strategy, in relation to its current and future demands for service.[9] Schendel and Hofer[34] describe six related major tasks in the strategic management process: (1) goal formulation, (2) environmental analysis, (3) strategy formulation, (4) strategy evaluation, (5) strategy implementation, and (6) strategic control. Inherent in this process is a realization that clinical laboratories need to analyze the external and internal environment, and opportunities for growth and development in new service markets, as part of a strategic planning process.[20] An environmental assessment includes scanning and analysis of external factors, such as economic trends; technologic trends; government, political, and legal trends; and present and potential competition.[20] This assessment yields strategic planning assumptions, target market definitions, and identification of threats and opportunities.[20]

Strategic planning is a related managerial activity that yields a good fit between the laboratory and its environment.[31] *Strategic planning* is the process of deciding on objectives for the organization, changes in these objectives, the resources needed to obtain these objectives, and the policies that are to govern the acquisition, use, and disposition of these resources.[2,18] Although many models for strategic planning exist, a functional strategic planning process for the clinical laboratory should include an environmental analysis, organizational strategic audit, and definition of the mission (goal formulation); development of general and specific objectives and resource planning; involvement of key personnel; and management in accordance with the objectives[1,16,18] (Fig. 3-1). Laboratory managers are

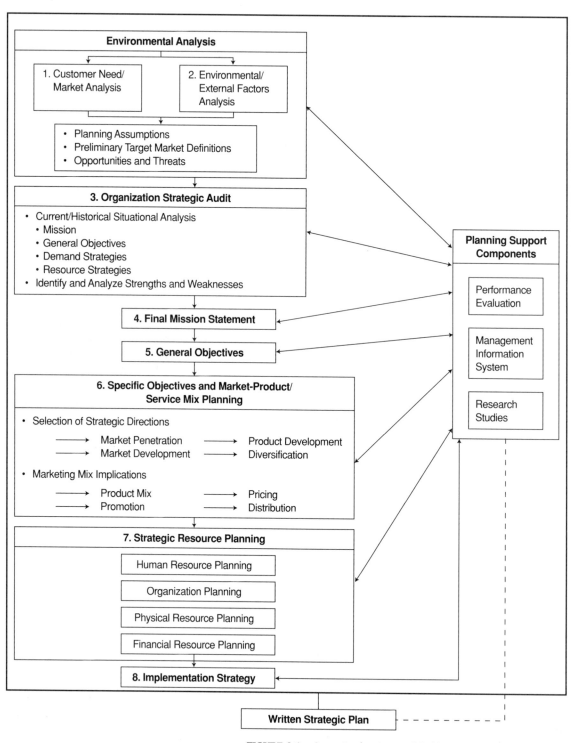

FIGURE 3-1. Strategic planning model. (© 1988, Steven R. Holmberg)

increasingly involved in strategic planning at the institutional level. Albers and Vice offer an example in Box 3-1 of a functional strategic planning process appropriate for use in a health-care facility.[1]

PLANNING AT THE DEPARTMENTAL LEVEL

The initial function of departmental management is planning. The laboratory manager must determine laboratory goals and objectives and the means for achieving them before he can organize, direct, or control the results. Scanlon proposes that a systems approach to planning is most effective, in that it allows the manager to adapt to changing situations, using feedback information during the process.[33] In the systems approach, planning is divided into the four phases listed in Box 3-2.

This systems approach emphasizes establishing a clear direction (goal or objective) before the laboratory manager begins planning strategies. When policies are set with the goal in mind, constraints are in place to guide the planning strategies prior to the major plan-development stage. The third step is characterized by a plan for completion of a project and short-range, interim plans. Finally, the details necessary for the plan's implementation should be specified.

Because planning is the initial function in all administrative activities, separating it from organizing and controlling functions is difficult. Figure 3-2 shows the relationship of organizational hierarchy to general planning and control mechanisms. The pyramid structure is typical when describing a hierarchy. The inverted pyramid reflects the degree of detail in each of the mechanisms listed in the planning and control structure. The laboratory director will generally deal with the institution's objectives and goals, one example of which might be to increase the scope of specialized chemistry procedures that the laboratory would perform in house, rather than send to a reference center. The administrative technologist deals with operational policies, the rules for action that will contribute to the successful achievement of goals and objectives. In the example just mentioned, perhaps the administrative technologist would establish policy regarding cost/test ratios to determine which special tests would still be sent to a reference center. The supervisory technologist is responsible for implementing procedures. Procedures are the sequence of steps to implement the short-range plans established by operational policy. In the achievement of this specific goal, the supervisor would undoubtedly have the responsibility for evaluating and implementing the special analytical procedures and procedures governing the staffing and instrumentation required. Finally, the technical and clerical staff deal with the rules that govern everyday testing

---

Box 3·1

Strategic Planning for the Health-Care Facility

I Strategic planning
   A. Review existing mission and goals using articles of incorporation, minutes of board meeting, and so forth.
   B. Develop baseline data.
      1. Assess market demand using population trends, demographic trends, hospital fee trends, regulatory trends.
      2. Estimate market share using trends, medical staffing trends, competition trends, and projected market share trends.
      3. Project resource use using data on admissions, outpatient visits, and average stay.
      4. Identify strategic issues, including geographic, competitive, resource, medical staff, and patient mix.
      5. Determine financial status, including payer-mix, inpatient capacity, and regulatory factors.
   C. Evaluate alternative courses of action, and identify strategic directions for various market segments.

II Developmental planning
   A. Do market segment analysis.
   B. Determine geographic alternatives.
   C. Configure programs.
   D. Determine financial feasibility.
   E. Design construction.
   F. Obtain certificate of need.

III Operational planning
   A. Identify management style, goals, and so forth.
   B. Establish operating budget.
   C. Establish capital budget.

IV Implementation of plans

V Monitoring of performance

VI Annual recycling or when significant new data are obtained

From Albers J, Vice JL: Strategic planning. Am J Med Technol. 49:411–414, 1983

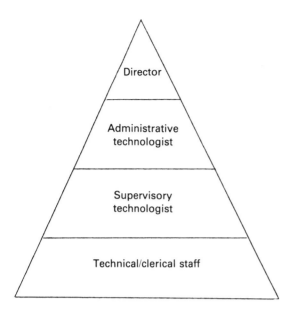

Organization hierarchy

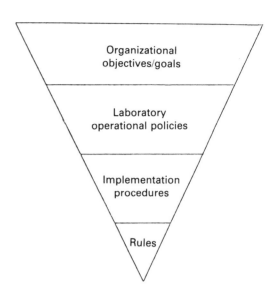

Planning and control mechanisms

FIGURE 3-2.   Laboratory planning and control structures.

and the performance of the newly established special chemistry analyses of the example. The mechanisms in this figure, then, serve a dual and overlapping role with regard to planning and controlling.

ESTABLISHING POLICIES AND PROCEDURES

Planning has sometimes been referred to as preparation for *where* the organization is going. Establishing policies and procedures addresses the question of *how* the

---

Box 3•2

Four Stages of Planning—Systems Approach

1. Establishing the goals and objectives for the laboratory
2. Formulating policies to carry out objectives
3. Developing intermediate and short-range plans to implement policies
4. Stating detailed procedures for implementing each plan

---

organization is going to achieve specific goals. As evidenced in Figure 3-2, planning mechanisms go from the abstract (general purpose objectives, strategies, goals) to the specific (rules). In between are the purposes, principles, and rules of action, known as policies and procedures, that guide an organization. Their purpose is to designate the aims and ends of an organization and the approximate means to be used in their accomplishment.* Laboratorians are familiar with the value of standard operating procedures for testing; these foster consistency of practice among employees and serve an educational purpose.[11,28] Similarly, management policies and procedures guide behavior and serve as a basis for evaluation.

Variations

Within the clinical laboratory, individual policies and procedures will vary according to purpose and application. Policies will vary in specificity. Some policies

---

* This section considers all those directives, both explicit and implied, that qualify as policies and procedures related to the clinical laboratory organizational operations. That is to say that the term *procedures* here excludes the analytical steps and accompanying information that are traditionally found in a laboratory testing procedure manual.[11,28]

should be stated in general terms to allow flexibility by professionals in the department. For example, a policy dealing with time off for continuing education may be written in general terms. By contrast, a procedure written to protect against hepatitis will usually be quite detailed. The importance of policies will also vary. Some will be common sense but must be written for the individual who does not always exercise this trait. In some cases, the level of determination of a policy may be to serve as a guideline only, such as the number of weekends each technologist may be required to work. Other policies will be "hard and fast," such as termination for being under the influence of alcohol while on duty.

Another aspect of policies and procedures that will vary is the timing or frequency. Some policies always apply, as in the case of reporting to work on time. Others are less crucial, such as the acceptable manner of dress if a technologist is called in for emergency laboratory testing in the middle of the night.

Origin

Policies and procedures may originate from various stimuli. One source over which laboratory administrators have little control is government regulation. An obvious example is the impact the Occupational Safety and Health Administration has had on clinical laboratory procedures for health and safety. At times, formal decisions from above in the organizational hierarchy will become the origin of a policy or procedure, as in the case of mandatory compensatory time for weekends worked. If a laboratory functions under a union contract, bargaining agreements become the basis of many policies. In addition, most institutions can point to at least one policy or procedure that originated from tradition. As an example, the allowance of a floating holiday traditionally taken on an employee's birthday suddenly shows up as a written policy stating that the day off must be taken on the employee's birthday. Finally, some policies are initiated through precedent.

Characteristics

There is no magic formula for writing a policy, but several key points are listed here. First, the policy must be reasonable. At times, laboratory managers become so engrossed in providing organizational guidance that this simple common sense component is lacking. If a procedure is not followed, it is usually because it is not understood or was not properly communicated. Understanding generally hinges on adequate two-way communication (discussion) before the policy or procedure is implemented. A policy or procedure also needs to

be flexible so that the policymaker has some latitude in its enforcement.

Some policies address the privileges of being associated with a particular institution or holding a specific position. The policymaker should be aware that such privileges may be perceived as rights. A prime example is the privilege to accumulate earned sick leave to be used in case of a major illness. The policy is laudable and functional until a healthy individual, about to leave the company, decides that it is his right to use his accrued sick hours as vacation days.

Policies and procedures for the operation of a clinical laboratory are typically developed in the form of a manual. A well-written, comprehensive policy and procedure manual can be an effective management tool to clarify management directives, reduce uncertainties, and save time and energy in dealing with personnel problems.[3] Consistent with the focus of strategic planning, the manual should begin with a broad objective, narrowing the focus to details for its accomplishment in the form of policies, procedures, methods, and rules. The example in Box 3-3 by Barros shows this narrowing and integration.[3]

DESIGN OF CLINICAL LABORATORY FLOOR PLAN AND WORK FLOW

An obvious example of integrating the planning, organizing, and controlling activities of laboratory managers is the design of laboratory facilities (see Chapter 17). Occasionally the laboratory practitioner has the opportunity to participate in the structural planning of a new laboratory facility. More frequently, a laboratory manager is asked to relocate a portion of the laboratory or to evaluate the efficiency of an existing section. In this planning, organizing, and controlling activity, several key pieces of information and techniques are useful.

Design of the clinical laboratory floor plan and work flow pattern contains both quantitative and qualitative elements. Frequently, concerns focus only on the amount of space available and not on how efficiently the space is being used.[30]

Design of Laboratory Space

The question of size in planning a laboratory is always a concern. Several factors need to be considered when determining the space required for an efficient laboratory. These include the scope of procedures to be performed, the intended operational approach for performing the procedure, the anticipated size of the laboratory staff, and the setting (eg, a teaching versus a nonteaching institution).[26]

Box 3•3

Creating an Effective Policy and Procedure Manual—Sample Entry

OBJECTIVE:

To provide optimum service in the laboratory department for both inpatients and outpatients

POLICY:

It is the policy of the laboratory to maintain 24-hour service 7 days a week for inpatient testing and 8-hour service 5 days a week for all outpatient procedures, unless special arrangements are made.

PROCEDURE:

1. Maintain sufficient laboratory staffing around the clock for all inpatient services.
2. Provide outpatient services between the hours of 8 AM and 4:30 PM Monday through Friday and 8 AM to noon on Saturday.
3. Schedule appointments for all outpatients.

METHOD:

1. Laboratory staff will be assigned to the following shifts: 7 AM to 3:30 PM; 3 PM to 11 PM; 8 AM to 4:30 PM; 11 PM to 7 AM.
2. Obtain approval from medical director or administrative director to schedule outpatient procedures outside the regular assigned hours.
3. Daily work schedules and job assignments will be posted 2 weekdays in advance.

RULE:

1. All employees will report for duty at time assigned. Deviations from these hours without prior approval will be considered cause for possible disciplinary action.
2. Three reported incidents of unexcused tardiness of more than 10 minutes will result in a written and verbal warning.
3. Five reported incidents of unexcused tardiness of more than 10 minutes will result in 1-day suspension without pay.
4. Additional reported incidents of unexcused tardiness will result in termination.

From Barros A: Developing an effective policy and procedure manual. MLO 17(6):29–33, 1985

Space Allocation

When either relocation or a new facility is planned, the laboratory manager is usually provided information on how much space is allocated for the laboratory. Several terms are essential to convert this information to meaningful figures. The term used to describe the total area based on outside location or building dimensions is the *gross area*. By contrast, the *net (useful) area* is the portion between the walls available for laboratory work space, excluding building support, mechanics (eg, ventilation, shafts for communication and transport, stairways), and support facilities (restrooms, custodial closets, storerooms). Another helpful term is *use factor*, which represents a percentage ratio of net useful area to gross area. The usual use factor for clinical laboratory facilities is 60%.

SCOPE OF SERVICES

The scope of procedures provided by the clinical laboratory reflects the type of hospital, facility, or population it serves. Even so, it is inadequate to project laboratory volume on the basis of the number of hospital beds or annual admissions. Such a projection does not include services provided for outpatient departments, dispensaries, special clinics, or emergency departments. In light of the skyrocketing hospital costs, the number of procedures performed for patients from some type of ambulatory care facility or department is bound to increase at a faster rate than other growth. By their nature, some types of hospitals, such as teaching medical centers with research programs, have increased tests over admission number predictions. Even daily census or percentage of occupancy figures are inadequate predictors owing to seasonal variations, competing providers of similar laboratory services, or the economic conditions of the community.

Laboratory Structural Design

Medical laboratories follow two basic structural designs: modular and open.[39] Both of these have advantages and disadvantages, and the choice of design has historically reflected the laboratory director's preference and philosophy of management. The key point is to recognize the positive and negative characteristics of each design to optimize efficiency and productivity. Indeed, it is possible to use a combination of the two designs within the same laboratory.

MODULAR LABORATORY DESIGN

Figure 3-3 shows the floor plan of a modular laboratory. The emphasis is on departmentalization, with a separate room for each laboratory division. This creates

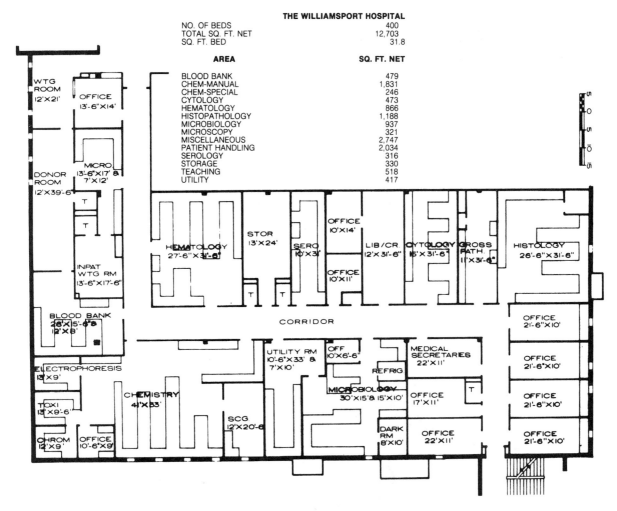

FIGURE 3-3. Modular laboratory design. (From Thomas RG: Manual for Laboratory Planning and Design, p 103. Skokie, College of American Pathologists, 1977. Reprinted with permission of publisher)

a degree of "turfdom." The separation of laboratories by walls has both good and bad effects on interdepartmental communication. Although discouraging needless visiting, the walls do not facilitate easy interaction among divisions when it is appropriate. Although there is little sharing of laboratory equipment in a modular design, there is also little encroachment of space. The modular design appears to be less flexible if expansion is needed, although most walls are removable. There is some merit to the separation of areas from a visibility standpoint to discourage interdepartmental checks and criticism during workload peaks and valleys.

The noise level is reduced in those laboratories where loud instrumentation is not used. The modular design promotes safety in that contaminated specimens can be localized, and in case of fire, the modules would contain the burning materials.

OPEN LABORATORY DESIGN

Figure 3-4 is an example of an open laboratory floor plan. With this design, many of the departments interface freely without dividing walls. For some laboratory administrators, this approach is more aesthetically

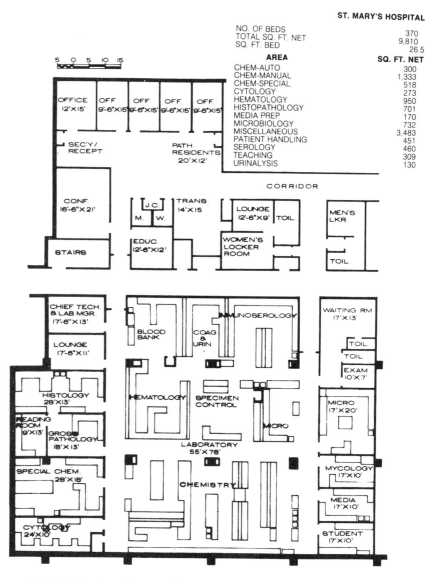

ST. MARY'S HOSPITAL	
NO. OF BEDS	370
TOTAL SQ. FT. NET	9,810
SQ. FT. BED	26.5
AREA	**SQ. FT. NET**
CHEM-AUTO	300
CHEM-MANUAL	1,333
CHEM-SPECIAL	518
CYTOLOGY	273
HEMATOLOGY	950
HISTOPATHOLOGY	701
MEDIA PREP	170
MICROBIOLOGY	732
MISCELLANEOUS	3,483
PATIENT HANDLING	451
SEROLOGY	460
TEACHING	309
URINALYSIS	130

FIGURE 3-4. Open laboratory design. (From Thomas RG: Manual for Laboratory Planning and Design, p 143. Skokie, College of American Pathologists, 1977; reprinted with permission of publisher)

pleasing because it gives the feeling of roominess. The open floor plan promotes interaction between departments and fosters the concept of "one big, happy family." This can have a negative effect if interaction between departments interrupts the daily routine. Visiting is less controllable, and it becomes obvious to all when a particular department is slow. At the same time, a department that is short of staff will feel unjustly busy if personnel cannot be shared. The open floor plan lends itself well to the sharing of equipment, and expansion is easily accomplished within the confines of the laboratory by simply rearranging several benches or reallocating a bench to the expanding department. There is less control of noise and safety hazards in the open design, and planning for both of these concerns is important if this floor plan is adopted.

Laboratory structural design should be consistent with the level of specialization and automation used. Many laboratories today are collapsing several automated areas (hematology, chemistry, endocrine) historically divided in a modular laboratory into a core laboratory.[5,24] The open laboratory design for a core laboratory is the more logical approach. In addition, current trends toward total laboratory automation and the use of robotics makes an open design more logical. Figure 3-5 shows a conceptual approach to movement of specimens and information in a primarily open design using robotics and total automation.[24]

Design of Laboratory Work Flow

Several other key planning, organizing, and controlling strategies deal with the flow of specimens into the laboratory and through the department for analysis and the return of the report to the requesting physician.[38]

Layout Flowchart

Physical layout has important effects on the efficiency of work procedures.[25] The layout flowchart allows the laboratory manager to study physical layout to eliminate unnecessary steps. Following is an example of the benefit of studying the layout work flow of complete blood count (CBC) and coagulation procedures within a hematology department.

Before the study (Fig. 3-6), specimens entered the laboratory by passing the supervisor's area to be logged in by the recording clerk. The CBC specimen then was carried to a cell counter in the far corner of the laboratory, judiciously placed so that it would be away from excessive traffic. The specimen then traveled to a sink area so that smears could be made and stained. Sometimes a routine test, such as a reticulocyte count or sedimentation rate, would briefly sidetrack the specimen before the differential was performed on the central island bench. The path of the CBC report, once the differential was complete, was relatively short, although the path of reporting immediate (*stat*) hemogram results from the cell counter followed the same trip across the room as the specimen originally followed. Coagulation procedures were also placed away from traffic, but this necessitated taking the specimen from the clerk's area, around the end of the central island bench to the far area of the laboratory, and then returning along the same route with the report.

A rearrangement of analytical equipment, which was done after the layout work flow was studied, is shown in Figure 3-7. The clerk responsible for logging in specimens and reporting results was moved closer to the specimen point of entry into the department. The supervisor was relocated to the corner alcove, because the routine specimen flow did not require his interaction. The path traveled by the CBC specimen was shortened considerably by placing the cell counter on the central island bench and relocating the coagulation testing on the same bench as the clerk. Reporting of stat hemogram values, CBC results, and coagulation procedures was facilitated by these relocations. Technical staffing was improved, too. The person operating the cell counter could perform stat coagulation tests with the instrument located directly behind him. The tech-

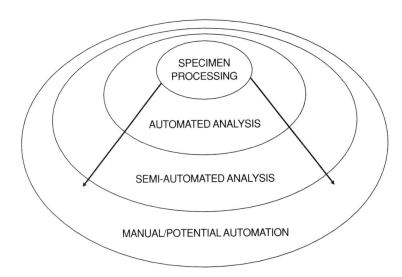

FIGURE 3-5. Schematic representation of a laboratory floor plan, organized based on automation levels.[24]

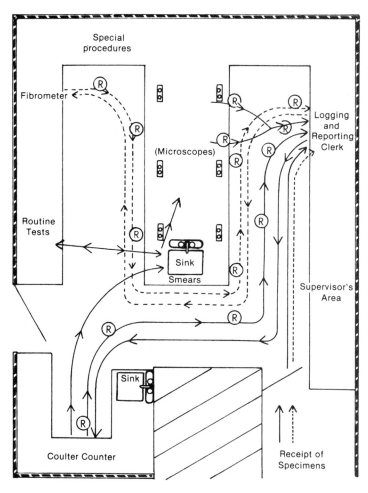

FIGURE 3-6. Laboratory layout flowchart before workflow study.

Key: —— Path of CBC with differential
      --- Path of coagulation tests
      Ⓡ Report Path

nologists performing differentials took advantage of the opportunity to stand up and stretch when taking stacks of completed CBCs back to the clerk for reporting.

Operational Flow Chart

Another helpful tool in assessing the efficiency of laboratory testing is the operational flow chart. The *flow chart* is a symbolic representation of a system broken down into its sequential component steps.[14] A process is first reduced to its basic steps, and these steps are then placed in proper sequence. Finally, the steps are graphically displayed in a flow chart emphasizing decision points and alternate pathways. This technique is especially useful if several individuals must share in the operation of a process. It can also be used to emphasize decision-making modes and describe the degree of responsibility and authority the technical staff has in deciding how a specimen is processed. Figure 3-8A shows some of the symbols frequently used in flow-charting, and Figure 3-8B is a flow chart for the process of urinalysis.[6]

Network Analysis

At times, a laboratory manager may want to add a time and efficiency dimension to the operational flowchart, which is best accomplished by using a network analysis

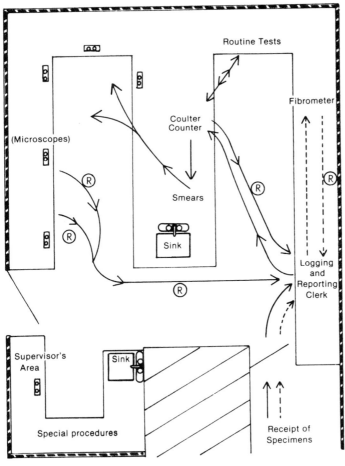

Key: —— Path of CBC with differential
 - - - Path of coagulation tests
 (R) Report Path

FIGURE 3-7. Laboratory layout flowchart after workflow study.

technique. Bennington defines *network analysis* as a "schematic and mathematical approach to the planning of a project which shows the relationships among different activities and how their timing will affect the overall project."[7] Several components of a project are evaluated, including the shortest possible completion time, activities with delay potential, and extra-effort-to-cost-benefit analysis.

The two most commonly used network analysis approaches are the program evaluation review technique (PERT) and critical path method (CPM). PERT is appropriate when one or more of the completion points must be reached at a specific time or in planning a project where a high degree of uncertainty exists (a totally new project, for example). The CPM technique, while similar, does not require a specific point completion time as in PERT.

The basis of network analysis includes construction of activities and events (Fig. 3-9). An *activity* is an operation requiring time between two events, such as drawing blood. An *event* is a time when one or more activities commence or are completed. For example, the receipt of the requisition in the laboratory (event) must precede the blood-drawing (activity). The *critical path* is defined as the chain of events and the total time all of these together require for completion of a project. The *noncritical path* is a chain of events leading to completion of the project but exclusive of some events in the overall project. *Float*

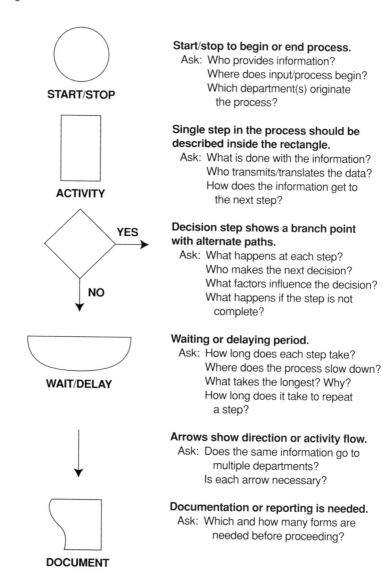

START/STOP

Start/stop to begin or end process.
Ask: Who provides information?
        Where does input/process begin?
        Which department(s) originate
        the process?

ACTIVITY

**Single step in the process should be
described inside the rectangle.**
Ask: What is done with the information?
        Who transmits/translates the data?
        How does the information get to
        the next step?

YES

NO

**Decision step shows a branch point
with alternate paths.**
Ask: What happens at each step?
        Who makes the next decision?
        What factors influence the decision?
        What happens if the step is not
        complete?

WAIT/DELAY

Waiting or delaying period.
Ask: How long does each step take?
        Where does the process slow down?
        What takes the longest? Why?
        How long does it take to repeat
        a step?

Arrows show direction or activity flow.
Ask: Does the same information go to
        multiple departments?
        Is each arrow necessary?

DOCUMENT

Documentation or reporting is needed.
Ask: Which and how many forms are
        needed before proceeding?

FIGURE 3-8.
(*A*) Flowchart symbols.[14]   **A**

is a term for spare time (slack) resulting from the difference between the times to accomplish the critical path and the noncritical path. Two activities can branch from a given event, thus creating concurrent activities within the project. Additional planning and evaluation tools can be found in Chapter 4.

LABORATORY ORGANIZATIONAL STRUCTURE

Organization in the clinical laboratory refers to structure and process.[8] *Structure* exemplifies stated relationships or framework, while *process* deals with interaction. The

three key elements of organization are the tasks to be performed, the individuals who are to perform the tasks, and the clinical laboratory as a workplace.

Organization of the Pathology Laboratory

Figure 3-10 is an example of an organizational chart for a clinical laboratory.[4] Note that this structure includes a core or central laboratory rather than multiple specialized sections. Although a standard fixture in most organizations, the chart serves only limited functions, one

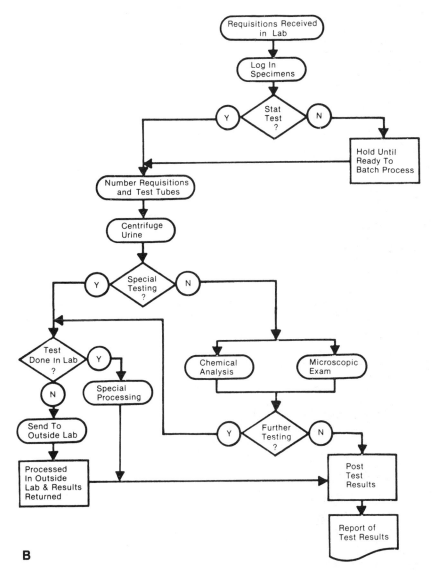

B

FIGURE 3-8. *(continued)* *(B)* Urinalysis flowchart. (From Bennington JL: Management and Cost Control Techniques for the Clinical Laboratory, pp 228, 232–233. Baltimore, University Park Press, 1977. Reprinted with permission of publisher)

of which is providing visualization of who is doing what and the chain of command. Townsend advocates the use of an organizational chart solely as an administrative tool—not for everyone's consumption.[40] As he has pointed out, organizational charts tend to demoralize people because nobody likes to think of himself as being below other people. Figure 3-11 shows the basic

functional titles included in the Clinical Laboratory Improvement Amendments of 1988 regulations, although other titles are frequently used.[36]

Organization plays an important role in the effectiveness of the clinical laboratory by defining the relationship between tasks, individuals, and the workplace. The basis for this relationship is authority, responsibility,

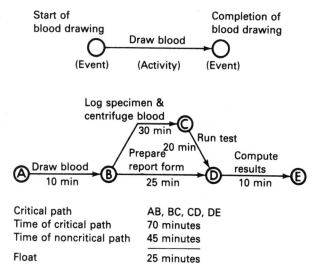

FIGURE 3-9. Network analysis—critical path method. (From Bennington JL: Management and Cost Control Techniques for the Clinical Laboratory, pp 242, 244. Baltimore, University Park Press, 1977; reprinted with permission of publisher)

and accountability. A laboratory manager possesses *authority* within the organization if he has the right to issue instructions that others are expected to follow. Authority is generally attached to a position, and its location on the organizational chart implies a degree of consent. *Responsibility* refers to the group of tasks or duties assigned an individual or position in the organizational structure, and *accountability* is the obligation to a higher authority for the successful fulfillment of assigned tasks. The organizational structure is a visual aid for evaluating each of these basics. For example, when investigating the difficulty a laboratory supervisor is experiencing in maintaining sufficient inventory (responsibility), the laboratory director may realize that the problem is in the purchasing system, which does not accept the supervisor's signature on a requisition (authority).

The organizational chart also attempts to show relationships between line and staff. In this organizational concept, a *line position* is one in which a superior exercises direct supervision over a subordinate. A *staff position* is advisory, supportive, or auxiliary. These terms were defined in industry, and health-care institutions seldom use the same connotation. When a laboratory manager speaks of his staff, he generally is referring to his technical personnel, who are serving in line positions. Individuals involved solely in academic instruction and research would be defined as staff to the functioning anatomic and clinical laboratories. Another component of the structure, more visibly staff, is the administrative section. Its role is supportive to the primary laboratory-testing function. There are times when line–staff conflicts occur, stemming primarily from a failure to define clearly the operational difference between the two.[23] This may produce a conflict when the rightful prerogative of a line supervisor is usurped by a staff administrator.

Sometimes it is helpful to map out the relationships in an organizational structure from several standpoints. Gallamore has contrasted the change in relationships and roles that occurs when both administrative and technical structures (in a highly departmentalized laboratory) are delineated (Fig. 3-12).[13] Consider the changing role of the laboratory manager in the two structures. In the administrative structure, he serves in a line position, while in the technical structure, his position is staff.

Organizational Design and Hierarchy

An organizational hierarchy is a multilevel, vertical structure signifying who outranks whom. In designing or evaluating a laboratory organizational hierarchy, several characteristics should be considered.

Departmentation or Specialization

The design of all organizational structures includes a division of labor. Overall goals are divided into activities. These activities are subsequently separated into departments to achieve a degree of specialization. In the medical laboratory, departments have reflected uniformity of technique (chemical analysis), uniformity of specimen required (whole blood for hematologic analysis), uniformity of function (administrative support), or uniformity of patient services (stat laboratory). In any large laboratory, it is obvious that specialization has

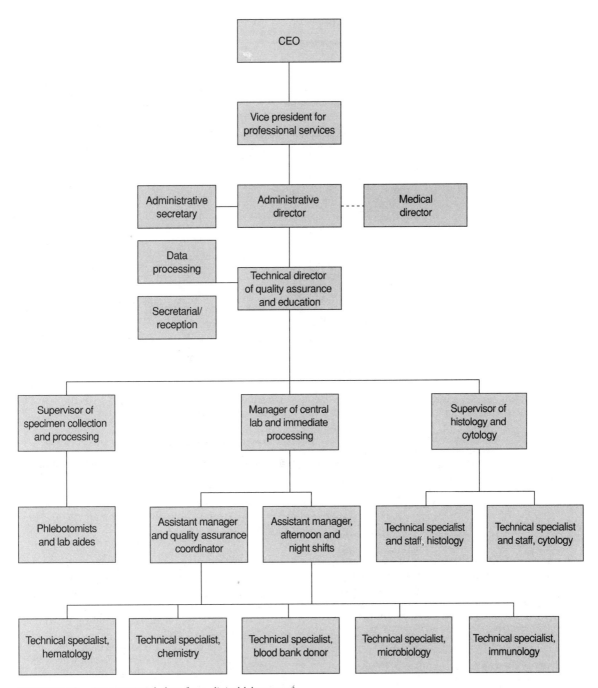

FIGURE 3-10. Organizational chart for a clinical laboratory.[4]

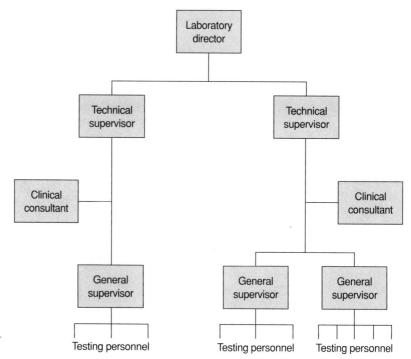

FIGURE 3-11. Laboratory performing high complexity testing.

a positive effect on efficiency. At the same time, the technical staff generally suffers from a degree of boredom with its limited scope of analytical procedures.

As noted previously, restructuring of clinical laboratories currently includes a trend toward a core laboratory with complementary specialized sections. This is consistent with the philosophy of a cluster organization.[27] Clusters are often designed around functional groups as shown in Figure 3-13.[16]

Scalar Principle

Organizational structures reflect a scalar chain or line of authority from the ultimate superiors in the laboratory (directors) down to the lowest rank, sometimes referred to as the chain of command. Authority throughout the hierarchy implies that decisions are being made at numerous levels.

Unity of Direction

If goals are to be achieved, coordination is essential. Unity of direction requires that a single laboratory manager be responsible for coordinating the activities necessary for achieving these goals and for the technical and support staff assigned to his department. By scruti-

nizing the organizational structure, it should be possible to eliminate overlapping managerial responsibilities.

Unity of Command

Not only must a single manager have coordinating responsibility for specific activities and personnel, he must also have the authority to carry these out. Another way of stating this concept is to say that a worker should receive orders from only one superior and be accountable only to him.

Span of Control

Effective control necessitates a limitation on the number of subordinates a manager is to supervise. Bennington states that four to six subordinates are appropriate.[8] The ideal number of subordinates probably varies with an individual manager's skills.

The concept of span of control is being challenged today as health-care organizations seek effective methods of "downsizing" or "rightsizing" their workforce.[10] Middle-management positions, specifically supervisory positions, are being removed in a delayering trend in response to economic pressures. A careful, reasoned approach to modifying the organizational structure requires an assessment of type and level of work done by

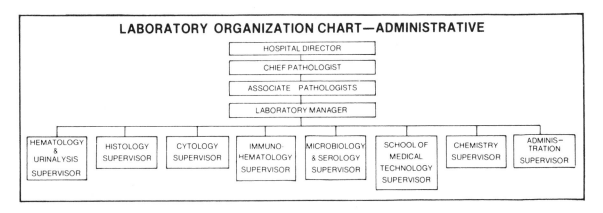

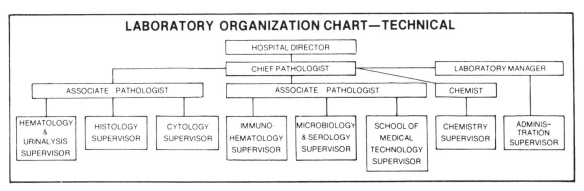

FIGURE 3-12. Laboratory organization chart—administrative versus technical structure. (From Gallamore C: The evolving role of the laboratory manager. Laboratory Management 13:45, 1975; reprinted with the permission of publisher)

subordinates, level of subordinate interdependence, subordinate and manger training, lateral communication channels, subordinate turnover (frequency of training), information systems technology assisting subordinates, and the number of performance requirements and measures.[10]

Depending on the institution and philosophy of the laboratory director, most organizational charts will fall into one of two basic designs. Figure 3-14 is an example of a flat organizational structure with few levels of hierarchy. By contrast, Figure 3-15 is a tall organizational structure with numerous levels. Without making a value judgment concerning which is better, consider some of their respective characteristics. The tall structure generally is used when there is increased specialization. Both the flat and tall structures exhibit the scalar chain of command, although the increased number of levels in the tall structure may prompt uncoordinated decisions and bypassing. The tall structure, by its inherent specialization, will generally permit a greater unity of direction. This can

be negated if an assistant chief technologist in the structure insists on having a say in the supervisor's coordinating decisions, thus making the unity of command ineffective. In this case, the technologists may think they must serve two masters. The flat structure is characterized by a broad span of control—many subordinates responsible to one superior—whereas the tall structure shows a short span of control. If the span of control is too broad, the manager may not have access to sufficient information to make quality decisions, or the technologists may complain that they cannot see their supervisor or get decisions made at all. If the span of control is too short, the manager may oversupervise by participating in day-to-day operations or offering unsolicited advice.

Organizational Myths and the Informal Structure

The organizational hierarchy, no matter how well designed, does not ensure total organization. Figure 3-16 shows the impact of the informal organization. It is not

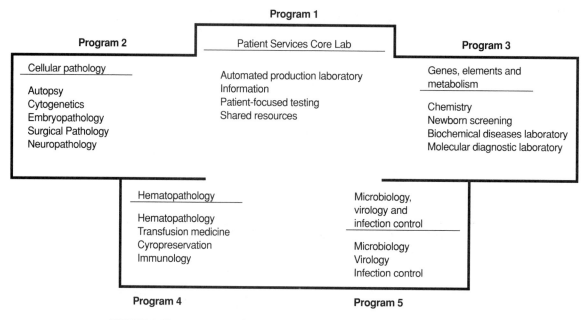

FIGURE 3-13.   Reengineered structure of BCCH/WH laboratory (functional alignment) (Reference 16).

always true that decisions are made by the manager, with orders flowing down and feedback information flowing up. The broken lines, indicating routes of communication in the informal structure, may be substantially different from those planned in the formal structure. The organizational chart may not show the true distinctions between line and staff or the influences that may affect decisions, as in the relationship between the administrative technologist and line technologist under Supervisor 3. Bypassing can occur, as reflected by the lines of communication and influence under Supervisor 1, whose assistant is totally missed. Supervisor 2 undoubtedly is affected by the influence two of his technologists have on his superiors, and it is certainly possible that the line technologist who influences the chief has more power in the structure than any other single technologist or supervisor. Lest one conclude that the informal organization is all bad, this simply is not the case.[32] Often information is communicated more abundantly and efficiently through informal channels than through those delineated in the formal structure. The informal organization is inevitable and has positive and negative consequences. The laboratory manager must be aware of its existence and impact.

REENGINEERING THE CLINICAL LABORATORY

Over the years, clinical laboratory managers have embraced various change concepts in a seemingly endless quest to gain greater efficiency while preserving quality. When clinical laboratories became cost centers under prospective payment reimbursement provisions,

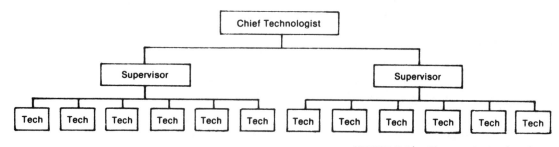

FIGURE 3-14.   Flat organizational structure.

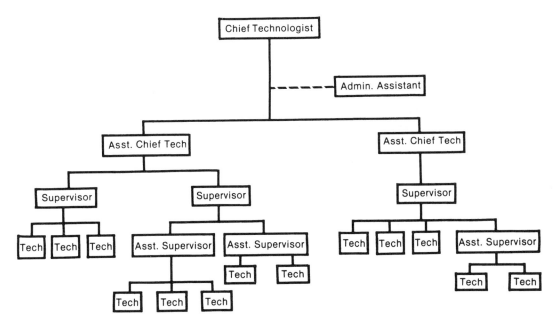

FIGURE 3-15.   Tall organizational structure.

streamlining of operations and rightsizing (a euphemism for downsizing) became popular change strategies. More recently, total quality management (TQM) and continuous quality improvement (CQI), an approach to quality management that focuses on meeting customer expectations, has taken the limelight for innovation. TQM/CQI emphasizes team or institutional performance to improve quality by looking at the design of systems or procedures as opposed to an individual employee's work.

All of these change concepts have dealt mostly with existing structures and processes. While improvements in efficiency and quality are possible with streamlining, rightsizing, and TQM/CQI, gains are lim-

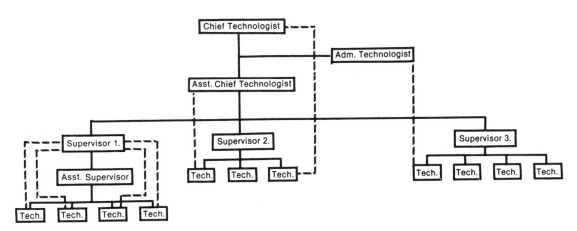

FIGURE 3-16.   Example of informal organizational structure. Broken lines indicate routes of communication and sources of influence not evident in the formal organizational structure.

ited to changes realized from adapting an existing system. Ongoing downsizing and restructuring reduces the number of people in the laboratory with a commensurate reduction in costs. However, the work does not disappear, and the people who stay are often overburdened. In some instances, the cost savings are only temporary as deleted positions are rejustified and reestablished based on work volume and a need to improve quality to the customer. New technology in the laboratory has also contributed to the belief that gains can be realized by restructuring. However, if you take existing processes that are not efficient and automate them with new technology, you end up with automated inefficiency.

Reengineering: Revolutionary Change

To realize major gains, major changes must be made. Enter the far more revolutionary change strategy of reengineering. Reengineering involves radically changing and reinventing the way work is done in the delivery of laboratory services.[21,22] Most large laboratories have built up layer on layer of bureaucracy and developed elaborate ways to process work. In some cases, these processes have become complicated and unwieldy. Few laboratories have stepped back to look at the entire laboratory services delivery system. Today, if a clinical laboratory was just beginning, managers might invent it in a totally different way.

Reengineering requires sweeping changes in management practices and organizational structure. Traditional vertical structures are replaced with a horizontal approach, which minimizes autocracy. Like TQM, reengineering uses interdisciplinary and interdepartmental teams to identify and solve problems but goes a step beyond in empowering employees to work in new arrangements. Employees close to the action are allowed to make key decisions. In short, reengineering redefines the way the laboratory uses technology and human resources.

Today, few clinical laboratories are reaping the benefits of reengineering. The majority of the literature on reengineering is found in the business literature. From the successes and failures reported there, laboratory managers can get a head start on preparing for reengineering.

Help shape the process.[17] Upper-level administration may lay down general guidelines and directions for a reengineering effort, but the laboratory management and staff will often play a role in determining whether it will succeed. Laboratory managers can help shape the reengineering process by suggesting selection criteria, interviewing, and evaluating candidates to serve on a steering committee. Identifying and dissemi-

nating literature about reengineering will also help prepare key staff who will serve as team leaders and team members in the process.

Create job statements and role descriptions that reflect the new laboratory structure. Existing position descriptions will not likely be useful for new positions created from reengineering. With reengineering, job statements are used as a standing point instead of position descriptions; roles are outlines as opposed to listing tasks; and work is structured around the customer rather than a specific function or department.

Devise a plan for working out compensation issues. The laboratory manager will need to work closely with the human resources department to structure pay scales and rewards commensurate with newly defined roles. This is crucial if the desired reengineering results are to be realized. Reengineering poses an opportunity to realign the position classifications of the laboratory to match better other high-complexity support services in the hospital.

Train the new work force.[17] A reengineered laboratory will have staff in roles that are new for them and for which they will require training. At the very least, training in team building, teamwork, and team decision making should be planned. Building trust in the new order will require emphasis over time.

Facilitate communication in the work force. Reengineering requires much change in the workplace, and change is always unsettling. Frequent meetings throughout the reengineering process to share the evolving plan and gather feedback will help quell the anxiety of change. Even brief printed pieces can be used to help staff understand how reengineering will benefit everyone in the future. Staff must realize that reengineering is not just another cost-cutting tool. Rather, it is a reinvention process about the quality of laboratory services provided to the customer, which ultimately affects the health of the institution and job security.

In summary, reengineering is a change strategy calling for reinvention of how laboratory services are provided. Some laboratories purport to be involved in reengineering when they are simply streamlining or tweaking existing operations. True reengineering focuses on change in core processes. Examples from the business world point to befits from reengineering, including better operational performance and improved basis for competition.

CONTROLLING OPERATIONS IN THE LABORATORY

The final management function of the laboratory administrator is controlling, that is, ensuring that plans are carried through the organizational and operational phases so that goals are met. Therein, the control process is closely linked to planning and organizational structure (see Fig. 3-2).

The control process involves (1) establishing standards, (2) measuring performance against these standards, and (3) correcting deviations from standards and plans.[7] Controlling involves locating operational weaknesses—those factors having a negative impact on the economical, effective, and efficient achievement of goals—and taking the appropriate action to ensure desired results.

Standards may be determined in several ways. Within the clinical laboratory, standards are mathematically determined to control the quality of any given analytical process (see Chapter 18). Standards may also be determined by experience or competitive operations, for example, in controlling the turnaround time acceptable for stat procedures. Finally, standards may be suggested or mandated by an accrediting body or governmental agency.

An excellent example of control within the clinical laboratory is the technique of self-study or evaluation preceding an accreditation inspection. The standards have been specified by the accrediting body. The operation of the laboratory is compared with these standards, and corrective action is implemented.

The clinical laboratory, by its complex nature, poses a problem of controlling medical data. Intralaboratory communications are essential for the correlation of patient results. Figure 3-17 is an example of a control mechanism for investigating patient results that are either abnormal (beyond established acceptable parameters) or have a questionable correlation. The use of such a communications form may prompt a chart review or discussion with the attending physician to ensure the release of quality data.

Control is also applicable in the management of human resources for the clinical laboratory. Personnel policies and procedures are the established standards against which performance is measured. Chapter 14 describes performance evaluation techniques and approaches. Control of deviations from established policy must be recorded to investigate the problem and take corrective action. Even many routine activities covered by personnel policy are best controlled using some form of documentation. Figure 3-18 is a general incident report form used to assist in recording deviations from routine, and Figure 3-19 is an example of staffing control by ensuring adequate coverage before an absence is granted and written documentation of the exercised policy.

The control process includes correction of deviations, a topic in itself when considering human resources. The single most important resource of the laboratory manager is his technical staff, and discipline (the

corrective phase of the control process) must be justly executed. The process is positively influenced if the supervisor creates an atmosphere in which employees abide by rules they consider fair. When necessary, discipline should be exercised in a gradual manner: first an oral reprimand, then written warnings, and finally suspension. The disciplinary sequence usually includes a statement and description of the problem, collection of facts, decision regarding the penalty and application thereof, and follow-up. Discipline should only be applied as a last resort. Indeed, the laboratory manager faces a dilemma when discipline is necessary. The climate of cooperation and trust is threatened. Douglas McGregor encourages the use of the "red hot stove rule" to preserve a cooperative and fair working environment. Under this rule, discipline is immediate, consistent, and impersonal. The manager must not procrastinate his decision to punish. The decision to punish must be made every time the deviation occurs, and the act should be punished, not the individual. This analogy between touching a hot stove and discipline allows no room for favoritism, waiting until punishment is more convenient, or applying a penalty inconsistent with the offense—all of which would promote unfairness.[37]

MANAGEMENT BY OBJECTIVES

Management by objectives (MBO) is a managerial process reflective of the planning, organization, and control functions. The MBO concept was first described by Drucker in 1954, and much research has been conducted on the process since that time.[41]

MBO is defined as a process whereby an employee and manager jointly define major areas of responsibility within the work setting, identify the commonality of organizational and personal goals, and establish a mutual understanding and acceptance of plans for future activities.[20,35]

Odiorne clarifies MBO as a set of procedural rules for management.[29] Figure 3-20 graphically displays a map of the MBO cycle. The key features of a typical MBO program are listed in Box 3-4.[15]

A key element in the MBO process is the definition of goals and objectives. *Goals* are general aims or purposes. *Objectives* are specific plans to achieve results through defined tasks within a certain time. For example, a goal may be "to increase the provision of appropriate procedures available on the midnight to 8 AM shift. The laboratory manager and hematology supervisor may jointly agree on the following objective:

To offer reticulocyte counts as a stat procedure during the midnight to 8 AM shift by retaining the technical staff covering these hours such that this pro-

UNIVERSITY OF NEBRASKA MEDICAL CENTER
CLINICAL PATHOLOGY
PATIENT RESULTS

INTRALABORATORY COMMUNICATION
ABNORMAL and or QUESTIONABLE DATA

TO: Dr. Frest (Clinical Pathologist)
FROM: Susan B. (Medical Tech.)
*PATIENT'S NAME: John Citizen *HOSPITAL NUMBER 012345
(and Initials)
PATIENT'S DOCTOR: Dr. Doctor INPATIENT: X
(and Initials) OUTPATIENT:
ROOM NUMBER 5433-1
DOCTOR'S TELEPHONE NUMBER 3033 WARD TELEPHONE NUMBER
*DATE/TIME 8-12-80
*REASON FOR COMMUNICATION:

↓ Anion Gap

*ESSENTIAL LAB DATA

Date	Time	TESTS 4-19 ANION GAP	8.4-10.4 CA++	6-8 TP	3.4-5.2 ALB	<3.1 GLOBIN		
8/6	0726			6.5	3.7	2.8		
8/12	0753	2	15.3					

ACTION TAKEN:

CONCLUSION: Malignant melanoma patient w/↑ Ca++

COMMENT: Admission diagnosis – malignant melanoma
Patient running ↑ Ca++
↑↑ proteins

*MINIMAL REQUIREMENT IN EMERGENCIES: COMPLETE THESE ITEMS

8-8-13
Date

Signature (Clinical Pathologist)

FIGURE 3-17. Control mechanism for abnormal or questionable laboratory data. (Reprinted with permission of the Chairman, Department of Pathology, University of Nebraska Medical Center)

CONFIDENTIAL REPORT OF INCIDENT (Not part of medical record)

Name and address of person involved. Give medical record number. Use addressograph if available.	IDENTIFICATION	SEX	AGE	TIME LOST (Employees Only)	NURSES STA. NO.
	☐ 1 - Patient ☐ 2 - Employee ☐ 3 - Visitor	☐ 1 - Female ☐ 2 - Male		☐ 1 - Yes (If unknown, check "No".) ☐ 2 - No	
	(19)	(20)	(21-23)	(24)	(25-29)

	INCIDENT DATE	REPORT DATE	INCIDENT		HOSPITAL CODE NOS.	
			SHIFT	TIME	STATE (2 Digits)	HOSP. NUMBER (3 Digits)
	(Digits Only)	(Digits Only)	☐ 01 - 1st ☐ 02 - 2nd ☐ 03 - 3rd	☐ A.M. ☐ P.M.		
(1 - 18)	(30 - 35)	(36 - 41)	(42 - 43)		(44 - 48)	

CONDITION BEFORE (Patients Only)	BED ADJUSTMENT (Not Bed Rails) (Patients Only)	LOCATION OF INCIDENT		NATURE OF INJURY (Injury sustained as a result of incident)
☐ 1 - Normal ☐ 2 - Senile ☐ 3 - Disoriented ☐ 4 - Sedated ☐ 5 - Unconscious ☐ 6 - Other ☐ 7 - Behavior	☐ 1 - Not Applicable ☐ 2 - Up ☐ 3 - Down	☐ 400 Admitting ☐ 410 Offices ☐ 420 Elevators ☐ 430 Corridors ☐ 440 Stairs ☐ 450 General Premises - Interior ☐ 460 Housekeeping ☐ 470 Dietary ☐ 480 Laundry ☐ 490 Eng. & Maint. ☐ 500 Patient's Room	☐ 510 Patients Bathroom ☐ 520 Nurses Station ☐ 530 Surgery & Recovery ☐ 540 Delivery, Labor & Recovery ☐ 550 Central Supply ☐ 560 Laboratory ☐ 570 Pharmacy ☐ 580 X - Ray ☐ 590 Physical Therapy ☐ 600 Emergency ☐ 610 Parking Lots & Sidewalks ☐ 620 General Premises - Exterior	☐ 100 Asphyxia, Strangulation, Inhalation ☐ 110 Burn or Scald ☐ 120 Chemical Burn ☐ 130 Concussion ☐ 140 Contagious or Infectious Disease ☐ 150 Contusion, Cut, Laceration ☐ 160 Fracture or Dislocation ☐ 170 Viscera Injury ☐ 180 Sprain or Strain ☐ 190 No Injury ☐ 200 No Apparent Injury ☐ 210 Other - Not Classified
(49)	(50)	(51 - 53)		(54 - 56)

INCIDENT CAUSE (57 - 58) If more than one cause, check predominating one and describe others in lower part of report.
*Do not use for employee or visitor incidents.

A - Falls	B - Medication		C - Other	
☐ 1 - Bed, Rail Up ☐ 2 - Bed, Rail Down ☐ 3 - From Chair or Equip. ☐ 4 - From Different Level ☐ 5 - On Same Level ☐ 6 - Fainting	☐ 7 - Patient Identification ☐ 8 - Dosage ☐ 9 - Route ☐ 10 - Unordered ☐ 11 - Duplication ☐ 12 - Omission	☐ 13 - Transcription ☐ 14 - Transfusion ☐ 15 - Wrong Medication ☐ 16 - Labeling ☐ 17 - Time Given ☐ 18 - Other ☐ 19 - I.V. or Injection Tech.	☐ 20 - Struck by Patient ☐ 21 - Struck by Equipment ☐ 22 - Struck Equipment ☐ 23 - Struck by Tool or Object ☐ 24 - Overexertion-Handling Pt. ☐ 25 - Lifting or Moving ☐ 26 - Loss of Personal Property	☐ 27 - Patient Care - Nurses ☐ 28 - Patient Care - Others ☐ 29 - Anesthesia ☐ 30 - Sponge, etc. Count ☐ 31 - Patient Identification ☐ 32 - Caught, In, On, or Between ☐ 33 - Misc. ☐ 34 - Needle Puncture

IF PATIENT	IF EMPLOYEE	IF VISITOR
Out-of-Bed Privileges? ☐ Yes ☐ No	Dept: _____	Reason for presence: _____
Cause for Hospitalization: _____	Job Title: _____	
	Date returned to work: _____	Home Phone: _____
Room No.: _____ Attending Physician: _____	☐ First Aid Only	Occupation: _____

GIVE BRIEF DESCRIPTION OF INCIDENT, INCLUDING PREDOMINATING AND CONTRIBUTING CAUSES. _____

_____

_____

EQUIPMENT INVOLVED: _____ MANUFACTURER: _____ SERIAL NO.: _____

STATE CORRECTIVE ACTION TAKEN TO PREVENT RECURRENCE. INDICATE IF FURTHER INVESTIGATION IS NECESSARY. _____

_____

List all patients in the room. Give names and addresses of witnesses. _____

_____

Was person seen by a physician? ☐ Yes ☐ No If "Yes", time seen: _____ A.M./_____ P.M.	PHYSICIAN'S NAME (PRINT)	PHYSICIAN'S SIGNATURE

PHYSICIAN'S FINDINGS _____

Name and Address of HOSPITAL	Name and title of person preparing the report.
	Supervisor's Signature

| (C - 2682 - H) 6-77 | HOSPITAL USE | CAT. 450707
PRINTED IN U.S.A. |

FIGURE 3-18. Incident report form. (Reprinted with permission of the Chancellor, University of Nebraska Medical Center)

UNIVERSITY OF NEBRASKA MEDICAL CENTER
ABSENCE REPORT
Submit to the Personnel Department to Report All Absences

Name _____   Date _____

Soc. Sec. _____   ☐ Monthly

Department Name: _____ Dept. No. _____   ☐ Bi-Weekly

I request that my absence of _____ hours from _____ thru _____ inclusive be charged to:

Vacation	☐	Leave of Absence	☐	Military Leave	☐	Work Comp. Injury	☐
Sick Leave	☐	Funeral Leave	☐	Jury Duty	☐	Other	☐
						Reason _____	

I have made arrangements with _____ or _____
                                    Supervisor   Staff Alternate
to discharge my duties and responsibilities during the period of my absence.

                          with
This absence is to be   pay.
                        without

FOR PERSONNEL USE ONLY

_____ _____ hours to be paid

PE-60 9/78

Signature of Employee

Recommended: _____
                    Dept. or Administrative Head

Approved: _____
                    Director of Personnel

FIGURE 3-19. Absence report form. (Reprinted with permission of the Chancellor, University of Nebraska Medical Center)

Box 3•4

Management By Objectives: Key Features

- The laboratory's common goals and the measures of success in meeting these are reaffirmed and considered, respectively.
- In light of past goal achievement, any revisions to the organizational structure are made to facilitate achievement.
- The supervisor and subordinate meet to discuss and set goals for the subordinate for a specified period of time (eg, 6 months). These goals reflect needs of both the organization and the subordinate.
- A joint agreement on the goals established and criteria for measuring and evaluating these goals is determined.

- At various intermediate times in the evaluation period, the supervisor and subordinate review the progress of the subordinate toward the mutually accepted goals. The supervisor's role is one of support, coaching, and counseling, rather than judging. Goals may be redefined or eliminated if they are no longer appropriate within the organizational context.
- A final evaluation at the end of the predetermined period measures the subordinate's achievement based on results accomplished, not on activities, mistakes, or organizational requirements.
- The performance of the entire laboratory is reassessed.
- From this point, the cycle is reinitiated.

(See reference 15)

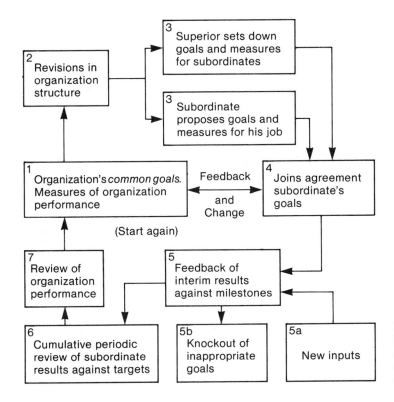

FIGURE 3-20. The cycle of management by objectives. (From Odiorne GS: Management by Objectives. New York, Pitman Corporation, 1972. Reprinted with permission of the publisher)

cedure will be performed with the same precision exhibited by daytime personnel by November 1, 19.

Based on this objective for the supervisor in light of organizational goals, a joint agreement between the supervisor and staff technologist on the midnight to 8 AM shift might be as follows:

> To perform reticulocyte counts routinely on the midnight to 8 AM shift with results not exceeding 5% variance from those obtained by day-shift personnel. This objective is to be reached by October 15, 19   following two in-service sessions and a structured period of reading and evaluating reticulocyte counts preanalysis and postanalysis by day-shift technical staff.

From this example, it is obvious that MBO can be implemented at any supervisor or subordinate level. MBO is not a panacea leadership process for involving subordinates in their work. While the advantages generally outweigh the disadvantages, several counterproductive problems can occur:

Heel-dragging participation. Both the supervisor and the employee must stretch their capabilities, rather than maintain the status quo.

Setting low standards (objectives). Some supervisors and subordinates set objectives well within reach, causing the employee always to appear favorable on evaluation and the department to appear full of overachievers.

Quantification. It is critically important that specific criteria be established for measuring achievement of objectives. It is difficult to define measurable criteria for some objectives, such as the improvement of morale.

REFERENCES

1. Albers J, Vice JL: Strategic planning. Am J Med Technol 49: 411–414, 1983
2. Anthony RN: Planning and Control Systems: A Framework for Analysis, p 16. Boston, Harvard Graduate School of Business Administration, 1965
3. Barros A: Developing an effective policy and procedure manual. MLO 17(6):29–33, 1985
4. Barros A: Reorganize your lab structure for productivity in the '90s. MLO 21(12):33–37, 1989
5. Bauer S, Teplitz C: Total lab automation: System design. MLO 26(9):44–50, 1995
6. Bennington JL: Flow charting. In Bennington JL, Handmaker H, Freedman GS, et al (eds): Management and Cost Con-

trol Techniques for the Clinical Laboratory, pp 225–237. Baltimore, University Park Press, 1977

7. Bennington JL: Network analysis. In Bennington JL, et al (eds): Management and Cost Control Techniques for the Clinical Laboratory, pp 239–257. Baltimore, University Park Press, 1977

8. Bennington JL: Organization and management. In Bennington JL, et al (eds): Management and Cost Control Techniques for the Clinical Laboratory, pp 31–42. Baltimore, University Park Press, 1977

9. Bezold C: The future of healthcare: Implications for the allied health professions. Journal of Allied Health 18:437–457, 1989

10. Blanchard MR: Delayering and span of control: A model to assess appropriate size during downsizing. Clin Lab Management Rev 9:430–439, 1995

11. Cordle DG, Floss AM, Strauss RG: A systematic and painless method for procedure manual review. Clin Lab Sci 9: 186–187, 1996

12. Fulmer RM: Supervision: Principles of Professional Management, pp 235–253. Beverly Hills, Glencoe Press, 1976

13. Gallamore C: The evolving role of the laboratory manager. Laboratory Management 13:45, 1975

14. Garza D: Reviving an old tool to target improvements. Clin Lab Sci 7:215–217, 1994

15. Gibson JL, Ivancevich JM, Donnelly JW: Organization Behavior, Structure, Processes, 3rd ed, pp 30–32, 366–367. Dallas Business Publication, 1979

16. Herbst DS, Dimmick JE: A model to begin reengineering the laboratory. Clin Lab Management Rev 9:396–403, 1995

17. Herbst DS, Dimmick JE: Strategies for a successful organizational transition. Clin Lab Management Rev 9:404–408, 1995

18. Holmberg SR: Strategic planning: A tool for the clinical laboratory. Clin Lab Management Rev 2:185–194, 1988

19. Holmberg SR, Logue LJ: A clinical laboratory environmental assessment and its implications for strategic planning: Part I. Clin Lab Management Rev 4:16–23, 1990

20. Holmbrg SR, Logue LJ: Developing an environmental assessment for effective clinical laboratory strategic planning: Part II. Clin Lab Management Rev 4:99–104, 1990

21. Johansson HJ, McHugh P, Pendleburg AJ, Wheeler WA: Business Process Reengineering: Breakpoint Strategies for Market Dominance. New York, John Wiley & Sons, 1993

22. Johnson E: Reengineering the laboratory: Strategic process and systems innovation to improve performance. Clin Lab Management Rev 9:370–380, 1995

23. Kast FE, Rosenzweig JE: Organization and Management: A Systems Approach, 2nd ed, pp 213–217. New York, McGraw-Hill, 1974

24. Markin RS: Clinical laboratory automation: A paradigm shift. Clin Lab Management Rev 7:243–251, 1993

25. Mayer RW: Designing a more productive laboratory. MLO 17(7):67–71, 1985

26. McCutheon G: Space allocation guidelines for the clinical laboratory. J Med Technol 2:772–777, 1985

27. Mills DQ, Friesen GB: Clusterss: A new style of organization. Clin Lab Management Rev 6:499–513, 1992

28. National Committee for Clinical Laboratory Standards: Clinical Laboratory Technical Procedure Manuals, GP2-R2. Villanova, PA, NCCLS, 1992

29. Odiorne GS: MBO: A backward glance. Business Horizons 21:14–24, 1978

30. Rappoport AE: Laboratory design. In Race GJ (ed): Laboratory Medicine, Vol IV (rev), pp 1–30. Hagerstown, Harper & Row, 1979

31. Reeves PN: Strategic planning revisited. Clin Lab Management Rev 8:549–554, 1994

32. Roseman E: Tune in to the informal organization in your lab. MLO 14(7):102–108, 1982

33. Scanlon BK: Management 18—A Short Course for Managers, pp 17–28. New York, John Wiley & Sons, 1974

34. Schendel D, Hofer CW: Strategic Management: A New View of Business Policy and Planning, p 15. Boston, Little, Brown, 1979

35. Snyder JR: Growth contracting: A step beyond performance evaluation. MLO 14(5):61–64, 1982

36. Snyder JR: Organizing the workforce. In Naeve RA (ed): Managing Laboratory Personnel: The CLIA and OSHA Manual, pp 1–29. New York, Thompson Publishing Group, 1994

37. Strauss G, Sayles LR: Personnel: The human problems of management, 3rd ed, pp 267–276. Englewood Cliffs, Prentice-Hall, 1972

38. Teeple KL, Snyder JR, Swanson F: Using planning tools for reorganization. MLO 19(4):59–64, 1987

39. Thomas RG: Manual for Laboratory Planning and Design (rev). Skokie, College of American Pathology, 1977

40. Townsend R: Up the Organization, p 116. Greenwich, Fawcett Publications, 1970

41. Weihrich H: Management by objectives: Does it really work? Bus Rev 28(4):27–31, 1976

4

Problem Solving—The Decision-Making Process

John R. Snyder • Bonnie R. Hendrix

Many specific managerial skills have an impact on the effectiveness of a laboratory administrator or supervisor; the most important is his decision-making ability. The decision is the core of administrative action. Any administrative activity—planning, organizing, directing, or controlling—requires the manager to be a decision maker. In fact, all organizational activity can be looked at as a series of decisions.

A great temptation for all managers is to rely on past experience and common sense as the basis for their decision-making skill. Unfortunately, this does not always suffice, because management in laboratory medicine evolves with nearly the rapidity of technical advances in the field. Decisions about personnel administration, electronic data processing, and method evaluation, to name just a few, are areas that require specific new judgment skills.[9] Today's laboratory manager faces an ever-changing environment. Scanlon summarizes this concern by stating that "decisions based solely on intuition and past experience are becoming less effective in dealing with organizational problems because things are changing at too rapid a pace and because yesterday's experience does not always mirror tomorrow's problem."[18] To decide means to pass judgment and determine a course of action. Perhaps the most complete definition is that managerial decision making is the selection of a preferred course of action from two or more alternatives after weighing the effects of the various alternatives in light of organizational goals. This definition adds two important facts: (1) consideration of the results if one alternative is chosen over another, and (2) the impact the chosen alternate will have in achieving organizational goals. These concepts are further delineated later in this chapter in the discussion of the problem-solving process.

AREAS OF CONCERN IN DECISION MAKING

Before attempting to make any management decision, there are several general areas of concern to which a laboratory manager must be sensitive:[5,6]

Quality of the Decision

To make a quality decision, the manager must determine whether he has all of the appropriate information available. Often the creative talents of several people are beneficial in generating possible alternatives. The manager may need to seek out information regarding specific skills necessary to complement a given alternative. The practice of "bouncing ideas off" peers, subordinates, and superiors is an excellent practice for gaining a broader point of view.

Acceptance of and Commitment to the Decision

This concern is fundamental to management, which must get things done through people. It is important to consider not only the degree of acceptance by the subordinates affected directly by the decision, but also the degree of acceptance at other levels of management within the organization. A group of employees' acceptance of a decision (with or without verbal and nonverbal reaction) does not ensure commitment. Commitment on the part of those who must implement the decision is essential. Sometimes commitment hinges on the attitude employees have about how the decision was made. There are times when it is appropriate to involve the laboratory staff in the decision-making process because it adds quality to the decision and increases the acceptance and commitment to the alternative chosen. Finally, consideration must be given to the acceptance the decision will receive outside the organization: How will other departments in the hospital be affected?

The Speed of the Decision

The time element must obviously be considered. If the decision needs to be made immediately, it is unlikely that staff can be involved. Even if it is not essential that the decision be a quick one, the laboratory manager must consider the length of time it will take to involve appropriate parties. If the decision process must be accelerated, there is generally a trade-off in quality and acceptance of the decision.

The Nature of the Value Judgments in the Decision

All decisions involve a value judgment in terms of what is beneficial or not beneficial and important or not important in projecting the probable outcomes of the decision. Chapter 10 describes these as hidden agendas for people attending meetings. The laboratory manager must recognize the impact these hidden forces may have on the acceptance and commitment to the decision. There are times when individual goals and organizational goals do not mesh because of differing value judgments. At these times, the manager must consider the nature of the value judgments when making a decision.

The Cost of the Decision

The use of organizational resources to make decisions costs money. This must be considered when the decision is reached, because the time of the people involved in the decision is an important component. Often it is difficult to quantitate the appropriate costs that will yield the best decision in terms of quality, acceptance, speed, and values.

DECISION-MAKING APPROACHES AND EFFECTS

There are many different "decision-making management styles," ranging from total dictatorship to total abdication. These are addressed here as approaches to decision making, because style implies a degree of consistency.

Management in the clinical laboratory is full of decisions. There are supervisors who think their managerial role is somewhat routine because few if any of their decisions would be considered major. In fact, all of the decisions they render are for routine situations, and hence they have a lack of concern about approaches to decision making. Perhaps these supervisors more than any others need to examine the decision-making process and the effect various approaches have on quality, acceptance, speed, value, and cost.

Making wise management decisions is not an intuitive skill. Supervisors who are new in their positions will attest to this. It is common for a fledgling supervisor to falter when faced with this newfound responsibility. This skill perhaps more than any other management skill requires an experiential learning period. Some laboratory managers never become good decision makers. Roseman categorized a variety of dangerous decision-making habits he observed in laboratory managers (Fig. 4-1).[14] If one considers first some pitfalls in the decision-making approaches, other more appropriate approaches may be easier to adopt.

The breathless decision, as the name implies, is made on the spur of the moment. While the laboratory supervisor cannot always prevent the need for a hurried decision, making too many is also a bad sign. These may signal a failure to plan, resulting in crisis management—putting out fires. Characteristic of the breathless decision is an oversimplification of the facts and a frantic effort to come up with *any* alternative, which ultimately becomes the decision.

Contrasted with the breathless decision are the trade-off and hold-off decision habits. The laboratory supervisor who practices the trade-off habit tends to solve the easy problems—find the ready-made and obvious solutions—but shelve the rest. Those that are shelved are put off so that the supervisor can avoid confrontation. This habit is an attempt to keep everything in harmony by trading off successful decisions (the easy ones) for half-successes or even failures. The supervisor who practices hold-off decisions looks at the trade-off habit and proposes that failures on tough problems are not necessary. If the decision is not made, then the situation will either resolve itself, or an obvious good alternative will surface. These supervisors work hard at postponing decision making by generating endless superficial alternatives. Unfortunately, this rationalizing of delay tactics tends to gather so much data that even relevant facts become hidden in a mass of irrelevancies. All of these dangerous decision-making habits are characteristic of the weak decision maker. Table 4-1 shows how decision making is related to the four basic functions of a manager: planning, organizing, directing, and controlling.[23] It also contrasts four typical decision-

Breathless decisions	
What You Do	Why
Act without thinking	Submit to time pressure
Limit alternatives	Succumb to emotion
Overreact	Avoid pain
Oversimplify	Avoid thinking
Solve the wrong problem	
Trade-off decisions	
What You Do	Why
Placate others	Seek harmony
Submit to authority	Focus on tasks, not goals
Solve easy problems	Think short-range
Tolerate partial solutions	Hope to reduce risk of failure
Repeat past mistakes	Desire to conform
Hold-off decisions	
What You Do	Why
Generate multiple, superficial alternatives	Fear of unknown
Gather irrelevant facts	Accept unworkable constraints
Fight the problem	Wait for more favorable conditions
Hop from problem to problem	Wait for someone else to act
Rationalize delay	

FIGURE 4-1. Dangerous decision-making habits. (From Roseman E: How to sharpen your decision-making. MLO 7:84, 1975; reprinted with permission of publisher)

making approaches along the spectrum from dictatorship to abdication.

Authoritarian

Some laboratory managers use the authoritarian decision-making approach with regularity. This manager views himself as a central authority, more knowledgeable than his staff because he has access to the big picture of the laboratory. His communication is one-way—down the organizational structure. He shuns opportunities to interact with his technical staff and pays little attention to their ideas, proposals, or suggestions for alternatives. Of the identified major areas of concern in decision making, this approach elicits a decision of the poorest quality, least acceptance and commitment, and least concern for value factors. The true worth of this approach lies in the speed at which a decision is reached. Because no one other than the laboratory

manager is involved, a decision is able to be rendered with speed.

Democratic

In a democratic society, the laboratory manager feels most comfortable attempting to reach decisions by majority vote. This does not mean that the manager polls the staff in his laboratory to determine the decision, but rather that he personally makes the decision after taking a straw vote. He perceives that this is best because the majority then will be committed to following through to implement the decision. The quality, acceptance, and staff feelings about this decision-making process are improved over the authoritarian approach, but those who spoke against the decision will generally feel ignored and disgruntled to some extent. The time taken to reach such a decision will be longer, because the manager has to poll his subordinates.

Table 4-1
Approaches to Decision Making

	Authoritarian	Democratic	Consensus	Laissex-Faire
Planning	All determination of policy is by the supervisor.	All policies are a matter of group discussion and decision, encouraged and assisted by the supervisor.	All policies are a matter of group discussion and decision with supervisor insisting that all members be satisfied.	Complete freedom for group or individual decision exists with a minimum of supervisor participation.
Organizing	The supervisor usually dictates the particular work task and work companion of each member.	The members are free to work with whomever they choose, and the division of tasks is left up to the group.	Division of duties and tasks is responsibility of all members of the group such that all members agree with structure.	The supervisor does not participate.
Directing	Techniques and activity steps are dictated by the supervisor, one at a time, so that future steps are uncertain to a large degree.	Activity perspective is gained during discussion period. General steps to group goal are sketched, and when technical advice is needed, the supervisor suggests two or more alternative procedures from which choice could be made.	General group discussion of techniques and activities occurs. All group members must agree on the approach to be followed. Supervisor actively seeks agreement through discussion, justification, and compromise.	Various materials are supplied by the supervisor, who makes it clear that he will supply information when asked. He takes no other part in work discussion.
Controlling	The supervisor tends to be personal in his praise and criticism of the work of each member, remains aloof from active group participation, except when demonstrating.	The supervisor is objective or fact minded in his praise and criticism and tries to be a regular group member in spirit without doing too much of the work.	The supervisor insists on uniform, harmonious peer review.	Supervisor makes infrequent spontaneous comments on member activities unless questioned, and no attempt is made to appraise or regulate the course of events.

(Adapted from White R, Lippitt R: Autocracy and Democracy, pp 26–27. New York, Harper & Row, 1960; by permission of Harper & Row)

Consensus

When the laboratory manager uses the consensus approach to decision making, he works hard at getting all members of his staff to at least partially agree with the decision made. He approaches the alternatives from a logical point of view and avoids arguing his own viewpoint. All staff members are encouraged to voice their opinions and to describe the reasoning behind their choice.[1] These differences of opinion are viewed by the manager as a help, rather than a hindrance, in decision making. He also avoids any conflict-reducing techniques, such as majority vote, averaging, or trading. Of the three decision-making approaches described thus far, the consensus format yields the highest quality decision, because everyone not only provides information and creativity, but also must explain the rationale for his favored alternative. The staff will feel good about the approach chosen, and this generally will result in increased acceptance and commitment.[17] However, this approach can be time consuming.

Laissez-Faire

The laboratory manager who uses this approach has nearly abdicated from his administrative responsibility. He sees his role as merely inputting into the decision process—a supportive effort—but leaves the planning, organizing, directing, and control of the process up to his staff. From this decision-making approach, it would appear that the laboratory manager is only a figurehead, with his staff in control. This is by far the least effective approach. If a quality decision is reached, it will usually be because of the presence of an informal leader. Most members of the laboratory staff will fault the manager for using this approach and will not feel satisfied with the process. With no manager directing, the wait for a decision to be made could drag on for extended periods.

Various levels of participation by subordinates in the decision-making process have a direct impact on the quality of the decision and how successful the manager will be in implementing the decision.[4,7,15] This is summarized in Figure 4-2. Resistance toward implementation is diminished with increased participation, but the trade-off is time.

No single decision-making approach is best for all situations. To be effective, a laboratory manager should vary his decision-making approach depending on the situation.[4,8] A laboratory supervisor may find the authoritarian approach to be best when making routine decisions about procedures, and certainly it is appropriate in an emergency situation. The democratic approach can be effectively used if the laboratory manager is deciding on a color scheme for new laboratory furniture. When deciding who should work various scheduled holidays, a laboratory supervisor can use the consensus method quite effectively. Abdicating, as in the laissez-faire approach, is perhaps only in order when decisions regarding the laboratory's annual holiday party are being generated.

Whether the approach is authoritarian, democratic, or consensus, the effective laboratory manager must always make the final decision.[12] He must make it as an individual and accept responsibility for it as an individual. If he relies solely on majority opinion or a consensus approach, he is not a manager; he is a presiding officer.

HUMAN FACTORS IN DECISION MAKING

Managers do not make decisions following any single pattern. Rather, they respond to a variety of complex factors, including economic, social, cultural, and politi-

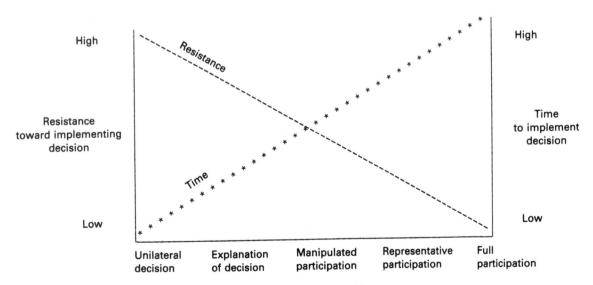

FIGURE 4-2. The effects of various levels of participation on the decision-making process. Participation lowers resistance to decisions but increases the time required to implement them.

cal pressures.[4] Another group of influences worthy of mention consists of the human factors that affect the manager's approach to decision making.[10] Robbins describes five such human factors and the impact each would carry.[13] The first has to do with the manager's personal value systems. The administrator's attitudes, biases, and personal beliefs, based on what society has told us is right or wrong, will have a significant impact on which decisions he considers major and on the array of alternatives that he will create. According to Robbins, the manager's perception of the situation will also play a role in decision making. The manager's judgment and creativity will reflect how he perceives the problem or situation requiring a choice. The third factor involves the limitations in human processing of information. Different managers have differing capacities for storing and sorting out bits and pieces of information related to the decision at hand. Rarely does the decision maker have all the information necessary far enough in advance to spend excessive time sorting out specifics, and this becomes the limitation. A decision maker is also conscious of and responsive to political and power behaviors relative to any given selection.[4] The manager may be concerned with warding off challenges to his decision-making power as a means of protecting his own self-interests. The fifth human factor affecting the decision maker is the constraint of time. A limitation on the time available for the manager to assess and study the situation before making a decision is characteristic of today's administrative environment. Hence, the decision maker, subject to an interaction of organizational influences and human factors, attempts to make the best possible choice. Obviously, the optimum decision is not always made. Sometimes the factors influencing a decision are so complex that analysis of the rationale is impossible. This phenomenon has been so widely substantiated that Rowe states it as a rule: "In any complex decision where personal or behavior factors apply, the individual's preference will dominate the results."[16]

QUANTITATIVE TOOLS FOR DECISION MAKING

Seeking selection of the best alternative is sometimes fraught with difficulties. There exist several quantitative techniques for better assessment of each alternative. These are briefly mentioned here, and the reader is encouraged to seek additional information if a technique appears appropriate for a given situation.

Queuing Theory

This technique is frequently called the waiting-line theory. Its objective is to balance the cost of having a waiting line against the cost of enough personnel to elimi-

nate that line. Queuing theory could be used to determine the number of phlebotomists required to draw blood in an outpatient clinic when the flow of patients varies such that lines occur at certain times.[19]

Linear Programming

When there exists a linear relationship between problem and objective, certain graphic, algebraic, or simplex techniques may be used. Linear programming is often used when two activities are competing for limited resources. This technique may be used when determining which of several chemistry-profiling instruments would be best for a given laboratory workload.

Probability Theory

This technique generally is used to assist the decision maker in reducing risk on the basis of statistics. In the blood bank laboratory, a statistical probability of the number of specimens requiring use of antibody identification panels may be used to predict the inventory of reagents necessary to avoid a stock-out or oversupply.

STEPS IN THE PROBLEM-SOLVING PROCESS

Problem solving and decision making are not synonymous activities. While they are similar, problem solving has several facets that separate it as a managerial skill from typical decision making. The primary difference is in determining precisely that for which a decision needs to be rendered. Figure 4-3 graphically describes a brief but comprehensive flow of events in the problem-solving process. Each of the steps in the problem-solving cycle could be expanded with substeps and detail similar to a massive decision tree. The simple, seven-step approach described here allows the manager the flexibility to modify when necessary but still have some basic guidelines to follow.

Step 1. Definition of the Problem

As in the treatment of disease, therapy is only effective if it is appropriate for the diagnosis. The manager must learn to look beyond the symptoms of the problem and focus on the real issue. Often a symptom, such as absenteeism, calls attention to the fact that a problem exists. Scanlon defines *symptoms* as "adverse events or things which are present in an operation but have not yet developed to the point of emerging as basic deviations."[12] The *basic deviations* are problems called "glaring mis-

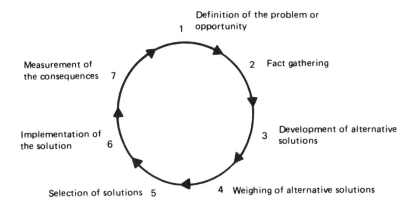

FIGURE 4-3. Flow of events in the problem-solving process. (From Knudson HR, Woodworth RT, Bell CH: Management: An Experiential Approach, p 239. New York, McGraw-Hill, 1973; reprinted with permission of publisher)

takes," as contrasted to *effect problems* (surface problems) or *causal problems* (root problems). The manager who focuses his attention on an effect problem is attempting to achieve a temporary solution, whereas addressing a causal problem should prevent recurrence of the deviation.

One pitfall that many managers encounter as they begin a problem-solving process is the temptation to hypothesize about what should have been done earlier so the problem would not have developed. Some problems will be inherited, some resulting from decisions made elsewhere in the organizational hierarchy, and still others from one's own doing. Regardless of the origin of the problem, the solution must still be made within the framework of the situation.

Step 2. Fact Gathering

Once the problem has been identified, the manager can begin to gather information needed for developing alternative solutions. Facts surrounding the decision situation are important to determine, as are constraints and assumptions. *Constraints* are factors that limit the scope of alternatives. *Assumptions* are applied to factors in an effort to simplify the problem and make it solvable. Fact gathering requires a search for pertinent information from people directly involved in the problem, from books and printed materials, from other people, and from experts and experimental work.

Step 3. Development of Alternative Solutions

The generation of possible solutions calls for creative thinking. Often when faced with this step, a manager will draw on his past experience; in most cases, this will be adequate. On the basis of similarities with and

differences from past experiences, the manager can adjust past alternatives that have proven successful. Past experience, however, can never be fully sufficient in developing alternatives; rather, its most useful purpose is to act as a guide. Today's manager must supplement his creativity by seeking information from others who have solved a similar problem or from individuals directly involved in the situation. It is wise to keep an open mind and not prejudge ideas as they are generated.

Step 4. Weighing of Alternative Solutions

This step requires the analysis of alternative solutions by stating the advantages and disadvantages of each possible course of action. For some problems, this may be a simple and straightforward task; for other situations, the analysis may be a complex and detailed procedure. This step also requires the consideration of each alternative as to how effectively it will accomplish the objectives and requirements of a satisfactory solution. The manager must consider the ramifications of each potential solution. Finally, consideration should be given the question of whether a chosen alternative will eliminate recurrence of the problem or generate another in its place.

Step 5. Selection of Solutions

Choosing the best possible course of action is obviously not an isolated event, but rather an integrated process. Considerable fact gathering and planning have already occurred. Even though alternatives have been scrutinized, any single approach is not always "best." There is generally more than one way to solve a problem, and when choosing a solution, trade-offs in quality, acceptance, speed, value, or cost may be necessary. When the decision is made, it is often wise to discuss it with someone who has considerable problem-solving skills.

Step 6. Implementation of the Solution

Of all the steps in the problem-solving process, the implementation step is usually the most time consuming. At the same time, even the best decision, if not properly implemented, is useless. This step is critical. As in the decision-making process, implementation must involve those who are directly affected by the solution to the problem. Scanlon identified three essential aspects of effective implementation[18]: (1) a questioning attitude concerning every detail of the decision and the development of necessary procedures; (2) a plan for communicating the decision to those involved and affected by it; and (3) participation by all levels—management and employees alike.

Step 7. Measurement of the Consequences

As depicted in Figure 4-3, once the solution to a problem has been implemented, the cycle is not complete. Evaluation of the consequences is appropriate. Not all decisions rendered will have the effect that was planned. An analysis of what occurred, whether predicted or not, provides an ever-increasing basis of experience from which future problems can be solved. Perhaps in the analysis and measurement of consequences, the problem-solving process will be started again. Problem solving as a management skill is probably best developed through repeated exposure with guidance in the laboratory setting. Consider the following problem described in Box 4-1 by a laboratory supervisor in a small laboratory.

The first step for the laboratory supervisor in this case is to define the problem. He must sort through a variety of symptoms surrounding the high turnover rate. He has ruled out job boredom and focused on staff salaries. The underlying problem, on the basis of information presented, is that the administration is unaware of the value—or is unwilling to recognize the value—of experienced technologists who require more pay.

In resolving this problem, there is considerable information to be gathered. The supervisor could survey the community to determine the standard for technologists' salaries and benefits. Certainly a record of the increased turnover would be essential. Some type of analysis of the cost of training or orienting a new technologist should be conducted. Perhaps the supervisor should document the feasibility of reducing the total

---

Box 4•1

Case Example: Problem Solving

I have a lot of trouble keeping experienced personnel. I know that the problem is not that our technologists are bored with their work but that they are dissatisfied with the amount they are paid. Our hospital has a policy of keeping salaries down by hiring inexperienced personnel for the laboratory rather than employing experienced technologists at rates that are competitive with other hospitals in the area.

Recently, I lost a technologist who had assumed a great deal of responsibility in running the laboratory. I had been trying to get the hospital to appoint her my assistant supervisor for a year, but they refused. Their reasoning was that it would cost too much money and that I did not need an assistant. Nevertheless, for a year she acted as my assistant without the recognition or money that would normally accompany this role. When I had to be away from the laboratory, I could depend on her to keep things running smoothly, but finally, when the hospital continually refused to raise her salary or give her a promotion, she left.

Last week, when I was sick for 3 days, the laboratory had a lot of problems that could not be solved by the inexperienced technologists who make up our staff.

What can I do?

---

staff if all technologists were experienced. Finally, some information should be gathered about potential legal ramifications of having nonsupervisory, inexperienced staff in charge.

Several alternatives could be developed and analyzed before a selection is made. This may include an attempt to resolve the problem within the laboratory, perhaps by trying a rotating supervisor in the absence of the designated management technologist. Perhaps a more comprehensive orientation is appropriate for the inexperienced technologists. The best solution may be a meeting with the hospital administrator describing the problem and presenting the data gathered. While it is generally difficult to explain the technical insufficiencies that result from inexperienced personnel, hospital administration can appreciate productivity figures and bottom-line profits and losses.

PROBLEM-SOLVING TOOLS

The advent of continuous quality improvement practices in laboratories today has led to use of a variety of problem-solving tools.[2] These are illustrated in Figures 4-4 and 4-5 from GOAL/QPC and are briefly described below.

Force field analysis enables identification of driving and restraining forces to analyze what helps or hinders movement. Examples of driving forces are profits, image, pride, improved sales, and less scrap and rework. Examples of restraining forces are high turnover, cost of redesign or reruns, and training.

Brainstorming is a group process in which members sequentially contribute their ideas one at a time in a rapid, free-flowing, and creative environment. Guidelines for implementation include recording ideas on a flip chart, discouraging criticism or negative comments, encouraging a volume of ideas, and accepting all ideas.

Cause and effect diagram (sometimes called a fishbone diagram) is a visual picture composed of lines and symbols showing the relationship between cause and effect. It helps to organize randomly connected causes and sorts out noncontributing causes.

Pareto diagram is a tool for identifying the true significance of data collected. The diagram highlights the factors responsible for the major number of defects in a process and the "vital few" and "useful many" pieces of data. Guidelines include deciding how data should be classified, using a check sheet to collect data for a time period, summarizing the data and arranging in the order of sequence from the largest to the smallest, and computing percentages. Approximately 80% of the observations will be attributable to only 20% of the categories observed (80/20 rule). The 20% are the vital few, and the rest are the useful many.

Action plan is a process tool that ensures that all the elements of your plan are considered. Basic questions to ask are who, what, why, when, where, and how. This tool allows management to advise and suggest before implementation takes place. Guidelines include using a facilitator draws the basic action plan on a flip chart, listing action steps and having the facilitator complete the chart as group consensus on each item is reached; gaining support and advice from management before implementation occurs; and being open to criticism and recommendation as the plan is strengthened.

Tree diagram is a tool used to map out the tasks that need to be accomplished to reach a goal. It lists the tasks sequentially, in order of completion, and develops the logical links between the interim tasks. It forces the team to examine all possible causes of a problem. This method is similar to the cause and effect diagram but may clarify complicated issues because of its linear de-

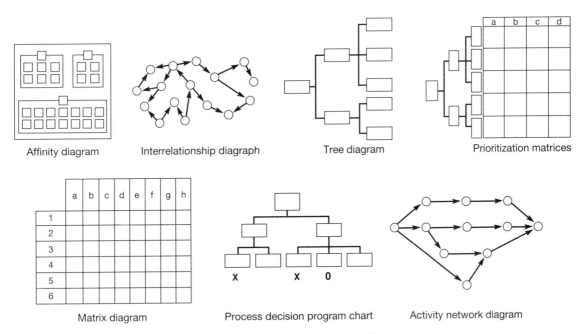

Affinity diagram   Interrelationship diagraph   Tree diagram   Prioritization matrices

Matrix diagram   Process decision program chart   Activity network diagram

FIGURE 4-4.   Problem solving tools illustrated. (Reprinted with permission from *The Memory Jogger Plus+ .*®, GOAL/QPC, 13 Branch St., Methuen, MA)

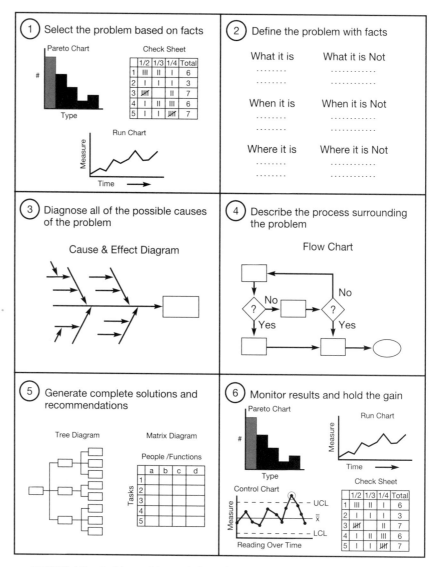

FIGURE 4-5. Problem solving with facts. (Reprinted with permission from *The Memory Jogger Plus+.®*, GOAL/QPC, 13 Branch St., Methuen, MA)

sign. Guidelines include developing a concise problem or issue statement, brainstorming for ideas, writing the ideas on cards or slips of paper, placing key issue cards or slips in the middle of the left edges of a flip chart, arranging the cards in the order of completion to the right of the issue card, and doing a reality check to look for missing steps.

Control chart is a time plot that also indicates the range of variation built into the system. The boundaries are marked by upper and lower statistical control limits. Control limits specify only what a process is capable of doing, not how a process is supposed to perform or what managers may expect to achieve. Points that fall outside the limits or into particular patterns indicate the presence of "special variation." Points that stay within the control limits indicate that most variation is coming from common sense.

Consensus is defined as group solidarity in belief

and involves general agreement and support for the final decision. Decision by consensus is difficult to attain and will take more time than voting, persuasion, or compromise. Guidelines include preparing your position for presentation, expressing your opinion and explaining it fully, expecting the group to listen attentively, modifying your position as new information and other positions are presented, and developing a group position that all can support.

Flowchart is a pictorial representation of all the steps in a process under study.[3] A flowchart should be made as detailed as practical so it can be used to analyze where bottlenecks occur, delays result, and waste accumulates (see Chapter 3).

Scatter diagram allows you to look at the relationship between two characteristics. The shape of the scatter of points tells you if the two factors are related. Points are plotted along an X and Y axis. Points are placed where the values of each pair intersect.

Affinity diagram gathers large amounts of language data, such as ideas, issues, and opinions, and organizes it into groupings based on the natural relationship between each item. Then, it defines groups of items. This is a creative rather than a logical process. An affinity diagram should be used when facts or thoughts are in chaos and issues are too complex to grasp. Traditional ideas are jolted by a whack on the side of the head (Box 4-2).

Interrelationship diagraph takes a central idea, issue, or problem and maps out the logical or sequential links among related items. It is a creative process that shows every idea can be logically linked with more than one other idea at a time. It allows for "multidirectional" rather than "linear" thinking. An interrelationship digraph should be used to correct sequencing of events; if the true problem is unknown and only symptoms are apparent; or with a complex issue in which interrelationships are difficult to identify (Box 4-3).

A *tree diagram* systematically maps out in increasing detail the full range of paths and tasks that need to be accomplished to achieve a primary goal and every

related subgoal. Use a tree diagram if a specific task is identified but needs clarification, implementation is complex and needs definition, or strong consequences exist for missing key tasks (Box 4-4).

Prioritization matrices prioritize tasks, issues, products, or service characteristics based on known weighted criteria using a combination of tree and matrix diagram techniques. Use a prioritization matrix if key issues are known but must be prioritized, resources for implementation are limited, or options generated have strong interrelationships (Box 4-5).

A *matrix diagram* organizes large numbers of pieces of information, such as characteristics, functions, and tasks, into sets of items to be compared. By graphically showing the logical connecting point between any two or more items, a matrix diagram can show which items in each set are related. It can also code each relationship to show its strength and the direction of the influence. Use a matrix diagram when "motherhood and apple pie" have evolved into defined tasks that must be assigned to the rest of the company, the "focused activities" generated must be tested against other things that the company is already doing, or a cumulative number score is needed to compare items (Box 4-6).

Box 4•3

Construction of an Interrelationship Diagraph

1. Assemble the right team.
2. Agree on an issue or problem statement.
3. Display completed cards.
4. Draw the relationship arrows.
5. Review and revise interrelationship digraph.
6. Select the key items in the finalized digraph.
7. Draw the final diagraph and highlight identified key factors.

Box 4•2

Construction of an Affinity Diagram

1. Assemble the right team.
2. State the issue clearly.
3. Generate and record ideas on Post It notes or index cards.
4. Display the completed cards.
5. Arrange cards into related groupings.
6. Create header cards that capture central ideas.
7. Draw the finished affinity diagram.

Box 4•4

Construction of a Tree Diagram

1. Choose the goal statement.
2. Assemble the right team.
3. Generate the major tree headings.
4. Complete the tree diagram under each major path.
5. Perform a reality check.

Box 4•5

Construction of a Prioritization Matrix

1. Define the primary goal.
2. Create the list of criteria to be applied to the options generated.
3. Rate the importance of each criterion by assigning a weighting number.
4. Compare all the options being considered to the weighted criteria.
5. Compare each option based on all criteria combined.

Box 4•7

Construction of a PDPC

1. Assemble the right team.
2. Determine the basic flow of proposed activities.
3. Select either the graphic or outline chart format.
4. Construct the PDPC using the selected format.

Process decision program chart (PDPC) maps out conceivable events and contingencies that can occur in any implementation plan. It identifies feasible countermeasure responses to these problems. This tool is used to plan each possible chain of events that needs to occur when the problem or goal is unfamiliar. Use a PDPC when the task is new or unique, the implementation plan is complex with multiple steps, stakes of potential failure are high, or the time schedule for implementation is critical (Box 4-7).

Activity network diagram is used to plan the most appropriate schedule for completing tasks and their related subtasks. It projects likely completion time and monitors all subtasks for adherence to the necessary schedule. This tool is used when the task is familiar with subtasks of known duration. Use an activity network diagram when complex tasks have multiple subtasks, simultaneous implementation paths can be used, and timeframes for completion of tasks are known and dependent on previous subtasks (Box 4-8).

Putting It All Together

These tools to assist in decision making and problem solving need to be carefully selected to yield maximum useful information.[11] Figure 4-6 shows sequentially the use of various tools as applied to a FOCUS-PDSA model.[22] This application to total quality management includes steps to *f*ind a process to improve, *o*rganize an effort to work on improvement, *c*larify current knowledge of the process, *u*nderstand process variation and capability, and *s*elect a strategy for continued improvement.

Box 4•8

Construction of an Activity Network Diagram

1. Assemble the right team.
2. Generate and record the tasks required to complete the project.
3. Sequence all of the identified activities based on a sequential flow or a simultaneous flow.
4. Assign a timeframe for completion of each task.
5. Calculate the shortest possible implementation schedule using the critical path method.
6. Calculate the earliest starting and finishing times and the latest starting and finishing times for each task.
7. Identify tasks with slack time, and calculate total slack time.
8. Review and revise the activity network diagram.

Box 4•6

Construction of a Matrix Diagram

1. Choose key options for a successful implementation.
2. Select the right team.
3. Choose the most appropriate matrix format.
4. Decide on the relationship symbols that will be used based on strength of the relationship and level of responsibility.
5. Complete the matrix.

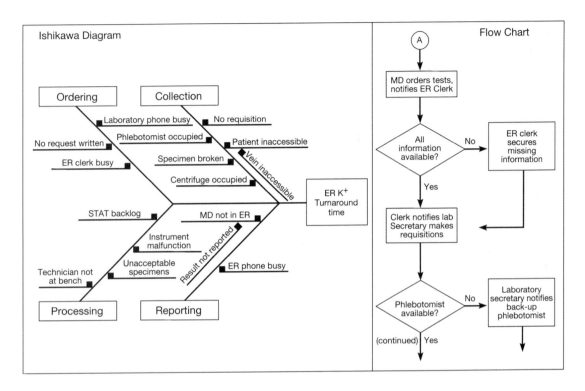

Check Sheet

Delays in production of Se K+ results from 1/1/91 to 1/7/91

Code/Delay Type		Mon	Tue	Wed	Thur	Fri	Sat	Sun	Total
A	Request not written by physician	I	I				I		3
B	Laboratory phone busy > 2 min.	I		I		II		I	5
C	Phlebotomists unavailable	III	II	III	III	II	IIII	III	20
D	Requisition not ready	II	I	I	I	I	III	II	11
E	Patient inaccessible	I	I	II	I		II	I	8
F	Vein inaccessible	I		II		I	II		6
G	Centrifudge busy	II		I		I			4
H	Specimen broken	II		I				I	4
I	STAT backlog	III			I		II	I	7
J	Technician not at bench	II		II		I	II	I	8
K	Unacceptable specimen	I	I		II		I	II	7
L	Laboratory secretary unavailable to report	III		I		I	I		6
M	ER phone not answered			I			II		3
N	MD not in ER	II		I		II		I	6
O	MD not answer page	I	I	II		II		II	8
P	Results not reported by ER secretary	II	I	II	I	III	II	II	13

FIGURE 4-6.   Example of applying problem-solving tools to improve serum potassium results to an emergency room (ER). (Simpson, KN, Kaluzny, AD, McLaughlin, CP. Total quality and the management of laboratories. *Clin Lab Management Rev* 5:453–454, 1991.)

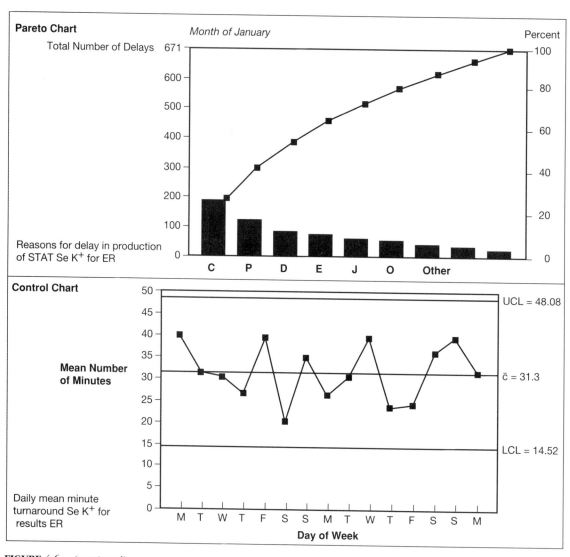

FIGURE 4-6. *(continued)*

CHOOSING A MANAGEMENT DECISION STYLE BASED ON THE SITUATION

It should be apparent at this point that decision making is an integral part of a laboratory manager's daily practice. Furthermore, there is little doubt that the effectiveness of a laboratory manager is largely based on his history of making the right decisions.

The clinical laboratory is a highly complex environment in which management decision styles may promote or detract from the effectiveness of the organiza-

tion. Although it is impossible to create a totally reliable formula for determining which decision style to use at which time, Vroom has proposed a normative model based on the complexities of any situation.[21]

The conceptual basis of the model rests on distinguishing among three classes of outcomes, which bears on the ultimate effectiveness of decisions. These include the quality or rationality of the decision, the acceptance and commitment on the part of subordinates to execute the decision, and the amount of time required to make the decision. The manager works through a decision tree (Fig. 4-7), answering a series of questions that will have an impact on decision effectiveness. The result is a descriptive management decision style based on the situation.

Problem Attributes Assessment

Vroom's model requires the laboratory manager to evaluate the situation and possible effects of differing decision styles using seven parameters called problem attributes (Box 4-9).

Types of Management Decision Styles

When the manager completes an evaluation of the situation by using the decision tree (see Fig. 4-7), he has identified the problem type. Using Table 4-2, he can then determine the acceptable decision-making method(s). These decision-making processes are keyed on the basis of autocratic (A), consultative (C), or group involvement (G), with the following variations:

AI—The manager solves the problem himself, using information available at the time.

AII—The manager obtains the necessary information from his subordinate(s), then decides on the solution to the problem himself. He may or may not tell his subordinates what the problem is in getting information from them. The role played by the subordinates in making the decision is clearly one of providing the necessary information to the manager, rather than generating or evaluating alternative solutions.

CI—The manager shares the problem with relevant subordinates individually, getting their ideas and suggestions without bringing them together as a group. The manager then makes the decision, which may or may not reflect his subordinates' influence.

CII—The manager shares the problem with his subordinates as a group, collectively obtaining

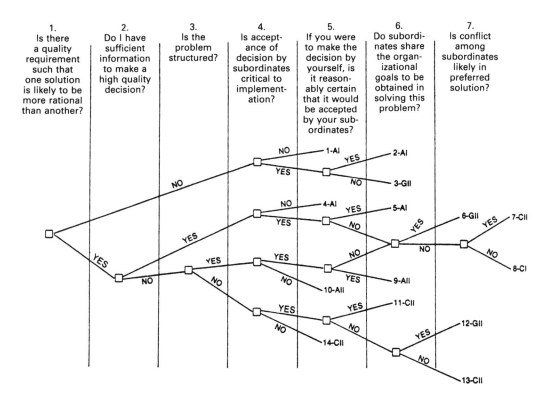

FIGURE 4-7. Decision process flowchart. (From Vroom VH: A new look at managerial decision making. Organizational Dynamics 1:5, 1973; reprinted with permission of publisher; all rights reserved.)

their ideas and suggestions. He then makes the decision, which may or may not reflect his subordinates' influence.

GII—The manager shares the problem with his subordinates as a group. Together they generate and evaluate alternatives and attempt to reach agreement (consensus) on a solution. The manager's role is much like that of a chairman. He does not try to influence the group to adopt

---

Box 4•9

Vroom's Model

1. Quality—the importance of the quality of the decision made. The manager must decide whether a quality requirement exists so that one solution is likely to be more rational than another.
2. Manager's information—the extent to which the leader possesses sufficient information and expertise to make a high-quality decision by himself.
3. Problem structure—the extent to which the problem is structured. The manager decides whether there is a planned approach based on previous experience. If so, this may provide a map for solving the problem at hand.
4. Acceptance—the extent to which acceptance or commitment on the part of subordinates is critical to the effective implementation of the decision.
5. Prior probability of acceptance—the extent to which the leader's autocratic decision can be expected to receive acceptance by subordinates. The manager evaluates the situation to determine whether he can be reasonably certain that a decision will be accepted by his subordinates if he makes it himself.
6. Goal congruence—the extent to which the subordinates are motivated to attain the organizational goals as represented in the objectives explicit in the statement of the problem. Essentially, the manager determines whether his subordinates want to solve the problem and whether they will achieve some personal goals in the process.
7. Conflict—the extent to which subordinates are likely to be in conflict over preferred solutions.

Table 4-2
Problem Types and the Feasible Set of Decision Processes

Problem Type	Acceptable Methods
1	AI, AII, CI, CII, GII
2	AI, AII, CI, CII, GII
3	GII
4	AI, AII, CI, CII, GII*
5	AI, AII, CI, CII, GII*
6	GII
7	CII
8	CI, CII
9	AII, CI, CII, GII*
10	AII, CI, CII, GII*
11	CII, GII*
12	GII
13	CII
14	CII, GII*

* Within the feasible set, only when the answer to question 6 in Fig. 4-7 is YES.

(Adapted from Vroom VH: A new look at managerial decision making. Organization Dynamics 1:2–7, 1973; adapted with permission of publisher)

his solution, and he is willing to accept and implement any solution that has the support of the entire group.

Consider the following case as an example of how Vroom's model can be applied to a decision-making situation in the laboratory:

You are the administrative technologist of special chemistry in a large commercial laboratory. The company's management has always been searching for ways to increase efficiency, especially in terms of turnaround time. They have recently installed a new computer using a modified on-line reporting system. To the surprise of everyone, including yourself, the expected decrease in turnaround time has not been realized. In fact, the time required from specimen entry to report availability has increased slightly overall, an increase in clerical report errors has been noted, and employee requests for transfer have resulted.

You do not believe there is anything wrong with the new computer system. You have had reports from other laboratories using the system, and they confirm this opinion. You have also had representatives from the firm that built the computer system go over it, and they report that it is operating at peak efficiency.

You suspect that some programming in the new computer system may be responsible for the problems. This view, however, is not widely shared among your immediate subordinates, who are four first-line supervisors, each in charge of a section, and the department's quality-control coordinator. The increase in turnaround time has been variously attributed to poor orientation of the technical staff, lack of an adequate system of financial incentives, and poor morale. Clearly this is an issue about which there is considerable depth of feeling and potential disagreement among your subordinates.

This morning you receive a phone call from the director of operations. He has just received your delayed report figures for the last 4 weeks and is calling to express his concern. He indicates that the problem is yours to solve in any way that you think best but that he would like to know by tomorrow what steps you plan to take.

You share the operations manager's concern with the increased turnaround time and know that your technical staff is also concerned. The problem is to decide what steps to take to rectify the situation.

Decision Strategy Analysis

Applying Vroom's model in this case, the administrative technologist attempts to answer the following diagnostic questions to assess problem attributes:

1. Is there a quality requirement such that one solution is likely to be more rational than another? YES (direct impact on efficiency).
2. Does the administrative technologist have sufficient information to make a high-quality decision? NO (unsure of exact problem).
3. Is the problem structured? NO (problem not solved before).
4. Is acceptance of the decision by subordinates critical to effective implementation? YES (implementation to be carried out by subordinates).
5. If the decision is made by the administrative technologist himself, is it reasonably certain that it would be accepted by his subordinates? NO (different decisions perceived as appropriate).
6. Do the subordinates share the organizational goals to be reached in solving this problem? YES (all concerned with problem).
7. Is conflict among subordinates likely in preferred solutions? YES (concerned that they are not faulted in the problem).

Using Figure 4-7, the administrative technologist identifies the problem type as 12; the management deci-

sion style indicated in Table 4-2 is GII. The problem should be shared with the supervisors and quality-control coordinator as a group. Together they should identify the problem, generate and evaluate alternatives, and attempt to reach a consensus agreement on the best solution. The solution agreed on by the whole group must then be implemented.

PROBLEM SOLVING AND DECISION MAKING WITH PROFICIENCY DATA

Analysis of proficiency survey results can often help in troubleshooting procedural problems and improve the instrument and procedure selection process.[20] Data from proficiency studies can aid both in the definition of the problem and in fact-gathering steps. Unfortunately, most laboratory managers peruse these data quickly to be sure that no obvious problems exist without gaining the maximum value of this decision-making and troubleshooting resource. With approximately 7,000 laboratories in the United States contributing to the CAP database, this resource can serve as a valuable technical and managerial tool for troubleshooting.

In most cases, if a problem exists with a procedure or instrument, it will be identified in the summaries of performance by all participants. For example, in recent slide tests for rheumatoid factor, more than 97% of the participants reported a survey specimen negative. However, most laboratories using one manufacturer's procedure reported the specimen positive, disagreeing with all other procedures and the consensus. The conclusion can be drawn that there is difficulty with this particular procedure.

The laboratory should compare its own unacceptable results with results on previous surveys to see whether the problem is an ongoing one. The unacceptable results should also be compared with daily quality control records for determining whether a systematic error exists. Because the CAP often includes values from very low normals to very high normals for each constituent, the laboratory should verify the linearity of each procedure.

Survey data can spotlight a number of specific problems. For example, evaluations of most urinalysis dipstick results are based on consensus of survey participants. Because the ketone portion of the dipstick is the first to become insensitive to trace amounts of a positive constituent, false-negative results in a particular laboratory may indicate that the sticks have been exposed to too much humidity and should be replaced.

No other resource provides as much information as the CAP's quarterly participant summaries about how a given method or instrument has performed in the hands of so many laboratories. For this reason, they are an excellent shopping guide. A laboratory can use them to compare its current instruments with products under consideration for purchase. Mean results give one a reasonable idea of an instrument's future accuracy, and coefficients of variation will reveal its future reliability or precision.

One chemistry analyzer consistently demonstrated accuracy and precision for blood urea nitrogen (BUN) when the proficiency sample was in the normal range. When an abnormal BUN of 51 mg/dL was tested, however, the acceptable range of responses (± 2 standard deviations) was 36 to 64 mg/dL.

If one is planning a purchase, one should personally check the product's track record against others in the survey.

REFERENCES

1. Birchall D, Wild R, Carnall D: Redesigning a way to worker participation. Personnel Management 8(8):26–28, 1976
2. Brassard M: The Memory Jogger Plus +. Methuen, MA, Goal/QPC, 1989
3. Garza D: Reviving an old tool to target improvements. Clin Lab Sci 7:215–217, 1994
4. Gill SL: Groups and decision making. Clin Lab Management Rev 9:464–476, 1995
5. Knudson HR, Woodworth RT, Bell CH: Management: An Experiential Approach, p 239. New York, McGraw-Hill, 1973
6. Laufer FN: Managerial decision-making in the laboratory. Clin Lab Management Rev 4:425–430, 1990
7. Likert R, Likert JG: A method for coping with conflict in problem-solving groups. Group and Organizational Studies 3: 427–434, 1978
8. McFarland DE: Management: Principles and Practices, 3rd ed, pp 75–133. New York, Macmillan, 1970
9. McFarland DE: Managerial Innovation in the Metropolitan Hospital. New York, Praeger Publishers, 1979
10. Michael SR: The contingency manager: Doing what comes naturally. Management Review 65(11):20–31, 1976
11. Moran J, Talbot R, Benson R: A Guide to Graphical Problem-Solving Processes. Milwaukee, ASQC Press, 1990
12. Ray JJ: Do authoritarians hold authoritarian attitudes? Human Relations 29(4):301–325, 1976
13. Robbins SP: The Administrative Process, pp 165–167. Englewood Cliffs, Prentice-Hall, 1976
14. Roseman E: How to sharpen your decision-making. MLO 7:84, 1975
15. Roseman E: The individual versus group approach to decision making. MLO 27(3):50–53, 1995
16. Rowe AJ: The myth of the rational decision maker. International Management August:38–40, 1974
17. Rubinstein SP: Participative problem solving: How to increase organization effectiveness. Personnel 54:30–39, 1977
18. Scanlon BK: Management 18: A Short Course for Managers, pp 35–49. New York, John Wiley & Sons, 1974
19. Schober A: We applied queuing theory to our outpatient lab service. MLO 9(12):69–77, 1977
20. Snyder JR, Glenn DW: Problem solving and decision making with proficiency data. MLO 18(2):46–49, 1986
21. Vroom VH: A new look at managerial decision making. Organizational Dynamics, pp. 2–7. New York, AMACOM, 1973
22. Welborn AL, Collins JB: Creating the environment for process improvement. Clin Lab Management Rev 9:477–489, 1995
23. White R, Lippitt R: Autocracy and Democracy, pp 26–27. New York, Harper & Row, 1960

5

Making the Transition to Laboratory Management

John R. Snyder • David S. Wilkinson

One of the most difficult hurdles for the new laboratory manager is the transition from staff responsibilities to administration responsibilities. Historically, most laboratory managers have been selected for promotion to a supervisory position based on their technical knowledge and skills or length of service in a particular institution. The transition to management includes new responsibilities, new demands and expectations, new duties, and new relationships. In a nutshell, the transition is a shift from doing clinical laboratory testing to managing the resources to provide laboratory services.

This chapter is strategically placed after those addressing the laboratory industry, regulations, management functions, and decision making and problem solving. To make a successful transition, the laboratory manager needs to understand the environment, the relevant laws governing service delivery, and some basic management processes and tools, in addition to the work that is performed in the laboratory.

This chapter is written in basic, practical language. Imagine standing at the portal of the laboratory for which you are about to assume managerial responsibility. It is your first day—you know only a few employees in the laboratory and have only the usual limited knowledge garnered during the interview. Where do you begin? How do you prepare to "hit the ground running?"

NEW RESPONSIBILITIES

A reasonable first step is to develop an understanding of the new responsibilities required of the position. Because personnel costs constitute the major portion of the laboratory budget, laboratory medicine is appropriately categorized as a labor-intensive industry. Some laboratory managers contend that the only manager who needs human relation skills is the line supervisor. This simply is not true. Figure 5-1 shows three management levels within the clinical laboratory and corresponding blocks of administrative skills needed and exercised. The bench-level supervisor must exercise a substantial number of technical skills in the performance of laboratory testing: instrument repair, troubleshooting, new procedure selection, and development. The laboratory director or administrator, conversely, exercises far fewer technical skills; rather, the emphasis shifts at this level to conceptual skills, such as long-range planning, goal setting, and innovating in response to change. The administrative technologist in the middle is required to exercise skills in both the technical and conceptual areas. Notice the block of interpersonal skills: All three levels of laboratory management need to be equally adept in this area. Human skills in a labor-intensive industry are of critical importance to managerial effectiveness.

A study reported by Karni and Seanger[12] queried managers and supervisors about the specific tasks to which they devote most of their time in a 1-year period. Table 5-1 shows a rank order of these management tasks. To make a successful transition requires competence in motivation, communication, time management, decision making, coordination, and training (Box 5-1).[29]

NEW DEMANDS

With the transition to a supervisory position, new demands are placed on the manager. In lieu of the demand for accountability of one's own work as a laboratorian, the new manager is now accountable for facilitating the

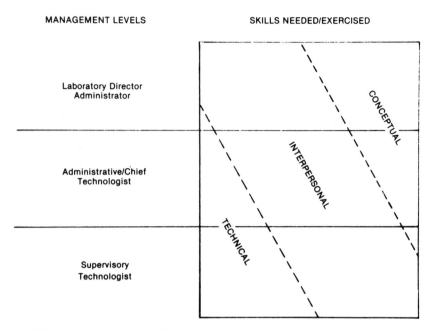

FIGURE 5-1. Leadership skills needed/exercised at various managerial levels. (Adapted from Beam LK: Relating people and tasks: Managing your administrative and instructional staff. In Langerman PD, Smith DH [eds]: Managing Adult and Continuing Education Programs and Staff, p 289. Washington, National Association for Public Continuing and Adult Education, 1979)

output of his employees to meet the demands of the employer. As shown in Figure 5-2, employer demands include expectations of cost containment, productivity, profit, and so forth.[29] Simultaneously, the manager faces demands from his subordinates, such as recognition, higher pay, and job satisfaction.[29] Umiker has accurately captured the dual demand situation in Figure 5-2 by illustrating it as a balancing act for the manager.[29]

NEW DUTIES

The new manager has a myriad of duties dramatically different from those required of a technical staff member as shown in Figure 5-3.[24] This illustration shows categories of duties. An understanding of financial management, for example, would be required to fulfill the duties of purchasing, billing, cost accounting, and budgeting.[24] However, a manager's responsibility for the human resource, for example, crosses many of the categories, including correspondence, education, personnel, and budgeting. Also, essential management skills like communication and motivation are not dis-

cretely isolated to a single category but permeate many duties.[18]

NEW RELATIONSHIPS

Beyond the demands and expectations noted previously, the new laboratory manager is faced with new relationships, as illustrated in Figure 5-4. The supervisor–subordinate relationship is highly complex and governed by state and federal laws and institutional policies and procedures.[16] This relationship affects both the efficiency and effectiveness of the laboratory's operation.[21] Trust and respect—in both directions—are essential for optimum productivity.[8] Sometimes new managers try to choose between being liked, a "nice guy," and being respected, a "formal" manager.[4] This dichotomy need not exist; new managers can acquire both if they involve employees, recognize them for their accomplishments, and view their new roles as facilitator and coach.[4]

A global measure of the quality of the supervisor–subordinate relationship is an assessment of work morale.[20] Good morale in the work setting is usually a

Table 5-1
Management Tasks to Which Clinical Laboratory Managers and Supervisors Devote Most of Their Time During a One-Year Period

	Managers		*Supervisors*
Rank	Tasks	Rank	Tasks
1	Communicate effectively (orally and in writing) with coworkers, superiors, subordinates, patients, and the public.	1	Communicate effectively (orally and in writing) with coworkers, superiors, subordinates, patients, and the public.
2	Develop a plan and objectives for laboratory unit/section.	2.5	Develop a plan and objectives for laboratory unit/section.
3	Prepare an operating budget.	2.5	Write procedures and policies appropriate for the laboratory and the institution.
4	Determine employee work schedules, including use of full-time and part-time employees, and proper mix of personnel by educational background.	4	Conduct performance evaluation, including correct grievance and termination procedures.
5	Purchase supplies, reference-laboratory services, or service contracts by appropriate means.	5	Establish and use a quality-assurance program to include statistics, proficiency samples, and check samples.
6	Perform productivity studies.	6	Understand and respond appropriately to the mission of the laboratory and the institution in which one works.
7.5	Understand and respond appropriately to the mission of the laboratory and the institution in which one works.	7.5	Recommend the purchase, lease, or rental of equipment based on methods, volume of work, costs of equipment, and reagents.
7.5	Prepare for and conduct meetings.	7.5	Purchase supplies, reference laboratory services, or service contracts by appropriate means.
10.5	Conduct personnel problem solving (eg, counseling and referral).		
10.5	Write procedures and policies appropriate for the laboratory and the institution.	9.5	Conduct personnel problem solving (eg, counseling and referral).
10.5	Prepare a capital budget.	9.5	Perform productivity studies.
10.5	Calculate costs per test, break-even analysis, and other fiscal parameters.		

Karni KR and Seanger DG: Management skills needed by entry-level practitioners, *Clin Lab Sci* 1988; 1:296–300.

sign of good working relationships; good work morale usually contributes to good work. However, work morale is affected by more than just the relationships between supervisors and subordinates; it is also influenced by the laboratory job itself, the work group, management practices, and economic rewards.[20] Morale is only a symptom; poor morale in not the root of a problem but rather a symptom of a problem.

Finally, the relationship that the new manager establishes with his immediate supervisor is important. In many ways, both of these positions in the organization share similar duties. Trust and respect between these two levels are equally important. Both the manager and his superior may have different leadership styles; they may respond to situations and circumstances differently. Fritz suggests "reading" the supervisor's behavior, seeking help, offering assistance when appropriate, and focusing on performance.[7] Because the laboratory manager is "closest to the action in the laboratory," he may sometimes think his supervisor is making a wrong decision about the laboratory. Bartolome suggests that rational and documented persuasion be used first to influence the supervisor before moving to more aggressive stages of confrontation or "going above the boss."[1] This will preserve trust and respect.

Box 5·1

Management Skills Required

Motivation: Creating a desire to achieve results
- Apply an appropriate leadership style.
- Eliminate dissatisfiers.
- Set an example.
- Coach and counsel.

Communication: Everyone knowing what he needs to know
- Encode messages.
- Select the right channels (memo, telephone, or intercom).
- Eliminate barriers to communication.
- Conduct meetings.
- Get feedback.

Time management: Making the best use of time
- Organize your own work.
- Delegate effectively.
- Establish priorities.
- Eliminate time wasters.

Decision making
- Establish rules, regulations, policies, and procedures.
- Seek expert advice.
- Make effective use of committees and meetings.
- Use planning and problem-solving techniques.

Coordination
- Coordinate machines and people.
- Coordinate laboratory activities with those of the medical staff, nursing service, emergency room, outpatient, and other departments.
- Coordinate laboratory shifts, departments, and sections.

Training
- Prepare new employees for their jobs.
- Teach technologists new procedures and new instruments.
- Support continuing education for laboratory employees.
- Participate in training programs for students, nurses, and others.

Source: Umiker WO: The Effective Laboratory Supervisor, pp 24–25. Oradell, NJ, Medical Economics Company, 1982

MANAGING VERSUS DOING

In years past, when a supervisor was needed, the common method was to evaluate the staff members within the department for the best-performing technologist. This individual was then appointed supervisor on the assumption that because he performed well at the bench, he would automatically make a good supervisor. Although it is true that a good laboratory supervisor must know most facets of the department for which he is responsible, he may or may not possess the potential for managerial skills. The new supervisor's perception of his responsibilities is a good indication of how successful he will become, as illustrated by the following case history adapted from Scanlon.[25]

A number of years ago, two medical technologists with essentially the same educational backgrounds, experience, and tenure in a large laboratory were placed in management positions at about the same time. As opposed to being paid for performing their technical specialty, they were now being paid for being technical administrators, or supervisors of departments in which clinical laboratory testing was performed. At the end of the first 6 months, one of them was experiencing considerable success and enjoying his new managerial job. The other was not so successful. He was experiencing problems in meeting schedules and test report deadlines, there was a degree of unrest among the technologists in his department, and he was becoming discouraged and frustrated. Higher level management was becoming concerned about the situation.

The first man had obviously adapted well to his new role. He realized that he was embarking on a new and different career within the laboratory organization and had adjusted accordingly. More specifically, whether it was because of his own insight or because he received help from his superior, he perceived his role and function to be different from what it used to be. Among the many things he did after being appointed a manager was to take inventory of the department in terms of the work that had to be done and the people he had available to do it. He concerned himself not only with the number of people available, but also with their individual skills and abilities, strengths, and weaknesses. He reviewed the work flow in the department and using this as a base, formulated priorities and schedules. Through individual and departmental meetings, he communicated to his people the teamwork approach to health care and the interrelationship that the department shared with other departments and the medical center as a whole. In addition, he gave his technologists a clear picture of where the department stood with respect to what was expected and the present status of performance. He shared and discussed with them some of the problems that he thought were inhibiting

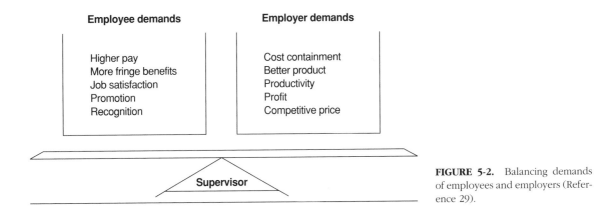

FIGURE 5-2. Balancing demands of employees and employers (Reference 29).

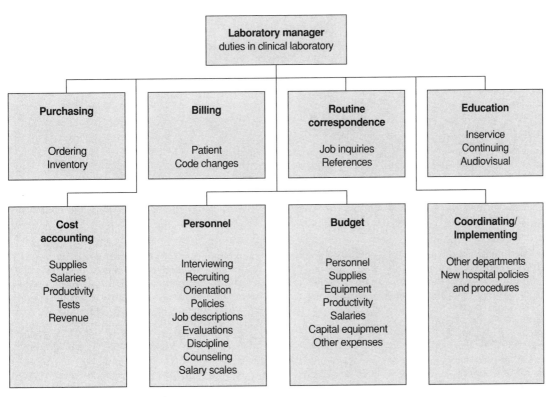

FIGURE 5-3. Managerial duties.[24]

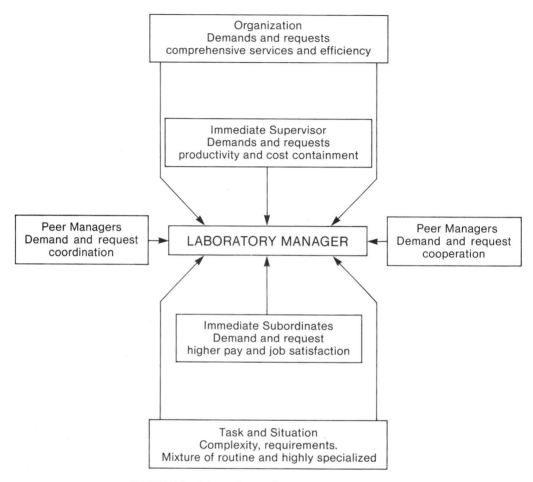

FIGURE 5-4. Relationships and variables to be perceived and balanced by a laboratory manager.

better departmental performance and obtained their ideas on what could be done to improve things. Beyond this, he took an active interest in each technologist individually and worked with him or her in a coaching capacity to set goals, help improve performance, and provide more satisfaction from the job. In other words, he *managed:* He planned, made decisions, organized, directed, and controlled.

The other man became somewhat overawed by his new role. As soon as he realized he was no longer expected to do actual laboratory testing, he became confused. He had to spend his time some way, so he began by making a point of checking every test result before it left the department. When he found an error, which he was bound to do, he was quick to call it to the attention of the technologist in question. He made

the corrections himself. He became convinced that more checking was needed; it almost became a challenge to find something wrong. This led him to spending more time to make sure things were done right. Frequently he would watch a technologist having trouble with a procedure so he could point out the flaw in the technique. He thought that all of the special procedures, research and development, and CAP check sample demanded his personal attention. Often he worked on these projects until late at night and on weekends. Because he became so involved in working alone on these "special" projects, that other responsibilities were neglected. Workload-recording reports and employee evaluations were not filed on time. At a laboratory supervisors' meeting, he was unable to give an adequate breakdown on the status of the entire department's work flow or comment on why the turnaround time in reporting of results was increasing. In addition, his staff assumed less responsibility for their work. They became passive. One of the more experienced technologists resigned, and two others requested transfers to other departments. This man was not *managing;* he was *doing.* He was doing what he had always done: practicing his technical specialty. In management, he had found something strange and different to which he could not adjust. He was not able to become a supervisor and gain satisfaction in the accomplishments of others. He could not let go of the pipet, the test tube, and all the other laboratory apparatus with which he worked. Eventually, he failed as a manager and returned to his specialty.

It is obvious from this case history that there is little direct relationship between technical and managerial skills. A manager requires a unique set of knowledge, skills, abilities, and attitudes. During this transitional phase, the new manager must recognize the shift from operational duties to supervisory duties. Inability to delegate is the most common downfall of the new manager.

The Manager's Circle of Influence

Although all levels of management have supervisory functions, supervisors are most often involved in laboratory management, so some additional attention to them is warranted. Successful supervisors are the key to successful laboratory administration.

The laboratory supervisor is undoubtedly the most significant member of the management team in influencing staff personnel. The supervisor's perception of his new responsibilities and his manner and attitude in dealing with his staff are important. Consider the effect of the supervisor's attitude (Fig. 5-5). Suppose a supervisor must find a way to schedule staff for holiday cover-

age of the laboratory; rather than discussing various options with his people, he arbitrarily assigns them, confident that they would merely fight among themselves if he did not. As would be expected, the staff begins to grumble over the decision. On the third scheduled holiday, the supervisor receives a call at home informing him that one member of his staff has called in sick. This had never happened before. In a rage, the supervisor reaffirms in his mind that this is typical of how inept the staff would have been in determining their own schedule and vows to continue making decisions without their input. The supervisor has fallen into the trap of this self-reinforcing cycle. His attitude about the staff dictated his manner of treating employees. How the employees were treated affected how they reacted. This reaction is reflected in their response or production, which in turn reinforces the supervisor's attitude. A vicious circle is created, one to which each supervisor should be sensitive.

The supervisor has the ability to create an environment conducive to effective and efficient operations. It is up to the supervisor to develop surroundings in which people will want to work to their full potential.[15] In the clinical laboratory, as in any organization, there are those who are only interested in picking up their paychecks. Most employees, however, would like to get something more out of their daily jobs. The supervisor has the responsibility for acting as a catalyst in causing efficient and rewarding performance. Fulmer has described six contributions that can be particularly important in creating an environment to encourage maximum accomplishment (Box 5-2).[9]

DELEGATION

What do managers do when they are having difficulty getting everything done at work or need to be absent? They delegate some tasks to coworkers. This takes some pressure off of themselves and motivates employ-

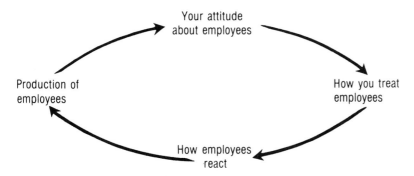

FIGURE 5-5. The manager's circle of influence.

Box 5•2

Creating a Productive Work Environment

1. A worker's job must define goals. These objectives must be carefully outlined and explained so that they are clearly understood by everyone involved. A person simply cannot work well toward an end that is not understood.
2. Surroundings should give workers a definite, clear idea of their roles in the organization. Not only must they understand goals; they must also recognize the kinds of personal judgment they can apply to the operation. In addition, the workers must have access to the information and tools necessary for the job.
3. The supervisor should try to remove any obstacles that might stand in the way of the worker's effective performance. If a supervisor cannot solve critical problems, he should ask for help from an immediate superior.
4. Ideally, the working environment should encourage personnel to do their jobs as the supervisors want them to be done. It must be clear that certain procedures are preferred because they are most effective.
5. The worker must have a sense of being a vital part of the organization, rather than a cog in a huge machine. The supervisor must always be aware that subordinates are people with needs and desires to be considered.
6. The supervisor should realize that some of his workers may have useful ideas for solutions to current problems. The working surroundings should stimulate them to express these ideas so that more answers can be found and more people can participate in making decisions.

minds as to the content and meaning of the contract's provisions:

1. Agreement on the scope of the job (responsibilities)
2. Agreement on the specific results the subordinate is to achieve (accountability)
3. Agreement on the time schedule
4. Agreement on the authority needed to carry out the delegation
5. Agreement on means used to measure performance (control and feedback)
6. Agreement that the superior and subordinate each accepts his part of the contract and will live up to it

Delegation is not an absolute panacea. Many of us have reasons for not delegating (Box 5-3). "It takes longer to teach someone to do something than do it myself." "It's never done quite as well when somebody else does it." Numerous management articles tell us how to fight the urge to do everything ourselves, but is delegation always appropriate?[28]

What Not to Delegate

Confidential Matters

All managers have access to a wide variety of information. Such data range from details that anyone can legitimately see to highly confidential documents protected by either institutional policy or state or federal law. There are also files that can be seen only by designated people.

Before you delegate a task requiring access to confidential information, stop and think about the sensitive nature of the information and to whom you are assigning the task. Suppose, for example, you needed to amass information classifying the types of disciplinary action taken against staff during the last 5 years. This is not a complex assignment; any competent laboratory clerk could collate this information with little effort. These records are private, however. In most instances, delegating this job would be wrong.

Crises and Staff Disputes

Ask any manager what job he or she could easily live without, and most will tell you that dealing with unforeseen crises is high on the list. Mediating a volatile disagreement between two parties is an equally undesirable task. As tempting as it might be to let someone else step in, the manager should handle these problems himself.

ees who might be getting bored with the monotony of their jobs.

On the surface, delegation appears to be a sound management strategy in any situation. If a manager wants to empower employees, he can delegate more authority and responsibility to them.[14] If you want your staff to grow professionally and personally, delegate.

An excellent way to get the full import of delegation is to treat it like a legal contract.[3] The "parties" (the supervisor and the subordinate in this instance) to the delegation (the contract) must reach a meeting of the

Box 5·3

Select Barriers to Effective Delegation

BARRIERS OF THE DELEGATE

1. An unwillingness to accept the task because of a fear of failure
2. Responsibility conflicts with the routine or priorities of the subordinate
3. Lacks experience, competence, and confidence.
4. Avoidance of responsibility
5. Overly dependent on the manager
6. An excessively large workload
7. Concerned with doing the wrong kinds of work—trivia
8. Disorganized

BARRIERS OF THE DELEGATOR

1. Lack of confidence in subordinate's knowledge and skill
2. Reluctance to relinquish responsibility
3. "It takes longer to explain it than do it" syndrome
4. Lack of time to train the delegate in the responsibility
5. Failure to delegate enough authority to accomplish the responsibility
6. Fear of not being needed if other people can do the job
7. Fear of loss of control or power
8. Feeling of imposing on others lack of legitimacy for the delegation process
9. "Perfectionist attitude"—"I'm the only one who can do it correctly."
10. Ego satisfaction—the manager shouldn't be doing the task but enjoys doing it and won't give it up
11. Lack of knowledge concerning the capabilities and potential of your personnel
12. Delegate is not present or available
13. A preoccupation with looking busy
14. A fear of being resented because it seems you are having others do *your* work

Resolving crises takes considerable time and experience. By their nature, crises are usually unplanned—the main reason why someone should not be sent in your place to take care of things. There is a good chance you will not have all the information that you need to delegate responsibility effectively to another.

Other Personal Matters

Certain other personnel matters also should never be delegated. You should always conduct the performance reviews of those who report directly to you, for instance. Evaluating how well one of your laboratorians is doing could probably be assessed by one of his or her colleagues; however, an effective performance appraisal requires establishing additional steps, either for remediation or development, necessary for an employee to become more valuable to the laboratory. No one can identify these steps better for you, nor should anyone be expected to.

Disciplining your employees is your sole responsibility. This is particularly true if disciplinary action might lead to termination. The laboratory manager must be directly involved in a progressive disciplinary action every step of the way. Otherwise, the likelihood is good that the employee will successfully grieve the process.

Finally, praise should never be delegated. Having Joe tell Mary she is doing a good job is not the same as when it comes directly from the manager. No doubt, there are other situations for which delegating responsibilities to someone else is inappropriate. This is just a sampling to help discern the appropriate situations from the inappropriate ones.

MANAGING TIME

In Chapter 1, the administrative process was described as managing three resources in the clinical laboratory: physical, human, and financial. All three of these resources are "external" to the manager. A discussion about making the transition to management would not be complete without a look "internally" at one of the most precious yet least understood and mismanaged resource—*time*.

Managing time connotes controlling the events that distance the manager from being productive.[6] Because distractions are a highly personal characteristic, managing one's time is in many ways managing oneself and the characteristics of the work environment that foster productivity. While the resource of time is a terrible thing to waste, everyone does it to some extent. For the laboratory manager, the ability to remain productive by managing time does not depend on how new or experienced a manager is; rather, it depends on how focused one is on preserving this resource.

Identifying Time Wasters

Time management is best approached from a problem-solving perspective. Because time is not an elastic or developable resource, one can only hope to make better

The time inventory process:

a. Do the inventory during a representative time period.
b. Note each task you do in detail, when you do it, and how long it takes; record tasks as you do them.
c. Make entries at regular time intervals.
d. Record interruptions and their sources.
e. Keep the inventory for at least one week; two weeks is preferable.
f. Summarize your findings on a time summary sheet and analyze them.
g. Do a new inventory every year or whenever your duties change significantly.

Time Inventory Sheet

Name: _____ Day: _____ Date: _____

Time		Activity	Interruptions		
Begin	End		P	O	Reason

A

Prioritizing tasks:

a. List activities
b. Estimate time to accomplish each
c. Prioritize—by letter and number
d. To get the most of your time:
   1) tackle the As first;
   2) handle the Bs an Cs later

The Plan Sheet
Date(s): _____

Priority	Activity	Estimated time to complete	Outcome/Status
A_ B_ C_	_____	_____	_____
A_ B_ C_	_____	_____	_____
A_ B_ C_	_____	_____	_____
A_ B_ C_	_____	_____	_____
A_ B_ C_	_____	_____	_____
A_ B_ C_	_____	_____	_____
A_ B_ C_	_____	_____	_____
A_ B_ C_	_____	_____	_____
A_ B_ C_	_____	_____	_____

B

FIGURE 5-6. Time management processes and forms. (*A*) The time inventory process. (*B*) Prioritizing tasks. (P, phone; O, other) (Sedlacek J: Time Management: A guide for Health Care Supervisors, Lexington, KY, University of Kentucky, College of Allied Health Professions, TIPS, 1989)

use of it as a limited or scarce resource. Time wasters can be classified as either internal—the result of some work habit or personal characteristic—or external—a pattern, practice, or characteristic of the work environment.

Sometimes its helpful to use time management tools to identify where one spends time; other times some simple armchair reflection is all that is needed. Figure 5-6 shows two forms with related directions for identifying time spent on various tasks and how to prioritize tasks. The time-inventory process provides a record of interruptions and their sources.[26] The prioritizing tasks form forces a rank order of what is to be done with an estimate of how long the activity might take.[26] Fringes[6] suggests the following troubleshooting technique: identify (1) person I see often, (2) how I waste their time, (3) how they waste my time, and (4) possible solutions. Common time wasters with suggestions for resolution are listed in Table 5-2.

Table 5-2 **Time Management Strategies**	
Internal Time Wasters	*Resolution Strategies*
1. Doing versus managing (ineffective delegation)	Practice delegating—ask yourself if someone else shouldn't be doing _____.
2. Personal disorganization	Conduct inventory process and prioritize tasks.
3. Procrastination	
* Socializing	Limit your visit to "howdy rounds."
* Reading low-priority items	Judge the return on time investment.
* Oversupervising	Try the management by exception approach.
* Running away—escaping	Time yourself on breaks.
4. Lack of planning	Set realistic deadlines; predict busy times, and schedule accordingly. Set goals and prioritize.
5. Inability to say "no"	Encourage staff to solve problems on their own. Provide help when needed, but make it a learning experience. Accept assignmens if you have sufficient time; learn to decline politely.
External Time Wasters	*Resolution Strategies*
1. The telephone	Have calls screeened. Return low-priority calls at same time each day. Keep up-to-date phone directory.
2. Drop-in visitors	Remove extra chairs from area. Rearrange work area so not facing traffic flow. If in an office, close door when not wanting interruptions. Limit drop-in visitors. Meet people outside your work area.
3. Paperwork	Conduct time inventory, and prioritize tasks.
4. Meetings	As leader, hold only when necessary. Choose participants carefully. Distribute an agenda prior to meeting. Start/end on time. As participant, identify role. Be on time. Bring materials. Help keep discussion on track.

THE FIRST SIX TO TWELVE MONTHS

The first 6 to 12 months in a new management position are probably the most crucial to continuing success. Just like first impressions, first managerial actions tell subordinates much about the new manager. For the manager promoted from within the institution, suddenly there are changed relationships with former peers. Some colleagues may be bitter if they also were hoping to be selected for the management position. In a different facility, the new manager may face a group of nervous staff members unsure of what their new boss would be like.

Do not expect a structural orientation to the new management role. There seems to be an assumption that if the new manager was qualified enough to be selected, he is capable of conducting his own orientation. Graham suggests that the new manager devise his own personal plan to learn the new position.[10] While acknowledging that a variety of missteps will be forgiven under the aegis of the manager being "new," the wheels are immediately in motion to determine credibility. First steps are crucial in developing the necessary trust and respect.

Graham recommends that in addition to looking and acting the part, the new manager should get to know everyone and find his way around the institution. Interviewing staff to learn the "lay of the lab" before effecting change can be accomplished with a service of open-ended questions:[10]

What works well and why?
What would you change; why and how?
What would you think is the number one issue and why?
What do you think the customer's perception of our service is and why?
What do you think the manager's role should be and why?

During the first 6 to 12 months in a new position, the manager should address seven basic points listed in Box 5-4. [13]

EDUCATING LABORATORY ADMINISTRATORS

Many laboratory supervisors and managers have been promoted into their positions without the benefit of formal management education; more often than not, their training has been received on the job.[5,19] Robbins has contrasted the concept of training to education.[23]

Training is the process of learning a sequence of programmed behaviors. We train bricklayers, television repairmen, typists, and hospital admission clerks. The activities of these jobs can be precisely defined, broken down, and analyzed and a "best way" determined. Training is the application of knowledge. It gives people an awareness of the rules and procedures to guide their behavior.

In contrast, education instills sound reasoning processes rather than merely imparting a body of serial facts. Education is the understanding and interpretation of knowledge. It does not provide definitive answers, but rather develops a logical and rational mind that can determine relationships among pertinent variables and thereby understand phenomena.

This statement might lead us to believe that laboratory administrators can be educated in the classroom alone. Although the classroom setting is adequate to introduce the principles of management science and the basic techniques of effective supervision, it does not provide a complete preparation for administrative responsibilities. The introductory experiences of applying these principles and techniques within specific situations are missing. We know that academic grades are incomplete predictors of success for performing laboratory analysis. The same is true of a classroom exposure to laboratory administration. There exists no substitute

---

Box 5·4

Assessment Strategies for the New Manager

1. Determine the expectations of your new supervisors.
2. Clarify your management philosophy and values to those who report to you. They should know what is important to you and what you expect of them.
3. Assess the people reporting to you; learn their strengths and weaknesses. Capitalize on your staff members' strengths, and help devise a plan to convert weaknesses.
4. Identify critical problems you have inherited. There are likely either not known or not known in detail at the start.
5. Set your agenda, both short term and long term, working with your key staff.
6. Revise structure, systems, and procedures as needed. Avoid changing only if it improves your ability to reach goals.
7. Be open to suggestions and ideas. One of your coworkers may have the solution to a critical problem or the great idea you've been struggling to develop.

for some type of trial experience or externship as part of the educational process. Indeed, if we were to survey laboratory administrators, it would be evident "that many outstanding administrators have never had a formal course in administration, whereas many incompetents have a long list of impressive academic accomplishments,"[22] as has been proven in industry.

Facilitating the development of technical managers requires an understanding of what technical managers need to learn and a sense of when they are most ready to learn.[16] When new supervisors were polled by Bittel to determine their feelings of need as they began new careers, the following results were obtained:[2]

89% wanted more knowledge of human relations
59% needed better communications techniques
40% felt deficient in personnel procedures and record keeping
39% needed help in operations planning
27% wanted better methods of staff development

Notice that most of the specified needs were for effective methods of dealing with people. This knowledge is not easily or simply obtained and probably is best realized through practice in the working setting. Once again, no substitute exists for experiencing these forces as part of the educational process.

CHALLENGES FOR TODAY'S LABORATORY MANAGER

A host of external forces has prompted clinical laboratories to change in recent years. Governmental intervention, cost-containment initiatives, prospective reimbursement, increasing competition, and societal demands for access to complex diagnostic services are just a few of the forces driving change. These changes, coupled with characteristics inherent in laboratory medicine, pose a significant challenge for the laboratory manager.[27]

Subsequent chapters dissect laboratory administration and supervision by functions and tasks in an effort to analyze thoroughly strategies for effective management. Before this dissection is begun, it is appropriate to recognize that management is a process and that functions and tasks overlap.

One helpful tool for understanding the interrelatedness of management function is a system analysis.[27] Leavitt proposed a systems model focusing on four interactive components or dimensions of an organization[17]: *task,* the mission, goals, and objectives of the laboratory; *structure,* characteristics of the organizational chart, including lines of authority and communication, division of labor, and work flow; *technology,* tools and instrumentation available for accomplishing

the goals; and *people,* laboratory employees' knowledge, skills, attitudes, and expectations. Figure 5-7 illustrates the interactive nature of each dimension with double-ended arrows. The systems model is helpful in viewing the laboratory from a holistic perspective and predicting how modifying one dimension of the system is likely to have an impact on other dimensions. For example, if the mission of the laboratory was expanded (task dimension) to include services to a health maintenance organization in the community, this change would probably have an impact on the work flow (structure dimension), the demands on testing equipment and data processing (technology dimension), and personnel requirements needed for the increased volume.

The figure displays selected negative characteristics of laboratory medicine influencing each of these dimensions that make managing a clinical laboratory difficult.[11] The task dimension is buffeted and responsive to demands in the marketplace for increased numbers of diagnostic procedures in opposition to cost-containment efforts. Managers are challenged to deal with the problem of poor image and lack of identity by laboratory staff in the structure dimension. In this dimension also, a lack of uniform personnel standards has technologists doing technician-level work, and vice versa. The organizational chart in many laboratories allows limited opportunities for career advancement. Rapid advances in the technology dimension have been a mixed blessing. While adding to the accuracy, efficiency, and cost-effectiveness of many analyses, they have prompted task repetition and significant variability between departments and settings. Laboratory work, even with advances in technology, remains stressful. Managers must also deal with dissatisfaction on the part of technical staff members when expectations for more challenging work are not realized and salaries remain mediocre in contrast to those of other health-care professionals. Interpersonal conflict among personnel often smolders as a result of allegiance to different professional organizations.

Although this list is far from conclusive, the sampling of characteristics discussed should be sufficient to heighten the awareness of the laboratory manager to the challenges inherent in administering the clinical laboratory. In addition, the systems analysis perspective shows how interactive the components of the clinical laboratory are.

Finally, as Leavitt[17] has pointed out, the managing process is an interactive flow of three variables: path finding, decision making, and implementing. The successful manager understands that the three variables are interconnected, and in the complexity described previously, he must be able to make decisions and im-

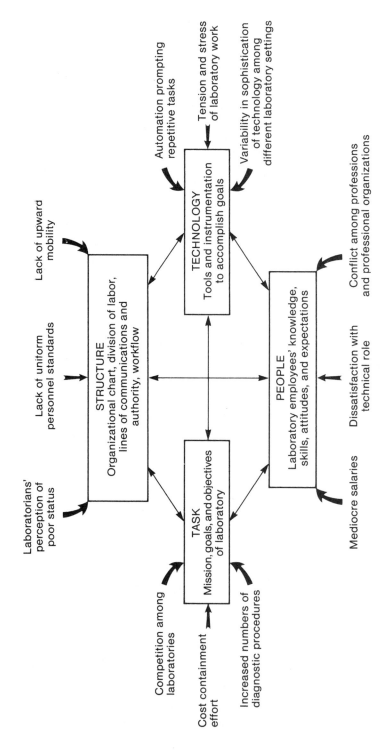

FIGURE 5-7. Select characteristics of laboratory medicine challenging laboratory managers.

plement them, often in the face of inadequate information.

BRIDGING THE GAP: AN APPROACH

Sufficient background is provided herein on the science of management to apply and develop a variety of managerial skills essential for effective laboratory administration. We have purposely avoided recording the research that led to the establishment of various principles. Accordingly, the development and differentiation of different schools of administrative thought have not been explored. The emphasis is on bridging the gap between the theory and the practice of clinical laboratory management.

REFERENCES

1. Bartolome F: When you think the boss is wrong. Personnel J 69(8):66–73, 1990
2. Bittel L: What Every Supervisor Should Know, 3rd ed, p 18. New York, McGraw-Hill, 1974
3. Challman S: Practicing Effective Delegation. Lexington, KY, University of Kentucky, College of Allied Health Professions, TIPS, 1989
4. Day D: Relating to employees—must the manager choose between being liked or respected? Clin Lab Management Rev 7:161–165, 1994
5. Florane RK: Marketability of medical technologists with a graduate degree in administration and supervision. J Med Technol 2:453–458, 1985
6. Fringes CS: Effective time management. MLO 20(7):43–45, 19
7. Fritz R: How to impress your boss. Clin Lab Management Rev 5:43–45, 1991
8. Fritz R: I'm your boss. . . why are you laughing? Clin Lab Management Rev 6:162–163, 1992
9. Fulmer RM: Supervision: Principles of Professional Management, p 6. Beverly Hills, Glencoe Press, 1976
10. Graham JE: A do-it-yourself orientation program for the new lab supervisor. MLO 25(4):38–41, 1994
11. Karni KR: Clinical laboratories—a survey. In Karni KR, Viskochil KR, Amos PA (eds): Clinical Laboratory Management: A Guide for Clinical Laboratory Scientists, pp 3–40. Boston, Little, Brown, 1982
12. Karni KR, Seanger DG: Management skills needed by entry-level practitioners. Clin Lab Sci 1:296–300, 1988
13. Kazemek EA: Steps to take when assuming a new management position. Clin Lab Management Rev 7:57–58, 1993
14. Ketchem SM: Overcoming the four toughest management challenges. Clin Lab Management Rev 5:246–263, 1991
15. King EC: A design for laboratory managers to encourage staff motivation. Laboratory Management 16(3):45–48, 1978
16. Lambert J: Becoming a HealthCare Supervisor. Lexington, KY, University of Kentucky, College of Allied Health Professions, TIPS, 1989
17. Leavitt HJ: Applied organizational change in industry: Structural, technological and humanistic approaches. In March TG (ed): Handbook of Organizations, pp 1144–1170. New York, Rand McNally, 1965
18. McBride K: Task analysis of medical technology administration and supervision. Am J Med Technol 44:688–695, 1978
19. McClure IL, Bayliss FT: Medical technologist supervisors: Are they prepared to manage? Am J Med Technol 44:97–111, 1978
20. Petrick JA, Manning GE: Work morale assessment and development for the clinical laboratory manager. Clin Lab Management Rev 6:141–149, 1992
21. Ramsey MK: What laboratory personnel like in supervisors. Clin Lab Sci 2:214–215, 1989
22. Relman AS: Cost control, doctors' ethics and patient care. Issues in Science and Technology Winter:103–111, 1985
23. Robbins SP: The Administrative Process. Englewood Cliffs, NJ, Prentice-Hall, 1976
24. Sattler J: A Practical Guide to Financial Management of the Clinical Laboratory, 2nd ed. Oradell, NJ, Medical Economics Company, 1986
25. Scanlon BK: Management 18: A Short Course for Managers, pp 3–4. New York, John Wiley & Sons, 1974
26. Sedlacek J: Time Management: A guide for Health Care Supervisors, Lexington, KY, University of Kentucky, College of Allied Health Professions, TIPS, 1989
27. Snyder JR, Hartzell RK: A systems analysis perspective for managing change in clinical laboratories. Lab Med 18:43–46, 1987
28. Snyder JR: When delegating is not the answer. MLO 25(5):7, 1994
29. Umiker WO: The Effective Laboratory Supervisor, pp 2–11. Oradell, NJ, Medical Economics Company, 1982

Part

II

Concepts in Managerial Leadership

6

Motivation—Managerial Assumptions and Effects

Diana Mass

In addition to sound leadership and organizational skills, a successful laboratory manager must also have the ability to motivate or instill self-motivation in employees. Because motivation must be directed toward a constructive outcome compatible with the goals of the organization, the prudent manager minimizes discrepancies between individual and organizational goals. Once this is accomplished, the manager will support and reinforce character traits that lead to the fulfillment of shared goals. This chapter examines some assumptions about human behavior, the theories of motivation that have evolved from them, and how managers can use those theories to motivate employees.

NATURE OF MOTIVATION

When different people perform the same job, invariably some do it better than others. If one can quantify each worker's contribution, one may find that the best person in each group is contributing two, five, or perhaps 10 times as much as the poorest performer. What causes these differences in performance? One answer is that these differences reflect individual differences in skill or ability. Another answer is that differences in performance reflect differences in motivation. At any given time, people vary in the extent to which they are willing to direct their energies toward the attainment of organizational goals. The problem of motivating workers is as old as organized activity itself, but only within the last half century has it been scientifically studied. This relatively brief period has seen the beginning of attempts to apply the tools of the behavioral sciences, particularly psychology, to the relationship between an individual's motivation and his or her work.[2,11,21]

Defining Motivation

Before examining the nature of motivation, the term must be defined. Motivation is not a simple concept, and its definition must refer to desires, goals, plans,

95

Box 6·1

**Four Essential Features
of Motivated Behavior**

1. Motivated behavior is purposeful, or goal directed.
2. The motivated individual expects that specific behaviors will lead to the attainment of goals.
3. Motivation is assumed to be selective or directional and requires that energy be involved to propel the individual to a level that enables the performance of the appropriate behavior.
4. Motivation involves the persistence of behavior over time so that effort can be sustained even if setbacks occur.

Jung J: Understanding Human Motivation. New York, Macmillan, 1978.

intents, impulses, and purposes. Some of these terms imply deliberate and calculated processes that involve reason, and others imply spontaneity. In general, the strength of a person's motivation depends on the strength of his or her individual motives. Motives are the causes that direct a given type of behavior. Thus, motives are the mainsprings of action.[11,12]

Motivated behavior has four essential features (Box 6–1). It is easy to see, then, that motivation is a complex concept, and an explanation thereof must include a discussion of personality, because the effectiveness of motivators varies among individuals.

Personality

Personality can be defined as the aggregate of an individual's behaviors. The development of personality is affected by many things: the individual's genetic and physical makeup; family size, composition, and style of interactions; the culture in which he is raised; the types of groups to which he belongs; the nature and amount of education; and so forth. The great number of possible combinations of these elements gives rise to individuals with different needs, and thus, a variety of motivation techniques is necessary.

Behavior constantly changes in response to the situations and the kinds of people one encounters. An individual's behavior is a function of personality. Components of personality include needs, drives, motivation, perceptual approaches, past experiences, atti-

tudes, values, and types of relations with others, all of which affect the individual's performance on the job.[12]

Motivation Process

The process of motivation is depicted in Figure 6–1. Because all behavior is motivated, either consciously or unconsciously, a cause-and-effect relationship exists. This phenomenon has often been called the path goals approach to fulfillment of unsatisfied needs. The first step in the path goals cycle involves the sensing or realization of an unsatisfied need. This is followed by establishing goals that are intended to fulfill the need and then developing behavior in an attempt to accomplish those goals. Motivation should not be confused with satisfaction. If action is viewed as a process, one can easily see that motivation describes the force that pushes people to perform, while satisfaction describes the feeling of contentment and achievement experienced after a goal is met. That is, people are motivated to seek satisfaction.[4]

Many of the early management scholars emphasized financial incentives as prime means for motivating individuals. Today money is still an important motivator; however, psychologists now agree that people seek to satisfy needs other than purely economic ones. There is a wide difference of opinion as to what these needs and their relative importance are. Most, however, take a pluralistic approach, which emphasizes that there are many different types of needs, each of which may be defined by the satisfaction it brings. Understanding that unsatisfied needs motivate people to alter their behavior to achieve their goals has led to the development of motivational theories. Four of the most well-known motivational theories are (1) the *need-hierarchy* the-

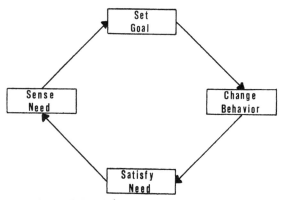

FIGURE 6–1. Path goals cycle.

ory; (2) the *two-factor* theory; (3) the *preference–expectation* theory; and (4) *theories X and Y*. A discussion of these theories and their relevance to today's organizational setting follows.

MOTIVATIONAL THEORIES

Need-Hierarchy Theory

One of the most widely adopted theories of human motivation was proposed in the early 1940s by Abraham Maslow. Maslow described a hierarchy of needs as a predictor and descriptor of human motivation. His theory of motivation is based on two premises: (1) Needs depend on what one already has. That is, needs that are not satisfied can influence behavior, but satisfied needs will not act as motivators. (2) Needs are arranged in a hierarchy of importance. When one need is satisfied, a higher level need emerges and demands satisfaction.

The various needs are described in a framework referred to as the hierarchy of needs (Fig. 6–2). According to Maslow, five general categories, or levels, of needs can be found in any individual: (1) physiologic, or survival, needs; (2) safety, or security, needs; (3) so-

cial needs; (4) esteem, or ego, needs; and (5) self-actualization, or self-fulfillment, needs.

These five categories of needs are arranged in a hierarchy ranging from the lowest order needs (physiologic) to the highest order (self-actualization). This hierarchy determines priority. According to Maslow, behavior is always determined by the lowest order level of need remaining unsatisfied, and unsatisfied needs are the important motivators. Therefore, when selecting effective motivators in the organizational setting, it is important to recognize whether a certain motivator is directed toward satisfying a previously unsatisfied need or one that no longer exists.[4,5,7,10,11,13,14,19,21] We can now examine the five need levels and relate them to a modern organizational setting.

Physiologic Needs

Food, clothing, and shelter constitute the primary needs, which are thus the prime motivators. In terms of the work environment, the satisfaction of physiologic needs is usually associated with money. What money can buy satisfies a person's physiologic needs. It should also be noted that money is useful not only as a satisfier of physiologic needs, but also as a satisfier of needs at any level.[4,5,7,10,11,13,14,19,21]

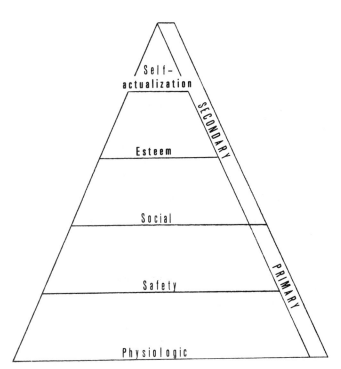

FIGURE 6–2. Hierarchy of needs.

Safety Needs

With the physiologic needs fulfilled, the next level of needs assumes priority. Safety needs include protection from physical harm, ill health, and economic disaster. In a work setting, this category has been broadened to include needs such as job security, medical insurance, and greater financial support. If an employee senses that management makes fair judgments regarding all subordinates, he is not likely to feel threatened. If, however, management's policies reflect favoritism and arbitrary discrimination, the employee may insist strongly on job security. This is evidenced by stronger demands from labor unions regarding job security and legal cases resulting from dismissal of an employee without sufficient justification. With regard to protection from physical harm, the Occupational Safety and Health Administration has been active in attempting to eliminate many of the dangerous elements of various jobs. Management's attention to safety to minimize these dangers serves as a strong motivator.[4,5,7,10,11,13,14,19,21]

Social Needs

After the safety and security needs have been satisfied, social needs have an influence on behavior. These include needs for giving and receiving affection and love; the need to accept, associate with, and be accepted by others; and the need to belong or to feel oneself a part of social groups. In essence, one needs to be liked by and to like one's coworkers. The fulfillment of social needs manifests itself in the formation of informal groups within organizations. Research has shown that in many cases, individuals seek affiliation because they desire to have their beliefs confirmed; that is, people tend to seek out others who share similar beliefs. Under proper direction, this natural activity can help in the formulation of a cooperative and constructive group. Unfortunately, management may fear that the group will develop consolidated attributes in opposition to the organization's goals. Hence, the social needs of the employee are often downgraded, leading to frustration and resentment.[4,5,7,10,11,13,14,19,21]

Esteem Needs

Maslow's fourth level consists of the esteem or ego needs, that is, the need to be recognized for what one does. This category includes the need for respect from others; the feeling of achievement, appreciation, recognition, and status; and, generally, a feeling of worthiness. These needs could be subdivided into two groups: self-esteem and esteem from others. Self-esteem refers to the development of self-confidence and self-respect. This often takes the form of mastery of an area of knowl-edge or competency in a technical skill. Currently, management's tool to help develop the employee's self-confidence usually takes the form of constructive appraisals of the employee. From the employee's viewpoint, knowing that a job is done well increases self-confidence. In addition, recognition by management and others leads to the development of self-respect.[4,5,7,10,11,13,14,19,21]

Self-Actualization Needs

The highest hierarchical need is for self-actualization, or self-fulfillment. Maslow defines it as the need "to become everything one is capable of becoming." In attempting to satisfy this need, an employee becomes less concerned about recognition and more concerned about the pleasure and sense of satisfaction obtained from performing a job. Self-actualization describes a potential for self-development. Unfortunately, rarely does an individual have the financial and emotional freedom to pursue ultimate self-development and total creativity.[4,5,7,10,11,13,14,19,21] In 1962, Maslow estimated that only 10% of self-fulfillment needs were satisfied, compared with 85% of the physiologic needs.[5] In keeping with his premises of a hierarchy, Maslow argues that the satisfaction of self-actualization needs is possible only after the satisfaction of all other needs in the hierarchy. As Maslow perceives it, the hierarchy-of-needs theory is applicable to most people in most situations. However, some individuals, because of their unique personality or situation, establish a different hierarchy of needs. For example, a great composer or artist might thrive on fulfillment of the higher level needs while caring little about his physical suste-nance.[4,5,7,10,11,13,14,19,21]

For the sake of definition, the needs are separated into five categories. In reality, however, they interact within the individual. Lower level needs never remain fully satisfied, and once the needs for esteem and self-actualization become important, a person seeks continuously for more satisfaction of them. In fact, people can never fully satisfy all of their needs. The need-hierarchy model essentially says that needs that are satisfied are no longer motivators. In essence, people are motivated by what they seek much more than by what they already have.[4,5,7,10,11,13,14,19,21]

Management's task in the application of this theory is to create situations within the organization that allow employees to satisfy their needs. Most organizations satisfy the lower level needs. Salaries and fringe benefits satisfy physiologic and security needs, respectively; interactions and associations on the job provide satisfaction of social needs. Typically, however, little opportunity exists for the satisfaction of higher level needs. Unsatisfied needs produce tension within the individual regardless of the level at which the need occurs. When an individual is unable to satisfy a particular need, frustration results.[13]

Frustration is a feeling that arises when one encounters certain kinds of blocks to need fulfillment. These feelings arise when the blocks seem insurmountable and when failure to overcome them threatens personal well-being. The reaction to frustration varies according to the person and the situation. Frustration can lead to behavior that is positive and constructive or negative and defensive. A useful model to describe the relationship existing between needs and constructive or destructive behaviors is shown in Figure 6–3.[4,13]

Figure 6–3 shows that unsatisfied needs contribute to tension within the individual, motivating a search for ways of relief. If one is successful in achieving a goal, the next unsatisfied need emerges. If attempts to satisfy needs are frustrated, a person may engage in either constructive or defensive types of behavior. For example, an employee who is frustrated in attempts to satisfy a need for recognition on the job may direct that frustration in a positive direction by seeking recognition off the job, temporarily satisfying the need and allowing job performance to remain intact. However, the organization will eventually be forced to deal with the need-frustration.

Conversely, destructive behaviors may consist of withdrawal, aggression, substitution, or rationalization. Withdrawal may be physical (quitting the job), but it is more likely that it will be internalized and manifested in apathy. Such individuals may have excessive absences or latenesses. Sometimes frustration leads to aggression. In certain rare situations, the frustrated employee may be aggressive toward his or her superior, but in most instances, the employee is more inclined to become aggressive toward other people or objects. Substitution takes place when an individual puts something in the place of an original object. For example, an individual's frustration in not getting a promotion may result in his or her trying to achieve leadership in

an informal group whose objectives are to resist and frustrate management policies.[4,13]

It is important for the manager to recognize and understand frustration. Frustration may occur when an employee has a strong need for esteem, but the job is such that it cannot satisfy this need. Management must restructure the job so that such needs can be met.

Two-Factor Theory

Maslow's need-hierarchy theory is a basic model on which many theories of motivation have been built. One of these is the two-factor (motivator-hygiene) theory developed by Frederick Herzberg in 1959 as a result of research to determine what affects employee motivation in work settings. The basic premise of Herzberg's theory is that employees are motivated to produce at high levels if they perceive that the result will satisfy their needs. Herzberg concluded that people's needs can be classified into two categories that are independent of each other and affect behavior in different ways.

Using a critical incident study, Herzberg interviewed 200 engineers and accountants. Each individual was asked to recount a time of feeling exceptionally good and a time of feeling exceptionally bad about his or her job and to describe the conditions that seemed to cause those feelings. The types of conditions that caused good feelings were rarely the same conditions that, when absent, caused bad feelings.

Good feelings were generally associated with the content of the job itself. Five factors seemed especially important: (1) opportunity for achievement, (2) recognition for accomplishment, (3) challenging work, (4) more responsibility, and (5) advancement. These factors, called motivators or satisfiers, contribute greatly to motivation and job satisfaction, but their absence from the organization does not necessarily prove to be highly dissatisfying.

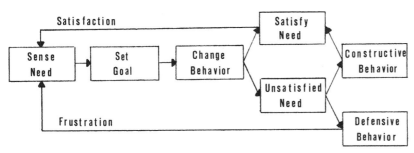

FIGURE 6–3. Behavioral response.

Bad feelings, conversely, were usually related to the environment surrounding the job. Lack of the following factors promoted dissatisfaction: (1) effective company policies; (2) competent technical supervision; (3) good interpersonal relations; (4) satisfactory salary, security, and status; and (5) appropriate working conditions. These environmental dimensions of the job are referred to as maintenance or hygiene factors because they are vitally necessary for maintaining a reasonable level of satisfaction. The term *hygiene* is used in the sense that proper hygiene prevents infection, and by analogy, good psychological hygiene prevents dissatisfaction. The accountants and engineers in the study expected these factors to be present and saw them as basic to the work situation. Their absence served as strong dissatisfiers, although their presence did little to promote good feelings. The hygiene factors are necessary prerequisites for motivation, but by themselves, they neither increase motivation nor cause satisfaction. Conversely, the hygiene factors, coupled with satisfiers, result in strong motivation of employees.[4,5,7,10,11,13,14,19,21]

Herzberg's theory suggests that job satisfaction and dissatisfaction are not opposites. Instead, the opposite of dissatisfaction is simply the absence of dissatisfaction. This distinction is important when related to levels of job performance. A neutral or zero point in performance levels exists when employees are neither dissatisfied nor satisfied with their jobs (Fig. 6-4). At this point, employees simply perform at the minimal acceptable level necessary to maintain their jobs and employment. What Herzberg emphasizes is that job satisfaction and dissatisfaction are influenced by different factors and exert different effects on employees. The hygiene factors tend to affect dissatisfaction, and their absence promotes performance below acceptable levels. Motivators tend to affect job satisfaction and motivation, and when they are present, they promote performance above acceptable levels.[13]

There is some similarity between Herzberg's and Maslow's work. While they both study what motivates human behavior, Maslow looks at the human needs of the individual, whereas Herzberg focuses on how job conditions affect the individual's basic needs. The relationship between the two theories is shown in Figure 6–5. Money and benefits satisfy needs at the physiologic and security levels; interpersonal relations and supervision are examples of hygiene factors that tend to satisfy

social needs; whereas, increased responsibility, challenging work, growth, and development are motivators that tend to satisfy needs at the esteem and self-actualization levels.

The basic advance of Herzberg's theory over Maslow's is that Herzberg distinguishes between maintenance and motivational factors. Herzberg shows that motivation derives mostly from the work itself and encourages management to build into the work environment an opportunity to satisfy the motivators by enriching the job. Job enrichment refers to increasing the scope of responsibility and challenge in work, not, Herzberg emphasized, simply increasing the number of tasks. It is a way for management to provide employees an opportunity to grow and at the same time receive achievement and recognition. It is a way to make the work itself a more rewarding experience.[4,13]

Expectation Theory

In 1964, Victor H. Vroom developed a motivational model that is more an explanation of the motivation phenomenon than a description of what motivates. The Vroom model views motivation as a process governing choices. According to this theory, an employee's motivation to perform effectively is determined by two variables, preference and expectation. Vroom believed that people subjectively assign preferences to all expected outcomes. In addition, he believed that the degree of motivation was a product of both the goals that people wanted to achieve and the degree to which they believed or expected that their own actions were instrumental in accomplishing their goals:

Motivation = Goal preference × Effectiveness of actions

Furthermore, Vroom proposed that the level of performance was equal to the product of the degree of motivation and the individual's own inherent abilities.

Performance = Motivation × Ability

If the two determinants of motivation nullify each other, there is no motivation, and the individual will not be motivated to increase performance. For example, if an employee values being promoted to departmental supervisor but realizes that even exceptional performance will not earn the position, the employee will not be motivated. Because there is no reason to increase

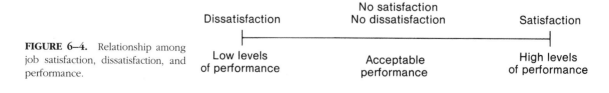

FIGURE 6–4. Relationship among job satisfaction, dissatisfaction, and performance.

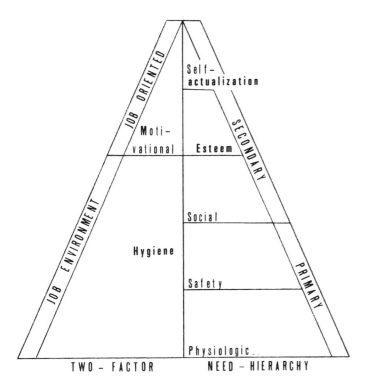

FIGURE 6–5. Comparison of two-factor and need-hierarchy theories.

performance, the employee does not. Vroom's model emphasizes that the motivational process is lodged within the individual. It depends on the individual having a specific, preferred outcome coupled with a belief or expectation that certain activities or behaviors will bring about the desired outcome. This model adds additional insight into the study of motivation because it attempts to explain how individual goals influence individual efforts.[5,7,10,19,21]

Theories X and Y

In 1960, Douglas McGregor published *The Human Side of Enterprise*, which attempted to demonstrate that management's basic attitude toward employees had a significant impact on employee job performance.[15] He described two basic management attitudes: theory X and theory Y. These attitudes are reflected in management styles based on different assumptions regarding human behavior (Table 6–1).[11,15] Theory X managers assume that employees are lazy, would rather be directed than left to their own initiative, do not want responsibility, and only seek safety and security. Theory X managers attempt to structure, control, and closely supervise their personnel. They believe that people are

motivated by money, fringe benefits, and the threat of punishment. These assumptions of theory X are similar to Herzberg's hygiene factors or dissatisfiers.

McGregor argued that the close supervision exercised by theory X managers resulted in less than satisfactory job performance. He believed that closely supervised employees would resist the restrictions and do only the required minimum. McGregor also believed individuals would not demonstrate any drive, initiative, or creativity to accomplish organizational goals under theory X management. Consequently, he proposed theory Y, a more positive set of assumptions regarding human behavior. These management practices are based on a more accurate understanding of human nature and motivation.[4,7,8,11,13,14,21]

Theory Y managers help their employees grow by allowing them to direct and control themselves. In this way, employees are able to satisfy their social, esteem, and self-actualization needs. According to McGregor, theory Y managers create climates that allow employees to achieve both individual and organizational goals, thus enriching all aspects of the job, as Herzberg advocates.

Theory Y thinking has given rise to the "participative" management style. Participative managers allow for decentralized decision making and delegate

Table 6-1
Theory X and Theory Y Assumption About Human Behavior and Motivation

Theory X	Theory Y
Work is inherently distasteful to most people.	Work is as natural as play if the conditions are favorable.
Most people are not ambitious, have little desire for responsibility, and prefer to be directed.	Self-control is often indispensable in achieving organizational goals.
Most people have little capacity for creativity in solving organizational problems.	The capacity for creativity in solving organizational problems is widely distributed in the population.
Motivation occurs only at the physiologic and safety levels.	Motivation occurs at the social, esteem, and self-actualization levels, as well as physiologic and security levels.
Most people must be loosely controlled and often ordered to achieve organizational objectives.	People can be self-directed and creative at work if properly motivated.

responsibility and authority to employees. The participative manager is a resource person for the employees, who exercise independent judgment in getting the job done. This style is most applicable when dealing with highly skilled employees (such as clinical laboratory scientists), when individual or group participation is advantageous, and when problems need to be solved. In the long run, this style of management elicits the greatest productivity for the organization.[7,13]

RESPONSIBILITIES OF MANAGEMENT

Because human motivation and behavior are extremely complex, it is not surprising that the theories are too simplistic to yield a model that is beyond reproach. Nevertheless, each theory does offer some insight into human behavior. It is management's responsibility to understand the shortcomings and strong points of each theory and synthesize the workable philosophies of motivation into concrete actions and policies.

Management Behaviors That Stimulate Motivation

Provide an Open Communication System

Individuals should be a part of the communication system and should be allowed to contribute to the decision-making process. In this way, the goals of employees will become integrated with the goals of management. An open communication system allows for trust, reciprocity, and growth on the part of individuals; at the same time, it decreases the effectiveness of informal groups and grapevines, which frustrate organizational goals. Part of good communication includes active listening. Active listening requires that managers give explicit responses to employees speaking to them. This process facilitates problem solving.

Provide an Integration of Individual Needs With the Organization's Goals

Organizational goals are met by employees who expect to meet their needs and are satisfied by their outcomes. A mechanism for accomplishing this is jointly establishing performance objectives. Individuals who understand the purpose of their work and are allowed to develop their job objectives will give their best efforts to achieving objectives, while at the same time developing strong feelings of identification with organizational goals. Management must be sure that the objectives are specific, clearly understood, and measurable. Objectives should be difficult but achievable. Objectives that are too easy or too difficult do not motivate people. Achieved goals build self-confidence and self-esteem. In addition, specific dates should be set for reviewing progress, because this process motivates employees to make reportable progress by the predetermined dates.

Delegate Responsibility and Authority

A good manager must trust others to accomplish organizational goals. Once employees demonstrate ability, they should be given the freedom to make decisions, implement actions, make mistakes, take corrective actions, and achieve goals without constant supervision. This process provides opportunities for enrichment.

Develop Employees' Self-Esteem

In general, the higher an employee's self-esteem, the better the employee performs. Management can promote employees' confidence in themselves by praising good work and expecting their best efforts. This can be accomplished by the application of the reinforcement principle: Reward behavior that is desirable, because people tend to repeat rewarded behavior. Following are additional points regarding this principle: Reward is most effective when applied immediately after behavior. Apply more reward at the onset of desired behavior than after the pattern is established. Ensure that the reward is acknowledged as such by the employee. For some employees, the reward may be a bonus; for others, it may be public recognition.

Maintain Contact

Successful leaders in any organization maintain personal contact with their colleagues. This allows for a better understanding of their personality characteristics, abilities, and potential capabilities. Through this contact, managers will understand the individual better and thus provide job enrichment opportunities that lead to job satisfaction.

Analyze the Problem, not the Person, and Take Corrective Action

Managers should never presume that performance deficiencies are attitude problems. If managers unwisely evaluate the person and not the work, then a lowering of self-esteem will result, which ultimately adds to the problem. If the problem is one of a personal nature, then active listening is required to solve the problem. When dealing with the negative aspect of an employee's performance, the manager should communicate in private and take corrective action. It is always important to maintain an employee's self-esteem.

It is management's responsibility to create an environment to encourage motivation. Furthermore, to apply the knowledge of motivational theory means to anticipate the factors most likely to have a motivational effect on work. An effective manager understands the employees' needs and endeavors to involve them in accomplishing the organization's goals.[16]

GROUP DYNAMICS

The major thrust of this chapter thus far has been directed toward understanding individual motivation as a means of improving an organization's productivity. When ideas and individual abilities are combined in a group effort, productivity increases.

Group Structure

Groups will inevitably form in any organization. For example, management might deliberately appoint several individuals to a committee charged with performing a specific function. This is referred to as a formal group. Conversely, an informal group is developed by several individuals who have shared mutual esteem and goals.

Groups, whether formal or informal, serve several functions. Formal groups allow the spreading of responsibility for decisions among many individuals and allow a broader range of participation in decision making. Additionally, they provide a formal division of labor to study specific problems and general issues. Finally, they arrive at more satisfactory and longer lasting decisions through discussion and compromise.

Informal groups allow the development of mutual benefit. Each individual possesses skills and knowledge and uses these to help other members perform their duties more satisfactorily. Additionally, informal friendship groups strengthen the individual's commitment to the organization, while reducing the level of unproductive competition. Thus, management should encourage group formation.

There are various assumptions about small-group behavior of which management must be cognizant. The following assumptions concerning group behavior will show how individuals act within groups and how groups function. This overview of group dynamics is presented to demonstrate the impact groups have on employee motivation and productivity.[7]

Motivational Assumptions

We can assume that the working group has an important psychological function. Development of feelings of satisfaction and competence can be profound, especially when they are reinforced informally by coworkers. A sincere and personal recognition of good performance by one's peers is often more meaningful than a general statement of approval by distant supervisors.

The second assumption follows as a natural outgrowth of the first. Most people want to be accepted by the people surrounding them and will work to gain their approval. The desire for acceptance stimulates people to interact cooperatively with each other, thus increasing the effectiveness of the group as a whole.[10] If the element of approval centers around positive or constructive behavior, it stands to reason that management should approve this type of group interaction.

The third assumption deals with the relationship of the formal group leader and the members. An effective leader knows that he cannot do all things at all times. The supervisor must rely on the group members working together to carry out directives so that the department operates smoothly, even in the supervisor's absence. In other words, it is assumed that the effectiveness of the group is related to the cooperative attitude of its members toward the formal leader.

The fourth assumption deals with the emotions of individuals. Suppressed feelings tend to eat away at an individual, rarely having a positive effect. It is generally assumed that an individual who is able to express emotion is likely to have better mental health. This presumably results in a better employee. However, great care must be taken with regard to how emotions are expressed. The ability to handle emotions objectively and rationally is a skill that is not developed overnight. Nevertheless, if group skills in this area are refined, the rewards can be staggering. Group morale and problem-solving capabilities can be greatly improved. Conversely, if emotions are vented irrationally, it is likely to have the opposite effect, causing disruption and conflict among the group members.

The fifth assumption of consequence to managers is that the previously discussed qualities are usually inadequately developed. Rarely in any group situation is there a perfect example of interpersonal trust, cooperation, or acceptance. Similarly, few people can claim to be in control of themselves in all aspects, at all times, in all situations; even the most level-headed occasionally lose their temper. Knowing that there is always room for improvement, management should strive to upgrade continually the positive aspects of human group behavior.

The sixth assumption states that resolution of problems is more effective and longer lasting if both sides involved are willing to work together. If management issues an ultimatum regarding a certain change without discussion or consultation with employees, the resistance will be pronounced. Conversely, if management and employees have the philosophy of working together with the goal of becoming mutually effective, resistance will be minimized.[6]

Clearly, these currently accepted assumptions regarding human group behavior are intricately involved in the motivational process. Thus, it follows that management must use leadership styles and managerial philosophies that benefit the individual and the organization.

MOTIVATING INTO THE 21ST CENTURY

In his book *The Third Wave*, Alvin Toffler[20] forecasts that workers will seek more responsibility and will have more commitment to work that fully uses their talents. In recent times, the economics of laboratory operation have led to cost-cutting measures that have, in many cases, created an increasingly mechanized work environment. A major consequence has been the underuse of the laboratory professional's talent, creating a negative motivational environment. One approach to circumvent this inevitable consequence is the use of self-

directed teams. A prototype of these teams has been described as quality circles.[1,3,9,17,18]

Established in Japan, quality circles have succeeded in harnessing the ingenuity and energy of the work force to the solving of problems within the organization. Fostered by management, quality circles involve employees voluntarily meeting in groups of 8 to 12 to identify, analyze, and provide solutions to problems in their work area. These individuals meet weekly, with their supervisor as the circle leader. Initially, the group receives training in techniques of problem solving, data gathering, and problem analysis. Solutions to problems are conveyed to management, which commits itself to responding to the circle within a stated length of time. Quality circles give the employee opportunity for involvement, participation in work improvement, challenge, and opportunity for personal growth.[1,3,9,17,18]

The benefits of quality circles or teams are rooted firmly in the motivational theories discussed in this chapter. Today's employee is viewed as one who brings a whole set of needs to the job and hopes to satisfy many of them on the job. Finding solutions to problems through a team approach provides personal and group gratification. The presentation to management offers individuals the opportunity to satisfy their highest goals of esteem and self-actualization as identified by Maslow. Through this interaction, the employee gains recognition.

The opportunity to do interesting and meaningful problem solving provides the work challenge described by Herzberg. Job enrichment through redesigning work routines is often limited by physical and other factors. Quality circles may not alter the entire job, but the effect of 1 hour a week involving Herzberg's motivators can have a dramatic effect on the other 39 hours.[1,3,9]

The design of quality circles or self-directed teams provides a vehicle for implementing McGregor's ideas by allowing employees to exercise self-direction and become more involved in working toward organizational objectives. Through quality circles, an employee gains the opportunity to be part of a team seeking common goals, matching his or her needs to the organization's goals. Quality circle solutions have produced savings that can be calculated in terms of increased production, cost-containment, and reduction in employee turnover. Improvements in attitude and morale have also resulted.[1,9]

The continued technologic and economic changes in the health-care field will no doubt take their toll on laboratory employees. Greater demands will be placed on laboratory professionals to increase their knowledge and maintain their skills, while dedicating their energies to improving productivity. This type of work environment may stifle motivation. However, employees want fulfilling and meaningful work experiences characterized by knowledge, care, respect, and responsibility. To ensure these outcomes, management must invest in the maintenance of human productivity. Laboratory management must consider how their employees' work can be enriched and the quality of their lives improved. The team concept provides an invaluable means to achieve these ends. Teams provide employees the opportunity to use their creative problem-solving, technical, and professional abilities in the identification and solution of problems. In these ways, teams serve a multibeneficial function: They enhance the quality of the employee, the organization, and health-care delivery in general. The team solution is a process of working smarter, not harder, that yields an increase in productivity—the key to financial security.[1,3,9,17,18]

SUMMARY

Management is encouraged to make the individual's job more challenging and responsible, thus allowing for individual advancement and growth. With the fundamental understanding that motivation is closely related to needs and individual personality, it is management's responsibility to create opportunities that allow satisfaction of those needs in a manner compatible with the individual's personality and the organization's goals. These must include attitudes, policies, and management styles that are supportive of the motivational process. If this is successful, management and employees will work together in a cohesive fashion to accomplish mutual goals and increase individual satisfaction.

REFERENCES

1. Baird JE Jr: Positive Personnel Practices; Quality Circles, Leaders Manual. Prospect Heights, IL, Waveland Press, 1982
2. Davis KR: Is Individual responsibility a radical concept in business? Clinical Laboratory Management Review Nov/Dec, 1979
3. Dewar DL: The Quality Circle Handbook. Ref Bluff, CA, Quality Circle Institute, 1980
4. Donnelly JH Jr, Gibson JL, Ivancevich JM: Fundamentals of Management: Functions, Behavior, Models. Austin, Business Publications, 1971
5. Filley AC, House RJ: Managerial Process and Organizational Behavior. Glenview, Scott, Foresman, 1969
6. Frech WL, Bell CH Jr: Organization Development. Englewood Cliffs, Prentice-Hall, 1973
7. Fulmer RM: Management and Organization. New York, Harper & Row, 1979
8. Gellerman SW: Management by Motivation. New York, American Management Association, 1968
9. Goldberg AM, Pegels CC: Quality Circles in Health Care Facilities. Rockville, MD, Aspen Publications, 1984
10. Gustafson DH, Doyle J, May JJ: Employee Incentive System for Hospitals. Washington, DC, U.S. Department of Health, Education, and Welfare, Publication No. HSM 72-6705, 1972 d425 msp109 tp 5-24-88
11. Hershey P, Blanchard KH: Management of Organizational Behavior; Utilizing Human Behavior. Englewood Cliffs, Prentice-Hall, 1972
12. Jung J: Understanding Human Motivation. New York, Macmil-lan, 1978
13. Koehler JW, Anatol K, Applbaum KL: Organizational Communication. New York, Holt, Rinehart and Winston, 1981
14. Labovitz GH: Motivational Dynamics Unit I: Mainsprings of Motivation. Minneapolis, Control Data Corporation, 1975
15. McGregor D: The Human Side of Enterprise. New York, McGraw-Hill, 1960
16. Meredith GG, Nelson RE, Nech PA: The Practice of Entrepreneurship. Geneva, International Labour Organization, 1982
17. Orlikoff JE, Snow A: Assessing Quality Circles in Health Care Settings: A Guide for Management. Chicago, American Hospital Publishing, 1984
18. Patchin RI: The Management and Maintenance of Quality Circles. Homewood, IL, Dow Jones-Irwin, 1983
19. Steers RM, Porter LW: Motivation and Work Behavior. New York, McGraw-Hill, 1975
20. Toffler A: The Third Wave. New York, William Morrow, 1980
21. Vroom VH, Edward LD: Management and Motivation. New York, Penguin Books, 1982

7

Laboratory Communications

Edward A. Johnson

A manager of any clinical laboratory facility must perform a variety of important management activities, such as planning, organizing, staffing, directing, and controlling. To carry out successfully such managerial responsibilities, the supervisor must have a clear understanding of two kinds of communication: interpersonal and organizational.

Interpersonal communication can be defined as a process of exchanging information and transmitting meaning between two individuals or in a small group of individuals.[13] *Organizational communication* can be viewed as a process by which managers develop a system to provide information and transmit meaning to large numbers of individuals within an organization and to relevant individuals and institutions outside the organization.[13] A supervisor who is able to deal effectively with his subordinates, peers, manager, and others within his organization recognizes that both processes of communication are essential to management because management is highly dependent on communication for its success.

INTERPERSONAL COMMUNICATION WITHIN THE LABORATORY

What does a clinical supervisor do when he communicates with his subordinates and others with whom he interacts in the process of managing his unit? To help provide an answer to such a question, two models related to the process of interpersonal communication are examined.[24] The focus is primarily on communication patterns between the supervisor and the subordinate, rather than between the supervisor and his peers or his superior.

A Simplistic View of Interpersonal Communication—Model I

One common way of representing the process of interpersonal communication is to view it as a source transmitting a message to a receiver, which results in some

action taking place (Fig. 7-1)[33] For example, assume that the administrative director of a laboratory thinks that he has several ideas for improving the work of the general bacteriology unit, and he wants these ideas implemented immediately. According to the model depicted in Figure 7-1, the director (the source) would convey these ideas both orally and in writing. The supervisor of general bacteriology (the receiver) would hear these ideas, and as a result of understanding them, would proceed immediately to implement them.

Any clinical supervisor who believes that the process of interpersonal communication functions in such a simplistic fashion is, of course, in for considerable difficulty in performing his job. Unfortunately, however, there are a number of supervisors today who do, in fact, subscribe to such a view.

The model depicted in Figure 7-1 simply fails to tell enough about the nature and complexity of interpersonal communication. It depicts what David K. Berlo refers to as a "conveyor theory of communication."[3] According to this theory, the process of interpersonal communication is viewed primarily as a transportation problem. In the example cited previously, the director is concerned only that the data move from point A to point B (see Fig. 7-1). Communication takes place when the director speaks to the supervisor of general bacteriology, but it cannot be assumed that *successful* communication automatically takes place whenever two individuals get together.[28,31]

A More Realistic Model of Interpersonal Communication—Model II

In reality, the process of interpersonal communication is much more complicated than that portrayed in Figure 7-1. The model presented in Figure 7-2 attempts to re-

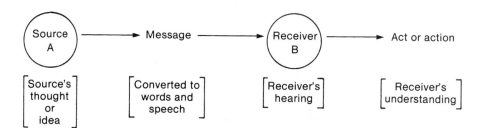

FIGURE 7-1.   A simplistic view of interpersonal communication.

flect the view of contemporary communication theory and to present in a more realistic fashion the major variables and relationships that characterize the situations faced by most supervisors of clinical laboratories. The model depicts the process of interpersonal communication as being dynamic, continuous, and complex. Each component of the model is discussed below separately. However, it is extremely important to recognize that these components are strongly interrelated.

Source

Interpersonal communication is generated by a source.[35] Interpersonal communication takes place because an individual wants to respond in some way to his environment.[20] For example, let us suppose that the supervisor of hematology is dissatisfied with the work of one of the medical technologists in his department. As the situation becomes increasingly more disturbing and uncomfortable to the supervisor, he seeks some way to convey his concern to the medical technologist. He is, in effect, responding to his environment and seeking to initiate some type of communication.[16,20]

Encoding

In interpersonal communication, the source (individual) engages in what is known as encoding. The *encoding process* takes place when the idea to be transmitted is transformed by the individual into written or spoken language.[20] When encoding, the source must search for appropriate ways to convey his meaning. If the message is not clear, the probability of communication failure will be high.

For example, if the supervisor of hematology cited in the previous example is to communicate to the medical technologist that he is dissatisfied with the medical technologist's work, he must translate his thought into language that the medical technologist can understand. The supervisor may succeed and select appropriate language, or he may fail and select language that is confusing to the medical technologist.

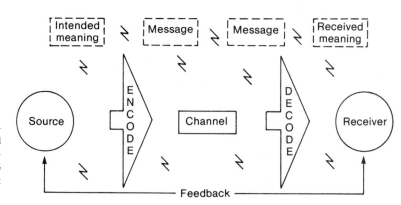

FIGURE 7-2.   A realistic model of interpersonal communication. (Adapted from Hicks HG, Arnold KK: Communication for supervisors. In Newport MG [ed]: Tools and Techniques, p 158. St Paul, West Publishing Co, 1976)

Message

The result of the encoding process is a *message*. The primary function of a message is to express the purpose of the source.[20] In a sense, a message is somewhat like a coin: It has two sides. There is the message as perceived by the source, and there is the message as perceived by the receiver. The two are not always the same.[35] For example, in the case of the supervisor of hematology and the medical technologist, the interpretation of the message may vary substantially because of the different perspectives of the two individuals.

Channel

A *channel* is the medium by which a message is transmitted[14]; it connects the source to the receiver. There are many types of channels; several may be appropriate for any given situation. Channels can be verbal (telephone calls or meetings) or nonverbal (letters, memoranda, and formal reports). Under the proper set of circumstances, any of the many types of channels can be effective.[35]

The channel decision is especially important, because it has implications for what type of encoding and decoding will be required and for the ultimate success of the communication effort.[35] The supervisor of hematology in the example cited previously could use any number of channels to transmit dissatisfaction (the intended message) to the medical technologist (Fig. 7-3). Some alternatives are discussed below[37]:

The supervisor may want to meet with the medical technologist and *tell* him that he is dissatisfied. In this case, the message is encoded in the form of direct verbal communication. The medical technologist must then decode the message, interpreting what the supervisor means. If the supervisor says, "I am dissatisfied with your work," the medical technologist may still have to decide, for example, whether that means that the supervisor likes to frighten the medical technologist now and then or whether he is on the verge of being fired.

The supervisor may decide to *telephone* the medical technologist about his dissatisfaction. In this instance, the supervisor encodes his message into an indirect verbal communication, and the telephone operates as a channel to the receiver.

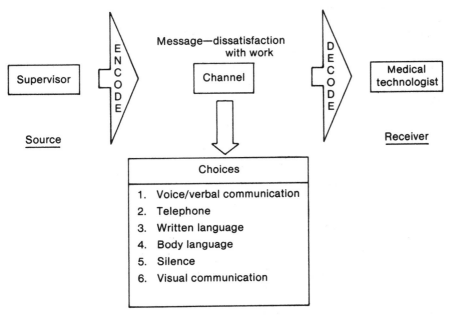

FIGURE 7-3. Some examples of channel choice. (Adapted from Wright J: The Communication Process: A Look at How Messages Are Sent, pp 13–19. Syracuse, Center for Instructional Development, Syracuse University, 1973)

If the supervisor wants to be more specific, he may choose to *write* his message in a memorandum, adding impact to his message, because the medical technologist will be able to look at the well-chosen words and reread them. In this case, the supervisor again encodes the message in written rather than spoken language.

Another way the supervisor could send his message would be to frown. He would be *using body language*, encoding his message into a frown, which the medical technologist might then decode as meaning that the supervisor is dissatisfied with the medical technologist's work. The medical technologist might not know the reason, so the message is rather vague, but it has nevertheless been transmitted.

Another possibility would be silence. When the medical technologist says, "Good morning," the supervisor might fail to respond. After a few mornings of this, the medical technologist might begin to get the message that the supervisor is dissatisfied. The message has been *encoded* into another form, still understandable to the medical technologist.

The supervisor could also use visual communication. He could enclose a "pink slip" with the medical technologist's paycheck. The medical technologist, understanding this as a dismissal notice, will most certainly receive the message that the supervisor is dissatisfied even before taking the time to read the words printed on the slip.

Decoding

For the process of interpersonal communication to function properly, the receiver must decode the message in such a fashion that he derives a meaning from it that is approximately the same as that transmitted by the source. Decoding is really encoding in reverse.[20]

It is not sufficient for the receiver to decode a message by simply attaching some meaning to it. Successful communication takes place only when the meaning that the receiver derives from a message is similar to that intended by the source. Failure to understand the intended meaning of a message is probably the greatest source of problems in interpersonal communication.[20]

Again using the example of the supervisor of hematology, the message, "I am dissatisfied with your work," may be decoded by the medical technologist to mean any of the following messages:

He must be dissatisfied because I was late three or four times during the past several weeks.

He must be dissatisfied because I was imprecise on the results of several blood workups during the past week.

He must be dissatisfied because I could not solve that problem he mentioned.

Differences in meaning occur because most sources and receivers have different backgrounds, experiences, values, needs, goals, expectations, attitudes, knowledge, and emotional constitution. Such factors determine the meanings that individuals give to certain words or actions. These factors can never be exactly the same for any two individuals; thus, no two individuals will ever attach precisely the same meaning to a particular set of words or actions. However, the greater the similarities among these factors, the greater the likelihood of successful communication.[20]

Feedback

Up to this point, the discussion has focused on communication of messages from the source to the receiver. Another important component of the communication process is feedback.

Feedback refers to a response from the receiver. In the process of providing feedback, the receiver encodes and sends a message through some channel to the original source, who is now in the position of being a receiver. In this way, the source can tell whether the original message did get through to the receiver. If the feedback indicates that the receiver understood the intended meaning of the message, additional communication can take place. If the message was unclear, however, the source might have to alter the encoding of the message until the feedback indicates that the receiver has understood the intended meaning.[20]

Looking at the case of the supervisor of hematology and the medical technologist, the medical technologist's reaction or response to the message, "I am dissatisfied with your work," will let the supervisor know whether or not the intended meaning was decoded. Suppose that the medical technologist did agree. If the medical technologist says, "I know; let's talk about it," he lets the supervisor know that he derived the intended meaning from the message. Conversely, if the medical technologist's response is, "What's the matter? The demands of your job must be getting to you," he is telling the supervisor that he did not derive the intended meaning from the message.

Feedback does not always have to be in the form of spoken or written words.[20] For example, if the supervisor sees a frown on the face of the medical technologist, he knows that the medical technologist either does not understand, disagrees, or is generally unhappy about the statement. If he sees a smile, he may think that the medical technologist assumes he is joking about what he has just said or is thinking about something that has nothing to do with his message. If he sees a blank face, he may believe the medical technologist is listening attentively or is bored. All of these facial expressions are part of feedback.

As we see how complex interpersonal communication can become, it is easier to understand why messages sometimes have a difficult time getting through.

Noise

In communication theory, noise has a broader definition than the typical one relating to loud sounds. It pertains to anything that may reduce the accuracy or fidelity of communication.[20] Noise is frequently inputted to the channel,[35] but it can be present in all of the components shown in Figure 7-2. Some illustrations of the impact of noise are provided below:[20]

Noise can exist if the source perceives an object or an activity in an incorrect way.

Noise can occur during the encoding process if the means selected do not adequately convey the appropriate mental perception of the source.

Noise can exist if the form or code of the message is not understandable to the receiver. This can take place, for example, if the source and the receiver speak different languages.

With respect to the channel, noise can prevent a message from getting through accurately. For example, it is extremely difficult to talk to someone in an exceptionally noisy environment.

Noise is present if the receiver does not decode the message correctly.

If the supervisor of hematology is dissatisfied with the medical technologist's work and wants improvement, he may select the wrong methods to encode his mental perception. If his laboratory is noisy, the message may not be heard clearly by the medical technologist. The possibilities for miscommunication are numerous.

The same components of this interpersonal communication system can be used to analyze the communication process between the physician requesting a laboratory test and the technologist.[22] Figure 7-4 displays the process from the sender, the attending physician, encoding the service request, channeling the message to the laboratory, where the request is decoded before the actual analysis is performed.[22] The communications loop is continued when the laboratory encodes the test result (report) for later interpretation by the

requesting physician. The channels of communication, whether in written format (ie, requisition and report forms) or verbal, are susceptible to comparable errors resulting from poor encoding, decoding, and noise.

INTERPERSONAL COMMUNICATION—A TRANSACTIONAL PROCESS

A useful way for a clinical supervisor to analyze interpersonal communication is through an awareness of the concepts associated with *transactional analysis* (TA). TA represents an attempt to understand human behavior based on how individuals interact and relate to one another.[4,5,19]

The subject of TA includes the following four components: (1) *structural analysis*—the analysis and understanding of the individual personality; (2) *TA*—the analysis of what people say to each other and how each responds; (3) *game analysis*—the analysis of motives, rewards, and tactics that individuals use to win in interpersonal communication; and (4) *script analysis*—the analysis of the patterns of habitual behavior or "scripts for life" that individuals consciously and unconsciously act out, making them winners, losers, delinquents, and so forth.[6]

Because of space limitations, the discussion that follows will focus on structural analysis and TA. However, the reader should become familiar with game analysis and script analysis by consulting Berne[4,5] and Harris[19] and the bibliography for this chapter.

Structural Analysis

According to TA, the personality of an individual contains three ego states: parent, adult, and child.

The *Parent ego state* contains the parts of an individual that behave in the same manner as the individual's mother, father, or guardian. All the rules and laws that the individual heard from his parents are recorded in the individual's Parent. All the "should do's," "shouldn't do's," "must do's," and "mustn't do's" are included in this state. At times, the Parent is nurturing and benevolent, whereas at other times, it is judgmental and critical. In either case, the Parent exerts a powerful influence on an individual. Many objections and excuses originate from this state.[1]

The individual's *Adult ego state* functions like a logical, computer-like, rational decision maker. It relies on facts to make decisions. It gathers, stores, and processes information from the Parent, Child, and Adult in an attempt to solve problems.[1]

The *Child ego state* in an individual represents what he was when he was young. It is the individual's

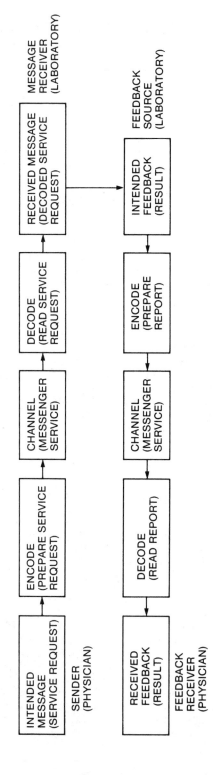

FIGURE 7–4. Communication process in the clinical laboratory.

emotions and feelings, his laughter and love, his fun making and creativity. It also contains the individual's fears, frustrations, moodiness, aggressiveness, and defensiveness.[1]

Although none of the three ego states is necessarily superior to or more desirable than the others, an important ground rule for a clinical supervisor is that successful transactions and effective communication between the supervisor and subordinate(s) in the laboratory generally can only take place when both parties are operating in their Adult states. This does not mean that the supervisor cannot transact with the subordinate's Parent or Child. However, when it comes to solving problems, the supervisor ideally should appeal to the subordinate's Adult.

Transactional Analysis

When a supervisor interacts with a subordinate, there are three basic types of communication transactions: (1) complementary transactions; (2) crossed transactions; and (3) ulterior transactions.

A *complementary transaction* can be defined as one that is "appropriate and expected and follows the natural order of healthy human relationships."[4] In such transactions, the source can usually predict the type of response that will be received. Complementary transactions involve only two ego states, and the stimulus and response vectors are parallel (Fig. 7-5). Another way of identifying a complementary transaction is that "(a) the response comes from the same ego state as that to which the stimulus is directed, and (b) the response is directed to the same ego state from which the stimulus is initiated."[36]

When the lines of communication are not parallel and do not meet the conditions cited previously, the *transaction is crossed.* Crossed transactions result in temporary communication breakdowns because the source receives a response that is unexpected (see Fig. 7-5).[36] Crossed transactions are not desirable. Effective communication can be increased only if the frequency

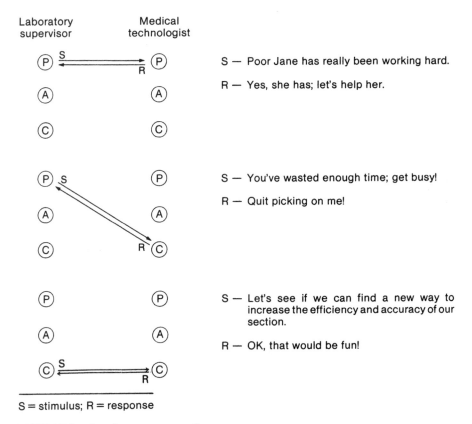

Laboratory supervisor / Medical technologist

S — Poor Jane has really been working hard.

R — Yes, she has; let's help her.

S — You've wasted enough time; get busy!

R — Quit picking on me!

S — Let's see if we can find a new way to increase the efficiency and accuracy of our section.

R — OK, that would be fun!

S = stimulus; R = response

FIGURE 7-5. Complementary transactions.

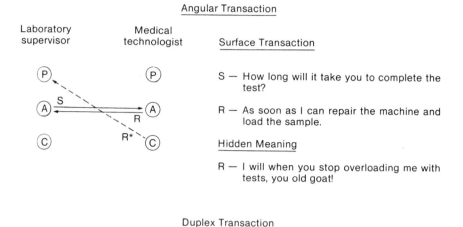

Angular Transaction

Surface Transaction

S — How long will it take you to complete the test?

R — As soon as I can repair the machine and load the sample.

Hidden Meaning

R — I will when you stop overloading me with tests, you old goat!

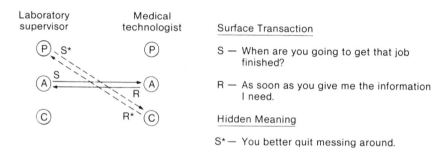

Duplex Transaction

Surface Transaction

S — When are you going to get that job finished?

R — As soon as you give me the information I need.

Hidden Meaning

S*— You better quit messing around.

R*— I will when you tell me what you want me to do, stupid!

FIGURE 7-6.   Ulterior transactions.

of crossed transactions is reduced. One method for eliminating crossed transactions would be for each individual to get in touch with each of his three ego states (Parent, Adult, Child) and respond to another individual's remark from the appropriate ego state. Another method would be for a person to become more or less locked into one ego state and respond from that frame of reference regardless of the stimulus behavior from another person.[36]

An *ulterior transaction* is generally more complicated than the two previous transactions because it involves more than two ego states and has a surface and a hidden meaning.[24] Such transactions can be angular (involving three ego states) or duplex (involving four ego states). In either case, multiple messages are communicated (Fig. 7-6).[26] Ulterior transactions tend to reduce effective communication and frequently weaken relationships between individuals. Because a person may not be aware of the mixed messages that he is

transmitting, this method of analysis should make him more likely to identify his own ulterior transactions. An important step toward eliminating ulterior transactions is to be able to recognize them when they occur.[26]

The premise of TA is that a supervisor of a clinical laboratory can eliminate or prevent many communication problems in his day-to-day relations with his subordinates if he learns to analyze his transactions. For example, if he learns to stay in the Adult, he is more likely to relate effectively to his subordinates than if he is locked into the Parent or Child response modes. TA is an important tool for clinical supervisors who want to improve interpersonal communication.

ORGANIZATIONAL COMMUNICATION SYSTEMS

Three formal types of communication are found in most organizations: downward, upward, and horizontal. An organizational chart (see Chapter 3), in addition to

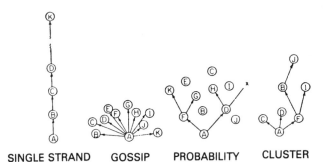

SINGLE STRAND   GOSSIP   PROBABILITY   CLUSTER

FIGURE 7-7. Grapevine methods of spreading information. (From Davis K: Management communication and the grapevine. Harvard Bus Rev 5:49, 1953)

showing lines of authority and accountability, is a diagram of an organization's formal communication network.

Downward Communication

This type of communication is probably the most frequently used channel in organizations.[24] It flows naturally from higher to lower levels of authority, and it has several basic purposes[21] (Box 7-1).

Downward communication also provides an opportunity for supervisors to spell out objectives, change attitudes, influence opinions, reduce fear and suspicion resulting from misinformation, prevent misunderstandings from lack of information, and help subordinates prepare for change.[24] However, that downward communication can be misused, especially if a supervisor does not allow for any significant feedback from his

subordinates. Just because a supervisor and a subordinate go through the *motions* of communicating with one another, this does not necessarily mean that they have actually communicated. Special efforts must be made on the part of a supervisor to make sure that instructions, orders, directions, and other types of downward communication are actually understood by subordinates.[20]

Upward Communication

The supervisor of any clinical laboratory facility who believes that downward communication is sufficient as an adequate channel for transmitting messages to subordinates will be in for a big disappointment. Most organizations provide, to some extent, for an upward flow of communication.[35] This is frequently called feedback.

Encouraging upward communication is not an easy matter, especially because it runs contrary to the usual higher-to-lower flow of authority found in most organizations.[20,24,32] Upward communication is important, however, and the supervisor of a clinical laboratory who encourages it will (1) obtain a better picture of the work, accomplishments, problems, plans, attitudes, concerns, and feelings of those in his unit; (2) be in a better position to identify individuals, policies, actions, or assignments that are likely to cause trouble; (3) strengthen the only device he has for tapping ideas and help from his staff; (4) receive better answers to his problems; and (5) help the flow and acceptance of his own downward communication simply because good listening makes good listeners.[24]

The research cited by Lewis clearly demonstrates that two-way communication (downward and upward) is more accurate for developing understanding than one-way communication (downward).[24] With two-way communication, the receiver has the chance to test the information being sent by the source, and the source can change the message immediately if necessary for the purpose of achieving a better understanding.

Box 7•1

Downward Communication: Basic Purposes

1. To provide specific task directives (job instructions)
2. To provide information designed to produce an understanding of the task and its relation to other organizational tasks (job rationale)
3. To provide information about organizational procedures and practices
4. To provide feedback to the subordinate about his performance
5. To provide information of an ideologic character to inculcate a sense of mission (indoctrination goals)

However, two-way communication requires more time than one-way communication, and it can cause the source to feel under attack in a psychological sense because the receiver can pick up mistakes or omissions and let the source know about them. Two-way communication can also be noisy and disorderly at times.

For the clinical supervisor who is interested primarily in speed, appearance, and the protection of his own seeming infallibility and power base, one-way communication is preferable, but the clinical supervisor who is interested in more accurate and valid communication will find that two-way communication can lead to more positive results.[24]

Horizontal Communication

Horizontal communication takes place between individuals who are at approximately the same level of authority in an organization.[20] It can be either formal or informal, depending on whether it is allowed for and shown on the organization chart.[24] The primary purpose of horizontal communication is to facilitate the solution of problems that arise from a division of labor and specialization.[20] The messages generally deal with task coordination, problem solving, information sharing, and conflict resolution.[14] For example, the supervisor of a special bacteriology unit and the supervisor of a general bacteriology unit in a certain clinical laboratory may find that the only way for a certain problem to be resolved is to have a closer coordination of the efforts of these two units.

One way to accomplish this coordination would be to use horizontal communication. Some problems could occur if only horizontal communication took place throughout an organization. The authority structure could possibly be abolished, and too many messages could flow in all directions without screening or filtering. As a result, a compromise between the rigidity of zero horizontal communication and the anarchy of total horizontal communication is generally supported by most supervisors.[24]

Informal Communication Systems

Upward, downward, and horizontal communication systems comprise only part of the total communication flow in any organization. Another important component to consider is the informal communication system.[11,20]

Informal communication systems exist in any formal organization, but they cannot be identified by looking at authority relationships on a formal organizational chart.[12] They result from the social interaction of employ-

ees. They do not have any official sanction, and at times they contain considerable scuttlebutt.[7] An informal communication system is frequently called the grapevine, because it moves back and forth across organizational lines (Fig. 7-7). It can be either beneficial or detrimental to an organization, depending to a great extent on the influence that a supervisor can exert on it.[20]

An informal communication system can be desirable because it provides insights into employee attitudes, it provides a safety valve for employee emotions, and it helps spread useful information. However, the dysfunctional aspects of such a system include its spreading of rumor and untruth, its nonresponsibleness, and its nonappearance on the organization chart, which contributes to uncontrollability. Two of its attributes that can work to either the good or detriment of an organization are its speed and influence.[24]

No supervisor in any laboratory facility should ever attempt to abolish such a system; it is a factor with which a supervisor must deal in the daily activities associated with managing his unit. The astute supervisor will attempt to understand it, analyze it, and consciously try to influence it.[12]

ORGANIZATIONAL AND INTERPERSONAL COMMUNICATION BARRIERS

If a clinical supervisor is to communicate successfully, he must learn what barriers or obstacles to effective communication stand in his way. Such barriers can be divided into organizational and interpersonal obstacles, although there obviously will be some overlapping.

Organizational Communication Barriers

Certain characteristics of any organization make communication especially difficult. Some of the more important ones are as follows[24]:

An organization is a system composed of overlapping and interdependent groups; as a result, if all things are somewhat equal, individuals will communicate more frequently with those who are geographically closest to them.

Subgroups within an organization demand and expect allegiance and loyalty from their members, and they have their own immediate goals and methods to achieve them. Thus, when a given message is communicated to several subgroups within an organization, each group may interpret a rather different meaning from the one that was transmitted.

Organizational groups represent different subcultures.

In a hospital setting, such subgroups as the clinical laboratory facility, the hospital administrative office, the emergency room, the nursing service unit, the radiology department, the dietary department, and the personnel department, establish and attempt to preserve their own value systems, idealized images, and traditions. Each group frequently develops its own jargon; for meaning to be transmitted between groups, then, each group must understand what the other group means when a certain word or phrase is used.

The members of an organization are composed of various systems of relationships (eg, work, authority, status, prestige, friendship). Each of these structures exerts an influence on the expectations that individuals have about who should communicate with whom and in what fashion.

In growing dynamic organizations, the relationships among members are in a constant state of change. Therefore, the problem for communicators frequently is to determine who is best to receive a particular message.

Interpersonal Communication Barriers

A basic problem in interpersonal communication is that the meaning that is actually received by an individual may not really be what the other individual intended to send. The source and the receiver are two separate individuals, and any number of barriers can distort the messages that pass between them. Examples of some of the more important interpersonal barriers are discussed below[31,32]:

1. A subordinate hears what he expects to hear. What a subordinate hears or understands when a supervisor talks to him is greatly influenced by the subordinate's own personal experience and background.
2. A subordinate frequently ignores information that conflicts with what he already knows or believes.
3. A subordinate evaluates the source. If a supervisor is perceived as trustworthy, friendly, and supportive, what is said is likely to be accepted and believed by the subordinate. Conversely, disliked or distrusted supervisors will find it difficult to communicate anything but the most banal facts to the subordinate. This represents an aspect of stereotyping.[9,18]

A subordinate who trusts a supervisor is more likely to accept the information that the supervisor provides than a subordinate who does not trust a supervisor. Trust building is important if the subordinate and the supervisor are to be able to participate in an open, honest fashion.

Research has confirmed that when there is trust between two parties, there tends to be a much lower level of misunderstanding between them. Perhaps this is so because there is less defensiveness and therefore better listening and better understanding. Perhaps it is so because to trust an individual, one must first know the other person, and when one knows and understands the other person, there is a greater tendency to empathize, if not move toward agreement. When the parties move toward agreement, communication naturally improves. Maybe there are fewer misunderstandings because when two people know each other, they can make their messages congruent with the other person's frame of reference.[9,18]

4. One dimension of stereotyping and evaluating a source is for a receiver to ignore "gray areas" and react in terms of "black or white," or right or wrong. For example, much of what is said by a supervisor who is distrusted by a subordinate will be ignored. Conversely, much of what is said by a supervisor who is trusted will be accepted as good and correct. This is called the halo effect. It occurs when a subordinate is not able to discriminate appropriately between the good and the bad that may be intermixed within a supervisor's comments.
5. In a strict sense, meaning cannot be conveyed from a source to a receiver; all that the source can do is convey words. However, the same words may suggest quite different meanings to different individuals. For example, it has been established that the word *run* has more than 800 different uses, the word *round* has more than 70 different uses, and the word *fast* can be just as confusing. In addition, the 500 most frequently used words have an average of 28 meanings per word.[24] This semantic problem is especially difficult when one is dealing with abstract terms, but even simple, concrete words and phrases can lead to communication problems. To a supervisor, "as soon as you can" may mean immediately; to a subordinate it may mean as soon as it can be done without delaying the subordinate's other work. Confusion can result even when words are selected with great care.
6. Emotions also play a role. When a subordinate is insecure, worried, or fearful, what he hears and sees will generally appear to be more threatening or distressing than when he is

secure. At the same time, when a subordinate is angry or depressed, he tends to reject what might otherwise appear to be a reasonable request or a good suggestion from his supervisor. Similarly, if the subordinate is in good spirits, he may not "hear" any problems or criticisms.

7. Subordinates learn to tune out many things. For example, certain statements that a supervisor makes may be ignored, actually never heard by the subordinate, because they sound so much like what the supervisor always says: "Work efficiently;" "keep busy;" "this test is stat;" "reduce costs." Thus, before a subordinate can hear a message, he must learn to discriminate between background noise (what is always being said by the supervisor) and what is significant and relevant new information worthy of attention.

Improving Organizational and Interpersonal Communication

Both organizational and interpersonal barriers can hinder and restrict the communication efforts of any clinical supervisor. Probably the most important step that such a supervisor can take to improve communica-

tion within his unit is simply to be aware of the complexity of the communication process. It cannot be taken for granted, and it must be performed as accurately as possible. An improvement in communication can be achieved through a greater knowledge of how the communication process functions. By being aware of and sensitive to how barriers can affect the process, the supervisor can take steps to minimize them.[20]

ORGANIZATIONAL COMMUNICATION: REQUISITIONS AND REPORTS

One of the most important organizational communications for the laboratory manager to analyze and improve is the test requisition–report cycle. Krieg illustrates this cycle as the meshing of two decision systems: (1) the attending physician making clinical decisions, and (2) the laboratory decision system by the technologist performing the specimen analysis (Fig. 7-8).[22] The potential for communication errors is great given the number of communication transactions.[15] Technology has reduced some communication errors (eg, bar coding and robotics have reduced some transcription errors and processing miscommunication[25] and computer requisitions with software designed to ensure appropriate use have improved the accuracy and diagnostic utility of requisitions).[34] In addition, it is possible to provide bet-

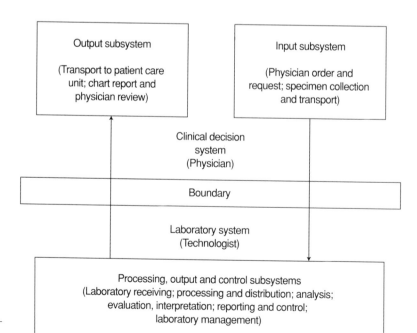

FIGURE 7-8. Physician–laboratory–physician communication loop.

ter communication from the laboratory back to the physician by improving the laboratory report.[27]

The College of American Pathologists inspection checklists (Box 7-2) pose the questions and guidance related to laboratory requisitions and reports.[8]

IMPROVING MANAGERIAL COMMUNICATION

Improving managerial communication depends on a number of skills. Some of the more basic skills include listening effectively, demonstrating empathy, monitoring feedback, and recognizing nonverbal cues.

Listening

Successful listening (like communication) is an active, dynamic process. If a clinical laboratory supervisor is to be an effective listener, he cannot be passive. He must actively attempt to grasp facts and feelings in terms of what he has heard, and he must be willing to help his subordinates work out any problems.[23,28] Alertness at every point of the communication encounter is a prerequisite for the supervisor and for the subordinate.[24]

Research indicates that most individuals listen at about 25% efficiency. In other words, an average person experiences a 75% loss of information over a short period of time because of poor listening skills. One of the primary reasons that listening-retention rates are so low is that the ability of the mind to think is four to six times as fast as the average person speaks (ie, 600–700 words per minute versus 125 words per minute). The receiver can easily tune in and out or divert his attention while the source is transmitting a message at a relatively slower speed. As a result, the receiver frequently indulges in a "skip-and-jump" listening pattern, pretending attention but giving way to distractions.[24] Because of this, most clinical supervisors will frequently face critical problems in terms of getting their messages through.

Some of the factors preventing the subordinate from being a good listener include the following:[13]

1. Faking attention when the topic is considered to be uninteresting (lack of interest)
2. Permitting diversion to take place because of emotional words or topics (evaluative or contrary attitudes)
3. Inefficient note taking (getting swamped with details)
4. Allowing environmental noise to continue (interruptions)
5. Listening only for facts and allowing the mind to wander (bad listening techniques)

There are, however, several things that a clinical supervisor can do to aid a subordinate's listening:[24]

1. He should tailor information on the basis of the subordinate's point of view.
2. He should phrase words and couch statements in language that is on the subordinate's level; however, he should not talk down to the subordinate.
3. He should transmit information, instructions, and directives in small units. Large amounts of data tend to be threatening, whereas small amounts of information are more likely to be accepted by the subordinate.
4. He should provide ample opportunity for feedback from the subordinate. In other words, he should find out what the subordinate has heard and what he has understood.

Listening is not something to be applied only when a supervisor is dealing with specific problems. It is a general attitude that a supervisor should apply when dealing with his subordinates. It is a matter of always being ready to listen to the subordinate's point of view and trying to take it into account before taking action.[32]

Skillful and effective listening is an art. It requires training and experience, and it can be learned through practice. Each supervisor must establish an approach that is comfortable for him and that is congruent with his personality, but it is recommended that he avoid using the same technique(s) with all subordinates and for all purposes.[32]

Regardless of what approach a supervisor does develop, however, the suggestions listed in Box 7-3 should prove useful.[13]

Listening can be contagious. If a laboratory supervisor wants his subordinates to listen to what he has to say, he must prove to them that he is an individual who consistently listens with understanding.[24]

Demonstrating Empathy

Empathy is sometimes defined as understanding, but it really goes beyond that. It includes understanding the feelings and the content of another individual's message. In a sense, empathy is seeing the world the way another individual sees the world or "getting inside the individual's skin and feeling the way that individual feels about something."[10]

A number of supervisors confuse empathy with sympathy. Sympathy goes beyond empathy and implies *agreeing* with what the other individual feels. Some supervisors are reluctant to develop the ability to empathize with a subordinate because they believe it implies that they are agreeing with the subordinate. Evidence suggests the contrary. Many people in a communication

(text continues on page 122.)

Box 7·2

College of American Pathologists' Inspection Checklists

REQUISITIONS AND SPECIMEN RECEIPT

☐ Is an appropriate specimen identification and accessioning system in use and consistently applied?
☐ Are specimens uniquely identified to minimize sample mixups, mislabeling, and so forth?
☐ Are there written criteria for the rejection of unacceptable specimens or the special handling of suboptimal specimens?
   Note: This question does not imply that all "unacceptable" specimens be discarded or not analyzed. If, for example, serum potassium is ordered and the blood sample is hemolyzed, there should be a mechanism to notify the requesting physician and to note the condition of the sample on the report.
☐ Is the disposition of all unacceptable specimens documented in the patient report or quality improvement records?
☐ Are all specimens accompanied by an adequate requisition?
☐ Does the requisition form include:
   Adequate patient identification information (at least name and location)?
   Note: A specimen code may be used for confidentiality if an alternative audit trail exists.
   Name and address (if different than the receiving laboratory) of physician or authorized person ordering the test?
   Note: This question refers to person(s) authorized by law to order tests or use medical information.
   Tests of assays requested?
   Time and date of specimen collection when appropriate?
☐ Is the time that the specimen was received by the laboratory recorded?
☐ Does the laboratory have a policy requiring oral requests for patient testing to be followed by an attempt to obtain written or electronic authorization within 30 days?

REPORTING OF RESULTS

   The laboratory must provide useful clinical data. Data must be legible, accurate, reported in clearly designated units of measurement, and reported to people authorized by law to receive and use medical information. Reference (normal) values should be indicated on the report.

Does the report form include:
☐ Name of patient?
☐ Patient identification number (hospital or laboratory)?
☐ When appropriate, name of ordering physician or physician of record?
   Note: In institutions where there are multiple ordering physicians or frequent changing of attending physicians, the ordering physician should be easily identifiable through a computer audit trail of other records of the test order.
☐ Date and time of specimen collection for appropriate specimen?
☐ Date and time of release of report (or if not on the report, are the date and time readily accessible when needed, as appropriate)?
☐ Reference (normal) values, for each reported test when possible?
   Note: Under some circumstances, it may be appropriate to distribute lists or tables of reference values to all users and sites where reports are received. This system is usually fraught with difficulties, but if in place and rigidly controlled, it is acceptable.
☐ Are results legible?
☐ Are copies or files of reported results retained by the laboratory in a manner that permits prompt retrieval of the information?

Box 7·2

(Continued)

Note: The length of time that reported data are retained in the laboratory may vary; however, the reported results should be retained for that period encompassing a high frequency of requests for the data. In all circumstances, a hospital laboratory must have access to the patient's chart when the information is permanently retained.

☐ Does the laboratory have procedures for immediate notification of a physician (or other clinical personnel responsible for patient care) when results of certain tests fall within established "alert" or "critical" ranges?

☐ Is there documentation of notification of the proper clinical individual of all critical values on any laboratory test?

☐ Except for special circumstances, are all referred specimens sent for analysis to laboratories accredited by the College of American Pathologists (CAP) or, in the case of hospital laboratories, to Joint Commission on Accreditation of Healthcare Organizations accredited laboratories?

Notes:

1. Special circumstances may allow exceptions to this requirement, (eg, for public health laboratories, such as a state health department laboratory or the Centers for Disease Control and Prevention).

2. "Referred specimens" include histopathology/cytology processing.

3. For *all* referral testing, the referring laboratory must verify that the reference laboratory is CLIA '88 certified for high-complexity testing in the specialty/subspecialty.

☐ Is the name and address of the laboratory that actually performed the procedure on the report, including referred specimens?

Note: The address of reference laboratories may be provided on the chartable report of the referring laboratory or available to the test requester in the referring laboratory's records. A reference laboratory includes any affiliated or special function laboratory that is separately accredited.

☐ For sample referred to another laboratory, is the original or an exact copy of the latter's report retained by the referring laboratory?

☐ Are referred test results reported by the referring laboratory as received from the reference laboratory?

☐ Is there a system whereby the identity of the analyst performing or completing the test and the date of the test can always be established?

☐ Has the laboratory defined turnaround times (ie, the interval between specimen receipt by laboratory personnel and results reporting) for each of its tests, and does it have a policy for notifying the requester when testing is delayed?

Note: This does *not* imply that all instances of delayed reporting for all tests must lead to formal notification of clinical personnel. Rather, clinicians and laboratory must have a jointly agreed on policy for when such notification is important for patient care.

☐ Are laboratory records and materials retained for an appropriate time?

Note: The following records must be retained for at least 2 years: specimen requisitions (including the patient chart or medical record only if used as the requisition), patient test results and reports, instrument printouts, accession records, quality control records, proficiency testing records, and quality improvement records. Instrument maintenance records must be retained for the life of the instrument. Serum and body fluid specimens should be retained for 24 hours. Blood films, permanently stained body fluid slides, and microbiology slides should be retained for 7 days. Any deficiencies noted by the inspector must be detailed in the summation report.

Source: College of American Pathologists: CAP Inspection Checklist, Laboratory General, pp 6–11. Northfield, IL, 1996

Box 7·3

Suggestions for Improved Listening

1. Stop talking; show that you can also listen.
2. Establish rapport with the subordinate. Put him at ease.
3. Indicate a willingness to listen to the subordinate. Look interested. Show empathy.
4. Eliminate distractions. Hold telephone calls, and select a quiet place to communicate. Do not engage in other activities.
5. Allow sufficient time for discussion. Listen patiently to the full message.
6. Keep your emotions under control. Do not get angry or lose your temper. Recognize and be sensitive to your emotional involvement in some topics, and try not to argue or criticize.
7. When you are not sure of part of the message, restate what you thought you heard in the form of a question. When you think that something is missing, ask questions.

situation are simply seeking understanding and do not necessarily demand agreement with their viewpoint. In fact, in many cases, a subordinate, once he has discovered that his supervisor really empathizes with (understands) his viewpoint, drops a difficult point or issue, or at least becomes less hostile and easier to deal with on that point or issue and on other matters.[10]

A clinical supervisor can show concern for a subordinate by standing in the subordinate's position, identifying with the subordinate's frame of reference, and helping to meet the subordinate's objectives. From this standpoint, empathy is an exceptionally strong component of effective communication.[2]

To empathize with a subordinate, a clinical supervisor should be able to answer a number of questions about the subordinate: [24]

1. What are his beliefs and values?
2. How does he see the world?
3. What disturbs and disrupts him?
4. Under what conditions will he accept or reject change?
5. Does he listen carefully and patiently to what is said, or is he more interested in who said it?
6. Does he weigh the evidence or simply go along with individuals he likes?

Answers to such questions cannot be obtained without the use of good interviewing skills, which are discussed more fully in Chapter 12.

Feedback

Any supervisor who does not provide for monitoring feedback from his subordinates will find his managerial and communication skills to be severely limited. If he does not encourage feedback from his subordinates, he may eventually become isolated or bypassed. A clinical supervisor who sincerely subscribes to the importance of feedback and wants to monitor it more carefully should find Table 7-1 especially valuable. What the table suggests is that certain cues, sent both from the subordinate and from within the supervisor himself, give the supervisor information concerning whether or not the subordinate and the supervisor understand each other.[29] These indicators represent danger signals, signs that the message may not be getting through. It is important for the supervisor to recognize these signals because they indicate that corrections are necessary.[29]

Nonverbal Communication

During the entire verbal communications process, the clinical supervisor and the subordinate communicate with each other in another way: nonverbally.[24,30] The nonverbal message a supervisor sends to a subordinate can cause the subordinate to tune out the supervisor, especially during the listening process. Beneficial or dangerous emotional environments can be created through nonverbal language, which can strengthen or destroy a subordinate's trust in a supervisor.[1]

A clinical supervisor must be able to recognize in a subordinate nonverbal cues, such as nervousness, confidence, anger, openness, rejection, or defensiveness. If the supervisor is not aware of these cues, he shows a lack of sensitivity to the subordinate's feelings. This can also lead to a reduction in trust.

Three of the more important areas of nonverbal communication are body language, voice intonations, and proxemics.[1] Body language is a significant component of nonverbal communication. It is important for a clinical supervisor to become aware of his own body projections and those of his subordinates. He can increase tension and decrease trust simply by projecting negative body language or by lacking sensitivity to a subordinate's body projection. Some of the major areas of interest in body language include the eyes, face, hands, arms, legs, body posture, and walk. These areas can be combined in different ways to indicate openness, evaluation, indifference, rejection, frustration, nervousness, or confidence.

Defensiveness, anger, or frustration on the part of a subordinate may be the direct result of a clinical supervisor's aggressive, dominant, or manipulative body lan-

Table 7-1
Sources of Feedback and Approaches to Monitoring It

Indicators*	Feedback From the Subordinate	Feedback From Within the Supervisor
Examples of feedback that indicate the subordinate does not understand the supervisor	Subordinate changes subject abruptly. Subordinate is apparently daydreaming or withdraws. Subordinate asks inappropriate follow-up questions. Facial expressions or posture showing discomfort Misinformation is shared with others Subordinate gives irrelevant answers, especially to probe questions. Subordinate shows signs of hostility.	Supervisor feels uncomfortable. Supervisor talks too much (excessively long statements). Supervisor repeats himself.
Examples of feedback that indicate the supervisor does not understand the subordinate	Subordinate's metamessage (words and voice or gestures) appears to be inconsistent with message. Subordinate's comments appear to be inconsistent with previous comments. Subordinate keeps repeating himself. Subordinate's voice or gestures show frustration (more intense or forceful). Subordinate begins to use a higher level of abstraction, more qualifiers, more pronouns.	Supervisor finds himself daydreaming. Supervisor interrupts repeatedly. Supervisor desires to argue or defend. Supervisor feels uncomfortable or confused.

* The indicators provided above are all examples of danger signals, indicators that the message may not be getting through. It is also possible to specify a set of indicators that the message *has* been received, but the danger signals are probably more important for the supervisor to recognize because they indicate that corrections are necessary.
(Adapted from Pyron HC: Communication and Negotiation for the Right of Way Professional, p 239. Culver City, International Right of Way Association, 1972)

guage. A deterioration of trust can result from such postures.

Additional meanings can be derived from changing voice intonations. Voice qualities generally account for the way a subordinate speaks his words. These include such factors as stress, resonance, speed, inflection, clarity, rhythm, and volume. Simple changes in such voice qualities can change the meaning of the same group of words. A lack of emotional sensitivity on the part of a clinical supervisor to voice tones can reduce trust between the supervisor and the subordinate.

One of the most important things for a supervisor to keep in mind when paying attention to the voice intonations of the subordinate is to concentrate primarily on changes in the subordinate's voice qualities. Some subordinates naturally talk fast, softly, or resonantly. When a subordinate changes his normal voice qualities, however, the subordinate is communicating something extra.

Another component of nonverbal communication is *proxemics*, the study of personal distance and territoriality. All individuals have various distances of interaction. For example, a supervisor can generally get physically closer to members of his family than he can get to subordinates in his unit. When he gets too close to

a subordinate, the subordinate will likely experience uneasiness and discomfort.

Research in proxemics indicates that there are four boundaries of interaction: the intimate (up to 2 ft), personal or casual (2–4 ft), social or consultative (4–12 ft), and public (12 ft or more).[17] During any interaction with a subordinate, a clinical supervisor probably would not want to work at all within the intimate space, nor initially within the personal space. The clinical supervisor can use proxemics to increase his trust with subordinates.

Knowledge about the entire area of nonverbal communication can increase the clinical supervisor's awareness of and proficiency in communication. The supervisor can become more sensitive to the subordinate's feelings, which can help considerably in building a trustful relationship.[1] Communication skills are critical tools that any clinical supervisor needs to interact with a subordinate in an open, honest, and constructive manner. These skills allow the supervisor and the subordinate to develop and maintain trustful relationships, and they enable the supervisor to determine whether he is communicating effectively with the subordinate and whether the subordinate is communicating successfully with the supervisor.

REFERENCES

1. Allesandra AJ, Davis JW, Wexler PS: Non-manipulative selling: Removing pressure and still getting the sale. California Real Estate 57:40, 1977
2. Berlo DK: Communicating Management's Point of View. A film from the Effective Communication Series. Rockville, MD, BNA Communications, 1965
3. Berlo DK: Meanings Are in People. A film from the Effective Communication Series. Rockville, MD, BNA Communications, 1965
4. Berne E: Games People Play: The Psychology of Human Relationships. New York, Grove Press, 1964
5. Berne E: Transactional Analysis in Psychotherapy: A Systematic Individual and Social Psychiatry. New York, Ballantine Books, 1961
6. Blubaugh JA: Advanced Communication Skills: Transactional Analysis for the Right of Way Professional (Workbook). Culver City, International Right of Way Association, 1978
7. Borman EG, Howell W, Nichols R: Interpersonal Communication in the Modern Organization. Englewood Cliffs, Prentice-Hall, 1969
8. CAP Inspection Checklists. Northfield, IL, College of American Pathologists, 1996
9. Communications in Right of Way Acquisition, Course 1, Student Reference Manual (old version), p 51. Culver City, International Right of Way Association, 1973
10. Communications in Right of Way Acquisition, Course 201, Student Reference Manual (new version), p 28. Culver City, International Right of Way Association, 1981
11. Davis K: Human Behavior at Work, pp 261–270. New York, McGraw-Hill, 1972
12. Davis K: Management communication of the grapevine. Harvard Business Review 5:43–49, 1953
13. Glueck WF: Management, pp 238, 249–250. Hinsdale, IL, Dryden Press, 1977
14. Goldhaber GM: Organizational Communication, p 40. Dubuque, William C Brown, 1974
15. Goslin LO, Turek-Brezina J, Powers M, et al: Privacy and security of personal information in a new health care system. JAMA 270(20):2487–2493, 1993
16. Grensing L: A three-stage formula to avoid miscommunicating. Clin Lab Management Rev 4:372–373, 1990
17. Hall ET: The Hidden Dimensions. Garden City, N.J., Doubleday, 1969
18. Hall J: Communication revisited. In Dupuy GM, Khambata DM, Ruth SR, et al (eds): The Enlightened Manager, pp 264–274. Lexington, MA, Ginn Custom Publishing, 1979
19. Harris TA: I'm OK—You're OK. New York, Harper & Row, 1967
20. Hicks HG, Arnold KK: Communication for supervisors. In New port MG (ed): Supervisory Management: Tools and Techniques, pp 157–170. St. Paul, West Publishing, 1976
21. Katz D, Kahn R: The Social Psychology of Organizations, p 239. New York, John Wiley and Sons, 1966
22. Krieg AF: Laboratory Communication, pp 3–24. Oradell, NJ, Medical Economics Co, 1978
23. Kumata H: Communication that gets results. Supervisory Management February:35 ff, 1966
24. Lewis PV: Organizational Communications: The Essence of Effective Management, pp 19–20, 38–41, 74, 91–120, 150–165. Columbus, OH, Grid, 1975
25. Maffetone MA, Watt SW, Whisler KE: Automated specimen handling bar codes and robotics. Lab Med 21: 426–443, 1990
26. Patton BR, Giffin K: Interpersonal Communication in Action, 2nd ed, pp 61–64. New York, Harper & Row, 1977
27. Payne N, Brigden M, Edora F: A redesign of RBC morphology reporting. MLO 28(4):60–64, 1996
28. Pearce CG: The managerial role in the speaker-listener exchange. Clin Lab Management Rev 6:308–313, 1992
29. Pyron HC: Communication and Negotiation for the Right of Way Professional, pp 237–239. Los Angeles, American Right of Way Association, 1972
30. Rosenfeld LB, Civikly JM: With Words Unspoken: The Nonverbal Experience. New York, Holt, Rinehart, & Winston, 1976
31. Strauss G, Sayles LR: Personnel: The Human Problems of Management, 2nd ed, pp 223–232. Englewood Cliffs, Prentice-Hall, 1967
32. Strauss G, Sayles, LR: Personnel: The Human Problems of Management, 4th ed, pp 162–170, 184–188, 266–271. Englewood Cliffs, Prentice-Hall, 1980
33. Thayer L: Communication and Communication Systems, p 23. Homewood, IL, Richard D Irwin, 1968
34. Winkel P, Statland BE: Using computers to TRAC, TRAP, TRIM. In Fitzgibbon RJ, Statland BE (eds): DRG Survival Manual for the Clinical Lab, pp 115–123.. Oradell, NJ, Medical Economics Books, 1985
35. Wofford JC, Gerloff EA, Cummins RC: Organizational Communication: The Keystone to Managerial Effectiveness, pp 25–32, 349. New York, McGraw-Hill, 1977
36. Woolams S, Brown M, Huige K: Transactional Analysis in Brief, p 17. Ann Arbor, Huron Valley Institute, 1974
37. Wright J: The communication Process: A Look at How Messages Are Sent, pp 13–19. Syracuse, Center for Instructional Development, Syracuse University, 1973

8

Leadership Styles and Group Effectiveness

John R. Snyder

The most comprehensive definition of management, perhaps, is that of the executives and academicians, which states that the process of management is the "guiding of human and physical resources into dynamic organization units that attain their objectives to the satisfaction of those served and with a high degree of morale and sense of attainment of the part of those rendering the service."[1] This directing function of guiding resources to achieve both organizational and personal goals is critically important. Guiding is often referred to as *leadership*. Leadership is a very complex activity. Many management authors and critics have defined leadership in different ways, several of which are offered throughout this chapter.

The relationship of the directing function to other managerial functions is embodied in the following definition of leadership:

Leadership is the ability to persuade others to seek defined objectives enthusiastically. It is the human factor which binds a group together and motivates it toward goals. Management activities such as planning, organizing, and decision-making are dormant cocoons until the leader triggers the power of motivation in people and guides them toward goals.[10]

Some authors have attempted to distinguish between the roles of managers and leaders.[7,22] In essence, all leaders are managers; not all managers are leaders, however.[12] Lombardi[40] has enhanced the definition of leadership by defining various roles that a leader plays in dealing with a changing work environment, such as health care today. Table 8-1 details these roles under four characteristics usually attributed to leaders versus managers: facilitator, encourager, enlightener, and activator.[40]

The general definition of leadership includes two key elements: the ability to motivate and the ability to focus efforts on goal accomplishment.[63] Managers have the authority to lead and direct, but they do not always have the power to influence and motivate.[35] This definition also includes a focus on the leader's or manager's ability to have the cooperation of staff workers to achieve organizational goals. Recall that one of the first steps in strategic management described in Chapter 3 is the definition of the laboratory's mission, goals, and objectives. The goals and plans for the laboratory need to be translated into departmental or divisional objectives if the laboratory is to achieve its mission. Likert referred to this critical leadership component as the "linking pin" function of the manager.[39] Figure 8-1 graphically displays the match between the creation of a mission statement, long-range goals, and strategic plans by top-level administration. These directives are mobilized by performance objectives at lower levels.[12,16,64] The laboratory manager plays a crucial role in linking his employees' efforts to where the organization and the laboratory are headed. In health-care institutions, like other multilevel organizations, goals and objectives are often formulated at the management team level (ie, in department head meetings). Too often these are not then shared with the staff who are ultimately responsible for implementation.

Within the clinical laboratory in the organizational context, there may exist two types of leaders: formal and informal. The formal leaders are those appointed to managerial positions of authority with responsibility for the laboratory analysis or functional tasks of those who report to them. Informal leaders may also be present, leaders whose influence is based on knowledge of the job, tenure with the laboratory, age, respect, or other characteristics. In some cases, conflict may arise when the two leaders in the same laboratory have different objectives for the same group of followers. Regardless of whether the functional leader is formally appointed or simply fills the role, still another definition of leadership sheds some light on this complex subject.[50]

Leadership is the process by which one person designates "what is to be done" and influences (in-

Table 8-1
Leadership Roles for the Change Process

Facilitator	Enlightener	Encourager	Activator
Communicator	Visionary	Listener	Planner
Advocate	Mentor	Perceiver	Arbitrator
Focal point	Counselor	Energizer	Orchestrator
Investigator	Developer	Rewarder	"Closer"
Voice of reason and validation	Role model	Legislator	Monitor
Sounding board	Presenter	Coach	Innovator

Source: Lombardi DN: The health-care manager's guide to managing change in challenging times. Clinical Laboratory Management Review 10:23, 1996

spires, commands) the efforts of others in order to accomplish specific purposes (objectives and work tasks).[50]

This definition contains four key elements: *acts, goals, influence,* and *acceptance.* Inherent in it is the fact that those who are to accomplish the task accept the leader's role and influence on them.

Early studies of leadership concentrated on the traits necessary to be an effective leader. Early hy-

potheses contended that a finite number of individual traits, whether intellectual, physical, emotional, or other personal characteristics, constituted effective leadership. Most of these physical, psychological, and sociologic traits were thought to be inherent and perhaps could be used to discriminate leaders from nonleaders. Many years of study have failed to pinpoint a single personality trait or set of qualities that was common to all leaders.[29] Rather, current philosophy suggests that

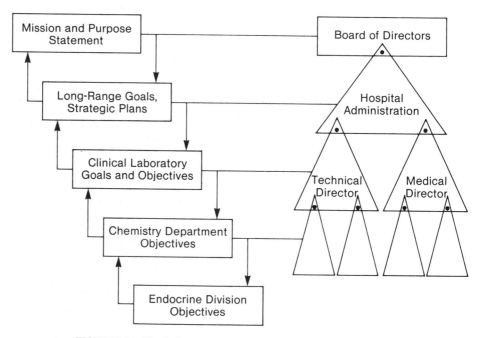

FIGURE 8-1. The "linking pin" function: involving employees in the goals and objectives of the laboratory.

leadership is a dynamic process in which there exists an interrelationship between the capabilities and inherent traits of the leader involved, the needs of the followers, and the characteristics and demands of the situation.[26,43] Schwartz has summed up the specific factors within these areas affecting leadership behavior as the size of the organization, the interaction and personalities of group members, the congruence of personal and organizational goals, and the level of decision making.[53]

The focus of this chapter is on leadership styles, the followers as a group to be effectively influenced, and situational variables. Because trait factors present at the time of birth are not the only determinants of effective leadership, a study of the various approaches to leadership with corresponding outcomes is appropriate.

MEASURES OF GROUP EFFECTIVENESS

Before considering leadership styles or leader behaviors, it is wise to identify the measuring tools that will indicate leadership effectiveness in dealing with followers. Gibson, Ivancevich, and Donnelly describe three measures of short-run organizational or leadership effectiveness, production, efficiency, and satisfaction, and two measures of intermediate or long-term effectiveness, adaptiveness and development.[20] *Production* reflects the ability to perform the quantity and quality of laboratory analyses required by the institution. This measure excludes efficiency, looking only at output items, such as test volumes and diversity of testing. *Efficiency* is defined as the ratio of outputs to inputs, focusing on the turnaround time for analyses, instrument downtime, technical staff unit production during a given block of time, and so forth. *Satisfaction* refers to the extent to which the laboratory is meeting the needs of its staff. A similar term, *morale*, reflects satisfaction as indicated by employee attitude surveys, absenteeism, turnover, and grievances. *Adaptiveness* is the ability of the laboratory section as a whole to respond to internal and external changes. There may exist a need to adapt practices or policies to alleviate problems associated with production, efficiency, or satisfaction. *Development* is a long-term measure of the ability to invest in the laboratory to enhance its operations. Examples of development measures taken to improve effectiveness include in-service programs, continuing education opportunities, and other growth-related activities. These measures of leadership effectiveness should be borne in mind by the reader during later discussions of leadership styles. Examples accompanying the styles should enable the reader to predict how these measures of leadership effectiveness would be influenced.

THE CLIMATE REFLECTING LEADER BEHAVIOR

Part of this complex issue of leadership is the joint function of the laboratory structure as an organization and its processes or procedures. This combination is termed the laboratory *climate*. The manager plays a key role in setting the working climate as defined (loosely or tightly) by the laboratory organizational structure and the usual mode of conducting the daily work.[20,30] The climate that the laboratory manager establishes, supports, or condones is, in turn, related to performance and job satisfaction. In a study of 300 scientists in 21 large research and development laboratories, Lawler, Hall, and Oldham report that process variables, rather than structural variables, have a greater impact on climate, and climate seems to have a greater effect on job satisfaction than on performance.[36]

Leader behavior analysis is the usual manner for studying leadership and group effectiveness. Three dimensions are fairly reliable indicators of the type of climate the leader is attempting to establish or foster: the degree of decision-making authority held by the manager, the manner of supervision, and the leader's interpersonal relationships.[50]

Degree of Decision-Making Authority Held by the Manager

The laboratory manager influences the climate by either involving subordinates in the decision process, soliciting their contributions before arriving at a decision, or totally excluding them. (The reader is referred to Chapter 4 for a discussion of the cost/benefit relationship in involving others in the decision-making or problem-solving process.) Because production was cited previously as one measure of group effectiveness, a study by Taylor[60] on the impact of management style, most noticeably "allowing input and participation in decisions," on staff productivity in 12 clinical laboratories is insightful. Although the study has some recognized shortcomings, including a nonrandom sample and absence of testing for factors other than management style that have an impact on productivity, Taylor did find a positive relationship. His study supports earlier research that found that productivity increases as the manager involves employees more in the decision-making process.

Manner of Supervision

This dimension of leader behavior refers to how closely a manager oversees the predetermined work of his subordinates. This includes not only monitoring the quality and quantity of work, but also specifically assigning tasks within the department. Some authors attempt to define this leader behavior further as "close" versus "distant" supervision or "direct" versus "indirect" supervision. Oversupervision can negatively affect the organizational climate; it is typified by the supervisor who "keeps pulling up the flowers to see how the roots are growing."[62] The technique of *management by exception* is based on the belief that staff can handle the majority of problems on their own (distant supervision). With this technique, the laboratory manager tells employees that two kinds of activities must be brought to his attention: (1) any unusual occurrence, special problem, or other event with which they cannot cope and (2) a defined list of specific deviations from the routine. In the first category, a technologist should perhaps alert the supervisor if calibration on a piece of instrumentation begins fluctuating more than is typical. In the latter instance, the supervisor may determine a list of abnormal results that should be called to his attention before being reported. In later discussions about leadership styles, an individual's supervisory climate is referred to as having differing emphasis on people or production concerns.

The Leader's Interpersonal Relationships

The climate of the clinical laboratory is definitely influenced by the nature of interpersonal relationships fostered by the manager between himself and subordinates. A manager may establish a "good buddy" personal relationship with each of his subordinates, or he may swing to the other extreme and have a totally nonpersonal relationship with his employees, treating them as he does the instruments and other assets of the department. Some laboratory managers foster a paternalistic relationship with their subordinates, referring to them as "my techs in the lab." The intent is usually one of protection and care for the subordinates in return for loyalty. The climate for each of these three interpersonal relationship examples would be different. A close personal relationship may foster erosion of authority, a strictly nonpersonal relationship may result in high turnover, and a paternalistic relationship prevents the development of self-reliance by group members.

These climatic influences are summarized in Table 8-2 as organizational variables and the characteristics that foster an organizational climate conducive to high productivity.[2]

The climate established by a leader's behavior has a major impact on the attitudes and sometimes the production of the laboratory. Much of the information related to communication and motivation in previous chapters and discussions about leadership styles later

Table 8-2
Factors Affecting Organizational Climate

Organizational Variables	That Require
Leadership processes	High confidence and trust
Motivational forces	Economic rewards based on compensation system developed through genuine participation
Communication processes	Free and valid flow of information at all levels
Interaction-influence processes	High degree of mutual confidence and trust
Decision making	Wide involvement in decision making and well integrated through linking processes
Control processes	Wide responsibility for review and control at all levels

Adapted from Argyris C: Management and Organizational Development, p 17. New York, McGraw-Hill, 1971; used with permission

in this chapter shed light on factors that influence the working climate and whether or not these promote good production by happy employees. Two past presidents of the United States spoke of leadership in such a manner as to incorporate the key element of climate. Eisenhower defined leadership as "the art of getting someone else to do something you want done because he wants to do it," while Theodore Roosevelt commented, "The best executive is the one who has sense enough to pick good men to do what he wants done, and self-restraint enough to keep from meddling with them while they do it."

THE LEADERSHIP ROLE OF MANAGERS AND SUPERVISORS

The clinical laboratory supervisor may be called on to assume a variety of leadership roles. In the following discussion, different viewpoints of the supervisor's role as postulated by Davis are linked to leadership functions.[11,61]

Often the supervisor is viewed as the key person in the laboratory because of his ability to facilitate or hinder significantly the production, morale, and flow of communications. As a key person, the supervisor serves as the hub of service in ensuring that laboratory tests are completed on time and the morale in the labo-

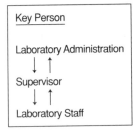

ratory is at an acceptable level. The key-person concept can be displayed graphically as follows:

Sometimes the supervisor belongs to neither the staff nor management, but rather is caught in the middle to interact with and reconcile opposing goals and objectives. The major function of this type of supervisory role is to identify and solve problems. This author, while still a fledgling supervisor, recalls the wise reminder of an early management mentor: "As a supervisor, you're not going to win any personality contests."

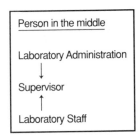

Some unfortunate supervisors are empowered only symbolically. Staff bypass them on their way to a higher level in the organizational hierarchy. The laboratory administration holds these supervisors responsible for the laboratory's performance but confines their authority. These supervisors appear powerless and ineffective as leaders, and the reason can be seen in the following diagram:

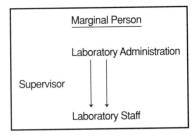

The legal status of most supervisors is that they are part of the administrative team. Often, the laboratory supervisor will be a "working supervisor," performing a mixture of both analytical and administrative responsibilities. With relation to their staff subordinates, these supervisors provide an initiating function of "thinking up" ideas, planning, and conceptualizing. An important concept about this role of the clinical laboratory manager is that as a supervisor of professionals, he serves as a leader among equals.

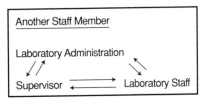

Some supervisors are expected to serve as staff specialists concerned with caring for the human side of the laboratory operation. The primary function of these supervisors as leaders is giving advice, information, or counsel.

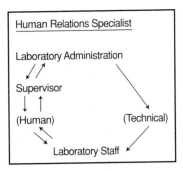

This discussion of the leadership role is not intended to categorize supervisors, but rather to show the differing perceptions with which a supervisor may be functionally considered. The supervisor has a unique position in the laboratory organizational hierarchy, synthesizing many parts of the roles described previously. He serves a key position in influencing productivity while being held accountable from above and below. While performing side by side with other technical professionals, he fills a leadership role that is best termed a leader among equals, responsible for maintaining the interpersonal relations and morale of the laboratory section. In summary, the laboratory manager's role is often supportive, similar to that advocated by Townsend: to carry water for the troops.[62]

Box 8•1

Bases of Power

Coercive power is based on fear. The supervisor who threatens to record negative incidents and place them in a subordinate's personnel file is exercising coercive power.

Reward power is based on the expectation of receiving tangible or intangible rewards. A laboratory supervisor might exercise reward power by offering to grant additional time off for volunteers who cover an emergency situation.

Expert power is based on special skills or knowledge. An assistant supervisor may influence the preventive maintenance practices of an entire department based on his special skills in trouble shooting certain instruments.

Referent power stems from a leader's ability to inspire by personality alone. This type of power is often referred to as charismatic power. An informal leader in the laboratory setting may move colleagues emotionally or psychologically through the use of referent power. For example, this leader may prompt an entire section to believe a particular policy is unfair by using persuasive personality skills.

Sanctioned power results from a leader's ability to negotiate and "trade off" favors. This is similar to reward power except that influence in sanctioned power can be exerted beyond the realm of one's duly authorized reward system. For example, a supervisor may influence the actions of other supervisors at a departmental meeting on the bases of premeeting negotiations to vote a particular direction on one item for a return-favor vote on another item.

Legitimate power is derived from an individual's position in the laboratory organizational structure. The supervisor, by designation, has legitimate power laboratory staff members. A supervisor may exercise legitimate power in assigning to cover the 3 PM to 11 PM shift every eighth week, for example.

Information power results from the control of some portion of the communication process or control of information itself. The laboratory administrator who refuses to disclose the percent salary increase to be granted on an annual merit review is exercising information power.

BASES OF POWER AND INFLUENCE

The ability to lead effectively implies acceptance by the followers of the leader's power. If one considers power in terms of who makes the decisions in a laboratory, the individual with power has the ability to limit alternatives of choice. In doing this, he has influenced the actions of those following.

The power to influence followers in the laboratory setting is not always a function of title or position, whether laboratory director, administrator, manager, or supervisor. Position-related power grants the manager only the authority to influence. Other personal and positional attributes provide the leader with a much stronger base of power. Bases of power are described in Box 8-1.[17]

The phenomenon of power plays a definite role in how effective a laboratory manager is perceived. Seldom, if ever, will the manager possess all forms of power just described. Recalling the managerial role as

Box 8•2

Trade-Off Areas: Using the Right Course

Quality of decision: What powers can be used effectively in arriving at the highest quality decision? Should expert power be used?

Acceptability of a decision: The use of which powers will prompt the most universal acceptance of a decision? Will legitimate power suffice?

Motivation of those over whom the manager has power: What effect on motivation will result from the use of certain types of power? Will coercive power be counterproductive?

Existing organizational relationships: What effect does the exercise of sanctioned power, for example, have on relationships now present in the laboratory?

Control of activities/responsibility: How might the supervisor's control of operations be affected by not totally exercising legitimate power in a particular situation?

Communication patterns: Will the use of information power, for example, adversely affect upward communication?

Need to maintain a position of power: Will the invitation to share leadership influence with others who possess different types of power threaten the manager's ability to exercise legitimate power at a later date?

a leader among equals, the astute laboratory manager will determine where the various types of power are held in the organization. The manager who relies solely on his legitimate power to influence subordinates will be a less effective leader than one who enlists the support of all staff members possessing power. For example, seeking the opinion of the staff member with expert power will increase the likelihood that the leader will be able to achieve group cooperation. Further, Reichman and Levy suggest that enlisting support decreases natural competitive tendencies and allows a compromise to achieve cooperation.[52]

Knudson, Woodworth, and Bell have described some of the trade-offs to be considered when a manager chooses not to exercise leadership influence through legitimate power.[33] The term *trade-offs* is not used here in a negative sense, but rather refers to those areas that may be affected when different power sources are allowed to exert influence. Trade-off areas are included in Box 8-2.

The ability to provide leadership that is effective in influencing group behavior often includes the application of some type of power. The laboratory manager needs to consider the cost/benefit result of exercising power personally or of inviting others with power to share in his leadership role. Regardless, the phenomenon of power is a real entity in the laboratory organization and deserves careful consideration.

FACTORS INFLUENCING LEADERSHIP STYLES

Historically, most laboratory managers have achieved administrative positions, whether first-line supervisory or directorship, without the benefit of advanced degrees in business or management. This does not imply, however, that these managers began without some form of leadership style. Earlier in this chapter, the concept of leadership based solely on intellectual, psychological, or sociologic traits was discounted. Undoubtedly, any reader can call to mind an example of someone he thought was an outstanding leader in the clinical laboratory or someone who was a particularly poor laboratory leader. A person's leadership style is defined through behaviors exhibited in the directing function that reflect assumptions and beliefs about the leader's position, his followers, and the salient components of the situation.[21] It may be informative at this point to investigate the influences that prompt the difference between an individual's effective (outstanding) or ineffective (poor) leadership style.

Leader-Influencing Factors

Much of what constitutes a leader's frame of reference from previous experiences influences his actions. This may include educational courses or seminars attended and the actions of past supervisors whom the individual perceived as outstanding leaders (role models). Past experiences also include the leadership methods a person has tried in the past after he has sorted out what was effective from what was ineffective.

There is little doubt that some personal traits influence a person's leadership style. His readiness to show fear or anger, for example, plays an influential role. His goals for himself, for his followers, and expectations of outcomes become a powerful influential force. How competent he feels as a manager influences his leadership behavior. This is supported by Mitchell, Larson, and Green, who report that leaders' perceptions of their own good behavior increases followers' ratings of leader behavior.[43]

In support of all the researchers who have attempted to isolate the trait or traits that comprise effective leadership, there does appear to exist an indefinable ingredient in leadership:

> There exists somewhere the gist of the manager, his soul, his philosophy of life, his basic approach to life and other human beings. This weightless component cannot be bought, sold, or built into an individual. If he *has* it, it can be nurtured and cultivated. If he doesn't have it, all the leadership training courses in the world can't make him a leader.[18]

Follower-Influencing Factors

The perceived characteristics of a group of subordinates influence a person's leadership style. The personality of the group may be perceived as openly receptive or adversely hostile, for example. Bias may be built into a leader's perception of his followers in such areas as the age of the personnel to be led. Contrast the belief that a group of subordinates is from the "old school," and therefore has to be told everything to do, with a "new school" philosophy, where the supervisor might want to ask everyone's opinion before making any decision. These types of assumptions influence an individual's leadership behavior.

Frequently, in the laboratory setting, a leader's behavior will shift with his perception of his subordinates' backgrounds and levels of development. The misconception exists that people who are less educated or are doing more routine tasks should be led differently from others with more education. For example, contrast the leadership style generally used with a group of phlebotomists or specimen preparation clerks with the leadership style used for a group of special chemistry technologists.

Situational-Influencing Factors

Undoubtedly the greatest number of factors influencing a leader's style has to do with his interpretation of the situation or problem.[28,30] The type of organization plays a substantial role: Supervisors lead differently if serving in a proprietary commercial laboratory than if working in a nonprofit hospital laboratory, government, or religious institution. The policies established within each of these differing environments limit or expand the leader's ability to influence the work climate. The size of the laboratory department will undoubtedly affect the leadership style as the manager attempts to deal with the span of control. Similarly, the nature of the communication process may cause the leader to be very close to his subordinates or very distant. Control, or lack thereof, of the departmental budget and the rewards system is often perceived as an influence dictating a leader's behavior with subordinates. Certainly the presence or absence of a union influences a leader's style. These concerns and others account for situational influences based on the characteristics of the institution that affect leadership style.[9]

Other situational factors as perceived by the supervisor regarding his position also influence the leader's style. A supervisor can only lead within the realm of his authority. It is possible to predict many laboratory supervisors' leadership styles on the basis of the pathologist's leadership style. It is unlikely that a supervisor will be very employee-concern oriented if his immediate supervisor is a pathologist whose interest is strictly in production. The supervisor's circle of influence would predict that these two styles would be in conflict. Finally, no discussion of situational factors would be complete without identifying time as a critical component that influences leadership style.

This is by no means an exhaustive list of factors that stimulate, detract from, or in some other fashion influence the basis for differing leadership behaviors. The factors identified are not all quantitative criteria. Lacerate verifies the fact that there is an important human angle in leadership styles to be considered.[38] This discussion is intended to prompt the reader to critical self-evaluation of the factors influencing his leadership style.

LEADERSHIP STYLES: THE LEADER DIMENSION

Theory X and Theory Y

Many behavioral scientists have attempted to study leadership behavior and its effects on subordinate productivity. Douglas McGregor's "Theory X–Theory Y" is perhaps one of the most well-known hypotheses.[42] According to McGregor, managers' assumptions about

human nature and human motivation influence their perception of the organization environment; this, in turn, prompts characteristic leader behavior. At one end of the spectrum are managers who focus on the aspects of superior–subordinate organizational structure with centralized decision making and strict external control. This leadership style is labeled *theory X*. The theory-X assumptions about employee behavior are summarized in Chapter 6, Table 6–1. Within the clinical laboratory, a theory-X manager assumes that most of his staff prefer to be directed, desiring as little responsibility as possible. In the theory-X manager's perception, staff members would rather have their supervisor exercise strict control in checking all results prior to reporting. The laboratory may be permeated by a feeling of fear, reflecting the leader's belief that staff members must be coerced to perform or intimidated into following the direction of the leader. Within the laboratory of the theory-X manager, all decisions for change are made in an authoritarian manner, seeking little or no input from staff members. As a rule, the theory-X manager also suffers from the lack of solicited information from staff members, because even crucial information that should be flowing up the organization is never communicated.

After concluding his description of theory X, McGregor questioned these assumptions of human nature in light of current levels of education and the democratic society in which we live. Drawing heavily on Maslow's hierarchy of needs (see Chapter 6), McGregor described an alternate theory of leadership called theory Y. The assumptions concerning human nature and motivation that characterize theory Y are listed in Table 6–1. A comparison of assumptions that underline theory-X and theory-Y leadership styles illuminates the two ends of the spectrum of manager behaviors as described by McGregor.

A laboratory that functions under theory-Y leadership most likely has all levels of laboratory professionals sharing responsibility for their activities. A subsection supervisor, for example, makes decisions regarding the selection and purchase of specific reagents for his area. Technologists share the responsibility with the supervisor for creating a holiday schedule and decreasing overtime in the laboratory. This reflects the assumption that the technical staff is creative and is willing to put these talents to use. Often the rewards system is directly linked with productivity and personal-growth goals. In this fashion, the theory-Y manager attempts to reward the full range of individual needs while recognizing that personnel can be properly motivated to accomplish organizational goals through the achievement of their own goals.

Lest one gain the impression from this discussion that theory X is "bad" and theory Y is "good," that simply is not the case. McGregor's definitions imply that most people under theory Y have the *potential* to be mature and self-motivated, given managers who are supportive, but a distinction must be drawn between attitude and behavior. Argyris recognized the difference between these two in his comparisons of A and B behavior patterns.[2,3] Theory-X assumptions are revealed in A-pattern interpersonal behavior and group dynamics. Theory-Y assumptions are reflected in B-pattern behavior. While it may be true that the best possible set of attitudes (assumptions) toward people may be theory Y, there may be some individuals who best function when the leader demonstrates type-A behavior. This, of course, will depend on the situation and the need to foster a more mature disposition of the employee.

Continuum of Leadership Behavior

McGregor has been widely criticized for the creation of a dichotomous, either-or situation. However, his work points toward two opposing poles in a continuum of leadership behavior.

Tannenbaum and Schmidt have defined the continuum by contrasting the use of authority by the leader of a group with the amount of freedom allowed the group regarding decision making (Fig. 8-2).[59] At one end of the continuum, the leader makes decisions without input from the group; at the other end of the contin-

uum, the problem is focused by the leader, but the followers play a major role in investigating alternatives and proposing solutions. The shift from autocratic leadership behavior at one extreme (theory X) is gradual as a leader changes behavior toward a more democratic approach (theory Y) at the other extreme (Box 8-3).

This continuum is often extended beyond the democratic pole to include a *laissez-faire* style. This style is one of abdication, the absence of formal leadership characterized by the lack of procedures and policies, with subordinates influenced only by informal leaders.

A well-known measurement tool to assess leadership patterns along this continuum was developed by Likert.[38] The four categories listed in Box 8-4 reflect characteristics of highest- and lowest-producing departments.

Likert's research supports the fact that a democratic leadership style, while not always being the most efficient, fosters higher productivity.[39]

Initiating Structure and Consideration—the Ohio State Studies

The Bureau of Business Research at Ohio State University, in attempting to identify various dimensions of leader behavior, considered two dimensions: initiating

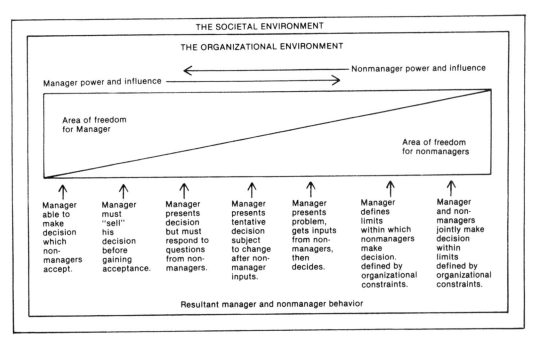

FIGURE 8-2. Continuum of leadership behavior. (Adapted from Tannenbaum R, Schmidt WH: How to choose a leadership pattern. Harvard Business Review 51:166, 1973; used with permission of the publisher)

Leadership Behavior Styles

Autocratic: The manager makes decisions alone.

Persuasive: The manager solely makes decisions, then attempts to influence followers by selling his idea, gathering support for his idea, and stirring enthusiasm among subordinates.

Consultative: The manager confers with subordinates to gather information, then makes the decision himself.

Democratic: The manager solicits not only information from subordinates, but also requests their involvement in the generation of alternatives and selection of a decision.

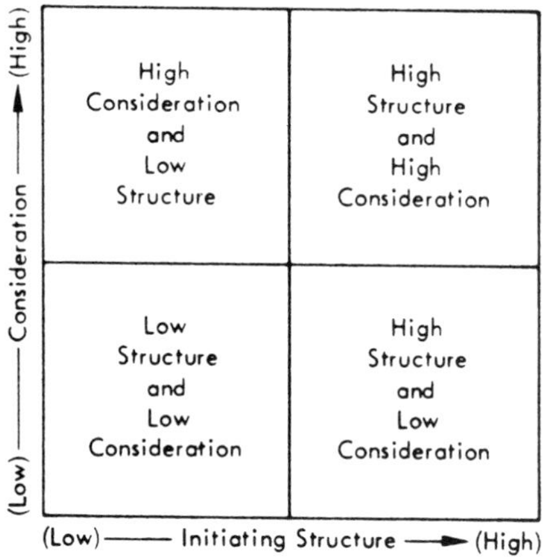

FIGURE 8-3. The Ohio State leadership quadrants. (From Stogdill RM, Coons AE [eds]: Leader Behavior: Its Description and Measurement. Research Monograph No. 88. Columbus, OH, Bureau of Business Research, The Ohio State University, 1975)

structure and consideration.[58] *Initiating structure* refers to "the leader's behavior in delineating the relationship between himself and members of the work group and in endeavoring to establish well-defined patterns of organization, channels of communication, and methods of procedures." *Consideration* refers to "behavior indicative of friendship, mutual trust, respect, and warmth in the relationship between the leader and members of his staff."[23] Two data-gathering devices, the Leader Behavior Description Questionnaire (LDBQ) and the leader Opinion Questionnaire (LOQ) were used to substantiate that these were, in fact, separate and distinct dimensions.

In assessing results from the LBDQ and LOQ, leader behavior was plotted on two axes, one for each dimension (Fig. 8-3). It was noted that a high score in one dimension did not preclude a high score in the other dimension. Laboratory managers exhibiting high consideration (relationship behavior) are leaders who are friendly toward their subordinates, who encourage a sharing of subordinates' concerns, who are willing to listen, and who are receptive to change. A laboratory manager characterized by high initiating structure (task behavior) is intent on making specific assignments with detailed guidelines telling subordinates exactly what is expected of them.

Blake and Mouton's Managerial Grid

While the Ohio State conceptual model examines leader behaviors predominantly perceived by others, Blake and Mouton's managerial grid measures the predispositions of managers in terms of (1) concern for people and (2) concern for production.[5] Although similarities in the two models exist in terms of relationship emphasis and task emphasis, the managerial grid stresses that this is an unnecessary dichotomy.[4] Rather than being mutually exclusive, Blake and Mouton contend that people and production concerns are complementary and must be integrated to achieve effective leadership.[4]

The managerial grid (Fig. 8-4) theoretically contains 81 possible positions or leadership styles. For discussion purposes, the focus usually centers around five basic styles (Box 8-5).

Blake and Mouton have used the concepts embod-

Effect of Leadership Styles on Productivity

1. Exploitative–Autocratic—typified by low trust, no participation
2. Benevolent–Autocratic—typified by condescension and token participation
3. Participative—typified by substantial trust and participation but with control and decision making retained by the leader
4. Democratic—typified by complete confidence and democratic decision making

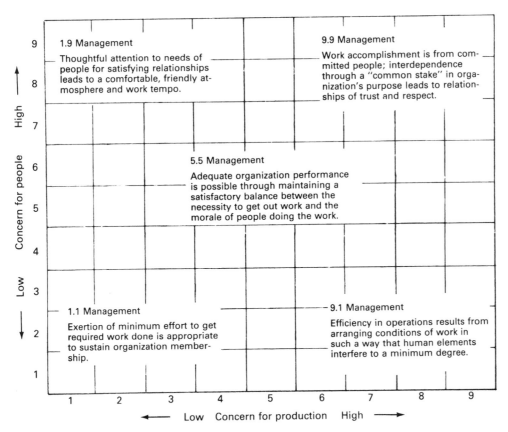

FIGURE 8-4.   The managerial grid. (From Blake RR, Mouton JS: The Managerial Grid, p 10. Houston, Gulf Publishing Company, 1964)

ied in the managerial grid extensively for organization and management development. A recent publication highlights the value of the grid concept after 20 years of experience with it by the authors.[6] They report that specific conditions in a manager's childhood experiences prompt his inclination to a given grid orientation. The advocated 9,9 team leadership is supported as the best possible orientation in terms of profitability, career success, and personal health. The publication outlines grid orientations that are correlated with heart attacks, asthma, ulcers, and cancer, among other diseases.

LINKING LEADERSHIP STYLE TO FOLLOWERSHIP

We have defined some dimensions of effectiveness and contrasted several leadership styles. A logical question arises: Is there a most effective leadership style? Leavitt provides the following answer:[37]

There is no such thing as the right way for a manager to operate or behave. There are only ways that are appropriate for specific tasks of specific enterprises under specific conditions, faced by managers of specific temperaments and styles.

The most effective leadership styles for a laboratory manager must include consideration of the leader's ability, the followers' motivations and characteristics, and the dimensions of the situation.[27,54,55] While the 9,9 team approach may seem the best possible for all situations, it is often difficult to sustain the team effort over time. The team approach is certainly preferred if the situation is one in which everyone has a stake in the outcome, such as the generation of policies and goals or overall evaluation of a laboratory section.

The 1,9 country club quadrant of leadership style is appropriate and, in fact, most effective when dealing with a situation in which motivation is based on personal interaction. External activities related to labora-

Box 8·5

Leadership Styles From Blake and Mouton's Managerial Grid

1. *1,1 Impoverished.* A laboratory manager with this leadership style has probably abdicated many of his responsibilities, encouraging subordinates "not to make waves" but to do the minimum to keep the laboratory going.
2. *1,9 Country club.* This leadership style would be reflected in the manager's inclination toward keeping the laboratory staff happy. Scheduled breaks are never violated, and frequent social gatherings take priority over laboratory productivity.
3. *9,1 Task.* The major emphasis by a laboratory manager with this orientation is one of work before all else. Development of a department with high productivity and efficiency is reflected in the manager's attitude that everyone is there, being paid, to work.
4. *Middle of the road.* This leadership style incorporates both a concern for the volume and efficiency of laboratory testing and concern for the morale of the department.
5. *Team.* A laboratory manager with this leadership style attempts to integrate laboratory and personal goals within the department. This manager enlists the participation of the staff in decision making and is a coach for the testing function (productivity) of the laboratory.

tory public relations, for example, often are not directly tied to the organization's reward systems. Consider the leading of a group of staff members in designing and implementing a weekend career day for high school students interested in becoming medical technologists. The most effective leadership style recognizes that the feeling of making a contribution toward the future of the profession is an intrinsic motivation. A leadership style emphasizing people concerns is the best approach.

Similarly, a 9,1 task orientation is appropriate and effective when deadlines are pressing. A laboratory manager may be faced with an emergency surrounded by chaos, for example. In this case, a leadership style reflective of an orientation toward work and immediate problem resolution is most effective. In addition to situations in which time is crucial, critical, or short, a task orientation is often appropriate for assigning very simple tasks.

Even the 1,1 impoverished leadership style may be appropriate for some situations. Consider a situation in which subordinates need to exercise flexibility and creativity, such as in certain types of problem resolution or research.[21] The wise manager will be there for support or assistance but does not attempt to influence the group's productivity. Often this leadership style may be appropriate for the administrative technologist when his subordinates (supervisors) are attempting to resolve problems within their sections. During his days as a newly appointed supervisor, this author recalls the leadership style exercised by his superior, the chief technologist: "You make the decision and I'll stand behind you, but you'd better be ready to come explain your rationale to me."

In real-life situations, it is often quite difficult to choose the most effective leadership style. Maintaining an optimum balance between concern for people and concern for production is at best a herculean task. An example follows in Box 8-6.

Participative Leadership

Many management authors support the 9,9 team approach to leadership as the ultimate style for which a manager should strive. The term participative leadership reflects the equally high emphasis placed on both production concerns and people concerns.

Many investigators have attempted to substantiate the value and acceptance of participative leadership.[41] Murnighan and Leung report that individuals led by a more-involved leader produce more than those led by a less-involved superior.[44] Cherrington and Cherrington contend that a participative leadership style for decision making yields higher efficiency and productivity.[8] Viola supports the participative leadership approach as fostering motivation among subordinates.[64] Still other advantages to the participative leadership style include the following:[47]

Subordinates have a closer identity with the organization.
There is less resistance to change.
Personal growth and development of subordinates are encouraged.
A wider range of experiences and ideas is solicited.[48]

However, implementing participative management in the laboratory is dependent on factors other than just the manager's desire to involve employees more in decision making. Snyder and Manuselis[56] studied the leadership and situational factors of 48 labora-

Box 8·6

Case Scenario: Leadership Dilemma

THE LEADERSHIP DILEMMA

I know a man who is a boss—not a big boss and not a very bossy boss. He does have a title on his door (Administrative Director of Laboratories) and plush carpet on his floor, and he takes his job very seriously and personally, which, of course, is his problem.

You see, when this administrator took courses in graduate school, he was taught that management was a question of profits and losses. Now he spends a great deal of time worrying about the cost-accounting of personnel problems—personal personnel problems.

Moreover, he says, it is going around. He keeps reading articles about "corporate irresponsibility" toward private lives. He hears how often an individual's work plays the heavy role in family crisis, but from where he's sitting...in a corner office looking down on the rest of the medical center...he sees something else.

He sees employees who want to be treated strictly professionally one moment and then treated personally the next. He sees the conflicts faced by his employees, but also the conflicts of being a boss. He is often in a no-win situation.

The administrator had three stories to tell me. The first was about his secretary. Last month when he interviewed her, he was warned by the personnel office to keep the questions strictly professional. On pain of lawsuit, he could not quiz her on her marital status or child care, so he stuck to the facts, just the facts—steno, typing, and work experience. Then, after hiring her, when one of her children got sick, he was expected to understand why she had to be home. He saw the situation this way: one month he wasn't allowed to ask if she had children; the next month he was supposed to care that they were sick.

Then there was the supervisor he wanted to promote. The technologist was clearly ambitious and good. The administrator had judged her on the basis of her work and management potential. He had groomed her and watched her. He had sent her away to attend management seminars, talked with her about taking on a higher level management position when one became available. Then he'd handed her the big promotion to Chief Technologist of the Stat laboratory, but the supervisor asked to be excused. She didn't want to make this change, because she just couldn't accept the responsibility for weekend and evening coverage. However, said the administrator, the supervisor had never described herself as inflexible on account of teenage children with extracurricular activities. Now, the administrator was to make allowances.

The third story was somewhat ironic, because it happened at the laboratory administration level itself. The administrative assistant in charge of personnel was a man who conducted the most careful, scientific, professional human resources program the administrator had ever seen. He screened people in and out of the laboratory, up and down the hierarchy, on the basis of multiple questions.

Now this man had just gotten custody of two small children. He had come in to ask for flexible hours. Under the circumstances, he wanted to know whether he could make some special arrangement that would help his personal life.

This particular administrator is not a Simon Legree, nor is he the sort of man who treats people like interchangeable plastic parts, so he adjusted to his secretary. He adjusted to his supervisor. He adjusted to the administrative assistant. He did it because a happy employee is probably a productive employee and all that.

He did it because a person's private life is a factor in his professional life and all that. He did it because he believed that a laboratory should be more flexible, to a point, but he feels a certain frustration. People want him to treat them professionally when it is to their advantage and personally when it is to their advantage. While he understands the family–work conflict, he also understands the conflict that comes with the title "boss."

Every day this administrator had to decide at what point the best interests of his employees conflict with the best interests of his laboratory. Where is it written, he asks, that institutions increasingly have to deal with personal personnel problems and issues? How do you balance the needs of the institution and the needs of the workers?

Sometimes this man is afraid that he's running a family agency instead of a medical center department. Other times he's afraid he's being a heel. The boss does not expect any sympathy. People don't sympathize with the boss anyway, he says, because it is hard to sympathize with someone who has the power to hire and fire you. He understands that, but the fact is that he's responsible for 150 lives and one departmental balance sheet. He takes both of these jobs very personally.

The dilemma is not resolved. The scenario is included here to heighten the awareness of the reader regarding the complexity of the leadership issue.

tory managers affecting participative management. They found that a manager's perceived leadership role, his leadership style, the number of employees for whom he was responsible (span of control), and the size of the institution (situation) contributed most to a participative management climate.

Participative leadership is a natural style for managers whose assumptions parallel theory-Y beliefs. Theory Y supports the concept that creativity is widely dispersed among subordinates, and participative leadership calls for input from staff members when making a decision or solving a problem.

Individual Temperaments

The group problem-solving technique just described highlights the value of many perspectives contributing to decision making. In the clinical laboratory, individual differences in terms of temperament (personality) can be either very useful or a sizable problem. To maximize the talent of individuals with different temperaments and minimize the disruption of conflicting temperaments, it is helpful for the laboratory manager to understand his superiors', peers', and employees' natural personality traits.[57]

Some managers would dismiss the value of learning about or even trying to accommodate differences in personality. Some laboratory managers would protest on the grounds that accommodation of personal temperaments diminishes treating everyone equally, while others expect that "professional behavior should equalize the differences that are natural in everyone as an individual." This brief discussion is intended only to introduce the foundation premises in temperament typology and provide enough examples of how this information is helpful to stimulate the reader's further study.[31]

The basis for most temperament assessment tools and personality classifications is Carl Jung's *psychological types*.[46] Jung's theory of psychological type included three pairs of opposing attitudes or functions: (1) attitude toward life; (2) perception or method of taking in information; and (3) use of judgment to reach a conclusion. Isabel Briggs Myers, author and proponent of the widely used Myers-Briggs Type Indicator assessment tool, added a fourth dimension, "orientation toward life."[45] Each of these continua is graphically displayed in Figure 8-5 with select characteristics of each type. While everyone uses both "ends" of the continua—for example, both sensing and intuition sources—to become aware of things, a natural preference for one kind of perception and one kind of judgment prompts individuals to use and develop more skills with one "set" of processes.

Extroversion/Introversion

Everyone falls somewhere along the continuum between fully extroverted and fully introverted. In general, the extrovert's interest flows mainly to the outer world of actions, objects, and people. By contrast, introverts focus more on the inner world of concepts and ideas. Research has documented that clinical laboratorians are predominantly introverts, a finding consistent with their characteristics, noted in Figure 8-5. The astute laboratory manager will note that while the extrovert technologist may not seem to "fit" the norm of the group, he has other gifts that make him valuable. The extrovert is the technologist of choice to plan the holiday season party, tour a group of high school students through the laboratory, and arrange a schedule of speakers for inservices. The extrovert will probably not do as well with a long, tedious technical procedure that requires maximum concentration.

Sensing/Intuition

The perception continuum contrasts two distinct ways an individual becomes aware of something. Those who prefer to perceive the immediate, real practical facts of experience and life are sensing types. Intuitive types prefer to perceive the possibilities, relationships, and meanings of experiences. Again, individuals use both methods of perceiving but are better at one and depend on it more. The sensing person really smells the coffee, sees the writing on the wall, and hears the music. The intuitive grasps for "the big picture" and relies on hunches and insight. A review of the characteristics of these two types (see Fig. 8-5) shows some noteworthy strengths of each—the sensing type will most closely follow the procedure manual when doing a laboratory analysis, whereas the intuitive type will be happy to learn how to use a new piece of equipment; for example—and some drawbacks of each—sensing types prefer not to take a research procedure and adopt it for use in the routine laboratory, whereas intuitives may make decisions on a "gut feeling" that is incorrect.

Because of the different preferences for perceiving information, intuitives need sensing types and vice versa. When putting together a committee to work on a problem or oversee the development of a new policy, the laboratory manager can capitalize on the gifts both types would add. For example, intuitives need sensing types to bring up pertinent facts, read the fine print in a union contract, and notice what needs attention most urgently. Sensing types need intuitives to bring up new

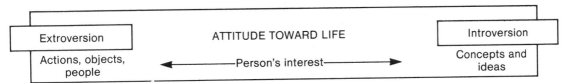

ATTITUDE TOWARD LIFE

Extroversion	Introversion
Actions, objects, people	Concepts and ideas

←————Person's interest————→

Extroverts:

Like variety and action.

Tend to be faster; dislike complicated procedures.

Are often good at greeting people.

Are interested in the results of their job, in getting it done, and in how other people do it.

Often don't mind the interruption of answering the telephone.

Often act quickly, sometimes without thinking.

Like to have people around.

Usually communicate freely.

Introverts:

Like quiet for concentration.

Tend to be careful with details; dislike sweeping statements.

Have trouble remembering names and faces.

Tend not to mind working on one project for a long time without interruption.

Are interested in the idea behind their job.

Dislike telephone intrusions and interruptions.

Like to think a lot before they act, sometimes without acting.

Work contentedly alone.

Have some problems communicating.

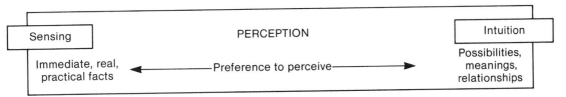

PERCEPTION

Sensing	Intuition
Immediate, real, practical facts	Possibilities, meanings, relationships

←————Preference to perceive————→

Sensing Types:

Dislike new problems unless there are standard ways to solve them.

Like an established way of doing things.

Enjoy using skills already learned more than learning new ones.

Work more steadily, with realistic idea of how long it will take.

Usually reach a conclusion step by step.

Are patient with routine details.

Are impatient when details get complicated.

Don't often get inspired, and rarely trust the inspiration when they do.

Seldom make errors of fact.

Tend to be good at precise work.

Intuitive Types:

Like solving new problems.

Dislike doing the same thing over and over again.

Enjoy learning a new skill more than using it.

Work in bursts of energy powered by enthusiasm, with slack periods in between.

Put two and two together quickly.

Are impatient with routine details.

Are patient with complicated situations.

Follow their inspirations, good or bad.

Often get their facts a bit wrong.

Dislike taking time for precision.

(continued)

(Part A)

FIGURE 8-5. Temperament dimensions and select characteristics. (Adapted from Myers IB: Type and Teamwork. Gainesville, FL, Center for Applications of Psychological Type, 1974)

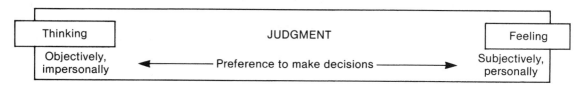

Thinking Types:

Are relatively unemotional and un-
interested in people's feelings.

May hurt people's feelings without
knowing it.

Like analysis and putting things
into logical order. Can get along
without harmony.

Tend to decide impersonally, sometimes ignoring people's wishes.

Need to be treated fairly.

Are able to reprimand people or fire
them when necessary.

Tend to relate well only to other
thinking types.

May seem hard-hearted.

Feeling Types:

Tend to be very aware of other
people and their feelings.

Enjoy pleasing people, even in
unimportant things.

Like harmony. Efficiency may be
badly disturbed by office feuds.

Often let decisions be influenced
by their own or other people's
likes and wishes.

Need occasional praise.

Dislike telling people unpleasant
things.

Relate well to most people.

Tend to be sympathetic.

Judgment	ORIENTATION TOWARD LIFE	Perception
Decisive, planned, orderly	←———— Preference to life ————→	Spontaneous adaptable, flexible

Judging Types:

Best when they can plan their work
and follow the plan.

Like to get things settled and
wrapped up.

May decide things too quickly.

May dislike to interrupt the project
they are on for a more urgent one.

May not notice new things that need
to be done.

Want only the essentials needed to
get on with a job.

Tend to be satisfied once they reach
a judgment on a thing, situation
or person.

Perceptive Types:

Tend to be good at adapting to
changing situations.

Don't mind leaving things open for
alterations.

May have trouble making decisions.

May start too many projects and have
difficulty in finishing them.

Want to know all about a new job.

May postpone unpleasant jobs.

Tend to be curious and welcome new
light on a thing, situation, or
person.

(Part B)

FIGURE 8-5. *(continued)*

possibilities, see how to prepare for the future, and supply ingenuity on problems.

Thinking/Feeling

This continuum, judgment, is the process of coming to a conclusion about something. The thinking individual prefers to make judgments or decisions objectively and impersonally by considering causes of events and where decisions may lead. By contrast, feeling types arrive at conclusions more subjectively and personally, weighing values of choices and how they matter to others. For the clinical laboratorian, the thinking end of the continuum is an expected and even learned approach based on the scientific method for work. This obviously is not always the stronger of the two approaches when dealing with interpersonal relationships as a peer or supervisor. Thinking types are analytical and logical and do not show emotion readily, characteristics that help them do some tasks like disciplining or terminating an employee and hinder them when faced with an employee or colleague who is upset. The feeling individual, in reaching conclusions based on a set of values and standards that take into consideration what matters to himself and others, is more people oriented and tends to be more sympathetic. When faced with interpersonal conflict, the feeling type will be the better listener but will have difficulty taking corrective action by talking to the person at fault in the conflict.

The laboratory manager should consider the strengths of both thinking and feeling types when planning a group activity because the two types are mutually useful. Feeling types need thinkers to hold consistently to a policy, stand firm against opposition, and reform what needs reforming. Thinkers need feeling types to persuade and conciliate, forecast how others will feel, and arouse enthusiasm.

Judgment/Perception

Opposite ends of the continuum for an individual's approach to life include the judging types, who prefer an orderly, planned, and controlled life, and the perceptive types, who tend to be flexible, adaptable, and spontaneous. Once again, both types have strengths and weaknesses. The judging types will see a project through to completion and be satisfied when a matter is settled, and perceptive types adapt well to changing situations and welcome new insights on a situation. However, judging types may reach a decision too quickly or not notice new things that need to be done, and perceptive types may start too many projects and postpone unpleasant jobs.

Readers should have, with this brief introduction, an appreciation of the natural differences in their supervisor, peers, and subordinates. The clinical laboratory work force is composed of "different drums and different drummers." With all the richness of the human personality, no two people are totally alike—a fact that makes individual differences best thought of as "gifts," or individual contributions. Clearly identifiable common threads are woven through each of us, however, and a knowledge of them can be useful in understanding how human behavior affects the accomplishment of work in the clinical laboratory. This knowledge is not to be used for stereotyping individuals on the basis of a few characteristics; rather, the types described here should be viewed as a template. Kindler notes that when managers handle differences well, they can identify underlying concerns, stimulate creative effort, reduce antagonistic feelings, correct misunderstandings, and guide commitment to needed change.[32]

LEADERSHIP AND THE SITUATION

Beyond the investigation of various leadership styles resulting from individual differences and the needs of the followers is the consideration of how the *situation* affects leadership effectiveness. Fleishman concluded that no single leadership style is most effective; rather, leadership effectiveness depends on the integration between task, power, personality, attitudes, and perceptions.[15] Tannenbaum and Schmidt, whose leadership continuum was considered previously, maintain that the successful manager is one who consistently and accurately assesses the situational forces determining the most appropriate leadership behavior.[59]

Research on leadership effectiveness in the late 1960s and early 1970s began to focus more on the effect of situational variance on leadership behavior, rather than on "situational determinants."[34]

Situational Leadership Theory and the Tridimensional Model

Hersey and Blanchard have added to the typical four quadrants of the Ohio model two additional situational dimensions. Figure 8-6 contains both a maturity of followers continuum and an effectiveness dimension, represented by the shaded, three-dimensional appearance.[26]

The maturity factor is part of Hersey and Blanchard's life-cycle theory. Maturity is considered in relation to a specific task to perform, rather than implying that an individual is mature or immature at all times. For example, a technologist may be very responsible (mature) in completing a particular laboratory procedure and somewhat irresponsible (less mature) in filling

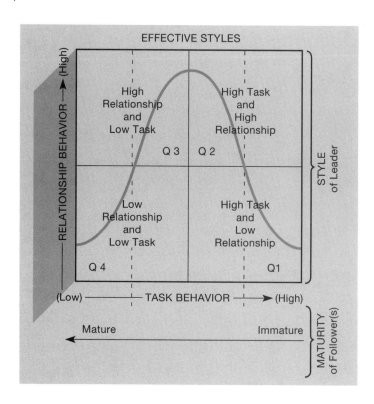

FIGURE 8-6. Situational leadership theory.

out all necessary forms to document preventive maintenance. This may require the manager to supervise more closely the technologist's report filing but exercise less supervision over specimen testing.

The life-cycle theory suggests that as the followers mature, the leader's behavior should change. This is displayed in Figure 8-6 as the line representing a curvilinear design between relationship, tasks, and other variables. The sequence proceeds from (1) high task–low relationship behavior to (2) high task–high relationship behavior to (3) high relationship–low task behavior to (4) low task–low relationship behavior. Consider the development of a new testing procedure to be added to a clinical laboratory's regimen. Early in the development, when the supervisor and staff technologists are attempting to modify a research design to make it practical for clinical application, the supervisor may need to exercise high task–low relationship behavior. Once the procedure is developed and implemented on-line, the supervisor can progress to quadrant 2 or 3 leadership behavior characterized by high relationship and low task emphasis.

The effectiveness dimension was first added by Reddin to the task-concern and relationship-concern dimensions.[51] This addition reflects the fact that a variety

of leadership styles may either be effective or ineffective, depending on the situation. With the third effectiveness dimension, eight possible combinations exist, as depicted in Table 8-3. Hersey and Blanchard's contribution to the effectiveness dimension is in the perceptions of followers, supervisors, and associates when these leadership styles are used. Table 8-4 contrasts some of these perceptions of leader behavior for effective and ineffective styles.

The Contingency Model

Fiedler postulated the first contingency model of leadership, supporting the premise that effective group performance is dependent on the leader's style of interacting with subordinates and the degree of influence and control allotted the leader by the situation.[14] An instrument was designed by Fielder to measure a leader's relationship or task orientation within the parameters of three situational criteria. The measurement tool contains 16 bipolar adjectives (such as efficient–inefficient) that the leader selects to describe an individual with whom he is least able to work. From this set of instructions, the title of the questionnaire, Least-Preferred Co-worker (LPC),

Table 8-3
Managerial Styles With an Effectiveness Dimension

Orientation	Ineffective	Effective	Leader Behavior
Q1 High task–low relationship	Autocrat	Benevolent autocrat	Telling
Q2 High task–high relationship	Compromiser	Executive	Selling
Q3 High relationship–low task	Missionary	Developer	Participating
Q4 Low relationship–low task	Deserter	Bureaucrat	Delegating

is derived. If a leader responds by selecting relatively favorable terms on the LPC, his orientation is toward establishing relationships. If the leader responds in unfavorable terms, he is considered task oriented.

The three situational criteria, or contingency dimensions, include the following:

1. Leader–member relations: how well the leader is liked, respected, and trusted
2. Position power: the amount of influential power the leader has in terms of hiring, firing, discipline, and control of the rewards systems
3. Task structure: the degree to which job assignments of subordinates are specifically defined (structured versus unstructured)

Fiedler reports that the more positive the leader–member relations, the greater the position power. Also, the more highly structured the tasks to be performed, the greater the leader's influence.

Figure 8-7 depicts eight situational conditions (I–VIII) correlated with task-motivated or relations-motivated leadership styles. If a laboratory manager is relations oriented, job performance will be better for situations characterized in IV through VII. On the other hand, productivity is enhanced by a manager with a task orientation for those situations described in I through III and VIII.

Both the tridimensional model and the contingency model support the premise that effectiveness of leadership style is dependent on situational variables,

Table 8-4
How the Basic Leader Behavior Styles May Be Seen by Others

Basic Styles	Effective	Ineffective
High task and low relationship	Seen as having well-defined methods for accomplishing goals that are helpful to the followers	Seen as imposing methods on others; sometimes seen as unpleasant and interested only in short-run output
High task and high relationship	Seen as satisfying the needs of the group for setting goals and organizing work and providing high levels of socioemotional support	Seen as initiating more structure than is needed by the group and often appears to be insincere in interpersonal relationships
High relationship and low task	Seen as having implicit trust in people and as being primarily concerned with facilitating their goal accomplishment	Seen as primarily interested in harmony; sometimes seen as unwilling to accomplish a task if it risks disrupting a relationship or losing "good person" image
Low relationship and low task	Seen as appropriately delegating to subordinates decisions about how the work should be done and providing little socioemotional support where little is needed by the group	Seen as providing little structure or socioemotional support when needed by members of the group

From Hersey P, Blanchard KH: Management of Organizational Behavior: Utilizing Human Resources, 3rd ed, p 107. Englewood Cliffs, Prentice-Hall, 1977 used with permission

THE SITUATIONAL FAVORABLENESS DIMENSION.

	I	II	III	IV	V	VI	VII	VIII
Leader–member relations	Good				Poor			
Task structure	High		Low		High		Low	
Position power	Strong	Weak	Strong	Weak	Strong	Weak	Strong	Weak
Most appropriate leadership style	T	T	T	R	R	R	R	T

T = Task-motivated; R = Relations-motivated

FIGURE 8-7. Fiedler's situational favorableness dimension. (From Fiedler FC: A Theory of Leadership Effectiveness. New York, McGraw-Hill, 1967)

such as maturity of the followers, relationship between the manager and his subordinates, the manager's power to influence, and the degree to which subordinates' tasks are structured.

DIAGNOSING THE SITUATION

At times it is helpful to have a tool that can be used to diagnose a difficult situation confounding the leadership efforts of the manager. Getzels proposed a theory of administration that considers management as a social process.[19] Within Getzels' model (Fig. 8-8), two dimensions operate simultaneously: an impersonal (normothetic) dimension and a personal (idiopathic dimension). The impersonal dimension consists of the institution with its roles (positions) and expectations (responsibilities) within the roles. The personal dimension consists of the individual selected to fill a position, his personality (knowledge and skills factors) in the role, and motivators required to alleviate needs. Conflict within the system may exist whenever there is a disharmony between the corresponding components of the two dimensions: role and personality. These may exist as an inter-role or intrarole conflict, interpersonality or intrapersonality conflict, or a combination role–personality conflict.

Role Conflict

Inter-role conflict occurs when two individuals clash over the boundaries of their job responsibilities, resources available, or "turfdom." An example might be a dispute over the priority for use of a refrigerated centrifuge shared by two technologists. Intrarole conflict usually occurs at the time a position is created if the responsibilities are not clearly or reasonably defined.

Personality Conflict

Rather than referring to the incompatibility of two co-workers, interpersonality conflict refers to a lack of shared attitudes, values, or interests in achieving organizational goals. For example, two technologists may have differing views on whether or not they should be required to perform phlebotomy as part of their daily routine. Intrapersonality conflicts exist when needs–disposition precludes achievement of expecta-

FIGURE 8-8. Getzels' social systems model of administration. (From Mattran KJ: Conflict management, organizational and personnel needs, performance evaluation. In Langerman PD, Smith DH [eds]: Managing Adult and Continuing Education Programs and Staff, p 351. Washington, National Association for Public Continuing and Adult Education, 1979. Used with permission of the publisher)

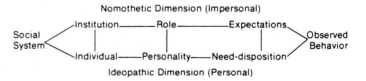

tions within a role: The performance of the closet drinker, for example, is affected by his habit.

Role–Personality Conflict

This is probably the most common form of organizational conflict. In this situation, an individual may not be qualified for a particular role (responsibility) or may be overqualified for the position and hence underused, or a change in the job requirements or personal preparation may bring about this conflict.

To demonstrate the utility of Getzels' model in diagnosing the situation, consider the case scenario outlined in Box 8-7.

This example is not an unusual situation to be faced by the laboratory manager. Using Getzels' model, the situation can be analyzed to identify the cause of the problem. In this case, the problem stems from a role–personality conflict in which the senior technologist feels he has outgrown his role on the basis of his newly acquired advanced degree. The problem is typical in that people frequently want to take on new responsibility with the completion of an advanced degree; this situation is referred to as "flexing newly credentialed muscles."

In this case, the manager was astute enough to diagnose the situation. At a counseling session, the perceived type of conflict was validated. The solution the manager chose to implement included an expansion of the role of the individual. This entailed delegating more responsibility to the senior technologist without expanding the hierarchical structure.

Fell and Richard point out the necessity for laboratory managers to be cognizant of the occurrence of role and personality conflict in their study of factors contributing to occupational stress of medical technologists and technicians.[13] Information gathered through situational diagnosis with Getzels' model should help uncover occupational stressors, such as role overload, role conflict, low participation, and role ambiguity, enabling the manager to minimize their effects.

Work Teams for the Clinical Laboratory

One of the more recent challenges for laboratory managers has been the trend toward development of work teams. Some institutions have assembled self-directed work teams in an effort to improve patient satisfaction and cut costs. Reorganization and reengineering efforts have lead to a "delayering" of laboratory organizational structures with a team functioning in place of a supervisor with subordinates.

From a leadership perspective, one might presume that work teams are simply an extension of participative management. Similarities exist. For example, participative management and work teams both empower employees to exert ownership and control, and both have reportedly increased employee performance, quality, and productivity. Differences exist, however, in the fact that true work teams require a change in organizational structure and the way work gets done.[65] Some employees mistakenly believe they are part of a "team" when they really are working cooperatively side by side. A true work team must function with a high degree of *interdependence* and work toward a jointly agreed-on goal.[65]

There are a variety of types of teams. Six types of teams with particular purposes have been identified by Harrington-Mackin (Box 8-8).[24]

Regardless of the type of team, common characteristics of effective teams are shown in Table 8-5.

Building a Team

Building a team is a complex but structured process. The clear first step is to identify who should participate

---

Box 8·7

Case Scenario: Personality Conflict

The laboratory manager of a large microbiology section directs a staff of 15 technologists who do most of the day-to-day testing for routine cultures and sensitivities. One of the senior technologists has recently completed an advanced degree in microbiology at a nearby university. During the time he was pursuing his studies, the laboratory supported his efforts through a 75% tuition-reimbursement policy and the special privilege of being released early from work in the afternoon to attend class.

Since completing the degree, this senior technologist has seemed unhappy at work, arriving late and often leaving early. There has been much bickering between the technologist and fellow staff members, especially with the recent addition of a senior technologist to specifically perform the mycology tests. General staff morale has slumped, it seems, and the manager has had to spend much time arbitrating disputes that most often involve the senior technologist of concern in this study.

Table 8-5
Characteristics of Effective and Ineffective Teams

Effective	Ineffective	Effective	Ineffective
Information		**Creativity**	
Flows freely up, down, sideways	Flows mainly down, weak horizontally	More options	Controlled by power subgroups
Full sharing	Hoarded, withheld	Solution oriented	Emphasis on activity and inputs
Open and honest	Used to build power Incomplete, mixed messages		
		Power Base	
People Relationships		Shared by all	Hoarded
Trusting	Suspicious and partisan	On competence	On politicking alliances
Respectful	Pragmatic, based on need or liking	Contribution to team	Pragmatic sharing Contribution to power source
Collaborative	Competitive		
Supportive	Withholding	**Motivation**	
Conflict		Committment to goals set by team	Going along with imposed goals
Regarded as natural, even helpful	Frowned on and avoided Destructive	Belonging needs satisfied	Personal goals ignored
On issues, not people	Involves personal traits and motives	More chance for achievement through group	Individual achievement valued without concern for the group
Atmosphere		**Rewards**	
Open	Compartmentalized	Based on contribution to group	
Nonthreatening	Intimidating		Basis for rewards unclear
Noncompetitive	Guarded	Peer recognition	Based on subjective, often arbitrary appraisals
Participative	Fragmented, closed groups		
Decisions			
By consensus	By majority vote or forcing		
Efficient use of resources	Emphasis on power		
Full commitment	Confusion and dissonance		

Source: Quick TL: Successful Team Building, pp 4–5. New York, American Management Association, 1992.

on the team. Teams develop in stages over a period of time. Quick identified five stages shown below:

Stage 1: *Searching*—The group is a gathering of employees until the question of "Why am I here?" and "What should I do?" are answered. Roles and tasks require delineation.

Stage 2: *Defining*—The group must define the task to be performed or objective to be reached. Conflicts and clashes are likely as personal agendas are modified to meet the organizational purpose of the group.

Stage 3: *Identifying*—At this stage, members of the team identify specific roles each will play (eg,

who will facilitate meetings). This stage constitutes a matching of task and personnel.

Stage 4: *Processing*—This stage occurs as the work of the team is accomplished. On-going evaluation of progress and interaction as a team is important.

Stage 5: *Assimilating/Reforming*—While teams with a limited responsibility (eg, task forces) will naturally complete their work and disband, a continuing team will change over time in membership and personality.[49]

Box 8-9 illustrates a sample series of team process steps.

This description of work teams is a brief overview

Box 8·8

Clinical Laboratory Work Teams

1. Organizational policy-making teams (multifunctional)—for example, an institution's quality council
2. Task force or cross-functional team—for example, a process improvement team to deal with turnaround time of laboratory testing
3. Department improvement teams (functional)—for example, to prepare for an accreditation site visit for the laboratory
4. Quality circles—for example, to address a problem crossing several departments or services
5. Self-directed work teams (functional)—for example, a team responsible for all patient care in a given area
6. Self-managed teams (functional)—for example, a section of the laboratory without an assigned supervisor in which the functions of planning, organizing, directing, and monitoring are shared among all staff

From Harrington-Mackin D: The Team Building Tool Kit. New York, American Management Association, 1994

Box 8·9

Sample Team Process

1. The team meets with the team manager to set team objectives for a specified period of time.
2. Members receive training on performance planning and evaluating.
3. Team members discuss and establish individual performance objectives and standards and methods of measurement.
4. The team determines how performance will be reviewed and submits plan and process steps to the team manager or human resources manager for review and approval. Options include the following:
   - All team members evaluate each other, and results are tabulated.
   - Two members of the team, one picked by the person being reviewed and one picked by the rest of the team, conduct and deliver the performance evaluation.
   - A chairperson selected by the team member being evaluated assembles a group of three or four people to evaluate performance.
5. Members receive training on coaching skills and conducting performance reviews and on how to receive and process feedback.
6. Throughout the project, the team participates in ongoing coaching and review. The team manager and supervisor and other teams provide regular feedback about the team's progress.
7. As the final review approaches, the team member completes a self-evaluation, and the entire team completes a written evaluation on the member. In addition, customer surveys and written evaluations from other independent teams may be added. All of the results are tabulated.
8. The two team members or any similar configuration (see item 4) review the information (self-evaluation plus others' evaluation), identify areas of congruence and incongruence, decide how closely objectives were achieved, and pinpoint areas for continued growth.
9. The evaluators meet with the team member and review the information, completing a final form that combines all the information. The evaluation includes the development of a performance plan, including new goals and skills for the duration of the project.

Source: Harrington-Mackin D: The Team Building Took Kit, pp 128–129. New York, American Management Association, 1994.

only. Establishing work teams is not a panacea for problems related to cost, efficiency, or bureaucracy. Managers need to be aware that team building requires support from upper administration, training of team members in roles and processes, and time—usually 3 to 5 years for a self-directed work team to be truly successful.[25]

Many of the barriers to implementing teams are similar to those encountered with delegation (see Chapter 5). Not everyone welcomes the opportunity to serve on a team. "Self-directed" does not mean that supervision is not required or that this is an inexpensive venture. Similarly, self-directed work teams do not lessen the amount of power held by the manager.

LEADERSHIP BEHAVIOR IN NEED OF CHANGE

Some subtle clues should alert the manager to the need for a change in leadership styles. This surveyed 1,000 supervisors and managers from 23 organizations, asking, "What would you say to your boss if there was one thing, if he would do it, that in your opinion would most contribute to the effectiveness of yourself and your work unit?"[54] The following is a rank-ordered list of responses:[61]

1. Share the company objectives with me.
2. Provide better, more honest communications.
3. Know my problems.
4. Set the objectives. Let me do the job my way.
5. Involve me in the decisions that affect me and my work unit.
6. Eliminate duplication of effort.
7. Back me up in personnel/grievance decisions.
8. Treat managers as if they were human.
9. Get rid of the deadwood.
10. Tell me what is expected of me.

These concerns provide a sound sketch of middle-management concerns when a change in the supervisor's leadership style is needed. Perhaps polling one's own subordinates would enlighten the reader to his own leadership style, and some changes might seem appropriate.

REFERENCES

1. Appley LA: The nature of management, film one in a series. In Supervisory Management Course—Part One. New York, American Management Association, 1968
2. Argyris C: Management and Organizational Development, p 17. New York, McGraw-Hill, 1971
3. Argyris C: Management and Organizational Development: The Path From XA to YB, p 12. New York, McGraw-Hill, 1971
4. Blake RR, Mouton JL: Managerial facades. Adv Manag J July:29–36, 1966
5. Blake RR, Mouton JL: The Managerial Grid. Houston, Gulf Publishing, 1964
6. Blake RR, Mouton JL: The New Managerial Grid. Houston, Gulf Publishing, 1978
7. Burden CA, Dorff PG: Understanding the leadership function: Leaders are not necessarily managers. Laboratory Medicine 18:327–329, 1987
8. Cherrington DJ, Cherrington JO: Participation, performance, and appraisal. Business Horizons 17:40, 1974
9. Crowley J, Rinker G, Neely AE, Anderson AS: Situational leadership for the laboratory. J Med Technol 3:303–306, 1986
10. Davis K: Human Relations at Work, 3rd ed, p 97. New York, McGraw-Hill, 1967
11. Davis K: Human Behavior at Work: Human Relations and Organizational Behavior, 4th ed, pp 120–133. New York, McGraw-Hill, 1972
12. Drucker PF: The Practice of Management. New York, Harper & Row, 1954
13. Fell RD, Richard WC: Health effects on job pressures. Lab World July:44–47, 1980
14. Fiedler FC: A Theory of Leadership Effectiveness. New York, McGraw-Hill, 1967
15. Fleishman EA: Twenty years of consideration and structure. In Fleishman EA, Hunt JG (eds): Current Development in the Study of Leadership, pp 1–37. Carbondale, Southern Illinois University Press, 1973
16. Frank ER: Motivation by objectives—a case study. Research Management 12:391–400, 1969
17. French JRP, Raven B: The bases of social power. In Cartwright D, Zander AF (eds): Group Dynamics, 2nd ed, pp 607–623. Evanston, Row Peterson, 1960
18. Fulmer RM: The New Management, p 336. New York, Macmillan, 1974
19. Getzels JW: Administration as a social process. In Halpin AW (ed): Administrative Theory in Education, pp 150–165. Chicago, Midwest Administration Center, 1958
20. Gibson JL, Ivancevich JM, Donnelly JH: Organizations Behavior, Structure, Processes, 3rd ed, pp 30–32, 366–367. Dallas Business Publications, 1979
21. Glassman E: A leadership skills program for scientist/supervisors. Laboratory Management 20(9):46–49, 1982
22. Goddard RW: Viewpoint: Leadership in the laboratory. Clinical Laboratory Management Review 5:70–72, 1991
23. Halpin AW: The Leadership Behavior of School Superintendents, p 4. Chicago, Midwest Administration Center, University of Chicago, 1959
24. Harrington-Mackin D: The Team Building Took Kit. New York, American Management Association, 1994
25. Harrington-Mackin D: Keeping the Team Going. New York, American Management Association, 1994
26. Hersey P, Blanchard KH: Management of Organizational Behavior: Utilizing Human Resources, 3rd ed, p 89. Englewood Cliffs, Prentice-Hall, 1977
27. Jago AG, Vroom VH: Hierarchical level and leadership

style. Organizational Behavior and Human Performance 18:131–145, 1977

28. Jenks JM: Speeding your growth with leadership skills. Clinical Laboratory Management Review 8:52–55, 1994

29. Jennings EE: The anatomy of leadership. Management of Personnel Quarterly 1(Autumn), 1961

30. Ketchum SM: Overcoming the four toughest management challenges. Clinical Laboratory Management Review 5: 246–263, 1991

31. Kiersey O, Bates M: Please Understand Me: Character and Temperament Types. Del Mar, Prometheus Nemesis Books, 1978

32. Kindler HS: The art of managing differences. Training and Development Journal 37(1):26–32, 1983

33. Knudson HR, Woodworth RT, Bell CH: Management: An Experiential Approach, p 326. New York, McGraw-Hill, 1973

34. Korman AK: "Consideration," "initiating structure," and organizational criteria—a review. Personal Psychology: A Journal of Applied Research XIX(4):349–361, 1966

35. Kouzes JM, Posner BZ: The credibility factor. Clinical Laboratory Management Review 8:340–353, 1994

36. Lawler EE, Hall DT, Oldham GR: Organizational climate: Relationship to organizational structure, process and performance. Organizational Behavior and Human Performance II, 14:139–155, 1974

37. Leavitt T: The managerial merry-go-round. Harvard Business Review July–August:131, 1974

38. Likert R: Management styles and the human component. Management Review 66:23ff, 1977

39. Likert R: New Patterns of Management, pp 113–115. New York, McGraw-Hill, 1961

40. Lombardi DN: The health-care manager's guide to managing change in challenging times. Clinical Laboratory Management Review 10:18–24, 1996

41. McDonnell J: Participative Management: Can its acceptance be predicted? Human Resource Management 15(2): 2–4, 1976

42. McGregor D: Leadership and Motivation. Boston, MIT Press, 1966

43. Mitchell TR, Larson JR, Green SG: Leader behavior, situational moderators, and group performance: An attributable analysis. Organizational Behavior and Human Performance 18:254–268, 1977

44. Murnighan JK, Leung TK: The effects of leadership involvement and the importance of the task on subordinates' performance. Organizational Behavior and Human Performance 17:299–310, 1976

45. Myers IB: Type and Teamwork. Gainesville, Center for Applications of Psychological Type, 1974

46. O'Brien RT: Using Jung more (and etching him in stone less). Training 22(5):53–66, 1985

47. O'Donovan TR: Can the "participative" approach to management help the decision makers? Hospital Management 112:16, 1971

48. Preston P: Encouraging creativity. Clinical Laboratory Management Review 5:5–14, 1991

49. Quick TL: Sucessful Team Building. New York, American Management Association, 1992

50. Rakich JS, Longest BB, O'Donovan TR: Managing Health Care Organizations. Philadelphia, W.B. Saunders, 1977

51. Reddin WJ: The 3-D management style theory. Training Development Journal 30(4):8–17, 1976

52. Reichman W, Levy M: Personal power enchancement: A way to execute success. Management Review 66:28–34, 1977

53. Schwartz D: Introduction to Management: Principles, Practices and Processes, pp 507–508. New York, Harcourt Brace Jovanovich, 1980

54. Scott WG, Mitchell TR, Birnvarum PH: Organization Theory: A Structural and Behavioral Analysis, 4th ed. Homewood, Richard D. Irwin, 1981

55. Singer HA: Human values and leadership: A ten-year study of administrators in large organizations. Hum Organ 35(1): 83–87, 1976

56. Snyder JR, Manuselis G: Factors affecting participative management in the clinical laboratory. J Med Technol 2: 532–536, 1985

57. Steger J, Manners G, Zimmer T: Following the leader: How to link management style to subordinate personalities. Management Review 71(10):22–51, 1982

58. Stogdill RM, Coons AC (eds): Leader Behavior: Its Description and Measurement. Research Monograph No. 88. Columbus, Bureau of Business Research, The Ohio State University, 1975

59. Tannenbaum R, Schmidt WH: How to choose a leadership pattern. Harvard Business Review May–June:162–180, 1973

60. Taylor JK: Participative management lifts lab productivity. MLO 18(4):46–50, 1986

61. This LE: A Guide to Effective Management: Practical Applications from Behavioral Science, pp 96–97, 108–11. Reading, Addison-Wesley, 1974

62. Townsend R: Up the Organization, pp 33, 86. Greenwich Fawcett Publications, 1970

63. Viola RH: Be a manager and a motivator. MLO September–October:131–136, 1974

64. Weihrich H: Management by objectives: Does it really work? Business Review 28:(4)27–31, 1976

65. Zenger J et al: Leading Teams. San Jose, CA, Zenger-Meller, 1994

9

TQM-CQI: Employee-Involvement Work Groups

Barbara L. Parsons • Dietrich L. Schaupp

During the last decade, rapid change swept through health care and exposed the laboratory manager to a wide variety of methods and programs designed to enhance organizational effectiveness. Some of these programs offer specific, short-term approaches, while others promote the benefits of long-term change.

Quality assurance programs, cost-containment programs, morale-enhancement efforts, and productivity-improvement programs are just a few approaches available to the manager. Although each method promises long-term improvement, after adoption and implementation, these programs often prove difficult to sustain. Some of these programs have achieved spectacular results; however, the majority have proved to be lackluster, sometimes destructive, and often costly during and after implementation.

Recent management thought extols the benefits of participatory group approaches for the health-care sector. Although participative management techniques have been on the management horizon for some time, only recently have they been applied in the health-care arena.

Among the more popular approaches to employee involvement are quality circles (QCs), quality of work life (QWL) programs, total quality management (TQM), continuous quality improvement (CQI), and autonomous work groups. From an employee-involvement perspective, these approaches are similar, but they differ in one respect: QCs, TQM, CQI, and autonomous work groups are more easily adopted to a nonunion setting, whereas QWL programs are more common in a union environment.

This chapter explores the feasibility of these approaches in a laboratory environment. Furthermore, it explains the background, function, and brief supervisory overview required to establish these approaches.

WHY EMPLOYEE INVOLVEMENT?

Although employee involvement is not foreign to the United States, it has more recently received considerable exposure as a Japanese import, with Japanese success in competitive manufacturing renewing America's interest.

It has been suggested that Japanese performance and productivity can be linked directly to the Japanese management style. Although the relationship is somewhat oversimplified, it is true that the Japanese have been strong advocates and practitioners of employee-involvement groups. Americans generally have been lukewarm to the idea. Americans have a long history of one-to-one management where the superior–subordinate interaction is the basic management unit. Furthermore, cultural differences between Japan and the United States are reflected in their respective management styles because most managers practice what is culturally "natural" to them. The Japanese style reflects a collective society, whereas American techniques have reinforced the virtues of individualism. Finally, American managers often do not really understand or know what employee involvement is. Our discussion addresses this issue.

Put simply, employee involvement means using employee groups to increase performance, quality, and productivity. Its roots lie in the American human-relations approaches so popular after World War II. Although it addressed worker satisfaction and group interaction, the human-relations approach stressed the employee's need for recognition and job security and a sense of belonging and importance.

An outgrowth of the human-relations approach emphasized the developmental aspect of human needs. It sought employee participation based on the premise that it would satisfy needs associated with personal development. This human-resources approach stressed employee self-control, self-direction, creativity, and innovation. It strove to create an environment that allowed employees to contribute to organizational goals and experience direct control of their work environment. Through an attitude of "ownership" or "control," employee productivity and performance were expected to increase.

The employee ownership–control argument is also the basis of the employee involvement approaches presented in this discussion. However, the techniques presented here stress group involvement as opposed to individual participation. Although there are participative schemes that involve employees on an individual basis, such as management by objectives, the major thrust of quality initiatives and autonomous work groups is that they use the group, not the individual, to achieve organizational goals. Furthermore, organizations that practice high-involvement approaches need more knowledge to manage these activities.

THE QUALITY MOVEMENT

Taylor

Although the concept of "total quality management" has only received attention in the United States since 1980, the development of processes to manage quality actually began around the turn of the century when Frederick W. Taylor, an engineer, developed a set of principles for improving the work of unskilled workers in the industrial setting.

Taylor applied a systematic approach to analyzing and defining work tasks, standardizing working conditions, tying rewards to success, and using skilled workers to achieve a positive financial impact through increased efficiency and productivity.

Shewhart

Others who followed Taylor continued to apply engineering, financial, and statistical methods for further impact on quality improvement. Walter Shewhart (1881–1967), a statistician with Bell Labs, applied sampling techniques to problem analysis in an effort to enhance control of production processes. He developed control charts to track performance so workers would have the ability to monitor their work and prevent loss and waste. He believe that total quality is a continuous cycle of four components: plan, do, check, and act.

Deming

Dr. W. Edwards Deming (1900–1993), a statistician and a student of Shewhart, further applied sampling technique to monitor process input and output to improve accuracy and consistency. Invited by the Japanese in 1947 to deliver a series of lectures on quality, Deming taught both the statistical principles he had refined and his 14 points as a "Charter for Management." Constancy of purpose, continual improvement, and profound knowledge were the three key components of Deming's 14 points.

Deming came to realize over the course of applying statistical techniques to quality improvement that quality is not determined by physical process alone, but by the actions and decisions of senior management. Therefore, quality does not come about simply by controlling the process and actions of workers, but by the decisions of managers who design the systems of work. He observed that managers determine markets, products, and services; select, train, and reward workers; allocate resources, tools, and equipment; and determine the physical facilities and work environment in which the processes take place. The role of the worker is limited to resolving limited problems directly under his control.

Deming believed that managers and workers have responsibility for minimizing variations in product or service and that the key to who does what is based on statistical diagnosis of systems and identifying which tasks are more efficiently and effectively controlled by workers and which tasks or decisions are more appropriately controlled by managers.

Juran

Born in 1904 and a contemporary of Deming, Dr. Joseph M. Juran assisted the Japanese in applying a management process that adapted the quality concepts and tools that had been successfully applied to production processes. By applying financial management concepts to managerial processes, Juran addressed a three-prong approach to managing quality: quality planning, quality control, and quality improvement. He suggested in his quality planning component that the customer be identified and his needs determined as a way of defining quality. Juran further advocates CQI through the use of project teams.

Crosby

In 1979, the Book *Quality is Free* established author Philip B. Crosby[1] as a quality guru. Of particular note are his emphasis on the cost of quality and his belief that management commitment is the most necessary component in a successful quality initiative. Crosby's approach further develops the concept of meeting expectations of the customer, doing things right the first time (a preventive strategy) and, using examples from health care, setting a performance goal of "zero defects." Crosby's approach to quality has been particularly challenging.

Feigenbaum

Originator of the concept "cost of quality," Dr. Armand V. Feigenbaum worked with managers to track the costs of failure and rework as a percent of annual sales. Having assessed these costs as somewhere between 10% and 40%, Feigenbaum espoused that every function in an organization has a responsibility for quality; this became known as total quality control (TQC). TQC includes product design, distribution systems, marketing systems, and customer support.

Summary

Quality control as a concept in manufacturing has progressed from designing efficient and effective physical systems of production, which explored the interaction of men and machines, to management systems involving planning and design to defining quality in the eyes of the customer. The common thread underlying all these approaches is to improve the process continually by controlling variations in the input–output transfer process. How that may be done is where employee involvement comes in.

Addressing quality issues not only dealt with production processes but raised issues of the "right way" to manage. Research has yet to identify the right way to manage but offers many approaches from which to choose. Selecting the right way for an organization to manage requires an examination of the type of product or service the business produces, the business environment in which the business operates, the values of the society in which it operates, and the characteristics and values of its work force.

The evolutionary process of management practice is a result of existing technology and the knowledge and values of society. Today's organizations are finding that some level of participation is required as an effective way to respond to customer needs in an ever-changing environment.

TOTAL QUALITY MANAGEMENT

As defined by Lisa M. O'Rourke,[2] TQM is "a shift in management philosophy that encompasses the mission and values, the involvement of leaders and managers in quality, the precise identification of customers and their requirements, the continuous improvement of critical processes, the measurement of performance and the development of an empowered and participative workforce."

Prevailing management thought suggests that quality is not determined exclusively by the employee, the shop floor, the caregiver at the bedside, or the laboratory technician who performs the analysis of the specimen. "Quality is determined by the senior managers of an organization, who by virtue of the positions they hold, are responsible for customers, employees, suppliers, and shareholders for the success of the business. These senior managers allocate resources, decide which markets the firm will enter, and select and implement the management processes that will enable the firm to fulfill their mission and, eventually, their vision."

The TQM model is based on the principles of meeting customer expectations, continuously improving work processes, and involving all employees to gain and maintain a competitive position in the marketplace.

Goal

The goal of TQM is to deliver the highest quality product or service for the customer at the lowest cost, while maintaining profit and economic stability. Management achieves its vision and mission by aligning its employees toward that mission, providing them with the skills to work in teams to identify and solve problems, and trusting them to do it.

Traditionally organizations have been designed around functional units. These functions focused on what the unit did with or to a raw material, an intermediate material, a specific kind of customer, a specific kind of service, or a specific product. The focus was on product management, and quality resulted from inspection of a completed task or product.

The focus of TQM is on the input–output transformation process, which puts quality into the planning phase to increase customer satisfaction, not identify what went wrong.

Management Support

Management must identify, select, and design a way to support the customer, the process, and the employees. Commitment to that support is provided through leadership, education, resources, communication, recognition, and evaluation.

- Leadership for such a significant organizational change must come from senior management.

The commitment to TQM comes not from the "right words," although they are important, but from the right questions and actions. What management *asks about* determines the real priority. What management *does* sets the performance example. Senior management must act as advocate, teacher, and leader. They must apply the tools and actively participate in and contribute to participative processes. They must become experts at leading change and receive ongoing training in problem solving and conflict resolution.

- Employee abilities must be aligned with the quality goal. Education provides employees with information about the organization (ie, mission, values, strategy, finances, market share), which brings them into alignment with management's philosophy and direction. Teaching employees the skills they need to impart quality to processes further supports the quality initiative and builds trust and commitment. Training often involves statistical analysis techniques, interpersonal skills, new technology, communication, leadership and facilitation, and setting objectives.
- Resources are necessary to support the quality effort and are reflected in time and money for meetings, travel, speakers, consultants, manuals and training materials, tools, and equipment.
- Communication processes must be enhanced and designed to be effective. New ways of gathering and sharing information must be identified. Information must be accurate, complete, and useful. Honest and open communication further builds trust and employee commitment that will result in quality decisions and actions.
- Recognition is necessary both as a way of communicating success and as a way of reinforcing and rewarding effort. It communicates what is important and identifies role models for others.
- Evaluation is contingent on data in the TQM process, not opinion. Customer needs and satisfaction provide objective and realistic information for assessing the organization's performance. Management must provide the tools and opportunities to gather meaningful data on which to base CQI decisions.

The Customer

Perhaps the most unique aspect of the TQM effort is the focus on the customer. Historically, quality focused on measuring outcomes based on a predefined set of specifications developed by owners, managers, or highly trained engineers who "knew what the customer wanted." Henry Ford, himself an owner and pioneer in automobile production processes, said, "The customer can have any color car as long as it is black."

With TQM, the shift is from product-driven organizations like Henry Ford's to market-driven organizations where the needs of the customers are the heart of every employee's job.

According to Karou Ishikawa, the best known of the Japanese quality prophets, "The customer is whoever gets your work next." His description requires that organizations recognize internal and our traditionally defined external customer. If we accept Ishikawa's definition, then suppliers to our processes become a part of the customer chain. The organization must clearly define their customers to identify customer needs so an effective work flow process can be designed that will deliver a quality service or product.

In the laboratory setting, the primary external customer is typically the physician who ordered the test or evaluation. However, the patient is also a customer of the process, as is the insurance carrier who reimburses the laboratory, the employer of the patient who subsidizes the insurance plan, or the managed care plan or health maintenance organization to which the patient belongs and for whom the laboratory provides services.

Internally, among the laboratory customers is the employee or staff physician who obtains the specimen, the clerk on the nursing unit who communicates with the laboratory, the technician who evaluates the specimen, and the nurse, physician, and other employees and clerks who receive documents and respond to the results. Although this may not be all-inclusive, literally anyone who uses the output of the laboratory process is a customer. That applies to each step and includes interactions of coworkers who become each other's customer.

While most people readily identify with the role of external customer, it is apparent that internal customers must also be serviced, even if it is only in the giving and receiving of accurate and timely information. In a fully committed quality effort, their needs and expectations are just as important in assessing laboratory output as the needs of the external customer; the underlying assumption being that a quality work flow process returns a quality outcome, and that outcome is influenced by the quality of every interaction and activity involved in converting inputs to outputs.

The concept of the internal customer introduces the supplier into the process. The supplier, whether it be the patient supplying the specimen or the organization that manufactures the equipment or the company who sells and services that equipment, impacts quality outcomes based on the quality of their inputs.

For example, a patient to whom proper instructions have *not* been given may appear for a particular blood screen that required him to fast for the previous 12 hours. When it is discovered that he did not fast, the expected outcome cannot occur. Time is lost, proper treatment is delayed, and the patient, the physician, and laboratory personnel are disappointed and frustrated. No matter where it occurred, the system was broken. Perhaps the need to fast was not understood by the office staff who communicated with the patient. Perhaps the physician neglected to mention it, thinking it was someone else's responsibility. Perhaps the patient did not understand what fasting meant and instead drove as "fast" as he could to his appointment that day.

The laboratory is both a customer and a producer in this process, and proper communication of laboratory (as customer) expectations to the suppliers (patient, physicians, staff) would have resulted in a quality outcome (a proper specimen evaluated and reported correctly) to the ultimate customer (the physician and the patient).

Work efforts in TQM organizations must be directed toward various internal customers, suppliers, and external customers, whether they are intermediate or the ultimate customer. What does the customer want?

Every health-care provider claims to be patient oriented and physician friendly, but few have developed and implemented a structured and scientific process for identifying the needs, expectations, perceptions, and satisfaction levels of the various external and internal customers that comprise the marketplace.

Most managers focus on what they think is important, *not* what customers think is important. Knowing what customers want and need saves wasted effort and resources and eliminates guessing and rework.

Tools available for assessing customer needs include various surveys, interviews, discussions, focus groups, site visits, observations, mystery shoppers, customer representatives, or teams and projects, conferences, complaints, letters, grievances, and any other sets of data and methods of information gathering that are meaningful.

In their book, *Taking the Mystery Out of TQM, a Practical Guide to Total Quality Management*, Peter Capezio and Debra Morehouse[3] state, "Quality begins and ends with the customer." They suggest that "to build a real quality advantage, everyone in the company needs to learn about their customers—who they are, why they use the products or services and how to keep them satisfied. First, last and always—customer requirements are the only true measure of quality. If you do nothing else this year, increase the ways and frequency of customer interface for employees throughout the company. Send everyone 'out to play' in the customers' playground and each person will return knowing a lot more about the 'game' and how to make the next moves."

Employee Involvement—Teams

Deming defined organizations as systems designed to serve customers. These systems are composed of processes and tasks that are linked together and affect one another. To excel at meeting customer needs, an organization must continually improve these systems. Employees are participants in the processes that result in customer-satisfying systems or organizations.

In TQM, employees are members of process-focused teams that study these processes methodically and find permanent solutions to problems. Putting employees in a team to problem solve accomplishes several things: (1) The diversity of experience and education of several individuals contribute to better understanding and decision making. (2) Meaningful involvement develops a sense of contribution and appeals to higher level intrinsic motivators like self-esteem and self-actualization. (3) Participants in designing a process of change are more likely to understand and adopt the change that translates into employee ownership. (4) Ownership significantly increases the desire for success.

The opportunity to participate in some team activity exists in virtually all modern organizations. They may be called task forces, quality teams, product improvement teams, self-governance, QCs, or other appropriate nomenclature, but they all require the same elements for success:

- *Roles* of the team must be clearly defined and understood.
- *Skills* necessary to function effectively must be identified and developed.
- *Participation* must be supported by the organizational culture.

Typically, a quality action team consists of five to nine people who share an issue or problem they are to resolve. Members are selected by management and can be drafted or volunteer. Because TQM focuses on a process and quality is seen as "holistic," many teams are cross-functional in their membership and problem-solving approaches. Management representation is desirable if processes that cross departments may be redesigned.

The role of the team is to work within the structured problem-solving process to diagnose and analyze problems, develop and implement effective solutions, and ensure that the solutions are ongoing through monitoring and feedback.

Selecting the "right" project is critical to the team's success and to the overall TQM effort. Most projects in the service industry focus on reducing response or cycle times, reducing cost, minimizing errors, and eliminating rework. Certain criteria must be considered when selecting a project:

1. The team activity should focus on a specific problem area that has been identified by the customer or customers.
2. The essential aspects of the problem should be measurable.
3. Data pertaining to the problem should be available.
4. Management must support the project with resource commitment.
5. The project scope must be manageable by the team.

Sources of project ideas include physician surveys, patient surveys, employee surveys, internal performance measurements, error rates, grievances, management suggestions, other units' customers, competitors, and so forth. Two general principles can be applied to quality problems: (1) 85% of quality problems are the result of faulty work processes, and only 15% are attributable to work error; and (2) 20% of our customers are responsible for 80% of our complaints.

This last rule, the Pareto principle, is often used by a team to determine priorities in focusing their efforts. A general rule of thumb for medical and patient-related services is to focus quality improvement efforts in the low frequency/high cost (risk) areas for the greatest return on the effort.

Many assessment and process tools are available to teams. A partial list includes brainstorming, flow charting, sampling, surveying, Pareto analysis, cause and effect analysis, histograms, scatter diagrams, control charts, and graphs. Because the principles of scientific management must be applied to quality improvement efforts, team education and training are vital to the success of TQM and CQI.

Team projects can last any length of time. Consideration must be given, however, to the amount and kind of data that are available, the previous experience of the team members, the nature of the problem to be resolved, and the amount of time allotted to team activities. Some kind of expectation should be set to prevent burnout and loss of interest. We have seen teams struggle for as long as 3 years working on problems that were ill defined and too global. Other teams have been quite effective in 3 months or less. Needless to say, the definition of the problem is a critical component of the amount of time required.

Facilitator

Each team has a team leader and a facilitator. The basic responsibilities of a facilitator include the following:

1. Communicating with teams, leaders, and the advisory group
2. Keeping records of team activities and progress
3. Implementing advisory group policy and communicating philosophy
4. Acting as a resource for team leaders in solving human relations problems
5. Assisting with training team members
6. Assisting team in selecting good projects
7. Operating the team on a temporary basis in the absence of the team leader
8. Reporting team progress to management and advisory council

A facilitator is an internal consultant, specializing in the quality process, who works with several team leaders. The facilitator knows problem-solving processes and tools and has well-developed leadership, communication, and group dynamics skills. Facilitators are typically chosen from the best employees and possess excellent work records and the respect of their peers.

Leader

The following are roles of the team leader:

1. Leading all team activities
2. Teaching problem-solving techniques to team members
3. Providing guidance for group activities
4. Ensuring proper communication with management, the advisory group, and the facilitator
5. Ensuring group record maintenance
6. Assisting with presentations to the advisory group

The team leader, to be successful, must be knowledgeable of the project area and possess skills for getting cooperation from multiskilled and multidisciplinary team members. It is helpful if the team leader comes from the unit most impacted by the problem to be solved.

For an understanding of how this structure (Fig. 9-1) operates in a hospital or laboratory, an explanation of each structural component is necessary.

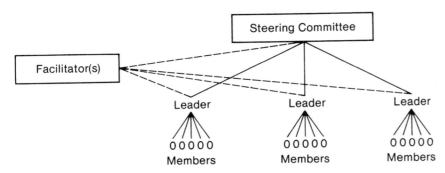

FIGURE 9–1. Quality teams structure.

Steering Committee

The steering committee functions as a board of directors. It establishes policies on implementation and administration of the program. It also sets program objectives and resources and, in general, provides guidance and direction for the program. The steering committee selects facilitators and meets regularly with them. The committee also attends management presentations. Representatives of the major organizational functions must be on the committee. If a union exists, representation should be solicited.

Should We Introduce Total Quality Management?

Before implementing TQM, one first must be aware that the process does take time and is costly. The cost factors cannot be ignored, because teams meet during work time. Most teams meet 1 to 2 hours a week. Management should ponder the following points before implementing a quality program:

- Is the existing managerial style compatible with a participatory management or employee empowerment philosophy required by TQM?
- What is the organizational history of previous programs (eg, management by objectives, cost containment, quality assurance, and hospitality training)?
- Is the organization willing to commit resources over the long-term tenure of the program?
- What is the organizational climate associated with employee morale, commitment, and flexibility regarding new programs?
- Will existing union(s) accept the process?

This list is not exhaustive, and other factors may be more pertinent to the reader's situation. These factors do, however, highlight specific concerns that should be considered before hastily undertaking such an effort.

Implementation

Once a decision to implement a quality management program has been made, it must be carefully orchestrated. In Japan, the introduction of QCs was compatible with a culture stressing collective decision making; in the United States, this is not the case. Some American organizations receive orders to implement participative quality initiatives from top management. They are encouraged, cajoled, or sometimes even pointedly told to implement the program. Often the program is introduced into the American organization with the hope that it will influence the organizational culture and indirectly change the QWL. In fact, it takes on the trappings of an organizational development effort with all the claims of success that often are difficult to substantiate even after several years. The claims of TQM are achievable, but it is a slow and arduous journey that demands planning and a culture receptive to employee empowerment. For example, a TQM/CQI program is not a panacea that will immediately erase a long history of strained management–employee relations. It can build new relationships that foster mutual problem solving and trust between participants. For successful implementation, consider the suggestions found in Box 9–1.

In general, conditions for successfully sustaining a TQM program hinge on organizational commitment and environment. In most cases, this means that the organization must make substantial efforts to educate organizational members about the process. The process requires that participants have access to information that in the past was considered confidential—for example, information dealing with quality, cost, and output are essential. Furthermore, the organizational climate must support a cooperative atmosphere that encourages open communication, sharing of information, and a genuine feeling of cooperative problem solving. Because some consultants would assert that this atmosphere is an end-result variable, the chicken-or-the-egg dilemma is an appropriate analogy. Without these conditions at the outset, implementation of the program is difficult; however, these conditions are the philosophic heart of a program that ensure a more participative approach to problem solving in the organizational environment. In any case, management must support and encourage openness and trust if the program is to succeed. These conditions reduce resistance to the program and allow implementation to proceed, usually in a sequential fashion (Fig. 9-2).

Pitfalls and Conclusions

The chief advantages of quality teams are obvious. If implemented correctly, the techniques can create major changes in employee attitudes and increase productivity and quality. However, they also can be costly, require constant management vigilance, and can deteriorate into a program identified more with management than with employees. In union situations, a TQM program can be criticized as having co-opted the union, reducing employees' influence over their work situation. A possible solution is a modified approach to employee involvement, QWL programs.

Box 9•1

Successful Total Quality Management Implementation Suggestions

Contain initial enthusiasm; be patient and let it evolve.

Allocate sufficient resources to train and educate; start with the board of directors and top administration, and work downward.

Provide an environment for open, honest, and positive communication.

Reassure, train, and encourage middle management with regard to the merits of a participative quality effort.

Allocate sufficient financial resources.

Publicize the program and its benefits.

Plan for scheduling problems and solve them.

Expeditiously implement the acceptable recommendations of the teams.

- Disseminate quality teams material
  ▼
- Research similar situation using quality teams
  ▼
- Discuss with impacted parties, all levels of management, union, and employees
  ▼
- Get outside help consultant
  ▼
- Establish steering committee
  ▼
- Identify baseline data points
  ▼
- Select facilitator
  ▼
- Develop implementation plan and secure approval
  ▼
- Develop or purchase training materials
  ▼
- Publicize program
  ▼
- Train management, staff, and quality team leaders
  ▼
- Start several pilot quality teams
  ▼
- Train participants
  ▼
- Shepherd pilot circle(s) to assure successful outcomes
  ▼
- Review and circulate pilot quality teams
  ▼
- Expand program and evaluate

FIGURE 9–2. Sequential implementation of a quality teams program.

THE QUALITY OF WORK LIFE APPROACH

The second major employee involvement approach is the QWL program. Although traditionally identified with manufacturing in the United States, QWL has experienced some appreciation in the service sector in recent years. Its adoption and adaptation to a health-care environment seems feasible, and it is for that reason that this approach is presented here.

The primary difference between QWL programs and other quality initiatives is the inclusion of the union as an active participant. Quality improvement programs can function in a union environment and often have the endorsement and encouragement of the union. It has a greater impact on work life in general because it legitimizes its efforts through union participation. QWL programs attempt to improve product quality or service, improve union–management relationships, and increase employee involvement. Most QWL programs have a structure similar to that of other team approaches, relying on problem-solving groups. However, the presence of a union introduces an extra dimension into traditional management problem-solving methods. Ordinarily, the traditionally adversarial collective bargaining relationship holds certain issues sacrosanct. Therefore, both union and management decide at the outset of QWL implementation which issues are untouchable. Usually, both sides agree that the collective bargaining contract remains in place, and management usually allows certain issues that traditionally were within the province of management to be addressed by the problem-solving teams. Generally, a QWL approach permits organizational problems to be divided into the three-legged stool of collective bargaining, management authority, and joint problem solving (Fig. 9-3).

Objectives

As depicted by the three-legged stool analogy, such an arrangement tends to categorize questions into collec-

tive bargaining (union) problems, management problems, or joint problems, representing each constituency's objectives. In reality, the objectives overlap, because the same people involved in the collective bargaining process also participate in the joint problem-solving (QWL) process. Each has entered the process with certain objectives: to reduce the adversarial relationship existing among the parties, gain popular support, increase influence in changing the work environment, and increase productivity or quality performance. Usually the broad objectives of the process are defined on a memorandum of agreement.

Because the QWL process will alter the traditional way of deciding and implementing change in the organization, the union and management negotiate an agreement that defines the objectives and boundaries of the process. Such an agreement may include the items listed in Box 9–2.

Organizational Structure

The organizational structure resembles that of TQM/CQI programs, except the QWL structure parallels and complements the traditional hierarchical structure. Steering committees are established, facilitators or coordinators are selected and trained, and work teams are established. Although the QWL program's structure

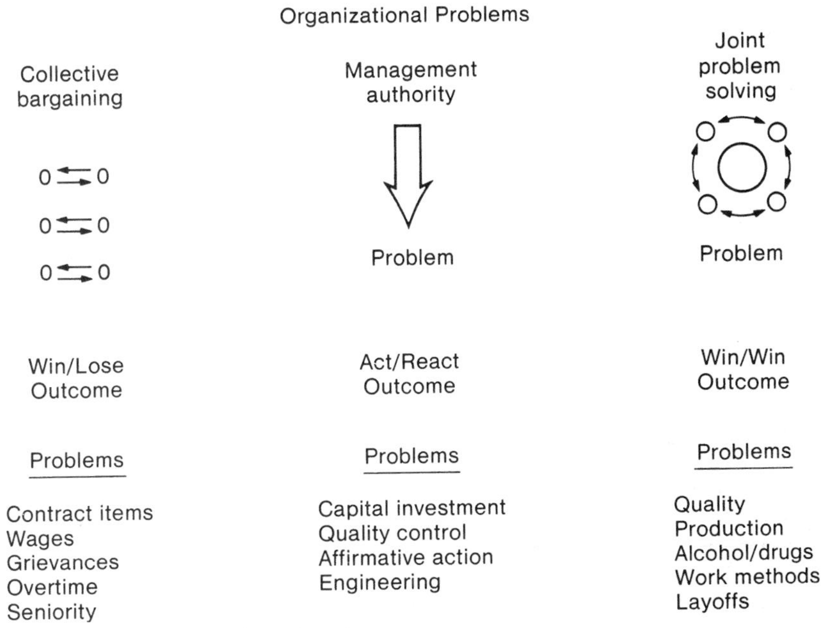

Organizational Problems

Collective bargaining	Management authority	Joint problem solving
0 ⇌ 0		
0 ⇌ 0	⬇	
0 ⇌ 0	Problem	Problem
Win/Lose Outcome	Act/React Outcome	Win/Win Outcome
Problems	Problems	Problems
Contract items Wages Grievances Overtime Seniority	Capital investment Quality control Affirmative action Engineering	Quality Production Alcohol/drugs Work methods Layoffs

FIGURE 9–3. The three-legged stool.

Box 9·2

Quality of Work Life Agreement Inclusions

Participation is voluntary.

Objectives are to improve the quality of work life (which may range from a better work environment for employees to greater performance in quality and productivity).

Collective bargaining issues will not be addressed.

Employee attitudes and morale will improve.

Jobs will be secured (through no layoffs) because of increased productivity or quality.

Both sides will have the right to withdraw from the agreement.

resembles a TQM program, the fundamental difference is *power*. The authority of a QWL program to implement

suggestions and influence outcomes is dramatically enhanced through the participation and legitimization of the union. The union is represented on the steering committee and in the role of the facilitator. The union comprises 50% of the steering committee membership and has equal representation in the position of facilitator; typically, one facilitator is selected by the union and one by management. Because union officers frequently are members of the steering committee, and facilitators are highly visible personalities with well-developed human-relations skills and generally accepted by all parties involved, the participants have a greater stake in ensuring the implementation of problem-solving suggestions. This mutual interaction of the union and management results in greater awareness of problems facing the organization and may lead to mutual trust as the process expands and is established throughout the organization. Work-team attitudes should progress from the adversarial win-lose to a cooperative outlook that fosters win-win solutions (Fig. 9-4).

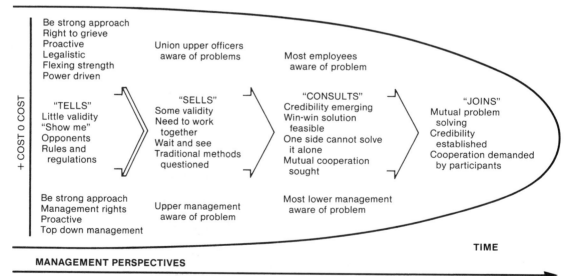

FIGURE 9–4.   Attitudinal evolution of quality work life (QWL) teams. (From Schaupp D, Elkin R: A model of communicating employee responsibility through labor-management participation teams in an organization in financial difficulty. In Chimezie AB, Osigweh Y [eds]: Communicating Employee Responsibilities and Rights, p 183. New York, Quorum Books, 1987)

Implementation and Training

The implementation process relies heavily on training. The intervention strategy most clearly identified with the QWL process is training, which takes two forms: (1) awareness training, which highlights the conceptual background and the need for the program, and (2) training in interpersonal relations and problem-solving skills, focusing on the QWL team. Training by outside consultants and by the coordinators provides the structure that allows the change process to take place. The awareness phase facilitates unfreezing of traditional attitudes. Team training for interpersonal relations and problem-solving skills encourages experimentation with the QWL concept. The positive outcomes experienced by work teams reinforce new attitudes about the process and the two collaborating parties, management and the union.

Examination of the training sequence and the progressive sequential implementation of the QWL process suggests three distinct, yet interrelated, training packages are appropriate (Fig. 9-5). Initially, management and labor must be brought together, preferably off-site, to familiarize themselves with the concept and to attempt to create cohesion between the two parties. The result of this meeting is a joint mission statement of commitment to the concept. Once the mission statement (memorandum of agreement) is completed, the parties select a steering committee with equal representation from both sides. Training is designed to help the steering committee set policy and function as a board of directors for the program. Usually the steering committee is composed of members who represent the leadership of the company and the union so that the need for training in policy formulation and implementation is minimized. Both groups are already familiar with that

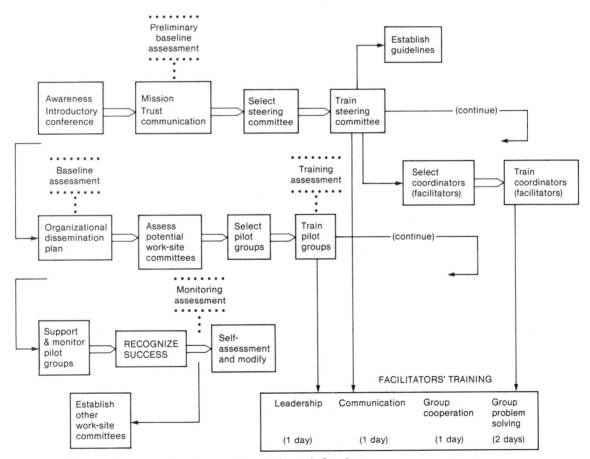

FIGURE 9–5.   Quality of work life (QWL) commitment/pilot study flowchart.

process. However, they usually are unfamiliar with joint problem-solving techniques, and this becomes a major element of their training. At this stage, coordinators are usually selected who attend the steering committee training. Finally, after the pilot teams have been identified, they are trained in group problem-solving skills.

The role of the consultant is very much in evidence during the start-up phase of the program. The initial awareness session and training of the steering committee are usually conducted by an outside consultant. Experience suggests that the two coordinators should conduct the initial QWL training in conjunction with the consultant. This "train the trainers" exercise is a significant factor in arresting any fears the coordinators might have regarding their impending role as trainers. Once pilot groups are in place, the coordinators monitor and evaluate their progress. Initial problems are selected that are relatively easy and solvable to help ensure initial positive outcomes. Thus encouraged, the pilot groups provide internal endorsement of the process and function as catalysts for further implementation.

Training Content and Mechanics

A salient objective of QWL teams is to bring decision making about work-related problems directly to the employees at the work site. Because this decision-making style is probably unfamiliar to most participants, training must include acceptance of the concept, the skills necessary to conduct joint problem solving, and the techniques required to implement the problem's solution. Changing old behaviors and habits is difficult for most adult learners who are not accustomed to a classroom. Therefore, training attempts to integrate the QWL work-team concept with the broad guidelines found in Box 9–3.

With these training prescriptions, the process can be introduced with positive results. The training material is designed to minimize note taking by trainees and is structured to present the essential idea yet allow for note taking should additional information evolve out of group discussion or "lecturettes." The objective is to create a feeling of ownership with the information that is discovered through the training process.

Pitfalls and Conclusions

Experience has shown that the sudden euphoria created during initial implementation results in "backsliding" to more traditional attitudes about institutional

---

Box 9·3

Guidelines for the Quality of Work Life Work Team Concept

Examples must be job specific.

Conceptual ideas must be "discovered" by the participants to enhance ownership by the trainees.

A lecture teaching format is minimized, and group activities are used wherever possible.

Role playing, group involvement, and group discovery are emphasized.

Skills are taught by using an on-the-job training format.

Off-site training is to be encouraged whenever possible.

---

training. Management especially tends to question the expected duration of training. Because most hospitals and institutions conduct training on organizational time, the cost can become problematic. The question often asked by administration is, "Can this process be reduced to 3 days or 2?" To accelerate the process, training often is much reduced in length and intensity over time—in some instances, by almost 50% in the first 6 months of implementation.

Management is aware of the "opportunity cost" associated with training and unfortunately sometimes is seduced by actions suggesting short-term cost-containment at the expense of long-term survival. On the basis of our experience, training still seems to be relegated to specific job-related skills training that stresses "how" instead of "why" things happen as they do in an organization.

Initial success also breeds complacency. Both parties sometimes lose sight of the fact that the QWL process, to be fully implemented in an organization with 700 employees, may take a minimum of 2 years. Both sides desire immediate improvement based on their own time agenda and criteria. Experience has further shown that the organization will have a greater chance for success if it retains an outside consultant who intervenes periodically to provide guidance and encouragement.

Overall, the feeling seems to be that the very least to be expected is significant improvement in communication through sharing of information. Some units experience significant cost reductions, increased morale, and noticeable changes in behavior, suggesting that collaboration occurs in a win-win atmosphere that benefits both sides for long- and short-term survival.

AUTONOMOUS WORK TEAMS

The third and final high-involvement team approach results in problem-solving groups that have significantly greater influence over their work environment than permitted by TQM/QCI, QC, or QWL programs. Although varied levels and degrees of employee prerogatives exist in the management of problem-solving teams, this approach stresses a philosophy that goes beyond the human resources viewpoint presently practiced by participation-oriented organizations.

Autonomous work groups or teams, as a management approach, strive to push knowledge, power, information, and extrinsic rewards to the lowest level of the organization. It is believed that this will increase productivity, employee commitment, and satisfaction. It is assumed that people can be trusted to make important decisions about their work, that their skills in making these decisions can be developed, and that greater organizational effectiveness will result.

Although most laboratory managers would agree with—and even identify with—these assumptions, autonomous work groups formalize them through an organizational structure that complements its philosophic base. Autonomous work groups seem a natural extension of group problem-solving approaches already used in an informal manner in laboratory settings. Variations of this model are used throughout the United States in manufacturing and service industries, with generally impressive results.

As described by Edward E. Lawler III, autonomous work groups are a radical departure from traditional management hierarchies but still fit philosophically with laboratory managers who practice participative management. This method is egalitarian in the sense that it attempts to give important decision-making powers to the individuals directly associated with a task. This means giving as much control as possible to individual work teams that determine almost all boundaries and objectives associated with the task.

A major tenet of this approach is that the team should have some voice in the selection of members, the arrangement of work flow, the establishment of standards for evaluation, and the supervision of quality control and productivity. As much as possible is delegated to the work teams. The teams are entrusted with responsibility to accomplish the activity or group of activities. This means that the teams must assume traditional management responsibilities for production goals, quality, purchasing, control of absenteeism, and performance appraisal. Although the limits and goals may change from team to team, responsibility for getting the job done rests with each team.

Structural Considerations

Because the philosophic basis of this approach is that work should be satisfying, challenging, and motivating, the team is cross-trained for all jobs under its authority. The thinking behind cross-training is that it allows mixing interesting jobs with routine ones and thus creates greater job flexibility. It instills responsibility not only for a specific job, but also for more broadly defined undertakings.

The work team concept can further be reinforced by a compensation structure that is skill based. Although all employees start at the base level of pay (for newly established units), they progress to higher levels of pay on the basis of skills acquired through cross-training. In most teams, for example, team members set standards for appraisal and actually evaluate their coworkers. Usually, all participants are salaried, and the team concept is strongly encouraged. For work teams to function properly, individuals require the knowledge of more than one job.

Other compensation options have been and are continuing to be developed. The challenge is to provide equitable pay based on team output while continuing to meet the needs of individuals. Some systems rely on bonuses based on output of the team, others base pay increases on profit sharing or one of its many forms.

Management

What happens to management? Management survives in a modified form. The management hierarchy is flattened as much as possible. In some organizations, work teams report directly to the unit or divisional manager. In other situations, the first-line supervisor is eliminated, and a key individual is selected by the team to maintain relationships with other lateral units or functional groups. Naturally, the work area and the tasks themselves ultimately determine the limitations of the team's managerial prerogatives.

In many of the newer organizations using a team approach, individual managers are encouraged to think in terms of facilitating organizational and team effectiveness by becoming coaches and counselors who are resources to the teams. Teams tend to need more leadership in the form of coaching, guidance, and direction than do individual employees. Managers begin to work more closely with suppliers in the process to improve availability of resources and remove barriers to the team's effectiveness. The role of the manager shifts from giving direction to providing direction by creating a vision of shared organizational goals.

Managers are still responsible for empowering the teams, building commitment, selling and supporting CQI, and facilitating information flow within and between teams.

Likewise, the staff often is greatly reduced. Because autonomous groups take on many of the duties of traditional support staff members, such as scheduling, purchasing, and inventory control, their function often is absorbed by the team. Not all staff roles are eliminated, but many become consultants to and trainers of teams, rather than decision makers. Increased training is encouraged, not only cross-training to master job-related activities, but also training to aid in self-development and career planning. Off-the-job training also is encouraged and supported.

Although there is no exemplary model that addresses all dimensions and problems encountered by autonomous work teams, the preceding description depicts what is happening in the United States.

Pitfalls and Conclusions

As with most innovative approaches, potential problems and pitfalls are abundant in autonomous teams.

A major problem often occurs with employee expectations: How much participation can be allowed? When does participation turn into permissiveness? What happens to individuals who do not fit into the team concept? What role should key individuals accept as pseudosupervisors? Because the team concept relies heavily on team participation and an understanding of group dynamics, how does an organization handle personnel unable or unwilling to learn interpersonal skills? These questions have not been answered, yet all the evidence suggests that organizations that have begun autonomous work teams also have expanded the program to include other teams.

However, the two most common problems with autonomous work groups appear to be (1) adequate time to meet and perform administrative duties and (2) interpersonal conflict. However, when autonomous work teams are working, productivity gains have been remarkable.

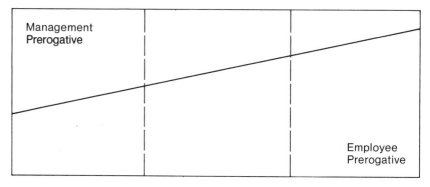

FIGURE 9–6. Employee involvement work groups. (Adapted from Lawler EE III: High-Involvement Management. San Francisco, Jossey-Bass, 1986)

CONCLUSIONS AND SUMMARY

The overwhelming trend in management in the United States indicates a wholesale adaptation of some form of employee-involvement work groups. Although the health-care industry has only recently experimented with participative quality programs, QWL and autonomous work group approaches seem compatible with health-care goals and existing managerial structures. Considering the industry's recent cost-containment emphasis and the general shift to a more competitive environment for clients and services, the health-care industry should seriously consider these approaches to enhance organizational effectiveness and long-run survival.

Depending on existing organizational parameters, managerial philosophy, and employee managerial relationships, some form of employee participation seems feasible (Fig. 9-6). Regardless of which approach is selected, enhanced employee satisfaction and morale are the universal outcomes. Increased productivity, better quality control, lower absenteeism, and lower turnover often accompany improved satisfaction and morale. The degree to which management is willing to empower its employees with managing their work environment determines which approach is selected. The techniques are available. It is up to management to use them for mutual employee–management gain.

REFERENCES

1. Crosby PE: Quality Is Free. New York, Mentor, 1979
2. O'Rourke LM: Exploring the possibilities: The first step in the total quality transformation. The Quality Letter for Healthcare Leaders 4(5):5, 1992
3. Capezio P, Morehouse D: Taking the Mystery Out of TQM. A Practical Guide to Total Quality Management. Franklin Lakes, Career Press, 1993

ANNOTATED BIBLIOGRAPHY

Aubrey CA II, Felkins PK: Teamwork: Involving People in Quality and Productivity Improvement. New York, Quality Press, 1988
    Six chapters of background and "how-to" go about setting up the participative process in an organization. Good section of four pages of references and additional readings. Easily readable; good figures and tables summarize context.
Capezio P, Morehouse D: Taking the Mystery Out of TQM: A Practical Guide to Total Quality Management. Franklin Lakes, Career Press, 1993
    Very practical and applied handbook that is easy to read. Contains questionnaires, surveys, checklists, and good examples.
Juran JM: Juran on Leadership for Quality, An Executive Handbook. New York, The Free Press, 1989
    Management perspective, good overview, easily readable Juran-applied management model.
Juran JM, Grjna FM: Juran's Quality Control Handbook, 4th ed. New York, McGraw-Hill, 1988
    Juran's quintessential, "everything-you-could-ever-want-to-know-about quality," worldwide. Handbook applications in detail; engineering-oriented format. Technical.
Peters T, Austin N: A Passion for Excellence. New York, Random House, 1985
    Examples of leadership excellence in real organizations and situations. Inspiring.
Ryan KD, Oestreich DK: Driving Fear Out of the Workplace. San Francisco, Jossey-Bass, 1991
    Must reading for anyone faced with a quality initiative. Focuses on the "people" motivation and how fear must be addressed before quality, productivity, and innovation can become a part of the organizational culture. Realistic and thought provoking.
Tanner AR, DeToro IJ: Total Quality Management, Three Steps to Continuous Improvement. Reading, Addison-Wesley, 1992
    Offers a systematic approach to applying quality to improve service. Simple, straightforward, easy to apply.
Walton M: The Deming Management Method. New York, Perigee Books, 1986
    Each of the 14 points explored in detail, and applied case studies presented.

10

Conducting Effective Meetings

Janie Brown Crane

Within organizational settings, meetings are essential to effective communication. Individuals must get together to function. They must share information, plan, solve problems, criticize, praise, make new decisions, and find out what went wrong with the old ones. The laboratory manager or supervisor who can conduct an effective meeting to further the objectives of the organization will be one step closer to becoming truly effective in his or her management and supervision.

MEETING PURPOSES

A *meeting* can be defined as that which occurs when three or more people get together with a leader to accomplish an objective. Meetings can be held for various reasons and with an equal variety of objectives. The departmental or staff meeting takes place when the chief calls his or her subordinates together to give them information, solve a problem, get information, or exchange ideas or for a combination of these. The committee or task force, composed of a chairperson and members, meets to accomplish an objective. Training meetings are held for a leader to teach knowledge, skills, attitudes, or a combination of these to a group of students.

More than 11 million meetings are held every day in the United States. It is estimated that middle managers spend 35% of their time in meetings, while the figure for top managers is 50%. Seven to fifteen percent of personnel budgets is spent on meetings, not including preparation time or training programs.

As one can see from these statistics, the meetings should play a significant role in attaining the organizational objectives as set forth. However, many people will voice the opinion that group meetings are held too frequently, take too much time, and do not achieve results. In one survey of 50 hospital administrators, meetings were listed by 34 people as time wasters and

were ranked fourth overall in a list of the biggest time wasters. (Meetings were listed right after telephone interruptions, drop-in visitors, and ineffective delegation.[2])

To avoid these negative attitudes, the laboratory manager or supervisor would be wise to ask, "Is this meeting really necessary?" before proceeding to schedule one. Because laboratory meetings are usually held for the common purposes of information giving, information getting, problem solving, attitude creating, or instruction, one should first examine other communication alternatives. The dissemination of information to employees can be in memo form. If the manager needs to gather information from employees, a questionnaire can be distributed to be returned to the manager, or information from individual employees can be solicited. For problem solving, the manager can again present the problem in memo form and request written suggestions and opinions from individuals. Attitude-creating communication would be more difficult in the written form, but a well-worded explanation or "pep talk" on paper is possible. Instructional communication could be accomplished through individual study followed by written examination, with practical training given on an individual student basis.

By no means is it expected that an organization could do without meetings. However, alternatives to meetings are practical under many circumstances. If the manager uses appropriate alternative methods as feasible, meetings could be held less often. Meetings that are held should be purposeful and necessary for objective accomplishment.

Meeting alternatives would not be wise choices whenever group face-to-face interaction is desired. If memos for information giving or getting require further explanation or the objectives cannot be easily understood, then a meeting should be held. Likewise, group interaction is often necessary for problem solving. This is especially true if members of the group, perhaps representative employees, can help to solve the problem or are needed to carry out the solution. If the manager must sell an idea, a policy, or a decision that has already been made, then an attitude-creating meeting may be the most beneficial communication form. Instructional meetings have the obvious advantage of uniformity, which individual instruction would lack. Group interaction also can save the manager time because he or she will have to present the material and answer questions about it only once.

After the manager determines that the meeting really is necessary, he or she can then ensure that it is a successful, effective one. By allowing an opportunity for interaction, meetings can build group cohesiveness and improve manager–employee relations while accomplishing the objectives.

PLANNING

The first and probably most important step toward conducting effective meetings is planning. It is estimated that 50% of a meeting's effectiveness comes from the mental preparation of the person who wants to have the meeting and the physical preparations made.[3]

The manager must realize that there is a vast difference between simply *scheduling* a meeting and *planning* for that meeting. The role of planning includes establishing the objectives, selecting the participants, distributing the agenda, making the physical arrangements, and considering the psychological forces at work.

It has been said that the better one understands that which he or she is trying to accomplish, the greater one's chances are of accomplishing it. Therefore, objectives should be clearly defined. "To look at overtime in the laboratory" should be rejected in favor of "To find a method of reducing overtime in the laboratory," if indeed it must be reduced. If the manager is holding an information-giving or information-getting meeting, he or she should state clearly what the participants are expected to understand or receive. "To have all participants understand the new dress code" would be better than "To explain the new dress code." Likewise, "To discuss possible causes of employee turnover" would not promote as much thought as "To have each participant contribute at least three possible causes of employee turnover for discussion." Whatever type of meeting the manager decides to hold, he or she should stay with the original objective. If participants are led to believe that they are making problem-solving decisions when actually the manager intends only to gather information to make an independent decision, the participants will soon learn that the manager does not mean

what he or she says and will become disillusioned with future meetings held by that manager.

Once the meeting objective(s) has been established, the manager must give careful consideration to who should attend, because often there is a direct connection between the participants in a meeting and the content and quality of decisions that come from it. If possible, all people who must ultimately approve, accept, or implement a decision should be involved from the beginning in making that decision. Naturally, if the manager is holding a staff or departmental meeting, then all of the designated representatives should be asked to attend. However, when calling a meeting for a specific reason, the manager should pick those who can accomplish the objective. There are several resource individuals who should be included. The person with all the facts is necessary. The idea person who can stimulate thinking and promote discussion is valuable, while the compromiser who is good at keeping the meeting on an even keel is an asset. Of course, the person who can approve the project because of informal power should be included and a key person who could be a barrier to the project. Representatives who could help sell the decision or project to others should also be included.

It is best if the manager can avoid surprise meetings. When possible, a 48-hour notice to the participants of when and where the meeting will be held, how long it will last, and why it is being held should be given. The distribution of the meeting's agenda at the time of notice will also improve meeting success. It must be noted here that objectives and agenda are not the same. Objectives are what is to be accomplished. The agenda consists of individual items to be discussed in consideration of the objectives. "Employee sick leave" would be the entry on the agenda with the objective clarified as "To find a method to reduce sick leave by 4 days/year/employee." The agenda items included at any one meeting should be related if possible and limited to fit into the designated timeframe. When distributing the tentative agenda in advance, the manager may find it helpful to ask for comments or additions before the meeting and to request participants to think about the problem(s) beforehand. The meeting will be better if the participants and the manager are prepared.

The physical preparations for a meeting should receive more attention than is usually given to them. If participants are unhappy about the chosen time, if the room and seating arrangements are uncomfortable, if the leader, chairman, or instructor cannot be easily seen or heard, then the meeting is off to a bad start with a dwindling chance of success. Making the physical preparations is as much the manager's responsibility as establishing objectives. He or she can decide on the basic physical plan and delegate the footwork to some-one else if there are many details to be handled.

The meeting should be scheduled at a time and place convenient for the participants. The manager may be free at 8:30 AM, but this may be a busy time for supervisors and others responsible for getting out the morning work. Therefore, the meeting should be held at a time when the participants are most likely to be relatively free of immediate obligations and can devote their full attention to the matters at hand. Also, the meeting place should be readily accessible. If it must be conducted at a place unfamiliar to the participants, the exact location and directions to get there should be provided.

Despite what many managers may think, the meeting room can be a critical factor. The room selected should fit the participants and be conducive to the type of meeting being held. The room should not be cramped, nor should it be too large. Unfortunately, within the laboratory, there may be only one or two choices of meeting places. For a special meeting, the manager may find it worthwhile to obtain a more desirable room outside the laboratory or to rearrange one of the usual meeting places to make it more suitable. Movable partitions or blackboards can be used to reduce the feeling of a too-large room, and chairs can be rearranged and tables removed from a too-small room. For an information-giving or instructional meeting, chairs should be arranged so that all participants can easily see and hear the leader.

A semicircle or U-shaped arrangement with the leader seated or standing at the edge of the open area is appropriate for information-getting and problem-solving meetings. (This also allows participants to see notes as they are written on the board by the recorder, as is discussed later.)

The meeting room should be adequately ventilated to avoid stuffiness and lingering cigarette smoke. If ventilation is not possible and the meeting will run longer than an hour, short breaks should be permitted. Breaks during long meetings allow participants to get some fresh air and give them a chance to collect their thoughts before the next phase of the meeting. Lighting should be adequate for seeing visual aids and note taking. A dark room may put people to sleep or at least hamper their ability to contribute and understand the material. The area should not be noisy. Extraneous conversations or noise from outside the room would definitely be distracting.

Visual aids may be beneficial to objective accomplishment. People retain about 10% of what is heard and 20% of what is seen but about 50% of what is both heard and seen.[1] However, aids are merely carrier devices for presenting ideas more effectively; the manager should not rely on them exclusively for making important points. If a visual aid is used, it should convey only one idea so that participants can keep their focus on the topic under discussion and not on the aid itself.

Just prior to meeting time, the manager or designee should check to make sure the physical preparations are complete. Electrical outlets for projectors and microphones should be tested, and lighting and seating arrangements should be checked. If needed, chalk for use at the blackboard, marking pens and paper for the recorder, and handouts should be ready. A meeting that is delayed or hampered because of the physical factors is likely to produce less than optimum results.

Finally, after the manager has completed the mental preparation and has made all of the physical arrangements, he or she should examine the psychological forces that will influence the progress and outcome of the meeting. This may be the most difficult aspect of planning, but a necessary one, especially for problem-solving and attitude-creating meetings. If the manager is aware of and has given consideration to the hidden agendas at work, the chances of conducting the meeting effectively will improve. The psychological forces that determine a person's behavior deserve more attention than can be given here; however, they are briefly discussed to help the manager understand the attitudes displayed and the positions expressed at a meeting.

An individual's hidden agendas are composed of external and internal pressures (Fig. 10-1). Pressure is not used here in the negative sense but as a feeling that has an impact on the group and its ideas. External pressures may be groups to which one is affiliated, such as unions, social organizations, or political groups; past commitments made that have an effect on current behavior; personal life forces; and forces that exist because of the person's relationship with the organization. Internal pressures are generated by the individual's own goals and aspirations. An example of these hidden agendas at work would be the different reactions of two participants to the problem of excessive overtime in the laboratory. One person might defend overtime on the basis of its necessity to provide proper patient service, when subconsciously that person is concerned about personal loss of income needed to support his or her family. On the other hand, another person might express beliefs that schedules and shifts could be rearranged to reduce overtime, when actually the concern is to protect his or her next-in-line position as a manager.

There is little the manager can do to control these hidden agendas. However, knowledge of the participants and awareness of the forces behind them will help the manager evaluate contributions made at meetings. Recognizing that everyone in the organization is influenced by a hidden agenda permits the manager to look beyond surface expressions or actions and attempt to determine the motivations underlying them.

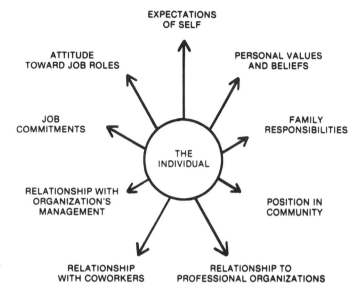

FIGURE 10–1.   Hidden agendas—factors influencing a participant's contribution in a meeting.

CONDUCTING THE MEETING

The manager should insist on prompt attendance and start the meeting on time. A delay in starting penalizes those who arrive on time and rewards latecomers. If staff meetings are known to start late, participants will soon stop coming on time, and more time will be wasted waiting for everyone to assemble. Interruptions other than extreme emergencies should not be allowed. If someone outside of the meeting can screen calls and take messages, the meeting will run more smoothly. When participants must come and go, it is distracting to others, and they must catch up on the discussion on their return, usually by whispering with a neighbor.

Participants should arrive at the meeting with the initial attitude of enthusiasm. This eagerness should have been generated by the manager during the planning phase when he or she notified participants of the meeting and its purpose, but it will wain unless the manager is able to maintain it. Leadership style, which is discussed separately, and ability to maintain control of the meeting once the participants are involved are important in keeping interest and enthusiasm.

The technique of conducting an effective meeting is essentially a technique of communication. In reference to this point, Benjamin Franklin is purported to have said, "If you state an opinion dogmatically, which is in direct opposition to my thought, and you imply no room for negotiation, then I must conclude in order to protect my own self-esteem that you are wrong, and I will immediately undertake to prove you wrong. On the other hand, if you state your opinion as a hypothe-

sis, with evidence of a willingness to discuss and explore, I will like as not undertake to prove you correct."

The wise manager will keep this in mind not only for himself or herself, but also for participant interaction. Each person should feel that his or her ideas are welcome, should be given credit for them, and even more importantly, that an occasional useless idea will not bring disgrace. The more opportunity participants have to incorporate their ideas and suggestions in a decision, the greater is their emotional ownership in it and the harder they will work to make it succeed.

As the meeting begins, the manager should clearly define the objective(s) and the method the group should undertake for its accomplishment. It is extremely important that the manager distinguish between *process,* how the problem is solved, and *content,* the problem and its solution. Once this is clearly established, it is still the manager's responsibility to see that the meeting stays on track.

If the meeting is for information or problem solving, the manager must elicit free and creative suggestions from the participants. To do so, criticism or comment, which might inhibit imaginative suggestions, should be withheld. Participant interaction should also be controlled to protect individuals from attack by others. If participants feel inhibited or that their ideas will be ridiculed, they will be less likely to contribute. When seeking information and involvement, it is better to use "overhead" questions so a volunteer can answer. The asking of direct questions should be used sparingly to avoid embarrassment if the participant does not know the answer. The manager should not dominate the meeting or allow one participant to dominate the discussion, because other participants will become resentful. Wandering from the agenda should not be allowed. The manager should expect and demand adherence to it. He or she should also be aware of and resist hidden agenda ploys. Socializing and allowing interruptions will cause the meeting to get off track. Unnecessary prolonging of a meeting causes participants to lose interest and hence should be avoided.

Although it is the manager's responsibility to stimulate and balance the discussion, healthy differences of opinion are not necessarily discouraged. A certain degree of conflict can play a constructive and positive role in fostering creativity and innovation. Some friction between participants creates an atmosphere conducive to the generation of fresh ideas. A conflict-free group may be static and operate at considerably less than capacity.

The manager's aim in reaching the objective should be to obtain a win-win solution through consensus. If it becomes apparent to the group that consensus cannot be reached despite meaningful discussion, then a decision made by the manager will be accepted more readily. At the meeting's conclusion, the manager should restate the objectives, summarize the accomplishments, thank participants for their contribution, and give assignments and announcements if appropriate. The participants should leave feeling glad that they attended. They will be more likely to accept and react positively to the decisions made if they felt the meeting was worthwhile.

The manager's job in conducting a meeting does not end when the meeting is concluded. The manager must now provide a record of what happened, follow up on decisions made, and evaluate the meeting to upgrade future ones.

A summary or minutes should be distributed if the manager wants the participants to have a record of decisions made and assignments given, if he or she needs to communicate with those who did not attend, or if the participants want a summary for their files or a clarification of what happened. The summary should state concisely the decisions made, the assignments and deadlines made, and any unfinished business to be taken up at another meeting. It should be distributed within 1 day of the meeting while it is still fresh in the participants' minds.

The manager must follow up to ensure that the decisions made are carried through and set deadlines for their implementation. Often decisions that involve policy changes or major operational changes will require another meeting to determine the implementation method, if time and resources did not permit that at the meeting in which the decision was made. If assignments to individuals were made, he should request progress reports at set intervals to ensure timely implementation of decisions.

The meeting should be evaluated. The real importance of a meeting must be judged by the results obtained from it; therefore, a meeting that produces no results fails and probably should not have been held in the first place. Opinions differ as to what constitutes a "productive" meeting. One set of criteria by which to judge the meeting would be to ask the following: Were the objectives accomplished? Were they accomplished in minimum time? Are the participants satisfied? If the objectives were not accomplished, the manager must investigate why. The information obtained may help to plan and improve the next meeting and better the chances of achieving objective accomplishment. If the meeting exceeded the established time limit, the manager must evaluate the process of the meeting. There may have been too many items on the agenda, or perhaps the manager's ability to maintain control needs improvement. It is more difficult to judge the impact and significance of dissatisfied participants. The manager must try to assess why they were dissatisfied. Meetings that leave participants unhappy or frustrated about the decisions made might cause them not to attend future meetings; to decide the manager is ineffective, thereby affecting future relationships; or to carry negative attitudes and low morale back to their jobs. If in evaluating the meeting, the manager cannot say that the meeting accomplished its objectives in minimum time with satisfied participants, he or she should seriously review all phases of planning and conducting a meeting so that the same problems will not recur. Table 10–1 summarizes the most common hurdles the manager must overcome to turn nonproductive meetings into productive ones.

AVOIDING NONPRODUCTIVE MEETINGS

Many of the solutions to causes of nonproductive meetings are straightforward and can be handled by the manager with practice once he or she recognizes their importance. Planning for the meeting is time consuming but can be accomplished efficiently if the manager takes all of the planning factors into account. After the meeting, the manager should be able to follow through by distributing minutes and establishing a method for implementation of any decisions made. However, as is the case for managers of almost any group or organization, laboratory supervisors will probably find actually conducting the meeting to be their downfall. Conducting an effective meeting is easier said than done. For practical purposes, this discussion is the problem-solving meeting, the one most likely to cause frustration in laboratory operations and employee relations.

Usually when a staff or special meeting is held, one or more entries on the agenda deal with a problem. Topics such as vacation coverage, physician overuse

Table 10-1
Causes and Solutions to Nonproductive Meetings

Causes	Solutions
Before the Meeting	
Lack of purpose	Hold meetings only when there is a definable, managerial purpose to be served in doing so.
Participants who do not want to come or are unprepared	Create enthusiasm—distribute agenda when giving notice; explain benefits of attendance; set convenient time and place in comfortable surroundings.
Lack of planning	Allow for and schedule appropriate planning.
Wrong participants	Include only those who are needed.
Not starting on time	Start on time.
During the Meeting	
Objectives unclear	Clarify objectives early in the meeting.
Participants disinterested, confused	Create enthusiasm—use understandable language; clarify as necessary.
Socializing, interruptions	Do not allow interruptions.
Wandering from agenda	Keep discussion under control.
Indecision	Keep objectives in mind, and work toward them.
Too much time spent on each subject; meeting too long	Set realistic time limits; keep meeting moving.
No summary	Summarize so participants are clear about what is to happen.
After the Meeting	
No minutes	Record and distribute minutes within 1 d.
Failure to follow up	Make assignments and check up on implementation.
Participants unhappy	Determine causes of dissatisfaction and correct for future meetings.
No meeting evaluation	Evaluate meeting to improve future ones.

of stat requests, and technologists' call-in policies are common examples. The typical way the problem is handled is played out in Box 10–1.

At this typical meeting, potentially good ideas are immediately judged, found to be faulty in some way, and then dismissed. The person who contributed an idea feels that he or she has been personally attacked and is more likely to tear down another idea if it is suggested by the person who attacked his or her idea. The meeting can easily get off track, good solutions can be ignored, and the meeting may end with the manager saying he or she will have to think about it. Participants leave not knowing what will happen, and the final solution to the problem may be less than satisfactory to all concerned.

To avoid these problems and conduct an effective meeting, the manager should consider the new interaction method as described by Doyle and Straus.[1] It is a method by which several people play roles that aid in separating the meeting process from its content, thus keeping the discussion focused on the objective. With this method, a facilitator is appointed who is neutral and nonevaluating. It is this person's job to make sure that participants use the most effective methods to accomplish their task in the shortest time. He or she helps the group decide on how they will solve the problem and then sees to it that they stay on track. It is also the facilitator's job to protect participants from being attacked by others. The group will need a short-term memory so everyone will record the same events in the same way. The recorder does this by writing the group memory on the blackboard or on large sheets of paper that are then posted on the wall in everyone's view. It is the manager/chairperson's and participants' responsibility to make sure that the facilitator does not manipulate the group and that the recorder's record is kept accurately. The manager/chairperson should keep the group focused on the agenda, set realistic time limits, and be aware of the organizational constraints when it comes to making final decisions (Box 10–2).

After the 10 ideas are amassed, the feasibility of each idea is discussed. The manager inputs advice if a possible solution could not be contained within the budget, within legal limits, and so forth. Because the ideas are recorded first and discussed later, participants forget who suggested what idea, and rejection of an idea is not taken personally. Because they are all on visual display, ideas can be combined until a workable solution is found.

If during the meeting, the facilitator or recorder wants to contribute as a participant, he or she can request of the manager to step out of the role temporarily, say what he or she has to say, and then go back to the role. If available, the manager can have individuals not involved in the problem-solving play the roles of facilitator and recorder.

At the conclusion of the meeting, the manager summarizes the decisions, states what will happen next, and then proceeds as discussed previously.

Portions of this imaginary meeting express another idea useful to the manager for problem solving. Even if the new interaction method is not used in its entirety, brainstorming is a useful tool. *Brainstorming* is a technique of problem solving in which a group of people gather and contribute ideas spontaneously, hoping to find the solution they could not find alone. Quantity of ideas is important, freewheeling is encouraged, and "piggybacking" (building on someone else's idea) is welcomed. Evaluation and judgment are reserved until all ideas are amassed.

Box 10•1

Typical Discussion of Problem at a Meeting

Manager: As everyone knows, Sam (*the only night-shift technician*) is quitting at the end of the month. It will take at least 6 weeks to hire and orient a new tech. How do you propose we cover during the interim?

Supervisor 1: Maybe a tech from each days-shift section could rotate onto nights for a week at a time.

Supervisor 2: There's no way I can have someone from my section rotate onto nights. I'll be short staffed because of vacations all summer as it is.

Evening Supervisor: (*getting off track*) I think we ought to hire two night-shift techs so we don't keep running into this problem every time someone on second or third shift quits.

Box 10•2

Sample New Interaction Method as Described by Doyle and Straus

Manager: As everyone knows, Sam (*the only night-shift technician*) is quitting at the end of the month. It will take at least 6 weeks to hire and orient a new tech. We need to discuss how to cover during the interim. Facilitator, how do we begin?

Facilitator: We could try kicking out some ideas for the recorder to write down. After we have a list of 10, we could mix and match them and come up with a workable solution. Does everyone agree: (*Heads nod in agreement.*) OK, then, let's try to come up with the 10 ideas in 5 minutes. Remember, no evaluation until the recorder has all 10 down. Ready? Who's first?

Supervisor 1: Maybe a tech from each day-shift section could rotate onto nights for a week at a time. (*Recorder writes down this idea.*)

Supervisor 2: (*jumping in*) There's no way I can have someone from my section rotate onto nights. I'll be short staffed because of vacations all summer as it is.

Facilitator: Wait a minute, Number 2, you may have a valid point, but we'll discuss the feasibility of each idea after we have them all listed. Who's next?

Evening Supervisor: Overtime might be a possibility. Some techs on second shift have expressed interest in it.

Facilitator: OK. Anyone else? We need eight more ideas.

In reality, brainstorming is difficult to practice. Because people are taught to evaluate an idea immediately, they hold back if they do not think their contribution will be accepted or if they feel they might be ridiculed. The manager may be able to overcome resistance to the brainstorming approach by having the group practice with an imaginary problem. Everyone must be aware that brainstorming does not solve the problem; it is only one step in the process.

EFFECTIVE LEADERSHIP

Most laboratory managers and supervisors are unschooled in communications. They have spent many years concentrating on the subject matter of their profession and have not had the time or opportunity to devote to developing communication skills. Also, many managers and supervisors have reached their present positions because of their technical abilities or their rapport with fellow workers and supervisors. A person who can function well at the technical and production aspects of a job does not necessarily possess the attributes necessary to handle the managerial duties of a supervisory position. Suddenly, on promotion or transfer from a staff technical position to a managerial or supervisory role, the individual is faced with problems and situations requiring good communication skills. It is no wonder that laboratory meetings held to give or get information, solve problems, give instruction, or sell decisions already made may be less than effective.

Meeting success rests heavily on effective leadership. In all meeting types, the leader (manager) has the same responsibility and accountability to conduct a productive meeting. He or she must be able to get things done through people. To do so, the leadership style must be adapted to fit the type of meeting to make the meeting as fruitful as possible. To provide information, an autocratic-type style is necessary for presenting and explaining directives without receiving any feedback. When collecting information, the manager will need to share the leadership to increase participation and stimulate the group to be able to gather as much data as possible. For decision making, the leadership is again shared because each participant's ideas are important to the final decision. Decision selling is a combination of the previous characteristics: autocratic with regard to the decision but shared leadership with regard to carrying out the decision. Meetings held for problem solving also involve shared leadership to use all resources available.

Another option for the manager to consider in leadership styles is to step down temporarily and allow someone else to chair the meeting if he or she has a stake in the decision. The conflict of running the meeting and having a personal stake in the outcome can lower participation and cause the process to control the content.

There are several basic "do's" and "don't's" to effective meeting leadership. Some have been discussed but merit reiteration. The Boy Scout motto, "Be prepared," is of prime importance. Without proper planning, there is no point in having the meeting. The manager should not bluff if he or she does not know the subject. Adequate research beforehand should alleviate this problem. Dominating the meeting discussion or allowing one participant to dominate will intimidate other participants, who will then be less likely to contribute. The manager should never appear to resent questions or comments or criticize individuals publicly. The impact of that type of behavior is evident. When giving technical information or holding a discussion with participants who do not know the background material, the manager must be sure to use language that is understandable. Maintaining tact while thwarting off-track discussions and side conversations will be beneficial to meeting progress. Finally, steering the participants to come to some positive conclusion so that they leave the meeting feeling that something has been accomplished is most important.

The more skillful one becomes at conducting meetings, the more critical one becomes of meetings. Therefore, the manager will find that effective leadership characteristics will be beneficial when attending meetings as a participant. The manager should know why he or she was asked to participate and be prepared to the fullest extent possible. The manager should arrive on time, stay on the subject under discussion, and remain open to the ideas of others. The manager should be able to identify with the leader's role and therefore not cause problems. On the contrary, he or she should be able to help the leader maintain control of the meeting by using leadership skills. As a listener, taking notes during the meeting will force the manager to keep his or her mind on the topic and be able to contribute more fully as a participant.

REFERENCES

1. Doyle M, Straus D: How to Make Meetings Work, The New Interaction Method, pp 4, 264. Ridgefield, Wyden Books, 1976
2. Kirkpatrick DL: How to Plan and Conduct Productive Business Meetings, p 29. Chicago, Dartnell Corporation, 1976
3. Lewis PV: Organizational Communications: The Essence of Effective Management, p 187. Columbus, Grid Inc, 1975

11

Management of Conflict and Change

Dietrich L. Schaupp • Barbara L. Parsons

Recently a sage remarked that the only truism about change is that it is constant. The same could be said about conflict. Both change and conflict have consumed the minds of some of the world's great thinkers, yet a casual survey of writings on management indicates that much more remains to be said.

Contemporary writing in both change and conflict suggests that the process is still not totally understood. This chapter provides a general discussion of what recent writers think about change and conflict and how this information might be used in the workplace.

At the outset we make several assumptions:

1. Change and conflict are inevitable in normal organizational behavior.
2. Responsibility for initiating change and maintaining an acceptable level of conflict lies with the laboratory manager.
3. The laboratory manager works toward the goals of the organization.

We will look at change and conflict from management's perspective.

CHANGE AND CONFLICT ARE NATURAL

The assumption that change and conflict are inevitable suggests that they are a natural outgrowth of the managerial process. Regardless of hierarchical level or specialty, a manager must perform the basic functions of planning, organizing, staffing, directing, and controlling. He or she is expected to manage these functions and at the same time, meet the organization's demands.

It is impossible to manage these functions without introducing change into the work environment. Change inevitably elicits some form of opposition, either from subordinates or from others directly or indirectly involved with the goals or objectives of the organization.

The novice manager often feels that the problems he faces are unique to his setting and situation. Although human relationships and the working environment do interact to create totally individual situations, the underlying causes and solutions to these problems are often very similar.

Once the manager realizes that change and conflict are a natural phenomenon in the management process, he can facilitate change and control conflict with minimal disruption and opposition. The effective manager will integrate the needs and desires of subordinates with the goals and aims of the organization.

THE LABORATORY AS AN ORGANIZATIONAL ENTITY

The medical laboratory exists to provide a service. In general, its staff performs a variety of anatomic and pathologic services that range from routine medical procedures to highly complex research. Whatever its specific responsibilities, the laboratory provides a valuable diagnostic function in the health-care process.

Because the laboratory is an essential element of modern diagnostic and therapeutic hospital services, it is usually an important subunit of the hospital's organizational structure. A hospital is composed of a triad: the governing board (also called the board of trustees, board of directors, board of councillors, or some other variation), the administrator, and the medical staff. Authority is organized along two lines: administrative and professional.

The governing board provides overall objectives and legal responsibility for the institution, but it is removed from direct participation in hospital operation. Administrative authority extends from the governing board through the administrator to the various department heads. Department heads include the controller, housekeeping manager, laundry manager, engineer, purchasing agent, laboratory manager, and so on.

The administrator relinquishes authority for direct patient care to the medical staff. Functions associated

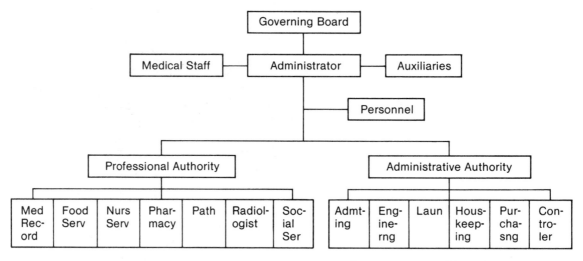

FIGURE 11–1. Typical hospital organization chart.

with providing patient care include nursing service, pharmacy, pathology, social service, medical records, and food service.

The administrative side of a hospital deals with day-to-day survival of the institution, and the professional side deals with patient care and treatment. This is a simplified view of a hospital, and the structure may vary depending on size and objective, but even this superficial overview makes it readily apparent that the administration of a hospital is difficult and complex.

As Figure 11–1 illustrates, the hospital laboratory is only one subfunction of the organized medical staff. It functions in harmony and competition with the other subunits in the organization while concentrating on its own objectives. It is usually subordinated to pathology, and its organization chart may resemble the one shown in Figure 11–1.

A medical laboratory may also be a separate entity that provides diagnostic services to medical institutions and physicians. In this instance, the laboratory is unencumbered by the multiple demands of the health-care process usually associated with hospitals. When it is a separate business, the laboratory has great autonomy and operates under the profit orientation of its owners. Whether part of a hospital or a separate financial entity, the medical laboratory is subject to change and conflict that will ensure its survival or demise.

Forces for Change

No laboratory functions in a vacuum. The laboratory must seek sustenance in the form of clients, scarce financial resources, personnel, and equipment to com-

plete its mission. To survive, it must be aware of its environment. A chief characteristic of that environment, and of all modern society, is change. The laboratory manager must possess the ability to recognize needed change and act accordingly.

Twenty years ago, few would have imagined that court rulings regarding medical malpractice suits would precipitate the onslaught of demand for laboratory services. A laboratory's external world is highly volatile. In general, any manager must acknowledge the four broad areas of change found in Box 11–1.

A closer look at the four areas of change reveals that factors affecting change also occur within the orga-

---

Box 11•1

Four Broad Areas of Change

1. The challenge of increased revenue production coupled with cost containment and high quality standards
2. The increasing trend for advanced education and training, coupled with employee aspirations for more interesting work and advancement
3. The accelerating demand for employee loyalty to the organization relative to the societal changes occurring in the marketplace
4. The problem of unionization and employees' demands for more rewards—financial and psychological—from their work environment

nization. For example, most middle managers are acutely attuned to personnel shifts that might affect their ability to manage their work groups. These changes may be drastic or subtle. In any case, the manager is aware that these forces exist and that he must deal with or diffuse them.

Most managers, after studying their internal and external environments, are able to distinguish between changes that will impede or enhance their ability to manage their own work unit. However, the ability to distinguish between the changes that are superficial or negligible and those that might have a major impact comes only with experience and knowledge of the process of change.

TRYING TO UNDERSTAND CHANGE AND CONFLICT

Faced with forces for change, the supervisor is caught in a dilemma. On one hand, based on his knowledge of the work environment, the manager realizes that there are compelling reasons for change. On the other hand, he realizes that organizations and the people in them tend to perform most efficiently under stable and predictable conditions. If the manager changes the work environment too much, he risks unexpected and detrimental outcomes. If he does not react to the demands of change, he may jeopardize the survival of his laboratory.

The laboratory manager must also function as a problem finder. He must not only react to change, but he must also identify and plan for change. He must realize that a planned program for change allows greater control and flexibility for the laboratory. To achieve control and flexibility, the manager must initiate change and function as an agent of change.

Change forces are not often of equal intensity or attractiveness; moreover, they are not always intense enough to be recognized nor attractive enough to prompt action. However, feeling compelled to make changes that are unwarranted is as dangerous as failing to recognize the need for change. Too much change may be as dangerous as too little.

A clearer understanding of change and conflict is possible with a motivational explanation. In the individual motivation process, needs create drives that lead to the accomplishment of goals. A need or deficiency is created where there is some form of psychological or physical imbalance. The need then manifests itself in some form of action or direction that is directed toward a goal that satisfies the initial imbalance. Although we recognize that such an explanation is clearly simplistic, it is a basic explanation of behavioral change.

Carrying the motivational model a step further, we find an explanation for conflict. Conflict occurs when

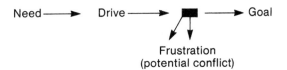

FIGURE 11–2. A simple model of frustration.

something or someone erects a barrier that does not allow attainment of the goal (Fig. 11-2). The barrier creates frustrations that may lead to a variety of defense mechanisms.

Conflict, then, occurs when an individual encounters some form of opposition in his motivational cycle. The barrier may be physical (outward) or psychological (inward). These frustrations are not necessarily negative from an organizational standpoint. For example, a manager who is rejected for promotion may not react defensively but may be spurred on to greater and better performance to achieve a denied objective.

So far we have implied that the individual process of change begins in the motivational cycle and is somehow linked with conflict. The cause–effect relationship between change and conflict is not that simple, however; most evidence today suggests that we still do not clearly understand this relationship.

The practicing manager is bombarded every day with a multitude of factors that he must evaluate before making a decision. We do not clearly understand how a manager weighs his decisions concerning strategy for action because individual values and perceptions vary. We will assume, however, that whatever course of action he pursues will take into consideration the long- and short-run survival of his work unit or laboratory. Therefore, we will assume that the change/conflict process within an organization or organizational subunit will be influenced, and to a certain degree managed, by the individual most responsible for its direction: the manager (Fig. 11-3).

Quite simply, the association between change and conflict generates some action or reaction that will ultimately change the human, technologic, or structural elements of the work unit to ensure its survival. However, the underlying managerial questions still remain: When should I change? How should I go about it? How does the change process work? To help the manager answer these questions, Edgar H. Schein offers the observations[10] in Box 11–2.

The Change Sequence

To manipulate change, the manager must understand the sequence of change. There is nothing so frustrating to a manager as to examine his action in retrospect and

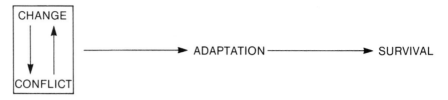

FIGURE 11–3.   Change/conflict survival model. (Adapted from Robbins SP: The Administrative Process, p. 343. Englewood Cliffs, Prentice-Hall, 1980)

conclude that he should have pursued a different course of action. It is easy to analyze actions in retrospect, but it is quite difficult to decide what should be done when confronted with external and internal forces for change. Understanding how far he has progressed through the change sequence can help the manager make that initial decision. Figure 11–4 shows one interpretation of this process.

The key to surviving in an organization is how well one reads the forces for change, not necessarily how actively one pursues change. Many managers are successful without being preoccupied with the change process. Also, many effective managers exert minimal influence on the functioning of their units, while others constantly initiate new programs and implement new procedures. To suggest that one style is correct and the other wrong would be foolhardy. Each may reflect the forces demanding change in their respective working units. Some units function effectively in a very turbulent environment, while others function better in a calm and stable environment.

Complacency can also be a problem. After initial attempts to improve his unit's efficiency, a manager eventually realizes that organizational barriers affect his ability to improve productivity and employee morale. Coupled with an organizational culture that discourages change, the manager often becomes complacent about the operation of his work unit and lapses into a management style that encourages the status quo.

The manager must possess curiosity, discontent, open-mindedness, and self-respect to be able to recognize the need for change.[1] He must understand and recognize the attitudes that are most conducive to change. The manager should question himself about how something can be done more effectively or why something happens. He should be dissatisfied with complacency or the "tried and true" method and seek ways to improve the functioning of his unit. A commitment to continuous quality improvement (CQI) fosters and supports a proactive manager.

The manager should be open to suggestions from sources other than his own experience and intellect. True open-mindedness is the realization that good ideas and suggestions also reside among subordinates. An effective change agent fosters communication from all levels of the hierarchy. TQM demands this participation.

Ultimately, the manager must have a genuine respect for his own abilities. Many managers ignore changes that evoke initial resistance when implemented. It is easier to submit to the status quo than initiate a procedure that might elicit short-run resistance. The successful manager overcomes the pressures to maintain the status quo by learning to manage the conflict of change effectively.

Having concluded that change is necessary, the manager must decide what type of change strategy

---

Box 11·2

Schein's Observations on the Underlying Managerial Questions

1. Any change process involves not only learning something new, but unlearning something that is already present and possibly well integrated in the personality and social relationships of the individual.
2. No change will occur unless there is motivation to change, and if such motivation to change is not already present, the induction of that motivation is often the most difficult part of the change process.
3. Organizational changes, such as new structures, processes, reward systems, and so on, occur only through individual changes by key members of the organization.
4. Most adult change involves attitudes, values, and self-images. The unlearning of present responses in these areas is initially and inherently painful and threatening.
5. Change is a multistage behavior modification cycle that is complex and requires a systematic approach.

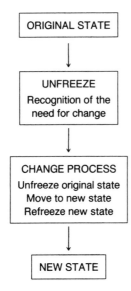

```
┌─────────────────────────┐
│     ORIGINAL STATE      │
└─────────────────────────┘
            │
            ▼
┌─────────────────────────┐
│        UNFREEZE         │
│   Recognition of the    │
│     need for change     │
└─────────────────────────┘
            │
            ▼
┌─────────────────────────┐
│     CHANGE PROCESS      │
│  Unfreeze original state│
│    Move to new state    │
│   Refreeze new state    │
└─────────────────────────┘
            │
            ▼
┌─────────────────────────┐
│        NEW STATE        │
└─────────────────────────┘
```

FIGURE 11–4. The change sequence.

should be used. The objective of the change process is the survival of the organization. Many recent change methods advocate a participatory approach, which involves both the management hierarchy and subordinates. This approach facilitates ownership and acceptance of the change process by the participating parties. Chapter 9 addressed TQM, CQI, and other participative processes that are effective in introducing organizational change. Many organizational-development, sensitivity-training, and management-development programs reflect this philosophy. Other change techniques exist and are discussed later in this chapter.

The Change Process

The change process is a difficult one. Trying to change individual human behavior is very hard. Changing the behavior of an entire work group is even more difficult, but it begins with changes in individuals. For individuals to internalize and accept change, a three-step sequence must occur: The individual must *reject* the old pattern or behavior, *move* to the new one, and ultimately *accept* the new behavior.

The first stage can be characterized as unfreezing the existing status quo. This step forces a person to unlearn or alter his way of thinking. He must be made aware of why his behavior may be ineffective, unproductive, or outmoded. This stage reduces the forces for resistance, and the person experiences doubt about his way of thinking. For example, medical technologists

might be given information about a new testing procedure that promises higher productivity. To overcome resistance to change, the technologist must be convinced that this procedure is superior to the existing one and that using the new procedure benefits him. In other words, he must be provided information by the manager to combat any resistance.

After a person rejects old behaviors, he must be persuaded to adopt new behavior. This starts the second step, the period of change or transition. At this stage, individuals should be willing to give the new procedure a try.

Through identification and internalization mechanisms, the manager can move individuals toward acceptance of new behavior. For example, the manager might reveal that the new procedure is used by other, very prestigious laboratories (identification) and suggest that his technologists try it to see how they like it (internalization). In this stage, the manager can facilitate the process by providing genuine two-way communication with subordinates. For example, he can provide information and guidance regarding the new procedure, but the employees should be encouraged to make suggestions and contribute to the change process. This might mean modification or reformulation of the procedure to meet the demands of the employees. The manager must also be malleable about the new procedure—after all, the objective of the process is the acceptance of the new procedure.

The third step is sometimes identified as the refreezing stage: The individual internalizes the new behavior, and it becomes part of his daily life. In our example, the technologists have accepted the new procedure. Reinforcement occurs through their own perceptions of its advantages and through information supplied by the manager about increased productivity, greater reliability, lower cost, and so on. It is important in this stage that the change is not extinguished. Tʰ environment must remain rewarding to the individuₐ who have adopted the change; if the environment doeₛ not continue to be rewarding, old behaviors may resurface. People tend to repeat behavior that is rewarding.

Diagnosing Resistance

Understanding the change process does not guarantee acceptance of change. In some instances, the most improbable changes initiated by management are embraced cheerfully by work units. In other instances, change programs have been initiated with disastrous results. Often, the programs that management thought would be accepted with enthusiasm fail badly. Why does one change strategy succeed, and others, with seemingly meritorious objectives, fail?

The answer may lie in change strategy selection and available information about possible resistance to the change. The manager must think through possible implications for the work unit before he implements any change that affects it. A manager must assess the change process in light of potential overt and covert resistance. Furthermore, he must consider the ramifications of the change itself.

Often, a change strategy is adopted because it seems to work somewhere else; however, what is feasible in one work unit does not guarantee success in another. The manager who bases change on his own environment has a greater chance for success. One way to increase the probability of success is to be aware of factors that might cause resistance to change. Although one could compile numerous factors, the obvious ones appear to be insecurity, social and economic costs, union intervention, and the reduction of autonomy.

Insecurity

Change inherently creates feelings of uncertainty and anxiety. Humans are creatures of habit. The person who has ample experience with and knowledge of one job procedure often exhibits inflexibility regarding a job change. It is quite logical that someone who has achieved status and recognition in a position would be threatened by a change in which the outcome is uncertain. An employee may feel threatened if he believes that changes may cause him to lose face or be inconvenienced. Many employees are "organization-wise." They think that management transforms "harmless changes" into more work, inconvenience, or loss of status. A good laboratory manager should never allow a technologist to equate change with insecurity. The field of laboratory medicine is dynamic; every professional who practices in the field of medicine must be continually exposed to change and made to feel comfortable with it.

Social and Economic Costs

Change may also demand social and economic costs. As employees orient themselves to their work environments, they establish elaborate social relationships with their coworkers and superiors. Cliques and informal work groups emerge. A sense of security, identity, and belonging exists with membership in a group. If change of one form or another threatens this relationship, workers will resist that change. For example, the introduction of a new testing procedure is often resisted by the people who are most familiar with the weakness of the old method. However, these people will attack the new procedure for a variety of reasons. The real reason, however, may be that the new procedure means different working hours, destruction of the existing work group, or the possibility of having to report to someone else. These negative responses are mere symptoms of the underlying social threat to the individual or the work group.

Likewise, the economic costs associated with change should be confronted. Individuals are extremely sensitive to anything that affects their income, especially if the income is a reflection of status or recognition. Economic costs may include replacement of an employee by more efficient technology or rejection of a new work schedule because it entails higher parking costs.

The Union

The relationship between union and management is the pivotal issue in the introduction of change. If both sides trust each other and there is harmonious cooperation, resistance to change is significantly reduced. The degree of resistance is often determined by past experiences, and it is critical that the manager understand the political dimensions of the union hierarchy. He cannot and should not expect to win approval of every proposal of plan of action that he presents to the union. Neither should a proposal be submitted only once if there is some possibility of finding a way to effect change that satisfies both sets of needs.

Reduction of Autonomy

An increase in control or accountability will usually be resisted by a technologist. No one likes to be evaluated if the evaluation takes the form of closer supervision or the reduction of discretionary decision making. Employees often interpret closer control as a lack of trust by management.

Likewise, if a work-related task that requires some form of judgment and skill is redesigned as a routine, repetitive task, the laboratory manager should expect resistance. This is especially true for tasks that have been assigned high status and prestige.

A Framework for Analysis

Diagnosis and Implementation

Before implementing a change process, a manager must have a clear understanding of what he wants to accomplish. Hersey and Blanchard indicate that the manager must have or be able to obtain the necessary skills to diagnose and implement the change process.[3] The success of a change process hinges on diagnosis and implementation skills.

In Hersey and Blanchard's model, diagnosis is the critical first step of any successful change process. The manager evaluates what is *likely* to happen if change does not occur, what *ideally* should happen, and what forces of resistance could block the actual from becoming the ideal. If there is a discrepancy between the actual and the ideal, the question, "Should I change something?" is answered—"Yes."

In reality, the answer may not be so simple. Hersey and Blanchard point out, for example, that the diagnostic phase is essentially an evaluation stage. The manager must correctly read the organizational and human variables that may impede or encourage the change process. For example, conflict in a work group may not be a problem if it does not impede group efforts to achieve the ideal or planned goals. Conflict might actually promote attainment of organizational goals through healthy competition. Only when it interferes with ideal goals does conflict become a problem. Naturally, if harmonious intragroup relations are a goal, conflict then becomes a problem. This approach forces the manager to think through what he wants to accomplish before he haphazardly introduces some change process.

The second step of the Hersey and Blanchard analysis is implementation. In this step, the laboratory manager uses the data from the first step and translates them into a systematic change process or strategem. The manager examines alternative solutions to the problem and then assigns appropriate strategems that will effect the change.

Hersey and Blanchard's approach can be condensed into six questions the manager should ask himself when contemplating change (Box 11–3).

These questions force the manager to think through the whole change process systematically. They provide structure and direction to the thought processes associated with organizational change. All too often a

manager takes corrective action without systematically diagnosing and analyzing the organizational and human changes that it might precipitate.

Leavitt categorizes organizational change approaches into structural, technologic, or people-oriented approaches.[5] The structural approach facilitates change through the formal rules, procedures, and guidelines of the organization. The technologic approach stresses the work flow, as exemplified by job descriptions and physical layout. People approaches favor training programs and appraisal techniques to change attitudes, motivational levels, and behavioral skills. Leavitt views the three approaches as interrelated: one does not change without affecting the other two.

Whatever viewpoint a manager chooses to follow, he must be an excellent diagnostician. The management prerogatives he possesses must be tempered by the realization that few of his managerial actions are isolated. However, a manager who considers too many variables and sees too many forces of constraint and resistance can render himself ineffective. Caution is important, but the manager serving as an agent of change quickly realizes that the change process is not for the fainthearted.

Some General Statements about Change Efforts

We have stressed that understanding the change process facilitates control of the process and lessens the chance that the manager will be overwhelmed by it. Also, we have strongly implied that the managerial role is probably the most effective and realistic change vehicle in the laboratory. Although third-party (consulting) relationships are effective, most situations must be resolved within limited time and financial frameworks. The role of an outside consultant is often not realistic or feasible. Therefore, we offer guidelines that might help the manager facilitate change.

Realize that mutual trust tends to facilitate change. If there are harmonious, trusting relations between the manager and his subordinates, the chance for successful change implementation is greatly enhanced. If, on the other hand, the organizational climate resembles that of an armed camp, a manager can expect resistance. Simply put, trust facilitates change, and lack of trust breeds resistance.

Create a climate that encourages and reinforces open, honest communication and supportive behavior. Also, acquire adequate resources to implement change; most importantly, be creative and adaptive. Naturally, it is helpful if all believe in the organization's goals and culture.

Only make changes that are necessary. Change is threatening and should be used with discretion.

Box 11·3

Henry and Blanchard's Approach When Managers Contemplate Change

1. What do I want to accomplish?
2. Should I change anything based on what I want to accomplish?
3. Is there a problem(s), and what are its parameters?
4. What possible solutions are available to me?
5. Which solution or strategy is the most appropriate?
6. How can I monitor and evaluate the change?

Employees may interpret frequently changed directives and goals as a lack of planning instead of judicious reaction to external and internal forces for change. Furthermore, constant change turns a stable work environment into one plagued by turbulence and uncertainty. Employees accustomed to a stable, predictable environment often resent changes introduced by management. Frequently changed work patterns or objectives can diminish commitment to organizational goals.

Do not be afraid to try something on a tentative basis. Nothing should be written in stone. Although some change processes must be very structured and inflexible, others should be tried on an evaluative basis. Not everything can be planned, nor will every result be anticipated. This is extremely important from the subordinate's viewpoint. Most employees are more willing to try something on a tentative basis than to be forced to make a change with little opportunity for modification. Resistance can often be overcome if employees know in advance that it is possible to negotiate changes.

Try to include employee participation in the planning stages of change. People tend to be supportive of change processes in which they are involved. A note of caution: It is foolhardy to include people in decision making who have neither the maturity nor the skill to make the decision. To do so establishes a dangerous precedent that the manager may not be able to satisfy in future decision making.

Be careful of upsetting established customs and traditions. Changes often appear revolutionary when viewed by the informal work group. The manager must be careful that change does not occur so quickly and intensely that insurmountable opposition to the change results. Sometimes a slower, evolutionary approach is just as effective, especially if the change attacks long-standing ways of doing things and threatens established interpersonal relationships and alliances.

Be aware of a "wallet mentality." If a change affects people's pocketbooks negatively, they tend to resist it. Technologic changes are resisted because employees perceive that the change will demand more of them in less time. They fear that such change will jeopardize their job security or overtime. The manager should anticipate these fears and attempt to assure employees that they will maintain their present levels of income.

Try to provide as much information about the change as possible. Although it is not always possible, try to implement changes with knowledge as the base of support. Most people want to know why a change needs to take place. Once the reasons are explained to them, most resistance evaporates. Some managers feel that the organizational merits of the change are sufficient to convince employees to adopt the change. Often, managers forget that selling the change to subordinates is necessary. Managers who hold that attitude

often find themselves blocked because employees perceive organizational merits in a completely different way than the manager. Withholding information can be especially troublesome when dealing with unions. It is probably wiser to share information regarding anticipated changes with the union than to surprise it. If the union can be brought into or identified with the change process, the process will tend to defuse this source of resistance.

Selection of a Change Stratagem

A Continuum

The selection of a change strategy depends on the diagnosis of the problem and the indicated remedy. The manager today is presented with a wide variety of procedures and must choose the one most feasible for what he wants to accomplish. The critical point, however, is the validity of the original analysis of the intended change. Selecting the correct change technique greatly facilitates the success of the change.

Numerous tactics and procedures are available to the manager; these methods represent a variety of philosophic orientations regarding the selection of a change process. To understand better how a manager can choose the best technique, it might be wise to examine two extreme orientations-to-change stratagems. One tries to overwhelm resistance, and the other tries to dissipate any resistance.

A strategy that tries to overwhelm resistance usually relies on hierarchical authority or power to impose the change. It is directive in nature and allows little input from the people who will be affected by the change, which is clearly planned and affects the total group or organization.

In this instance, change is often swift and complete. Opposition might be anticipated, but the manager's power to impose the directive is greater than the power of the forces resisting it. Naturally, the change may sustain itself if hierarchical powers or efforts diminish or disappear.

Often, the manager imposes some change that he realizes will be unpopular, but he tries to convince his subordinates that if they try the change, they will see that it was the right move. An example of this was the federal government's imposition of civil rights laws on a population that strongly resisted it. The feasibility of such an approach is strongly tied to the manager's past record and power to effect such changes, the time he has available to impose the change, and the general preference of the subordinates regarding implementation style.

When the Civil Rights Act was passed, the population was aware that the federal government had the power to implement such legislation and had done so in the past. The federal government settled on a timeframe and chose a style legitimized by the federal system. Such an approach is certainly feasible in the workplace.

At the other end of the continuum is the "bottom up" or participatory approach. In this approach, the manager uses tactics designed to win over the opposition. Such an approach is used where acceptance of the change is important. Subordinates are brought into the decision-making process and are strongly encouraged to contribute to diagnosis, analysis, and implementation of the change. Such an approach usually requires more time and, by the very nature of its style, is less specifically planned than a directive approach. Employees are less threatened and tend to become part of the change process. This generates commitment, motivation, and a sense of achievement among most participants.

Because the change is not forced on the employees, it tends to have a much longer staying power than a hierarchically imposed change. The objective is the evolution of a behavioral change, not the imposition of one. Again, the organizational climate and the manager's prevailing style are critical variables. A well-liked manager who projects a certain amount of personal power tends to have greater success with this approach than one who is not trusted and uses an authoritarian approach to problem solving.

Depending on the actual environment of the change process, either approach is feasible. Selection of the appropriate strategy is clearly dependent on how well the manager has diagnosed the change problem. Both strategies can be superimposed on a continuum developed by Kotter and Schlesinger.[4] They have investigated methods for dealing with resistance to change and have identified four situational variables that should be considered before choosing a change strategy. Their strategic continuum, adapted to our needs, and the situational factors are shown in Figure 11–5.

Kotter and Schlesinger point out that change efforts based on inconsistent strategies invariably run into problems. A quickly implemented change that is not well-thought out or planned tends to run into unanticipated problems. Likewise, a rapidly implemented change strategy that involves a large number of people usually stalls in its own inertia and takes on fewer participative characteristics with time. According to Kotter and Schlesinger, successful change efforts are located on the strategic continuum in relation to their four situational variables[4] (Box 11–4).

The Kotter and Schlesinger strategems are listed below and summarized in Table 11–1. Each strategem has been illustrated in a manner that will identify the appropriate context for its use.

Education and Communication

This approach is feasible when inaccurate or inadequate information creates resistance to change. It is especially appropriate when the manager needs to create

Strategic continuum	
OVERWHELM	WIN OVER
Fast	Slower
Clearly planned	Not clearly planned at the beginning
Little involvement of others	Lots of involvement of others
Attempt to overcome any resistance	Attempt to minimize any resistance
Key situational variables	
The amount and type of resistance that is anticipated	
The position of the initiators vis-a-vis the resistors (in terms of power, trust, and so forth)	
The locus of relevant data for designing the change, and of needed energy for implementing it	
The stakes involved (e.g., the presence or lack of presence of a crisis, the consequences of resistance and lack of change)	

FIGURE 11–5. Change continuum and situational variables affecting choice of strategy. (Adapted from Koiter J, Schlesinger LA: Choosing strategies for change. Harvard Bus Rev 57:111, March 1979)

Box 11•4

Four Situational Variables Affecting Change on the Strategic Continuum

1. The type and degree of anticipated resistance. The greater the degree of resistance anticipated, the more the initiator will move to the right in selecting a strategy to win over or minimize the resistance.
2. The amount of power and trust the manager is given. The less power he has, the more the manager is forced to select a strategy to the left of the continuum; conversely, the greater his personal power, the more he can afford to move to the right.
3. Data and energy needed to implement and design the change process. If the manager requires commitment and data from individuals who might resist the change, it behooves him to involve them in the design of the change effort. Likewise, if he has the power and information to overwhelm any resistance, then a strategy on the left side of the continuum is feasible.
4. The stakes involved. If a short-run crisis exists and the survival of the firm is in jeopardy, then a move to the left on the continuum is warranted. Likewise, if radical action is not called for and the problem involves many people, a win-over strategy from the right side of the continuum is reasonable.

Table 11-1
Strategies for Dealing with Resistance to Change

Approach	Applicable Situations	Advantages	Drawbacks
Education plus communication	When there is a lack of information or inaccurate information and analysis	Once persuaded, people will often help with the implementation of the change.	Can be very time consuming if many people are involved.
Participation plus involvement	When the initiators do not have all the information they need to design the change, and others have considerable power to resist	People who participate will be committed to implementing change, and any relevant information they have will be integrated into the change plan.	Can be very time consuming if participants design an inappropriate change
Facilitation plus support	When people are resisting because of adjustment problems	No other approach works as well with adjustment problems.	Can be time consuming, expensive, and still fall
Negotiation plus agreement	When someone or some group will clearly lose out in a change, and that group has considerable power to resist	Sometimes it is a relatively easy way to avoid major resistance.	Can be too expensive in many cases if it alerts others to negotiate for compliance
Manipulation plus co-optation	When other tactics will not work or are too expensive	It can be a relatively quick and inexpensive solution to resistance problems.	Can lead to future problems if people feel manipulated
Explicit plus implicit coercion	When speed is essential, and the change initiators possess considerable power	It is speedy and can overcome any kind of resistance.	Can be risky if it leaves people angry at the initiators

commitment among the people who resist change because of misinformation or lack of information about the change. Although such a strategy appears simple, it can be time consuming if a large number of people are involved. It will have a greater chance of success if the "teacher" and the "pupil" trust one another. The assumption here is that communication and logic will prevail.

Participation and Involvement

Bringing subordinates into planning or implementation of change is an excellent method when the manager does not possess the expertise or knowledge to implement the change himself and the resisters have significant power to impede his efforts. As discussed previously, participation often generates commitment by the participants to the change process. This approach can also result in time-consuming compromises that do not fit the organizational needs. It must be handled carefully because once a decision has been made by the group, it is difficult for the manager to push it aside.

Facilitation and Support

This works best with problems that deal with adjustment to the change process. It helps people adjust to change by facilitating their reaction to the change and by being supportive as the change occurs. It tries to reduce anxieties and fears by providing time for reflection, educational training, or additional counseling. This approach is time consuming and expensive and requires a certain amount of patience on the part of the manager. It tries to smooth the disruption by allowing time for coping with change. Like the others, however, it is not always successful.

Negotiation and Agreement

This strategy is feasible when someone has to lose or give up something, and that person possesses a significant amount of power to resist the change. Under these conditions the manager might barter or offer something to gain compliance and avoid major resistance or create commitment. This sometimes is an easy way to get compliance, but it can become expensive. If individuals or groups understand that the manager is willing to negotiate, they are likely to comply only when something is offered in return. It can establish a dangerous precedent.

Manipulation and Co-optation

When all other methods do not work or are too expensive, the manager may resort to covert change tactics. The manager manipulates the situation to evoke com-pliance. He may selectively release important information or orchestrate events that endorse his change efforts. Another kind of manipulation is co-optation. The manager might ask a key individual to participate in the design of the change process. This creates the appearance of endorsement or identification, rather than participation. Either of these tactics can be inexpensive and quick but also very dangerous. If people perceive that they are being manipulated, the manager runs the risk of having all his actions perceived as covert attempts to influence. If discovered, he destroys his trust and may create doubt about his motives when changes occur in the future.

Explicit and Implicit Coercion

If speed is essential and the manager has considerable power, he might resort to coercion. Fear can be used to gain compliance, as can direct or implied force. A manager sometimes uses this approach when other techniques and methods have failed. It is effective if the manager can overwhelm his resistance, but it can be risky. Most people strongly resist such tactics. If a manager is going to attack resistance by force or fear, he must know he can win. If he loses, the defeated manager will have a long way to go to regain power.

What are the implications of this for the laboratory director? A variety of change methods are available to the manager, although much of the literature today tends to advocate and endorse a participative approach to change (refer to Chapter 10). We agree with this trend. As suggested in the discussion of developments in the next decade, the work force will be highly educated, mobile, and specialized. For this reason alone, a manager should consider strategies located on the right side of the continuum. In general, people do not want to be ordered and directed; this invariably generates resistance and resentment. The immediate and long-run effects are better served if, when possible, the chosen strategy involves the people affected by the change. People like to feel that they have some control over their work environment. Likewise, a win-over philosophy tends to build bridges of trust between people.

Conflict and Conflict Management

No matter how carefully a manager chooses his strategy, conflict still occurs during the change process. We have implied that functions associated with the management process invariably lead to conflict. This conflict is rooted in the individual's motivational need–drive–goal cycle: When someone or something erects a barrier that blocks or opposes goal attainment, frustration results. This encourages the individual's development of defense mechanisms, and these mechanisms may be a cause of conflict.

Conflict has been defined as "any kind of opposition or antagonistic interaction between two or more parties."[7] Conflict also has a conceptual basis. If conflict is perceived, conflict exists; if it is not perceived, it does not exist. This means that conflict can be latent or overt, accurate or inaccurate. The point is that conflict is a matter of individual perception.

This perspective can be expanded to include conflict situations between individuals, groups, and organizations or any combination thereof. It is not difficult to imagine that incompatible interests and goals among different parties can result in some form of conflict. Thus, conflict can occur internally or externally.

The managerial role requires not only an understanding of conflict but also an ability to control and direct it. Because the manager must live with conflict, he must also be able to manage it. To manage it, however, requires understanding the conditions that foster conflict in an organization.

Sources of Conflict

What conditions nourish and breed conflict in an organization? The formal organization attempts to specify in advance the nature of human relationships in that organization. No matter how carefully planned and executed work-oriented behavior might be, the very existence of a formal organization seems to ensure conflict. Individuals want to control their own work environments, and this need for self-determination is often a basis for work-related conflict. Following is a discussion of several common underlying causes for organizational conflict.

Scarce Resources

Most organizations have a common resource base from which resources are reallocated to the various units and subunits of the organizations. Everyone wants the biggest part of the resource pie. The scarce resource could be anything: time, equipment, money, employees, or other items. Because each unit sees its mission as the most important or most critical, its members sometimes resort to extreme measures to secure the scarce resource. When this happens, conflict usually occurs. Often individuals or groups will present biased or exaggerated evidence to ensure the "proper" allocation of resources.

Values

The health-care field attracts highly competent, specialized individuals. Each employee in a hospital brings with him many years of training and his own perception

of what professional behavior should be. Because a hospital is a complex organization staffed by many diverse professionals, it is easy to understand why professional value orientations may differ. A nurse may need immediate results from tests performed by medical technologists, but he may be unaware that the technologists also have other, more critical, work to perform. The two groups often misunderstand one another's duties and responsibilities and the work pressures associated with them. Furthermore, the nurse functions in a line relationship, the medical technologist in a staff role. Unfortunately, each group often misinterprets the actions of the other, and neither seems to understand the hierarchical limitations and relationships regarding their respective responsibilities and authority.

Ambiguous Organization

Organizational conflicts often result because of undefined or overlapping duties and responsibilities. Organizations usually try to prevent this by developing job descriptions and organization charts that clearly define the roles of separate groups and individuals. Because of the dynamic nature of most organizations and the less formal daily interactions that develop, overlapping duties and responsibilities exist. This results in political behavior such as bickering and complaining about one party's jurisdictional responsibility to another. When the manager observes such behavior and cannot attribute credit or blame to one party over the other, more definitive jurisdictional responsibilities may be needed.

Dependence

Conflict often occurs when one party is dependent on another. For example, during a flu epidemic, a physician will order certain tests for a patient, and these tests will be sent to the laboratory for analysis. After a period of time, the physician might urge the nurse to contact the laboratory about the test results. The laboratory is now besieged with extra work because of the epidemic and reschedules the work flow accordingly. A misunderstanding may result based on the laboratory's perception of the doctor's impatience, the nurse's numerous telephone calls for the test results, and the hospital manager's strict inflexibility with overtime pay.

Communication

Communication barriers are often the cause of conflict. The most obvious example occurs when two parties use such specialized jargon that communication ceases. Physicians often explain diagnosis to patients in such technical language that patients are too intimidated to admit a lack of comprehension. When this happens, communication ceases. It is important to express the information clearly and in a way the intended audience will understand.

Interpersonal Conflict

A common conflict in organizations is the clash of incompatible personalities. Although a manager might try to segregate the individuals, educate them about their perceptions of one another, and preach tolerance and understanding, some personalities affect each other the wrong way. There are interpersonal conflict situations that are so one-sided that the other party does not know conflict exists. Some people become highly dissatisfied when their roles are compared with the role of another person, for example, when someone is promoted or receives an increase in pay not granted to coworkers. The organization may unwittingly foster such dissatisfaction by encouraging excessive competition for promotion or merit increases.

Different Viewpoints on Conflict

Managers hold three different viewpoints about conflict.[8] Some managers see conflict as primarily destructive, signaling a breakdown in the management process. Others tend to look at conflict as natural and inevitable and will learn to live with it. Finally, some view conflict as an essential variable in the continued survival of the organization. They feel that the laboratory manager who admits that resolving conflict and clarifying misunderstanding consumes much of his time may be functioning very effectively in his role as manager.

Traditional Viewpoint

The classical management theorists look on conflict as the malfunctioning of the management process. If the manager had planned, organized, or controlled his work unit better, conflict would not occur. If conflict does occur, it is an indication that the manager is not correctly performing his job. It also assumes that conflict is dangerous and should be resolved by management as soon as possible. The management of conflict means that better planning has to be initiated, the hierarchical structure should be used to resolve conflict, and conflict should be avoided when possible. Under this approach, the causes of conflict are analyzed and resolved by removing the cause of conflict. This is a classical management approach to handling conflict, and it still is prevalent in many organizations.

Behavioral Viewpoint

The behavioral viewpoint holds that harmony and tranquility do not necessarily mean high productivity. This perspective has it that conflict is not all bad and that there actually are some constructive aspects of conflict. All organizations are recognized to have built-in conflict situations, and it is assumed that the manager's duty and responsibility is to accept and manage it. This viewpoint warns the manager, however, that making or allowing too many waves could result in outcomes detrimental to the organization.

Interactionist Viewpoint

This viewpoint argues that there might not be enough conflict in organizations.[7] Although the negative and destructive aspects of conflict are recognized, it is also believed that organizations sometimes need conflict as a stimulus for adaptation and survival. The manager is not only concerned with reducing and resolving conflict, but also with stimulating it.

With this viewpoint, conflict may be functional or dysfunctional. If it furthers the goals of the organization, it is functional; if it hinders organizational performance, it is dysfunctional. Simply put, it states that organizations need to be responsive to their internal and external environments to survive. If a manager becomes too complacent or snuffs out the forces that facilitate change, there is great danger that the organization will lack the adaptability necessary to survive in today's highly competitive world. Furthermore, it views conflict as an integral part of the change process.

A re-examination of our initial model on conflict and change shows that we agree with this viewpoint. While his model displays conflict as the determinant for change, it is our belief that there is not enough empirical evidence to state that conflict causes change. They are, however, closely interrelated, and this relationship is the catalyst for organizational adaptation and ultimately organizational survival.

We believe that the interactionist viewpoint is a realistic one. It not only incorporates much of the thinking from the other two viewpoints, but it allows growth and change to occur and makes the manager directly accountable for this process. It is inconceivable to us that a formal organization will not encounter conflict if it is responsive to its internal and external environments. It also appears realistic that adaptation and survival of the organization require the subordination of individual interest to that of the organization. This means that the stimulation of conflict initiated by the manager may disturb some employees.

We are cautious, however, of endorsing behavior that stimulates conflict. Once conflict is introduced into the work setting, it is our belief that the "conflict" is often difficult to control and contain.

The Japanese Viewpoint

It is fashionable to adapt or adopt Japanese management styles to an American setting. Some well-managed American firms have adopted a Japanese orientation to conflict, which seems to correspond to many of our own viewpoints on conflict and change. The Japanese approach to conflict holds that conflict is inevitable in organizations, but uncontrolled conflict is considered intolerable. Conceptually, a Zen approach to management stresses harmony and tranquility. The Japanese believe that harmonious relationships are the underpinnings of effective management. This does not mean that competition should be avoided, only that conflict should be avoided. Conflict and change should be managed through approaches that stress cooperation through participative intervention techniques.

Participative intervention techniques, such as quality circles, task groups, labor–management committees, and productivity programs, all resemble a "bottom up" form of management. The individual as a member of a group is asked to participate in a change process or problem-solving situation that solicits commitment, creativity, and acceptance. The emerging viewpoint among many well-managed organizations is the importance of organizational harmony for successful implementation of change and the management of conflict.

Conflict Diagnosis and Coping Techniques

Much of what has already been said in our discussion about the diagnosis and implementation of various change processes also holds true for conflict techniques. Selection of an appropriate technique to deal with conflict depends on an accurate analysis of the conflict situation in the first place.

Conflict does not usually appear overnight. It often festers without the knowledge of the recipient party. Furthermore, conflict usually passes through several progressive stages before it manifests itself to others[6] (Box 11–5).

The parties may be at different stages of the conflict cycle, which complicates management of conflict. For example, one person may be manifesting conflict behavior while the other is still trying to figure out what is happening.

The manager must have a keen sensitivity to and understanding of his work environment to deal effectively with conflict. He must not only be alert to potential conflict situations and know how to handle them, but must also know when to encourage conflict.

Box 11·5

Progressive Stages of Conflict

1. Latent conflict. At this stage, the basic conditions for potential conflict exist but have not yet been recognized.
2. Perceived conflict. The cause of the conflict is recognized by one or both of the participants.
3. Felt conflict. Tension is beginning to build between the participants, although no real struggle has yet begun.
4. Manifest conflict. The struggle is underway, and the behavior of the participants makes the existence of the conflict apparent to others who are not directly involved.
5. Conflict aftermath. The conflict has been ended by resolution or suppression. This establishes new conditions that will lead either to more effective cooperation or to a new conflict that may be more severe than the first.

Knowing how to prevent conflict situations means understanding the underlying causes of conflict. A laboratory manager must be able to diagnose potential problems and structure situations to prevent them. People generally disagree about facts (perception of the present situation or problem), goals (how each party would like things to be), methods (the best way to achieve the goal), and values (the qualities and beliefs each thinks is important); the manager must be able to deal with these disagreements.[11]

For example, teaming two individuals with divergent viewpoints as to what constitutes a fair day's work creates a potential conflict situation. It should not come as a surprise that disagreements will occur between the two. A manager must be alert to these potential disagreements and carefully think through his managerial actions.

No matter how carefully the manager has analyzed a situation, open disagreement between parties can occur. The manager must ask himself what causes the conflict. Was each party exposed to a different informational base? Has the same information been perceived differently by the opposing parties because of past experience? Have the parties been put in a situation or role that forces them to take opposing positions?[11] The answers to these questions define the parameters of the conflict situation. Only after the manager has attempted to clarify the parameters can he effectively influence the opposing parties to select the appropriate mode of conflict resolution or reduction.

It is generally understood that it is easier to resolve differences caused by misunderstanding or lack of information than differences caused by opposing values. Likewise, certain conflict resolution modes are more effective with one type of conflict problem than with others. Table 11-2 presents some of the more common conflict resolution techniques and briefly describes their strengths and weaknesses. Selection of the appropriate technique depends on the resources available to the manager, the stage of the conflict cycle, the consequence of doing nothing, the timing of the intervention, the power of the hierarchy, and the manager's leadership style.

Often the manager must exercise his leadership function in the role of supportive facilitator or counselor. Here his function is not to resolve the conflict himself, but to bring the opposing parties together and let them resolve the conflict. He acts more as a referee than a judge. He interferes only to explain and define the variables, issues, and boundaries of the conflict. Likewise, he makes the parties understand that it is their responsibility to resolve the conflict, not his.

This requires a certain amount of skill on the part of the manager because this type of conflict management usually results in some form of verbal confrontation. Some common sense rules (Box 11–6), however, help the manager maintain a facilitating role.[9]

The manager must provide a constructive climate for the confrontation and prevent it from deteriorating into a destructive, name-calling feud. He can, for example, allow for a cooling-off period if one of the sessions becomes too heated. Likewise, he may reveal new information about the situation. However, his most important objective should be to keep the resolution session going and on track. Many managers are uncomfortable in the role of facilitator because they feel a strong sense of accountability and responsibility for the outcome. These managers feel that they would have

Table 11-2
Conflict Resolution Techniques

Technique	Brief Definition	Strengths	Weaknesses
Problem-solving (also known as confrontations or collaboration)	To seek resolution through face-to-face confrontation of the conflicting parties. Parties seek mutual problem definition, assessment, and solution.	Effective with conflicts stemming from semantic misunderstandings. Brings doubts and misperceptions to surface.	Can be time-consuming. Inappropriate for most non-communicative conflicts, especially those based on different value systems.
Superordinate goals	Common goals that two or more conflicting parties each desire and cannot be reached without cooperation of those involved. Goals must be highly valued, unattainable without the help of all parties involved in the conflict, and commonly sought.	When used cumulatively and reinforced, develops "peace-making" potential, emphasizing interdependency and cooperation.	Difficult to devise.
Expansion of resources	To make more of the scarce resource available.	Allows each conflicting party to be victorious.	Resources rarely expandable.
Avoidance	Includes withdrawal and suppression.	Easy to do. Natural reaction to conflict.	No effective resolution. Conflict not eliminated. Temporary.
Smoothing	To play down differences while emphasizing common interests.	Points of commonality stressed. Cooperative efforts are reinforced.	Differences not confronted and remain under the surface. Temporary.

(continued)

Table 11-2 continued

Technique	Brief Definition	Strengths	Weaknesses
Compromise	To require each party to give up something of value. Includes external or third-party interventions, negotiation, and voting.	No clear loser. Consistent with democratic values.	No clear winner. Power-oriented—influenced heavily by relative strength of parties. Temporary.
Authoritative command	Solution imposed from a superior holding formal positional authority.	Very effective in organizations because members recognize and accept authority of superiors.	Cause of conflict not treated. Does not necessarily bring agreement. Temporary.
Altering the human variable	To change the attitudes and behavior of one or more of the conflicting parties. Includes use of education, sensitivity, and awareness training, and human-relations training.	Results can be substantial and permanent. Has potential to alleviate the source of conflict.	Most difficult to achieve. Slow and costly.
Altering structural variables	To change structural variables. Includes transferring and exchanging group members, creating coordinating positions, developing an appeals system, and expanding the group or organization's boundaries.	Can be permanent. Usually within the authority of a manager.	Often expensive. forces organization to be designed for specific individuals and thus requires continual adjustment as people join or leave the organization.

functioned more effectively had they resolved the problem in the first place. However, allowing the participants to resolve their own problem forces them to think through the problem and the parameters and consequences associated with it. Once a solution has been resolved, they are more committed to it than to one imposed by the manager.

ENCOURAGING CONFLICT

So far we have been concerned with the prevention and resolution of conflict, but in some instances, the encouragement of conflict makes good management sense. Conflict is an essential component of the adaptation and survival of the firm. Furthermore, some evidence suggests that conflict spurs greater productivity

and that decision-making characteristics are enhanced by it. Likewise, many practicing managers realize that stress and conflict are sometimes the only feasible solutions to lackadaisical and complacent attitudes. Conflict is the basis of competitive techniques found among work groups who require self-motivation.

The question remains, however, of when to initiate conflict stimulation. Although there is no specific criterion for determining when conflict should be introduced into the work environment, Robbins has compiled a list of 10 questions that are appropriate for managers to ask themselves (Box 11–7).

According to Robbins, a positive answer to one or more of the questions suggests a possible need for conflict stimulation.

Likewise, Robbins has identified three broad categories for stimulating conflict among individuals and

Box 11·6

Common Sense Rules to Help the Manager Maintain a Facilitating Role

Review past actions and clarify the issues before the confrontation begins.

Communicate freely; do not hold back grievances.

Do not surprise the opponent with a confrontation for which he is not prepared.

Do not attack the opponent's sensitive spots that have nothing to do with the issues of the conflict.

Keep to specific issues; do not argue aimlessly.

Maintain the intensity of the confrontation, but ensure that all participants say all that they want to say. If the basic issues have been resolved at this point, agree on what steps will be taken next toward reaching a solution.

Box 11·7

Robbins' List of 10 Questions for Managers to Ask Themselves When Initiating Conflict

1. Are you surrounded by "yes men"?
2. Are subordinates afraid to admit ignorance and uncertainties to you?
3. Is there so much concentration by decision makers on reaching a compromise that they may lose sight of values, long-term objectives, or the company welfare?
4. Do managers believe that it is in their best interest to maintain the impression of peace and cooperation in their unit, regardless of the price?
5. Is there an excessive concern by decision makers not to hurt the feelings of others?
6. Do managers believe that popularity is more important for obtaining organizational rewards than competence and high performance?
7. Do managers unduly want consensus with their decisions?
8. Do employees show unusually high resistance to change?
9. Is there a lack of new ideas forthcoming?
10. Is there an unusually low level of employee turnover?

Robbins SP: Conflict management and conflict resolution are not synonymous terms. California Management Review 21(2): 67–75, 1978

groups (Box 11–8). Manipulation of the communication channel, for example, allows the manager to control information for functional purposes. Holding back information not only enhances the power of the manager but also increases hostility among the work group. Lack of information regarding merit increases or transfers may create stress situations that result in greater productivity. Likewise, a strategically planted piece of information can often create uneasiness and lay the groundwork for a major policy change. It is an excellent strategy for testing the new policy. Although the use of such techniques may appear unethical to some managers, more seasoned managers already consciously or subconsciously use such tactics. It is not really a matter of what kind of manipulation is used but of degree.

Changing structural variables can increase hostility. For example, increasing the size of an organizational unit can generate conflict by strengthening bureaucratic tendencies. Transferring several task-oriented individuals into a work group recognized as complacent can also create conflict.

Finally, the manager can alter personal behavior factors. The classic example of such a tactic is to put an authoritarian, dogmatic, and inflexible individual into a leadership role with a flexible, compatible work group. Likewise, changing the status or altering the privileges of an individual or group can cause dissatisfaction. Even such simple steps as revoking parking privileges or invoking a uniform dress code can generate discord.

It should be obvious that using these tactics can be dangerous. To do so involves gamesmanship and shows disregard for individual sensitivities and feelings. Many managers resort to such tactics anyway, because they realize that a manager cannot satisfy the needs of all employees all the time. Often individual aspirations and needs must be sacrificed for the survival of the unit or organization. This does not mean that a manager should be callous to the needs of his subordinates, but that he should be aware that he represents and serves two constituencies: his subordinates and his organization. A manager electing to serve only one is usually ineffective.

Some General Statements About Conflict

The logical approach to conflict management is a contingency one. Whether a manager stimulates or resolves

Box 11•8

Three Categories for Stimulating Conflict

Manipulate communication channel:
  Deviate messages from traditional channels.
  Repress information.
  Transmit too much information.
  Transmit ambiguous or threatening
    information.
Alter the organization's structure (e.g., redefine jobs, alter tasks):
  Increase a unit's size.
  Increase specialization and standardization.
  Add, delete, or transfer organizational
    members.
  Increase interdependence between units.
Alter personal behavior factors:
  Change personality characteristics of leader.
  Create role conflict.
  Develop role incongruence.

conflict is a matter of the variables surrounding the conflict situation. It is doubtful that only one method of conflict resolution can resolve the problem. There is no universal cure-all when it comes to conflict-resolution techniques. The selected technique must conform to and be compatible with the parameters and variables identified in the diagnostic stage of the analysis. A manager does not mirror his perceived expertise with that mode, rather than what is appropriate for the situation. We tend to repeat behavior with which we are comfortable, but that action is not sufficient for all situations.

Much of the literature today, especially that found in textbooks, advocates a humanistic approach to conflict management, such as the increasing collaboration as a change objective. In itself, this approach is admirable. Most managers, however, do not have the time and resources to deal with it effectively. Furthermore, many of them may be afraid of it, probably with some justification.

Recent research indicates that a participation approach is not as feasible in large systems as it is in small ones and that power equalization may be necessary for collaboration to occur. Furthermore, interdependency between conflicting parties may better facilitate the problem-solving approach. Likewise, in situations of great conflict, unconditional collaboration may be naive.[12]

Problem-solving techniques require some basic assumptions to be successful. The conflicting parties must desire a mutually acceptable solution. Couple this with trust in the other party, a belief that cooperation is better

than competition, the idea that opposing opinions are not only healthy but legitimate, and the basic conditions for successful confrontation and problem-solving are met.[2] The objectives of such an approach certainly are noble, although the conditions that facilitate its success are somewhat more difficult to achieve. The point is that collaborative problem solving is just one tool available to the manager for resolving conflict.

The manager is always confronted with the problem of choosing a conflict-handling mode that is compatible with his desired outcome. Regardless of the technique selected, someone often has to pay the price with regard to satisfaction, personal and organizational resources, and influence. There are costs and benefits associated with each technique; they should be considered before a choice is made.

A note of caution should be interjected for managers contemplating stimulating conflict. The danger associated with the various stimulating techniques is found in the nature of the conflict itself. Although the objective of the conflict may be to increase the effectiveness and efficiency of the organization, the costs to the organization may be substantial. The danger is that the manager may lose control of the situation. The manager must be careful that he does not ignite a flame that could consume him in the process of conflict stimulation.

Because of time constraints, or a crisis situation, or other techniques have failed, a manager may resort to a hierarchical, authoritative solution. If a manager uses his positional power to impose a resolution, the participants may feel that his actions are arbitrary, personal, and discriminatory. The manager who opts for such a solution should have the support of higher level management.

A FINAL NOTE

Change and conflict are intertwined, and an understanding of the two concepts is essential for good management. The degree of effectiveness a manager achieves in handling these two concepts depends to a great extent on how effectively he diagnoses the conditions and parameters surrounding them. The ultimate framework for analysis will be each manager's individual value system.

We believe that the desire of most employees for greater involvement in their work environments strongly endorses a participative approach to management of conflict and change. Participative approaches are not only more effective, but will invariably reap high standards of quality and efficiency.

Our faith in participation is based on the premises that the size of most laboratories is well suited for participative schemes, that most laboratories are either relatively autonomous subunits within a larger system or independent stand alone units, and that a harmonious climate in laboratory fosters efficiency and effectiveness more than any other approach to change and conflict. Coupled with the increased educational and professional expertise in today's laboratories, employee involvement techniques are worth considering.

However, the manager is faced with a variety of other options concerning conflict and change management. Should he sacrifice self-interest over the collective good or individual expectations over organizational ones? Should he stress the rational, the efficient, or the humane solution?

Acknowledging these dilemmas does not make the selection of the appropriate change process or conflict resolution any easier. However, the reader now has the ability to ask questions that will orient him to the process of choice. Ultimately, the answers must come from within the manager himself. With the techniques and stratagems presented here, the flexible manager now possesses a repertoire of skills to help him find those answers.

REFERENCES

1. Bennet AC: Improving the Effectiveness of Hospital Management, pp 162–166. New York, Preston Publishing Co, 1972
2. Filley AA: Interpersonal Conflict Resolution, pp 60–69. Glenview, Scott, Foresman and Co, 1975
3. Hersey P, Blanchard KH: Management of Organizational Behavior: Utilizing Human Resources, 3rd ed, pp 273–284. Englewood Cliffs, Prentice-Hall, 1977
4. Kotter J, Schlesinger LA: Choosing strategies for change. Harvard Bus Rev 57:112–113, 1979
5. Leavitt HJ: New Perspectives in Organization Research. New York, John Wiley and Sons, 1964
6. Pondy LR: Organizational conflict: Concepts and models. Administrative Science Quarterly 12:296–320, 1967
7. Robbins SP: Conflict management and conflict resolution are not synonymous terms. California Management Review 21(2):67–75, 1978
8. Robbins SP: Organizational Behavior, pp 287–289. Englewood Cliffs, Prentice-Hall, 1979
9. Rue LW, Byars LL: Management: Theory and Application, p 252. Homewood, Richard B. Irwin, 1977
10. Schein EH: Organizational Psychology, 3rd ed, pp 243–244. Englewood Cliffs, Prentice-Hall, 1980
11. Schmidt WH: Conflict: A powerful process for (good or bad) change. Management Review 63:5–8, 1974
12. Thomas KW: Conflict and collaborative ethic. California Management Review 21(2):58–59, 1978

ANNOTATED BIBLIOGRAPHY

Bridges W: Managing Transitions; Making The Most of Change. Reading, Addison-Wesley Publishing Co, 1991
Very good "how to" approach that offers the manager a process for dealing with change. Introduces new change concepts and living with change.

DuBrin AJ: Contemporary Applied Management. Plano, Business Publications, 1985
An excellent summary of current management concepts and techniques. It presents practical behavioral science-oriented techniques for managers and professionals.

Duck JD: Managing Change: The Art of Balancing. Harvard Bus Rev November-December:109–118, 1993
Offers a discussion of management's role in the introduction of organizational change, consideration for communication, human resources, trust, and the use of a transition management team.

Filley AC: Interpersonal Conflict and Resolution. Glenview, Scott Foresman & Co, 1975
This book addresses the problem of interpersonal conflict and presents techniques and methods for conflict resolution and management. It is a good supplement for workshops on understanding and handling personal conflict.

Harvard Business Review. Boston, Graduate School of Business Administration, Harvard University (bimonthly publication)
Although it has a general orientation, this journal often presents articles of interest to the health professional, such as articles that have wide applicability for laboratory management.

Hersey P, Blanchard KH: Management of Organizational Behavior: Utilizing Human Resources. Englewood Cliffs, Prentice-Hall, 1988
This is a general text on management, emphasizing a behavioral approach. Although not specifically targeted for laboratory administration, it provides an excellent overview of current management thinking and should be an invaluable guide for the health professional who has not had formal management training.

Lippitt GL: Visualizing Change: Model Building and the Change Process. La Jolla, University Associates, 1973
This is a model-oriented text dealing with change. Although conceptual in orientation, it provides a broad discussion of change and includes an excellent bibliography.

Pritchett P, Pound R: Business as Unusual; The Handbook for Managing and Supervising Organizational Change. Dallas, Pritchett & Associates, Inc, 1988

Pritchett R, Pound R: High Velocity Culture Change; A Handbook for Managers. Dallas, Pritchett Publishing Co, 1993
These two handbooks offer down-to-earth wisdom to managers and employees that inspires acceptance and ownership of change. Worth the comfort of knowing you are not alone.

Robbins SP: Managing Organizational Conflict: A Nontraditional Approach. Englewood Cliffs, Prentice-Hall, 1974
This book discusses conflict from an organizational perspective. It is essential reading for practitioners who view the survival of the organization as paramount. It provides an excellent explanation of constructive conflict from a management orientation.

Vecchio RP: Organizational Behavior. Chicago, Dryden Press, 1988
A board survey of behavioral concepts applicable to managers in general. Although targeted for college audiences, it is an excellent source book for laboratory managers.

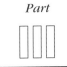
12

Interviewing and Employee Selection

Stephen L. Wilson • John R. Snyder

In our competitive health care environment, the need to make wise hiring decisions has never been more important. The most important resource of any manager is his personnel.[38,41] The clinical laboratory is no different. Any clinical laboratory must be cognizant of the current realities of the health-care delivery system in which managed care will be an increasingly predominant model of delivery. Clinical laboratories in hospitals will be providing services in an environment in which third-party payments will be more carefully controlled and administered. Laboratories in ambulatory care sites, health maintenance organizations, and preferred practice organizations can expect to be similarly affected. Overall, fewer resources will be available for laboratories, which will be expected to provide high-quality services with fewer personnel than in previous years. Working smarter and more efficiently requires special attention to the hiring and selection of personnel. Laboratory medicine is a labor-intensive service, as evidenced by the percentage of budget allocated to salaries. Effective procedures for hiring are critical for three reasons: (1) an employee's performance affects the performance of other staff in the laboratory; (2) recruiting, hiring, and training are expensive and time consuming; and (3) legal requirements, such as the Americans With Disabilities Act of 1990 and the Age Discrimination in Employment Act of 1967, must be followed in recruitment and hiring of staff.[39] For this reason, a good deal of time and effort should be devoted to planning for an effective and efficient staff. This chapter covers personnel administration aspects of recruiting, interviewing, selecting, transferring, and promoting in the clinical laboratory.

Turnover of personnel in the laboratory was a problem that plagued many institutions a decade ago. Karni, Studer, and Carter reported annual job turnover among clinical laboratory personnel in a large Midwestern city in 1970, 1975, and 1980 to be 20%, 19%, and 15%, respectively.[14] It is evident that during the 1980s, diagnosis-related groups (DRGs) played a major role in reducing turnover by limiting the opportunities for relocation. In a 1987 survey of 200 laboratories, 85% had experienced a 3% to 7% decrease in full-time equivalent positions.[41] Beyond reduced staffing levels, hiring practices have changed somewhat in response to prospective payment, including a trend toward hiring more generalists. Anticipated increases in the numbers of technician-level workers replacing technologists in clinical laboratories have not materialized as predicted. Perhaps the slim pay differential between the two levels of technical personnel, usually only $1,500 to $4,000 per year, does not merit hiring staff with fewer problem-solving and disease-correlation skills. Other aspects of personnel have also been affected by DRGs: "The tight economic climate has forced laboratory managers to demand more work from fewer workers, and in many cases it has resulted in smaller salary increases, salary caps, reduced benefits, and postponement of workplace improvements."[41]

In addition, the seasonal peaks and valleys in laboratory volume often complicate the staffing picture, which in turn is reflected in recruiting, interviewing, and selection activities. A supervisor must plan in advance for the usual attrition (normal resignations and retirements). Erratic ups and downs in staffing volume, expedient hiring, and substantial overtime are all indicators that a problem may exist either in the selection process or in the work setting.[43] Retraining and constant orientation of new personnel are costly in terms of operational efficiency and quality of results.[31]

RECRUITMENT

The role of the laboratory supervisor must be to take a strong, positive leadership role in recruitment and retention of staff.[1] The current environment in health care makes staff recruitment a tough balancing act. The supervisor must be proactive enough to anticipate vacancies and the need to recruit but conversely must be aware that some staffing adjustments may be necessary as hospitals and facilities re-engineer their organizations.

The group of applicants from which a manager may select is variable. A laboratory supervisor cannot assume that the right employee will come along just when needed. Many rural and some metropolitan areas experience shortages of qualified laboratory personnel on a continual basis. Declining enrollments in clinical laboratory science educational programs may herald more severe laboratory manpower shortages for some institutions. Therefore, it behooves laboratory administrators to recruit in advance of staff vacancies and follow up all requests for information concerning the availability of current and future positions.

Recruitment of laboratory personnel relies primarily on newspaper and professional journal advertising. As competition for certified practitioners has heightened, some institutions have prepared enticement packets describing promotional opportunities, personnel benefits, and community educational and recreational advantages. Others have prepared elaborate slide or tape recruitment programs that can be taken to professional meetings and college campuses. Professional recruitment agencies are an expensive option, although they usually are successful in securing applicants. Perhaps the most rewarding recruitment of

bench-level staff is the result of efforts directed at the professional educational programs. Some institutions encourage potential employers to meet with their students through a placement option. Regardless of the tactic used, the need for recruitment activities as part of the interviewing and selection process is becoming more evident.

A strong laboratory staff is the result of years of perceptive hiring.[40,42] The long-term health of the department is not ensured if the employees are too similar in experience, age, job development, and promotability. Often it appears less costly and more efficient to recruit from within an institution's own educational program, but beware the phenomenon of in-breeding. Hiring too many of one institution's graduates for too long may be detrimental. The introduction of new perspectives is always healthy. The infusion of new blood keeps the laboratory system from growing stagnant, repetitious, and overly reliant on internal judgment. Optimally, there should be a mix of newcomers and old-timers, because too many hard-driving, overly ambitious outsiders can be almost as destructive as too many long-term "old fogies."

HUMAN RESOURCES PERSONNEL

Most hospitals and large facilities have developed effective, professional human resources departments. Within these units are skilled support personnel who can provide valuable assistance to laboratory supervisors in the hiring process. These organizations establish policies that define the role of the human resources department in the recruitment and hiring process. For instance, job descriptions and advertising may be channeled through the department to ensure compliance with federal and state regulations. Applications and resumes may be collected and reviewed by human resources personnel, and they may be involved in communicating, at least initially, with the applicant pool. The supervisor should work closely with the organization's human resources personnel about expectations for filling vacant positions.[1] These professionals can provide invaluable assistance in the hiring process and ensure that the supervisor follows proper legal and administrative procedures when filling a vacancy.

LEGAL ASPECTS OF INTERVIEWING AND EMPLOYEE SELECTION

Legal issues are increasingly involved in employee recruitment and selection in health-care settings. Society is no longer forgiving of human error in the delivery of care. Hospitals and other clinical health-care professionals are held to a higher standard because of the level of care that is expected by the public. Legal precedent has established that hospitals enter into an implied contract with patients that care will be delivered by competent, responsible professionals.[7] In a situation in which an employee may have erred and as a result harmed a patient, the employing hospital or clinical facility could be found to be liable if (1) the harm or injury was foreseeable; (2) the employer hired and placed an employee in a job that was beyond his or her competence, creating the conditions for an error to occur; and (3) the employer should have known that the person employed was not qualified for the position.[26] Clearly, the need to hire laboratory personnel wisely and carefully is important to the success of the clinical laboratory.

During recent years, a variety of federal and state laws have been enacted to ensure equal employment opportunities for all individuals.[13] The provisions of these laws apply to daily employer decisions of recruiting, hiring, promoting, training, and terminating.[35] Moreover, these regulations extend to selection procedures.[35] Devices used to select an employee for employment, such as written tests, seniority systems, interviews, and application forms, are subject to scrutiny under these laws.[15,32] A brief summary of the major regulations that apply to employee selection follows.

Title VII

Title VII of the Civil Rights Act enacted by the Congress of the United States in 1964 is the major legislative effort to guarantee equality to all people. The act was amended by the Equal Opportunity Act of 1972 and the Pregnancy Discrimination Act of 1978. Title VII forbids employers of more than 15 people from limiting, classifying, or segregating employees in such a way that would deprive any person of employment opportunities or adversely affect his status as an employee on the basis of that individual's race, color, religion, sex, or national origin.

Although Title VII is often associated with women and minorities, several other groups have been included by subsequent legislation. These are the handicapped (Rehabilitation Act of 1973 and the Equal Employment Opportunity for Handicapped Individuals Act of 1980), veterans of the Vietnam conflict (Vietnam Veterans Readjustment Act), and people between the ages of 40 and 70 (Age Discrimination Employment Act of 1967).[16,17]

The original emphasis of Title VII was on protection of the individual from discrimination in employment. The act also emphasized opportunity, based on the equal-treatment test. Nevertheless, certain minorities still suffer from discrimination. The unemployment rate for African Americans continues to be twice that for white people.[35] Women employed full-time have a median annual income less than men.[11] Because of these inequities, a movement to redefine discrimination in terms of outcomes, rather than opportunities, began. This movement emphasized the statistical *effects* of employment practices on minority groups, rather than the violation of individual rights.[22,24]

Affirmative Action

Affirmative action programs are based on the effects of discrimination. President Johnson, in 1965, instituted an executive order (executive order 11246) calling for equal opportunities to be applied to all aspects of the personnel process. These orders applied to all contractors working for the federal government. This action greatly improved on the affirmative action orders of the Kennedy administration (executive order 10925, 1961), which were at best symbolic. However, it was not until 1968 that goals and timetables became a part of these programs. In a later executive order, President Nixon clarified the meaning of affirmative action (executive order 11749, 1969). Additionally, he added provisions ensuring that recruitment efforts would be extended to all sources of job candidates by requiring employers to make use of the present skills of employees, to provide programs to upgrade their skills, and to participate in school and government efforts to improve community conditions affecting the employees. These executive orders were part of an effort to equalize the percentages of minorities in federal or federal contract employment and apply only to government employees; they are distinct from the provisions of Title VII.

Many different state and federal laws determine who must adopt affirmative action programs. Any employer holding federal contracts or subcontracts totaling more than $2,500 must have affirmative action programs for the handicapped; if the contracts total more than $10,000, the employer must have a program including women, African Americans, Hispanics, Asians, Native Americans, and Vietnam veterans. Since federal research grants are considered to be contracts, almost all university-affiliated hospitals are bound by these orders. Many states have similar regulations. Employers who have been found by the courts to have discriminated in the past (under Title VII) may be required to institute affirmative action programs.

Affirmative action is a plan for positive steps that an employer will take to ensure equal opportunity. It cannot be viewed as a standardized program that must be accomplished in the same way at all times by all employers. There are three basic elements in an affirmative action program[43] (Box 12–1).

There are several criticisms of affirmative action. Some see it as a quota system that imposes unfair burdens on white men and leads to reverse discrimination. However, the goals of affirmative action programs are clearly defined and distinct from rigid, inflexible requirements or quotas. Quotas are specifically prohibited, as illustrated in the Supreme Court's decision in *Bakke v. The University of California at Davis* (1978) and *Weber v. Kaiser Aluminum* (1979). Goals are simply statements by the employer that the number of minority individuals employed will reach the level that would be achieved by drawing from the labor pool without bias.

Other critics contend that affirmative action programs lead to lower standards, implying that the relative qualifications of candidates will be ignored at the expense of mandatory percentages, resulting in preferential selection. Preferential selection in actuality occurs only in the infrequent situation of equally qualified candidates where a minority candidate is given preference or when, in the process of ranking, positive credit is given for minority status. A recent ruling by the Supreme Court in *Johnson v. Transportation Agency, Santa Clara, California* (1987) has further emphasized that employers who voluntarily set hiring and promotion goals to improve representation of women and members of minority groups where a "manifest imbalance" exists have some protection against claims of discrimination by nonminority men. In this case, a male employee charged "reverse discrimination" when a woman with slightly fewer qualifications was promoted to the job he was seeking. Although it is too early to ascertain the total impact of this ruling, it should not be construed as a quota system. Rather, institutions are able to modify their affirmative action plans to allow consideration of sex and race where a "manifest imbalance" exists.

By focused recruiting and employee development, larger numbers of well-qualified minorities can be brought into the labor market, resulting in a larger, more diverse pool of talent. Additionally, as equal opportunity goals are reached, the number of reverse discrimination conflicts will decrease.

Because affirmative action has been in existence for a relatively short time, it is still too early to assess the full potential of these programs in terms of measurable practices, such as changes in outreach, interviewing, skill-upgrading programs, promotion reviews, and employee selection, and the effect they will have on the goal of achieving full integration.

Discrimination is deeply ingrained in our society. Fry recently published a study that predicts that affirmative action programs will not achieve full integration for minorities until the year 2013. The future success of affirmative action programs will not depend on formal programs, but rather on our society's commitment to end discrimination and improve the status of disadvantaged groups.

THE EQUAL EMPLOYMENT OPPORTUNITY

Commission

The effectiveness of Title VII and affirmative action programs depends largely on employers' willingness to comply with the law. When employers do not comply, the Equal Employment Opportunity Commission (EEOC) and the courts determine what constitutes violation of the law and set the penalties for noncompliance. The EEOC was formed in 1965 as the enforcing arm of the Civil Rights Act. It is a compliance agency whose investigative powers are evoked by the charges of discrimination filed by an aggrieved person or EEOC commissioner. The state governments have similar agencies commonly referred to as fair employment practices commissions to regulate similar state statutes. Affirmative action programs, being executive orders, are under the jurisdiction of the Departments of Justice and Labor (Office of Federal Contract Compliance) and the Civil Service Commission.

The EEOC has identified three aspects of discrimination:

·Box 12•1

Three Basic Elements to Affirmative Action

1. The employer's current work force is analyzed to determine whether the percentages of minorities employed are similar to the percentages available in the labor pool who possess the basic job-related qualifications. When substantial disparities are found, an analysis is made of the selection process that is operating to exclude the minority individual.
2. A statement of hiring and promotion goals and a timetable for correcting deficiencies are established.
3. A plan for attaining the goals and a system for regularly monitoring the effectiveness of the affirmative action program are implemented.

1. Disparate treatment
2. Disparate impact
3. Perpetuation of past discrimination

Disparate treatment is the most easily understood type of discrimination. The employer simply treats some people less favorably than others because of age, race, color, religion, sex, marital status, or national origin. Disparity in treatment includes failure to recruit, hire, transfer, or promote minority group members on an equal basis with white people. Usually it must be proved that disparate treatment is a matter of practice and that the differences are "racially premised." Statistical evidence showing a difference in treatment is relevant only to prove that the employer regularly made discriminatory decisions, not to support the contention that a work force is racially unbalanced.

The disparate-impact doctrine is designed to prevent unintentional discrimination resulting from apparently neutral practices. A case of discrimination can be proved by showing that an employment practice has a disparate effect between white men and any protected group. If disparate effect is shown, employers must prove that such practices result from business necessity or are unrelated to the employment status of the employee allegedly discriminated against.[26]

Perpetuation of past discrimination is sometimes built into an employer's hiring and promotion practices, especially when he uses a merit or seniority system for promotion or selection. These procedures exclude minorities because past discrimination has resulted in their lacking the necessary skills, education, training, or job attitude. The objective of Title VII is to remove barriers that have operated in the past to exclude minorities. This is usually accomplished by the modification of seniority systems and by the recruitment of minorities into training and continuing education programs that influence selection for promotion.

Many employers are finding that the issue of discrimination is far from academic. There are hundreds of cases in the federal courts, and many of the court decisions have cost employers a great deal of money. In one case, Standard Oil Company of California agreed to a $2 million settlement as restitution for laying off 160 older employees during a reduction in force.[2] An employer who fails to comply with EEOC guidelines can be subject to judgments under Title VII calling for significant back-pay awards; if the employer is a federal government contractor, he can be barred from receiving any additional government contracts. Under Title VII, the employee has the right to bring a civil suit against the discriminating employer. However, the employee must give notice to the EEOC that he intends to bring suit 60 days before he files. During this period, the

EEOC usually conducts an investigation of the alleged discrimination and attempts a reconciliation between the employer and the employee. In cases where there is strong evidence of discrimination, the EEOC will actually bring suit against the employer. If the EEOC does not bring suit, the employee still has the right to bring his civil suit. The employee may seek legal and equitable remedies, usually wages lost because of the discrimination. The employee may even recover damages for pain and suffering, or the employee may ask for retroactive seniority as restitution for past discrimination.

Additional Legal Considerations in Hiring

Several recent legal actions have had a considerable impact on how prospective employers must assess applicants. House Rule 4154, amending the Age Discrimination in Employment Act, extends protection under the Act to workers in the private sector and to most state and local government employees older than 70 years. The amendments eliminate mandatory retirement for workers over age 70. The new amendments also require that employers cannot discriminate against any individual over 40 years in terms of paid benefits or continued employment. Although this law became effective January 1, 1987, there was a 7-year exemption for implementation of these amendments for state and local government employers when dealing with public safety employees, such as police, fire fighters, prison guards, and tenured college professors. This has caused some consternation on the part of employers who feel they will have less power to determine the composition of their work force. They fear the potential for discrimination suits brought by an older worker can be an increasing problem for which they are ill prepared. Also, there is some concern that a "gray-haired work force" will, potentially, create morale problems for other workers.[18] These concerns can be minimized by creative use of retirement plans. In summary, age cannot be a discriminating factor in the hiring process, and potential applicants must be assessed on the basis of individual merit.

On June 1, 1987, the Immigration Reform and Control Act of 1986 took effect. This legislation prohibits employers from knowingly hiring or continuing to employ illegal aliens. Personnel departments in institutions will most likely handle the responsibility of checking potential employees' identity documents, such as a driver's license with photograph, and work eligibility records such as a social security card or certificate of United States citizenship.

THE HIRING PROCESS

Carefully conducted hiring processes generally mean that those selected will be aware of the job responsibilities and eager to accept the responsibilities. These individuals will be more likely to make a commitment to the goals of the organization and to remain for an extended time. A careful hiring process will ensure that all applicants are given equal consideration for the position, thus protecting against possible complaints of discrimination or prejudice. Conversely, a poorly conducted hiring process may result in an inadequately prepared individual or one who does not fit with the needs of the position. Poor screening may have failed to bring to light problems such as absenteeism or chronic lateness. Perhaps most important is the possibility that a well-qualified candidate was not given a proper review, resulting in a hiring decision that is costly for the clinical laboratory in terms of poor service and perhaps morale problems with other staff.[48] There are at least five possible steps in the hiring process (Box 12–2).

Review of the Completed Application or Resume

The screening of the resume and job application is important as a preinterview activity. Together, both provide a professional history of the candidate that will provide the basis for the interview. These materials should be checked for evidence that the applicant's education and work experience fit the needs of the laboratory. They should be reviewed for evidence of stability and commitment as seen through relatively long terms of employment. Any gaps in work experience should be noted, along with an understanding of the progression in job levels that has occurred for the candidate in previous employment. Items such as breaks in employment, level of progression, and job responsibilities should be addressed during the interview.

Box 12·2

Five Possible Steps in Hiring

1. Review of the completed application or resume
2. Telephone contacts with candidate pool
3. Preliminary and final reference checks
4. Conducting the interview
5. Selection and notification of candidate

THE APPLICATION FORM

In the process of interviewing candidates for employment, the employer gathers preliminary information about the applicant's potential for success in a given position by use of an application form. Because the application is often used as a screening tool to eliminate at an early stage unqualified individuals from consideration for employment and because eventual hiring decisions are made on the basis of answers given on the application, it must conform to Title VII of the Civil Rights Act: Questions appearing on the form must be established to be related to legitimate occupational qualifications. Further, it must not have a disparate impact on minorities by the use of qualifying factors that disproportionately screen out protected groups in favor of white male applicants. With the exception of questions pertaining to an individual's arrest record, Title VII does not specifically forbid the inclusion of non–job-related items. However, when the employer is charged with discrimination, the burden of proof (of the business necessity of the question) rests with the employer. In a study published by *Fortune* magazine on May 8, 1978, it was found that some 99% of the employers studied included at least one inappropriate question on their application form; 38% included more than 10 inappropriate items.

The investment of time and effort in preparing an application that is unbiased will be rewarding in terms of obtaining suitable employees and avoiding charges of discrimination and consequent costly legal proceedings. A good method to use when designing such an application is to make up a worksheet containing the information needed about an applicant before a decision to hire is made and the information needed for recording purposes after the applicant is hired.[38] This list will vary for each job description. Accordingly, specific applications must be tailored for specific jobs. Then list the reasons the information is needed. This will help determine whether the information is job related. Using this information, prepare an application with the points listed in Box 12–3.

It is probably best to discard any question if there is even a remote possibility that it cannot be justified by these criteria. In some cases, merely rewording an inappropriate question will make it acceptable. Table 12–1 identifies acceptable and unacceptable questions.[13] Questions may be established as an occupational qualification by conducting research to validate the item as a predictor of success for a specific position. Also, such research can be used to substantiate that the item does not have a disparate impact on any protected group. Some information that you may need for the record or statistical purposes and that cannot be asked on the application can be obtained after hiring. Such

Table 12-1
Eliminating Discrimination From Pre-employment Interviews

Subject	Lawful Questions	Unlawful Questions
Race or color	None	Complexion or color of skin; coloring
Religion or creed	None	Inquiry into applicant's religious affiliations, church, parish, pastor, or religious holidays observed
National origin	None	Inquiry into applicant's lineage, ancestry, national origin, descent, parentage, or nationality; nationality of applicant's parents or spouse; mother's tongue
Sex	None	Inquiry as to sex; how to be addressed (eg, Mr., Mrs., Ms.)
Marital status	None	Asking if the person is single, divorced, or married; name or other information about spouse; ages of your children, if any.
Language	Inquiry into languages applicant speaks and writes fluently	Inquiry into native language. Inquiry into how applicant acquired ability to read, write, or speak a foreign language.
Education	Inquiry into applicant's academic, vocational, or professional education and the public and private schools attended	
Experience	Inquiry into work experience	
Relatives	Name of applicant's relatives, other than a spouse, already employed by this company	Names, addresses, ages, number, or other information concerning applicant's spouse, children, or other relatives not employed by the company
Notice in case of emergency	Name and address of person to be notified in case of accident or emergency	
Military experience	Inquiry into applicant's military experience in the Armed Forces of the United States or in a state militia; inquiry into applicant's service in particular branch of United States Army, Navy	Inquiry into applicant's general military experience
Organizations	Inquiry into applicant's membership in organizations that the applicant considers relevant to his or her ability to perform the job	List of all clubs, societies, and lodges to which the applicant belongs
Birth control	None	Inquiry as to capacity to reproduce, advocacy of any form of birth control, or family planning.
Age	Are you over 18 years of age? If not, state your age.	How old are you? What is your date of birth?
Disability	Do you have any impairments, physical, mental, or medical, would interfere with your ability to perform the job for which you have applied?	Do you have a disability? Have you ever been treated for any of the following diseases...?
Arrest record	Have you ever been convicted of a crime (give details)?	Have you ever been arrested?

(continued)

Table 12-1 *continued*		
Subject	*Lawful Questions*	*Unlawful Questions*
Name	Have you ever worked for this company under a different name? Is any additional information relative to change of name, use of an assumed name, or nickname necessary to enable a check on your work record? If yes, explain.	Original name of an applicant whose name has been changed by court order or otherwise; maiden name of a married woman; name and dates, if previously worked under another name
Address or duration of residence	Applicant's place of residence and how long he has been a resident in this state or city	
Birth place	None	Birth place of an applicant; birth place of applicant's parents, spouse, or other close relatives
Birthdate	None	Requirements that the applicant submit birth certificate, naturalization, or baptismal record; requirement that applicant produce proof of age in the form of a birth certificate or baptismal record
Photograph	None	Requirement or option that applicant affix a photograph to employment form at any time before hiring
Citizenship	Are you a citizen of the United States? If not a citizen of the United States, do you intend to become a citizen of the United States? If you are not a citizen of the United States, have you the legal right to remain permanently in the United States? Do you intend to remain permanently in the United States? Have you ever been interned or arrested as an enemy alien?	Whether an applicant is naturalized or a native-born citizen; the date when the applicant acquired United States citizenship; requirement that applicant produce naturalization papers or first papers; whether applicant's parents or spouse is naturalized or native-born citizens of the United States; the date when parents or spouse acquired citizenship.

Box 12•3

Application Preparation Points

1. Do the questions conform to Title VII of the Civil Rights Act, EEOC guidelines, *Guidelines on the Employment Selection Process* (available from local offices of the EEOC)?
2. Do the questions relate specifically to the job that the applicant is seeking? Can it be proved to be an occupational qualification or an absolute business necessity?
3. Do the questions violate the applicant's right to privacy?
4. Will the questions disqualify a disproportionate number of minorities or protected group members? Are there any valid studies that indicate that these items are valid predictors of occupational success?

EEOC, Equal Employment Opportunity Commission.

information includes photographs for identification purposes, age, sex, race, marital status, and so forth.

It is a good idea to include on the application a blanket statement indicating that you are an equal employment opportunity/affirmative action employer and are not interested in receiving information that may be construed to be discriminatory in nature. The application should include a statement signed and dated by the prospective employee, indicating that he has not falsified any information on the application. This is necessary in the event you wish to terminate the employee for such reasons. If you intend to check references, you will need the applicant's signed permission for this.

As a final check for the validity of your application, you may want to submit it to the local offices of the EEOC for their advice and approval. An application example is shown in Figure 12–1.

The application is often your first contact with prospective employees. For this reason, it should, in addition to gathering vital information, make a positive statement about the employer. Because it is a vital part of the employee selection process, the use of the most appropriate application will be to the employer's best interest.

TELEPHONE CONTACTS WITH CANDIDATES

When trying to verify a pool of qualified applicants and to have more complete information, it may be useful to conduct a preliminary telephone screening process in which potential candidates are called and the requirements of the position are discussed further. This may be particularly useful when the position offered is of a general nature that would attract a number of different applicants. Telephone screening can determine the real interest and qualifications of an applicant. Additionally, salary requirements, the working situation, and supervisory responsibilities can be clarified. A telephone screening process can be a useful and cost-effective way of defining the applicant pool by sorting out disinterested or unqualified applicants.

REFERENCE CHECKS

Depending on what information is made available through the application and resume, the supervisor may choose to contact references before or after the interview. It is usually the norm to follow up with a reference check after the interview; however, important information can be obtained through preinterview reference checks that assist with questioning during the interview. Reference checks are important because how a prospective employee has performed in the past is a good predictor of how he will perform in the future. However, the nature of information that can be obtained from a former employer has been rigidly limited by various state and federal regulations designed to protect the applicant.

The major restriction is the applicant's written permission to contact the people he has listed as references. Any inquiry as to the person's previous salary, scholastic aptitude, or work habits violates his right to privacy. Information supplied concerning the applicant's lifestyle may indicate race, national origin, or other protected-group status and thus may be discriminatory and violate the applicant's civil rights under Title VII. Moreover, any previous employer or supervisor who gives deleterious information is subject to charges of slander by the applicant. As a result, some employers have established a "no reference" policy or limit references only to specific information, such as dates of employment and job title.[28] This can seriously limit the prospects of gaining accurate, reliable information on applicants. One important option is to insist on the applicant signing a document giving permission to conduct an appropriate background check. There should be a signed release for each employer reference to be checked.[21]

The purpose of the reference check is to validate the applicant's employment record, which can be accomplished through a telephone call, personal visit, or written reference. There are differing views on how to check reference information. Having written documentation from a previous employer has definite advantages, while telephone checks provide much easier and quicker access. The use of the telephone with follow-up by fax may be most efficient. Signed releases and summaries of discussions can be quickly transferred between parties. To minimize legal complications and maximize the effectiveness of information gained in the process of checking, references should be limited to (1) obtaining information related only to the job, including title, duties, and performance related only to evaluations and other information on the record and (2) verification of employment dates, salary history, attendance record, and reasons for leaving.

In general, avoid asking for opinions or subjective assessments because these are not verifiable. However, be sure to check gaps in the applicant's work record; check all appropriate academic and certification credentials noted by the applicant, and question thoroughly any information received from the reference that is in any way different from that given by the applicant.[21]

It is important to validate the information supplied to you by the applicant (dates of employment, position) with the employer's record. Any discrepancies found do not speak in the applicant's favor.

(text continues on p. 212)

Employment Application

This application form must be completed, signed and dated in order for you to receive employment consideration at The Ohio State University. You may also wish to submit a resume to provide additional information. Your application must be submitted to the Staff Employment Services Office, 53 W. 11th Avenue, (614)292-5304, for Classified Civil Service positions; to the Professional Employment Services Office, 2130 Neil Avenue, (614)292-9380, for Administrative and Professional positions; or to the Office of Hospital Human Resources, 1654 Upham Drive, (614)293-4995, for University Hospitals and College of Medicine positions. At the time of employment, the University must verify your citizenship and work authorization.

THE OHIO STATE UNIVERSITY IS AN EQUAL OPPORTUNITY/AFFIRMATIVE ACTION EMPLOYER

PLEASE TYPE OR PRINT WITH A BLACK PEN

Identification

Name: _____
               (Last)   (First)   (Middle)

Address: _____
               (Street/P.O. Box)

_____
               (City)   (State)   (Zip Code)

Telephone Numbers: _____
               (Home Number)   (Message Number)   (Business Number)

Social Security Number: _____

Work Preferences

What type of work are you seeking? _____

Where do you want to work? (check one)   ☐ Columbus campus   ☐ Regional campus: _____   ☐ University Hospitals

What appointment would you accept ?   ☐ Full-time   ☐ Part-time   ☐ Intermittent   ☐ Seasonal   ☐ Temporary

What shift would you accept?   ☐ Days   ☐ Evenings   ☐ Nights   ☐ Weekends   ☐ Rotating

Date available to start: _____

Education

Please Circle Last Year of Formal Education Completed:	Grade and High School 1 2 3 4 5 6 7 8 9 10 11 12		College Fr So Jr Sr 5 6 7 8	Other 1 2 3 4	
	Name and Location of School	Degree Received	Program or Major Coursework		Grade Average
Last High School					
College, University, Business, Technical or Military Schools					
Graduate School					

FIGURE 12–1.   Sample employment application form.

Experience (List all employment)

Current or Most Recent Position		Dates of Employment	
		From (Mo./Yr.)	To (Mo./Yr.)

Employer	May we contact this employer? ☐ Yes ☐ No	Department

Address		Supervisor

Phone	Final Salary	☐ Full-time ☐ Part-time ☐ Summer ☐ Temporary

Description of duties, responsibilities and equipment operated

Reason for leaving _____

Previous Position		Dates of Employment	
		From (Mo./Yr.)	To (Mo./Yr.)

Employer	Department

Address	Supervisor

Phone	Final Salary	☐ Full-time ☐ Part-time ☐ Summer ☐ Temporary

Description of duties, responsibilities and equipment operated

Reason for leaving _____

Previous Position		Dates of Employment	
		From (Mo./Yr.)	To (Mo./Yr.)

Employer	Department

Address	Supervisor

Phone	Final Salary	☐ Full-time ☐ Part-time ☐ Summer ☐ Temporary

Description of duties, responsibilities and equipment operated

Reason for leaving _____

FIGURE 12–1. *(continued)*

Experience (continued)

Previous Position		Dates of Employment From (Mo./Yr.)	To (Mo./Yr.)
Employer		Department	
Address		Supervisor	
Phone	Final Salary	☐ Full-time ☐ Part-time ☐ Summer ☐ Temporary	

Description of duties, responsibilities and equipment operated

Reason for leaving _____

Previous Position		Dates of Employment From (Mo./Yr.)	To (Mo./Yr.)
Employer		Department	
Address		Supervisor	
Phone	Final Salary	☐ Full-time ☐ Part-time ☐ Summer ☐ Temporary	

Description of duties, responsibilities and equipment operated

Reason for leaving _____

Certification and Statement of Understanding

I certify that all of the information furnished in this employment application and its addenda are true and complete to the best of my knowledge. I understand that the University may investigate the information I have furnished, and I authorize any person, firm, or organization to supply any information about me concerning any past employment, military duty, convictions, or personal information to The Ohio State University and I release any such person, firm, or organization from any responsibility in disclosing such information. I realize that any misrepresentation or false information included in the application materials or provided in the interview process can lead to the withdrawal of an offer of employment or to termination from employment. I understand that any future offer of employment may be conditioned upon the results of examinations, physical or other, as may be necessarily required by the University. The University will pay the reasonable cost of any examination which may be required.

Signature _____ Date _____

FIGURE 12–1. *(continued)*

The Ohio State University Hospitals
and
Arthur G. James Cancer Hospital & Research Institute
Employment Addendum C Form

The Ohio State University Hospitals and the Arthur G. James Cancer Hospital and Research Institute are drug free workplaces. Individuals offered employment are required to successfully complete a pre-employment physical which includes drug testing. If found positive for illicit drugs, after informing the applicant, the application will be removed from hospital employment consideration.

Name: _____ **Social Security Number** _____
Last   First   Mi

1. How did you learn of employment opportunities at The Ohio State University Hospitals or the Arthur G. James Cancer Hospital & Research Institute? _____

2. List any professional or technical licenses or certificates related to the type of employment you are seeking (e.g., Paramedic, Animal Technician, RN, LPN, Stationary Engineer) and indicate license number and expiration date.
    _____
    _____
    _____
    _____
    _____

If you are applying for a position that requires operating a motor vehicle, please complete question **3. a, b, c.**

3. **a. Yes No** Do you have a valid driver's license?

    Issuing State:_____   Number _____
    Expiration Date: _____

    b. Yes No Do you have a valid commercial driver's license?

    Issuing State: _____   Number _____
    Expiration Date: _ _____ _____

    c. Yes No Do you have a valid chauffeur's license?

    Issuing State: _____   Number _____
    Expiration Date: _____

4. **Yes No** Are you a former employee of The Ohio State University, University Hospitals, or the Arthur G. James Cancer Hospital & Research Institute?
    If **yes**, list date of resignation and your name at time of resignation _____

5. **Yes No** Are you currently enrolled as an Ohio State University student for more than 10 credit hours?

6. **Yes No** Are you under the age of 18? If **yes**, submit a copy of your school board work permit.

7. **Yes No** Are you a citizen or permanent resident of the United States? If **no**, what is your visa type and I-94 expiration date? _____

8. **a. Yes No** Are you a veteran of active military service in the U.S. Armed Forces? If **yes**, what branch of service? _____

    b. Yes No Are you submitting a copy of your DD214? This is required in order to receive military service credit for classified civil service positions.

(Continue on reverse)

The Ohio State University
Form 11118—Rev. 12/93

FIGURE 12–1. *(continued)*

9.   **Yes   No**   Have you ever been dismissed from a position for delinquency or misconduct? If **yes**, give details in COMMENTS section.

Question 10 is asked only with reference to the bona fide requirements of the position(s) being sought. **A "yes"** answer will not jeopardize your candidacy unless the question is related to the duties of the position.

10.   **Yes   No**   Have you ever been convicted of a criminal offense? If **yes,** give details in COMMENTS section. (You may omit any offense adjudicated in a juvenile court and any traffic violations for which a fines of less than $50.00 was paid—except if you are applying for positions which require driving.)

          COMMENTS
A.   Indicate details regarding any **"yes"** answer to questions 9 and 10 of this addendum.

_____
_____
_____
_____
_____

B.   Indicate all **equipment** you operate which may be utilized in the positions for which you have applied. This would include all office equipment, copiers, typewriters, word processors, computers, as well as machine tools, vehicles, cleaning equipment, construction equipment, electronic equipment, etc.

_____
_____
_____
_____
_____

C.   Indicate any comments you have regarding your **training, education, qualifications, and skills** (typing speed, computer software package, etc.)

_____
_____
_____
_____

NOTARY SECTION - TO BE COMPLETED AT TIME OF INTERVIEW

I solemnly swear (or affirm) I am the individual named in this application and the information given herein is true and complete to the best of my knowledge.

Signature of applicant before a notary public: _____

Subscribed and duly sworn before me according to Law, by the above named applicant this _____ day of _____, 19____, at _____, County of _____, and State of Ohio.

                                              _____
                                              Signature of Notary Public

          (Seal)

                                              _____
                                              Official Title & Expiration of Commission

FIGURE 12–1. *(continued)*

See reverse side for instructions

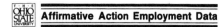

Affirmative Action Employment Data

The Ohio State University is an AFFIRMATIVE ACTION/EQUAL OPPORTUNITY EMPLOYER. In an effort to meet its affirmative action, nondiscrimination objectives, and in order to comply with federal and state laws, regulations and guidelines, you are urged to complete this form by providing the information requested below. Please note that provision of this information is voluntary and, if provided, this information will be handled confidentially. Failure to provide this information will not subject you to any adverse treatment. Please print or write clearly using a pen. See additional information and instructions on reverse side.

SECTION I — APPLICANT INFORMATION

Name _____

      last   first   middle

A. Sex: ☐ **1.** Male   ☐ **2.** Female

B. Race/Ethnicity:
- ☐ **1. Black, Non-Hispanic** — A person having origins in any of the Black racial groups of Africa.
- ☐ **2. American Indian or Alaskan Native** — A person having origins in any of the original peoples of North America, and who maintains identification through tribal affiliation or community recognition.
- ☐ **3. Asian or Pacific Islander** — A person having origins in any of the original peoples of the Far East, Southeast Asia, the Indian sub-continent, or the Pacific Islands. This area includes China, Japan, Korea, the Philippine Islands and Samoa.
- ☐ **4. Hispanic** — A person of Mexican, Puerto Ricn, Cuban, Central or South American or other Spanish culture or origin, regardless of race.
- ☐ **5. White, Non-Hispanic** — A person having origins in any of the original peoples of Europe, North Africa or the Middle East.

C. Are you disabled?   ☐ **1.** Yes   ☐ **2.** No

Disability means any person who (1) has a physical or mental impairment which substantially limits one or more major life activities; (2) has a record of such impairment; or (3) is regarded as having such an impairment. If you are disabled, we would like to include you under our Affirmative Action Program. Accordingly, it would assist us if you would tell us about: (1) any special methods, skills and procedures which qualify you for positions that you might not otherwise be qualified for because of your handicap, so that you will be considered for any positions of that kind, and (2) the accommodations which we could make which would enable you to perform a job properly and safely. You may provide the requested information below and/or on attached pages.

_____

_____

_____

D. Are you a Vietnam-era Veteran?   ☐ **1.** Yes   ☐ **2.** No

A Vietnam-era Veteran is any veteran of the armed forces who, between August 5, 1964 and May 7, 1975, served on active duty for at least 181 consecutive days, or who was discharged sooner because of a service-related disability.

E. Have you been determined to be a "special disabled veteran"?   ☐ **1.** Yes   ☐ **2.** No

F. What prompted you to apply to The Ohio State University?
- ☐ 1. Notice in University Personnel Postings.
- ☐ 2. Personal contact (name of contact) _____
- ☐ 3. Notice in professional journal (name of journal) _____
- ☐ 4. Newspaper advertisement (name of newspaper) _____
- ☐ 5. Placement service (name of placement service) _____
- ☐ 6. Other (please describe) _____

G. Date of birth: _____

          month   date   year

APPLICANT: DO NOT WRITE BELOW THESE LINES

SECTION II

This section must be completed by the department if the applicant has applied directly to the department for a current, specific job vacancy.

H. Position Title _____

I. Position Posting Number _____

J. Department _____ **K. Department No.** _____

L. EEO Job Category _____

The Ohio State University
Form 9488, Rev. 10/88 Stores 53757

FIGURE 12–1. *(continued)*

THE OHIO STATE UNIVERSITY
AFFIRMATIVE ACTION EMPLOYMENT DATA

Applicant Information

1. The University is requesting the information in Section I on the reverse side of this form in an effort to meet its affirmative action, non-discrimination objectives. In addition, federal and state laws, regulations and guidelines require that the University collect information concerning its applicants for employment. (If you receive this form in the mail, please return it in the enclosed business reply envelope addressed to the Office of Affirmative Action).

2. Provision of the information on the reverse side of this form is voluntary. Failure to provide this information will not result in any adverse treatment of you as an applicant or as an employee if you are hired.

3. The information you provide will not be forwarded to an employing department. This information *will remain confidential* unless:
   a. You provide the information to an employing department voluntarily, or
   b. You are a disabled applicant, in which case the University *may* need to inform:
      (1) Supervisors and managers regarding restrictions on the work or duties of disabled individuals, and/or regarding necessary accommodations;
      (2) First aid and safety personnel, when and to the extent appropriate, if a disability condition might require treatment; and
      (3) Governmental officials investigating compliance with respect to the Rehabilitation Act of 1973.

University Employment Services Offices Information and Instructions

1. Each of the University's employment services offices (Professional Employment Services, Staff Employment Services and the University Hospitals Human Resources Office) shall provide this form, together with the employment application, to *all* applicants for employment at the University.

2. Completed copies of this form will *not* be available to employing departments. The forms will be retained for the purpose of compiling information regarding the composition of the applicant pool, and to assist the University in the evaluation/enhancement of its affirmative action recruitment efforts.

3. In an effort to assist in the recruitment, selection and/or accommodation of disabled applicants, the employment services offices may provide certain applicant information to the individuals listed above in item 3.b.

Department Information and Instructions

1. Please provide this form, along with the appropriate business reply envelope (addressed to the Office of Affirmative Action) to *all* applicants for a current, specific job vacancy who have not been referred by one of the University's employment services offices. Persons expressing interest in general employment possibilities, and not in a specific vacancy, should *not* be provided a copy of this form by the department until they become candidates for a specific job opening.

2. Complete Section II of this form *prior* to providing the form to an applicant.

FIGURE 12–1. *(continued)*

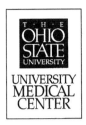

To the applicant: Please supply the name and address of a previous employer for reference purposes and sign your name. Thank you.

REQUEST FOR REFERENCES:

TO: Name: _____

                 Company: _____

                 Address: _____

              City/State/Zip: _____

REGARDING: _____
                 Applicant Name   Social Security #

                                                                      /   /
              _____   _____
                 Signature   Date

To the employer: The person named above has applied for a position as a _____
at The Ohio State University Hospitals and has given your name as a reference.

Your answers to the following questions will help us evaluate this individual's candidacy.

Position Held: _____

Dates of Employment: _____ to _____

Quality of Work: _____

Attendance Record: _____

Reason for Termination: _____

Eligible for Rehire?   YES   NO   If not, please explain: _____
_____

Additional Comments: _____

SIGNATURE: _____

TITLE: _____

DATE: _____

Thank you for your cooperation.

PLEASE FOLD TOP PORTION INSIDE

FIGURE 12–1. *(continued)*

Other information can be gleaned from the employment record. An individual who has a record of short stays with employers may indicate a lack of stability, which should be assessed further in an interview. Advancements in job position, attendance in training programs, or participation in continuing education by the applicant suggest positive qualities that can be further evaluated in the interview.

Although reference checks are a limited source of information concerning a prospective employee, they remain a vital part of the selection process. In the clinical laboratory, an individual's credentials are critically important for ensuring the quality of laboratory results. One of this chapter's authors recalls an incident in which a chemistry supervisor was hired on the basis of his self-stated academic preparation equivalent to a doctoral degree. The individual at the time appeared to be a godsend in the middle of a crisis following several evening-shift resignations. Months later, after the manpower shortage had been alleviated, technical problems arising in the laboratory prompted the chief technologist to check references on the new chemistry supervisor. The resulting information revealed academic preparation perhaps equivalent to the baccalaureate level but without the degree. Reference checks, therefore, as evidenced by this example, play an important role in the interviewing and selection process if quality is to be maintained.

CONDUCTING THE INTERVIEW

An interview is essentially a conversation between two people that permits a give-and-take exchange of information and ideas. Even though the interview process has not been shown to be particularly reliable, it is still the primary process by which employment decisions are made.[18] An employment interview should have structure and purpose to gather information, give direction, or motivate. The interview serves two basic functions.

First, it provides the opportunity for the employer to get to know the applicant. The applicant's qualifications for the job, background, and previous employment records are analyzed and discussed. Subjective information concerning maturity, personal appearance, attitudes, potential, and other pertinent areas is gathered. Second, the interview gives the applicant essential information about the nature of the job, hours, benefits, continuing education and training programs, and opportunities for advancement. Further, it creates an early feeling of mutual understanding between the employer and the applicant. A good initial relationship not only gives a positive impression to the most valuable prospective employee, but also is the basis for a lasting rapport between management and the employee.

The major advantage of the interview is that it is more flexible than a written interaction. It is particularly useful because it allows the interviewer to probe for more information than is on the written application.[12,23] The interview process has five separate but overlapping stages: (1) warm-up, (2) getting the applicant to talk, (3) drawing out, (4) information, and (5) forming an opinion.

The *warm-up* stage allows the interviewer to put the applicant at ease and to begin to develop a rapport in a relaxed atmosphere for the interview. This is important because most applicants are somewhat apprehensive. At this point, it is helpful to initiate a constructive atmosphere through a few general social remarks or similar interactions. The interviewer should create an atmosphere of sincere and genuine interest, recognizing the applicant as worthy of attention. An applicant who is at ease is far more likely to provide candid self-expression and an accurate assessment of attitudes, feelings, and ideas.

In the second stage, the interviewer must *get the applicant talking*. The interviewer must clarify the purpose of the interview quickly, explaining its function in terms that can be readily understood. The interviewer must have formulated goals and purposes for the interview, primarily from a review of the completed application and other pertinent information that has been gathered about the applicant. A good first question is extremely important to trigger the applicant's flow of conversation. This question should be one with which the applicant will probably be comfortable. For instance, asking an open-ended question, "I see that you have worked as a chief technologist at Memorial Hospital for the last 3 years. Can you tell me what you enjoy most about your job?" This allows the applicant to set the pace of the conversation.

In the *drawing-out* stage, the applicant is encouraged to describe further his or her background, qualifications, and other attributes he believes support his candidacy. During this stage, the interviewer should use various questioning techniques to learn as much as possible about the applicant. This is a critical time for the interviewer to assess as accurately as possible whether the applicant has appropriate knowledge, skills, and attitudes for the position. Information that is missed at this stage probably will not be retrieved later. Some critical interviewing techniques are reviewed later in this chapter.

In the *information* stage, the interviewer presents a picture of the institution and the specific job for which the applicant has applied. A part of this process necessarily involves selling the position and laboratory to the applicant. The best qualified applicants generally have choices among positions, and they are comparing the benefits and challenges of this position with other potential opportunities.[46] The best features of the job should be emphasized along with promotion and training opportunities, fringe benefits, salary, and other relevant information that would attract the applicant. Scheduling a tour of the laboratory can provide an excellent opportunity for the applicant to view the work setting and meet potential coworkers. This allows laboratory staff to meet a possible new employee. Their impressions can provide the interviewer with additional data with which to make a hiring decision. It allows the applicant to ask any questions about his perceived role and gives the interviewer clues about his real interest in the position, aspirations, and future goals.

The last stage of the interview is when an *opinion is formed*. This is usually done after the applicant has left the office and when constructive note taking can take place. Generally, it may be appropriate to take a few notes during the interview; however, major observations and analyses should be delayed until after the applicant has left. The interviewer must assess the applicant's qualifications against the requirements and conditions that have been identified for the position.

Interviewing Basics

The interview process should be structured to determine if the applicant has the qualifications to perform the responsibilities of the position and the overall fit of the applicant to the job and the organization. Also through this process, the applicant should better understand the position and should know if it provides the challenge and satisfaction desired. A few basic planning techniques can help the manager conduct an effective interview.[5,9,19]

INTERVIEW PREPARATION

The interviewer should take ample time to plan the process by carefully reviewing the job description. The interview should be scheduled so that there is ample time to conduct a quality, interactive process with the applicant and to ensure that there is a sense that ample time was spent with the applicant. The interview requires preparation by the interviewer. Both the requirements for the position and applicant's resume should be reviewed, and questions should be prepared that are relevant. If a tour is to be conducted, be sure that the appropriate people are alerted and available to meet with the candidate.[46]

ANALYSIS OF THE RESUME

Careful review of the resume for analyzing the applicant's experience and abilities is extremely important before the interview. The resume detail is the applicant's chronologic work record and other data useful in determining whether the candidate seems appropriate for the position. Through careful analysis, questions can be formulated for the interview. A review of the resume should determine, for instance, the chronologic record of the person's employment, educational qualifications, service to the profession, community activities, and other information that profiles the applicant. The reviewer can also pinpoint potential areas of concern, such as lapses in the work record, numerous job changes, lack of advancement, and other data to be investigated during the questioning portion of the interview.

INTERVIEW ENVIRONMENT

The interview process is a complex task involving screening and evaluation of much verbal data from the applicant; thus, a quiet atmosphere with minimal distractions is advantageous. Also, the interviewee will feel more comfortable in a setting that is private, free from phone calls or interruptions from staff. It is also important for the interviewer to create an environment without bias that may distort perceptions.

STRUCTURED INTERVIEW

In any interview, the interviewer must proceed in an organized fashion, generally proceeding in reverse chronologic order from the applicant's current position and covering prior work and educational preparation. All of this information will give the applicant an opportunity to demonstrate qualifications for the position and identify such items as career progress, job stability, overall motivation, and salary history. To be fair to candidates and ensure that consistent data are collected, a common set of questions should be generated and used with all the interviews. Try to group questions around common themes. For instance, questions centered on job skills and knowledge could be clustered while supervisory experience and academic preparation should be grouped together in other sections.

COMMUNICATION SKILLS

Communication during the interview process should be as simple and nonthreatening as possible. The interview is designed to determine the match between the applicant's experience and training with the duties and responsibilities of the position. The questions posed by the interviewer should not be complex but should be structured to elicit useful information. Many times, interview questions are relatively ineffective, resulting in a waste of time and only providing an opportunity for an applicant to provide answers that please the interviewer. More sharply defined questions that challenge the interviewee and may provide more useful information might include "What responsibilities do you now have in the laboratory that reflect your ability to perform this job?" rather than the more common question, "What are your responsibilities now?" Also ask questions that attempt to gain an assessment of experiences and performance. Asking for specific examples of job-related accomplishments challenges the interviewer to relate past performance to future performance and can provide useful information for the interviewer.[3]

Questions might be framed, "You say that over the past 5 years you became directly responsible for the supervision of four laboratory technicians. How did you use this responsibility to improve clinical performance in your area?" An understanding of some basic questioning techniques enables the interviewer to be more precise in the data-gathering process. Types of questions typically used in the interview process include those defined in Box 12–4.

Effective use of questioning techniques is an interviewing skill that maximizes the gathering of information about the applicant.[12] The development of questioning techniques takes concentrated practice; however, with time, the interviewer should be able to develop the interviewing process to the point that a considerable amount of critical information is gained during a relatively short interview period.

Box 12•4

Qualification Interview Questions

Has the applicant attended any manufacturer's workshops for this particular instrument?

Does the applicant have any experience in working with the particular instruments?

Has the applicant evaluated procedures in the past?

How has the applicant responded to an open-ended question dealing with the appropriate approach for determining the impact of an interfering substance?

INTERVIEW TERMINATION AND FOLLOW-UP

The interviewer establishes the conclusion of the interview when he decides that all the relevant information is gathered and the purpose of the interview has been achieved. The interviewer should summarize the major points and tie up loose ends brought out at the interview. As at the beginning, casual social comments are an appropriate way to wind down the interview. Often, the last words of the interviewer are remembered longest. In particular, the interviewer should express an appreciation for the opportunity to talk to the applicant. It is appropriate in closing to give the applicant some idea of how the interviewer has assessed the applicant's qualities. It is also appropriate for the interviewer to indicate how he will be communicating with him after the interviewing process has been completed. The applicant should be provided with a realistic date by which he can expect to hear from the employer. On the other hand, if the candidate appears to be unsatisfactory, the interviewer should clearly indicate that the applicant may not be matched with the job.

Misunderstandings can lead to charges of discrimination. At the conclusion of the interview, the interviewer must ensure adequate follow-up by considering results, updating employment records, and other routine procedures, such as contacting the personnel department. Some information gathered in the interview may not be as easy to quantify. Writing up notes taken during the interview clarifies impressions or ideas and emphasizes the applicant's strong or weak points.

Limitations of Interviewing

Anyone with supervisory responsibilities eventually becomes involved in the interviewing process. Successful interviewing is a challenge; however, interviewing skills can be mastered by simple training, exposure, and practice. Although much of the success of the interview is based on the skills and discipline of the interviewer, there are some limitations inherent in all interviews.

First, it is important to emphasize that there are certain questions that may not be asked during an interview. These are the same as those prohibited on the application form (see Table 12–1). For instance, race and color are never acceptable standards for hiring, and no questions should be asked that relate to these areas. Although recent court rulings indicate that institutions may hire on the basis of sex or race when there are clear inequities, it is never appropriate to focus on such areas as part of the interview. Questions related to sex are always to be avoided. For instance, questions related to marriage ("Are you married?" "Do you have any children?") or spousal relationships ("Where does your husband work?") are inappropriate and should be avoided. Questions can be asked in such a way as to gain relevant information but not infringe on the applicant's right to privacy.[18] For instance, it is discriminatory to ask a woman about who will take care of her children. However, if the position requires the ability of the applicant to work extended hours during peak periods of time, a question may be asked such as, "At certain times of the year, we have especially heavy workloads, and overtime may be required. Is there anything that would prevent you from performing this part of the job satisfactorily?" Questions related to national original, religion, age, and arrest or conviction records are all inappropriate as well.

The second limitation of interviewing is that the reliability of the interview is markedly lower when the interview is unplanned, aimlessly directed, and vague. In this situation, the interviewer is likely to rate applicants inconsistently: The same applicant might receive different ratings in two interviews with the same interviewer. A thorough knowledge of the job description; a firm set of qualifications, including standards for each level within a position; and a systematic plan for assessing each applicant increase the interviewer's reliability.

Team interviewing is another method that increases reliability. Often, individual interviewers do not rate applicants similarly; pooled judgments more successfully assess the applicant. It is a good idea to have as a member of the interviewing team a person who has current information on the job vacancies, wages, and benefits (eg, laboratory manager, personnel representative). An interviewer's lack of knowledge in this area may discourage valuable applicants. The interviewing team should also include individuals with the necessary technical skills to assess the applicant accurately (eg, bench technologist, technical supervisor). Team interviewing can be accomplished in a conference or by progressive interviews.

The third limitation of the interviewing process consists of the degree to which the interviewer intervenes in the interviewing process. When the interviewer dominates the conversation, useful information cannot be gathered. When the interviewer fails to listen or give mental attention to what is being said, important information will be missed, and the value of the interview will be limited. The interviewer should encourage the applicant to speak freely. He should not only listen, but also attempt to comprehend the speaker's intent. The interviewer should avoid interrogating the applicant by overuse of statements beginning with "what," "when," "where," and "why." Placing the applicant in a stressful situation will limit information exchange and frighten valuable applicants away.

A fourth limitation of interviewing is created by the interviewer through attitudes, biases, and prejudices that influence the appraisal of the applicant. These are responses over which the interviewer has little control and which can never be totally eliminated. A good interviewer, being aware of these weaknesses, can discount them in his assessment of the applicants. One common interviewer bias is called the "halo effect." The halo effect occurs when a single characteristic of the applicant dominates the interviewer's judgment in other areas. For instance, the fact that an applicant may have graduated from the interviewer's college may dominate the interview and may overshadow the applicant's limited job experience. The halo effect can also take a negative form. For instance, an applicant's appearance or dress (having a beard, wearing jeans) may create an initial negative impression about the applicant that will unfairly bias the overall assessment.

Another interviewer problem is the lack of flexibility. The interviewer who asks the same questions and in the same order with no variance cannot accurately evaluate the applicant's responses. Optimum information can be exchanged only through thoughtful, individualized probing.

Finally, the interview is often limited by the interviewer's decision to hire too early in the interview process. Immediate decisions based on such preliminary information as personal appearance and general manner, rather than experience and training, can cause job-related problems later.

In summary, the interview process is a complex task requiring effective communication skills; careful attention to constructing a planned, organized interview; appropriate use of questioning techniques; and a genuine desire to select the best qualified applicant on the basis of the candidate's knowledge, skills, and attitudes under fair and open competition.

THE SELECTION PROCESS

Once the interviews are completed, the supervisor is faced with sorting out the information gathered and making a selection. This decision will affect many facets of the supervisor's realm of influence and responsibility. A common pitfall in the selection process is the assumption that the personal judgment of the hiring laboratory manager is sufficient to determine an applicant's qualifications. Some managers attempt to make a selection based on *body chemistry*—a feeling of whether a person is right for the job. Reliance on personal feelings has caused the downfall of many individual laboratory supervisors.

Input should be solicited from all those involved in the interviewing process; this will increase the value of the selection decision. The final decision of which applicant to hire, however, must be the responsibility of the immediate supervisor. Unfortunately, no single formula applies to screen out those not well suited for a position and select the most qualified applicant. One of the most successful approaches is to list the qualifications necessary for the vacant position (based on specific tasks and the job description) with a corresponding semiquantitative evaluation. One category of qualifications may address the academic preparation and work experience relevant to the position. For example, if the job description calls for major responsibilities in the repair and preventive maintenance of particular instrumentation, qualification items may include those found in Box 12–5.

For nearly all applicants, regardless of the specific job description, a category dealing with individual work characteristics and interpersonal relations skills would be appropriate (Box 12–6).

Semiquantitation of these qualifications can be accomplished by establishing a numerical scale (perhaps 1–10) for each item. This will force critical evaluation of those components essential for a given position and assist in ranking the applicants. One inherent problem with this approach is the weighting of the characteristics. Avoid selecting someone whose extremely high ratings on academic preparation and work experience shadow some problems recorded as low ratings in the area of interpersonal relations. Particularly noteworthy is guarding against hiring a career-entry staff member on the basis of academic performance. A study by Firestone, Lehmann, and Leiken found that characteristics other than academic ability are more important predictors of the professional success of medical technologists.[8]

Finally, a manager should not be afraid to hire someone perceived as being more capable than he is. The success of many administrators is largely dependent on their ability to draw together a group of highly skilled individuals and to unify their expertise to create an exceptional team.

Once a decision to hire has been made, both a letter of offer and letter of rejection must be framed. Because of legal concerns, both must be carefully written and increasingly, as a matter of policy, they may have to be reviewed and approved by the human resources department. The letter of offer should clearly and accurately convey the details of the job offer. Any misrepresentation or misinterpretations can create a poor employment relationship from the beginning. The applicants not selected should receive a letter of rejection that is positive but brief. The supervisor should never attempt to write, in an effort to be helpful, an analysis or extensive commentary on why an applicant was not hired. To do so only invites potential legal problems.

TRANSFER AND PROMOTION

When vacancies occur in staff and supervisory positions, transfers and promotions may be viable alternatives to outside recruitment and selections.[37] Increasingly, this may be the case as institutions downsize, and employees are encouraged to search for other opportunities within the laboratory. The clinical laboratory would seem to provide substantial breadth for transfer. It may appear to technologists that transferring from one department to another in the clinical laboratory as a lateral move is an excellent option based on their current generalist education. Unfortunately, technologic advances in the laboratory make such transferring a less than optimal situation if the laboratory is departmentalized. If a laboratorian has not worked within the department to which he wishes to transfer, a considerable amount of retraining will be necessary.

At times, employees will request transfers to different departments or different specialties within a department. The transfer in this manner plays a vital role in providing an alternative for the individual who assumes a situation with no upward mobility. A staff technologist may request a transfer to get around a blockage in his career ladder aspirations or as a means of seeking greater challenge in technical responsibilities.

Transfers are a managerial tactic used at times to cope with incompatibilities between a given position and the employee holding it. A transfer may effectively resolve a problem situation in which an employee is not capable of performing the required tasks or has developed personal friction in dealing with his supervisor or peers. Frequent remedial transfers from department to department when conflict arises among the staff are not advised. This results in a glossing over of serious problems. Rather than postpone the resolution of these problems with a transfer, the problem needs to be identified and handled directly.

Promotion to a supervisory position or selection of a supervisor from outside warrants special consideration. Few technologists are adequately prepared to assume managerial roles solely on the basis of career-entry education. However, such responsibilities are often expected soon after completion of the entry-level degree.

A recent study by Peddecord and Taylor of the education, training, and experience of supervisory personnel in interstate laboratories found most supervisors to be prepared at the baccalaureate level and having more than 10 years of experience.[29] Historically, technologists have been promoted on the strength of their technical expertise and tenure in the laboratory, and less emphasis has been placed on their managerial skills.

Box 12·5

Qualification Items

Leading questions: This type of question tends to lead the applicant to a predetermined answer. These have no place in the interview and should be avoided. If they are used, the amount of information obtained is minimal, and the answer only tends to confirm what is implied in the question. For example:
"You obviously don't like working at Metropolitan Hospital, do you?"
"You really haven't had much experience related to this position, have you?"
"You seem to have had some problems at your lab job, haven't you?"

Open-ended questions: Questions that are open ended cannot be answered with a yes or no. They require more explanation and provide the interviewee with an opportunity to offer unsolicited information or clarify comments. While such questions allow the interviewee to control a portion of the interview, they also create an environment in which the interviewer is able to glean a great deal of information:
"You've heard the description of the job, could you now tell me how you think you fit into it?"
"If you were to take this position, how would it fit into your future ambitions?"
"Can you tell me your reasons for leaving your last job?"
"As you can see, the job of senior medical technologist at this hospital has some problems attached to it; how do you think you would help solve these problems and make the laboratory more productive?"

Direct questions: These questions can be answered with a "yes," "no," or one-word answer. In general, such questions should be avoided because little constructive information is gained.[10] The best use of these questions is when you want to gain specific information, rather than a general explanation. The questions should be quick and to the point and are most effective when followed by open-ended questions.
"What is your current salary? What salary considerations do you feel are important in the position for which you are applying?"
"Having seen the laboratory, are you still interested in this position? What do you think you can do to make the laboratory more productive?"

Probing questions: Probing questions are designed to delve more deeply into the interviewee's answers. These are particularly useful in eliciting specific examples of what the interviewee has done and why.[23] There are a number of different situations in which probing questions are appropriate. For instance, in response to a short incomplete answer, the interviewer may want to delve more deeply to gain more specific information.
First question: "Have you gone to any continuing education programs recently?"
Applicant response: "A few."
Probing question: "Can you describe these programs for me?"
Some probing questions may be used where there is need for further clarification or to explain a response that was unclear or did not make sense in the context of the question.
First question: "What do you think you would enjoy most about being the supervisor of the laboratory section?"
Applicant response: "The job looks really challenging."
Probing question: "What would you enjoy about the challenge?"
Sometimes a probing question will be channeled more directly to focus on a perceived feeling or attitude that has been identified by the interviewer. Thinking that it is important to amplify on it, the interviewer may want to probe more deeply in an attempt to ascertain the true frame of reference of the interviewee.
First question: What particularly appeals to you about the technologist position for which you are applying?"
Applicant response: "It seems like the kind of position in which I could work independently from others without any of the usual hassles with the other technologists."
Probing question: "What kinds of hassles have you experienced when working closely with others?"

Hypothetical questions: These questions provide the interviewer excellent insight into the problem-solving thought processes of the applicant. Good hypothetical questions will pose a potential problem and ask the interviewee to propose a solution. These provide an opportunity for the applicant to demonstrate insight, experience, and innovation.
"If this laboratory is going to maintain its present level of activity, some entrepreneurial ventures are going to have to be pursued. Do you have any ideas as to how we might be able to expand our services or scope of testing offered?"
"The job you are applying for requires a lot of interaction with hospital management who have so far been insensitive to problems that cost-containment measures have caused us. Do you have any ideas about how we might be able to help them better understand the laboratory operation?"

Box 12•6

Individual Work Characteristics Interpersonal Reasons Skills Interview Questions

How closely supervised does the applicant need to be? Is he able to plan and organize his own work?

Is the applicant able to make sound decisions?

What is the applicant's predicted ability to get along with even the most troublesome fellow laboratorian in the department?

Promotion from within may be an ideal approach for filling supervisory positions that have been vacated. The techniques described previously concerning interviewing and selection still apply. Laboratory administrators should encourage the maintenance of good individual evaluation records to identify achievers with growth potential. A wise manager will maintain an ongoing, informed grooming process for possible candidates for future promotion. This is best accomplished by delegating some supervisory responsibilities and counseling the potential leader when appropriate. Some institutions maintain rather elaborate *career-ladder tracks* for employee improvement in preparation for promotion opportunities of the future.

The use of career ladders can be an effective means of developing a more productive staff.[4,25] Such staff development plans offer employers an opportunity to realize professional advancement and job satisfaction without changing institutions. Other job enrichment opportunities, such as participatory decision making and contact with other patient service representatives, help prepare staff technologists for promotion.[5,33,45]

Of significant importance is the degree of support and assistance provided the newly promoted individual. Despite the fact that the new position probably carries increased responsibilities, management must not make the promotion a "sink or swim" transition.

While the benefits of promotion to the individual and the organization are obvious, the process is not without problems. The mere existence of the promotion policy creates what is perhaps the most difficult situation—the employee who is unlikely to be promoted. The laboratory supervisor has the responsibility of not only watching out for and developing potential staff for promotion, but also helping those not promotable to accept their fate. An individual unsuitable for promotion must not be allowed to take for granted that he is in line for various promotions on the basis of longevity.

After several occasions of being passed over, a problem is likely to develop that might result in serious charges of favoritism. The most effective tactic to use in dealing with the employee unlikely for promotion is a one-to-one discussion about the responsibilities of the new position long before a decision is made. The supervisor should attempt to point out the incongruities between the employee's abilities and the requirements of the new position. Perhaps guidance can be provided to help the employee supplement his background or improve his performance to prepare himself for eventual promotion.

Another promotion-related problem is the employee who does not want to be promoted. Laboratory administrators are frustrated from time to time by the employee with excellent potential who lacks the desire for advancement. This person has reached the limit of his ambition or perceived ability. Most often, refusal of promotion by laboratory personnel hinges on the employee not wanting to take on additional responsibility or problems associated with the new position. This should not be held against the employee. A discussion of the benefits to the organization and promotable employee may assist in convincing him to try the new responsibilities. If the employee still declines the promotion, administration must look elsewhere.

Promoting an employee always involves a degree of risk. The new position undoubtedly has responsibilities for which the candidate has not had the opportunity to display competence. Most people have observed a leader who was promoted beyond the level of his competence. So widespread is this phenomenon, in fact, that it has achieved the distinction of being termed the *Peter Principle:* "In a hierarchy every employee tends to rise to his level of incompetence."[28] The effect of this phenomenon on the staff is likewise interesting: "Employees in a hierarchy do not really object to incompetence *(Peter's Paradox).* They merely gossip about incompetence to mask their envy of employees who have pull."[30] The promotion of an individual may yield an incompetent employee at a key level in the organizational hierarchy. Therefore, the promotion process must be undertaken with great care.

REFERENCES

1. Brown N, Chellin V: Recruitment and retention leadership. J AHIMA 64(8):60–63, 1993
2. Business Week, p. 91, February 24, 1975
3. Camp RR, Hermon MV: The employment interview: Avoiding the traps with effective strategies. Cl Lab Mgt Rev. Nov/Dec:500–513, 1993
4. Crane VS, Jefferson K: Clinical career ladders: Doing more with less. Health Care Supervisor 5(3):1–11, 1987
5. Crystal JC, Deems RS: Redesigning jobs. Training and Development Journal 37(2):44–46, 1983

6. Famularo JJ (eds): Handbook of Human Resources Administration. New York, McGraw-Hill, 1986

7. Fenton JW Jr, Kinard JL, David FR: Negligent hiring and retention: Some evidence of hospital vulnerability. H Care Mgt Rev 16(1):73–81, 1991

8. Firestone DT, Lehmann CA, Leiken AM: Predictors of career advancement for laboratory professionals. Lab Med 17: 759–762, 1986

9. Galassi JP, Galassi MD: Preparing individuals for job interviews: Suggestions from more than 60 years of research. Personnel Guidance Journal 57(4):188–192, 1978

10. Hallas G: Honing hiring skills. Contemporary Long-Term Care. Apr:38–41, 1991

11. Hoffman NM, Martin BG: Affirmative action: What does it really mean? MLO 11:49–57, 1979

12. Hopkins JT: The top twelve questions for employment agency interviews. Personnel J 58(5):379–381, 1980

13. Iry TR: Keeping the employment interview legal. MLO 13(11):97–115, 1981

14. Karni KR, Studer WM, Carter SJ: A study of job turnover among clinical laboratory personnel. Am J Med Technol 48: 49–59, 1982

15. Kraft JD: Adverse impact determination in federal examinations. Pub Per Mgt 7(6):362–367, 1978

16. Lehr RI: Employer duties to accommodate handicapped employees. Labor Law Journal 31(3), 1980

17. Linenberger P, Keaveny TJ: Age discrimination in employment: A guide for employers. Personnel Administration 24(7):87–98, 1979

18. Linney BJ: Interviewing from the organization's perspective. Physician Exec 19(1):46–49, 1993

19. Makin P, Robertson 1: Selecting the best selection techniques. Personnel Management. November:38–42, 1986

20. McConnell CR: The Effective Health Care Supervisor. Rockville, Aspen Systems, 1982

21. McConnell CR: How dangerous is truth in employment references? H Care Superv 12(2):1–16, 1993

22. McQuire JP: The use of statistics in Title VII cases. Labor Law Journal 30(6):361–370, 1979

23. Micheals DT: Seven questions that will improve your managerial hiring decisions. Personnel Journal 59(3):199–224, 1980

24. Miller EC: An EEO examination of employment applications. Personnel Administration 25(3):63–81, 1980

25. Miller K: How rotation can help boost productivity. MLO 19(l):53–58, 1987

26. Munchus G: Check references for safer selection. HR Magazine. June:75–77, 1992

27. Norwood JM: But I can't work on Saturdays. Personnel Administration 25(l):25–30, 1980

28. Parks DG: Employment references: Defamation law in the clinical laboratory. Cl Lab Mgt Rev. Mar/Apr:103–110, 1993

29. Peddecord KM, Taylor RN: Education, training, and experience of supervisory personnel in interstate laboratories. J Med Technol 2:114–118, 1985

30. Peter LJ, Hull R: The Peter Principle. New York, William Morrow, 1969

31. Pigors P, Meyers C: Personnel Administration: A Point of View and a Method. New York, McGraw-Hill, 1977

32. Portwood JD, Koziara KS: In search of equal employment opportunity: New interpretations of Title VII. Labor Law Journal, 30(6):353–359, 1979

33. Rosland FA: A study of job enrichment preferences among medical technologists. J Med Technol 2:127–130, 1985

34. Sawyer S, Whatley AA: Sexual harassment: A form of sex discrimination. Personnel Administration 25(l):36–44, 1980

35. Sherman M: Equal employment opportunity: Legal issues and societal consequences. Pub Per Mgt 7(2):127–137, 1978

36. Sikula AF: Personnel Administration and Human Resources Management. New York, John Wiley and Sons, 1976

37. Simon WA: A practical approach to uniform selection guidelines. Personnel Administration 24(11):75–80, 1979

38. Smith RE: Successful People Management: How to Get and Keep Good Employees. Toronto, Macmillan, 1978

39. Solomon RJ: Legal considerations of medical-practice employee selection. Arch Ophthalmol (112):324–328, 1994

40. Stockard JG: Rethinking People Management: A New Look at the Human Resources Function. New York, AMACOM, 1980

41. Strauss G, Sayles LR: Personnel: The Human Problems of Management, 3rd ed. Englewood Cliffs, Prentice-Hall, 1972

42. Sweet D: The Modern Employment Function. Reading, Addison-Wesley Publishing Co, 1973

43. Terry GR: Supervision. Homewood, Richard D. Irwin, 1978

44. Tune L: DRGs three years later: Lab staffing trends mixed. Clin Chem News 13(6):l–2, 1987

45. Umiker WO: Job enrichment: Whose responsibility is it? MLO 14(11):58–64, 1982

46. Umiker W: Selection interviews of health care workers. H Care Superv 6(2):58–67, 1988

47. Zahsin EM: Affirmative action, preferential selection, and federal employment. Pub Per Mgt 7(6):378–393, 1978

48. Zinober JW, Maier C: Selecting the best to be the best: How to gain a competitive edge for your organization, Part I. Cl Lab Mgt Rev. Nov/Dec:483–488, 1993

ANNOTATED BIBLIOGRAPHY

Dann JD, Stephens EC: Management of Personnel: Manpower Management and Organizational Behavior. New York, McGraw-Hill, 1972

Part 2 of this reference, entitled "The Employment of Manpower," provides a concise look at determining the demand for manpower, recruitment, selection, testing, and interviewing.

Famularo JJ (ed): Handbook of Human Resources Administration. New York, McGraw-Hill, 1986

This comprehensive book covers all aspects of personnel management with current information. Part 4 has several chapters devoted to recruitment, selection, and placement of personnel.

Flippo EB: Principles of Personnel Management, 4th ed. New York, McGraw Hill, 1976

Part 3 of this book discusses job analysis, recruitment and hiring, and tests and interviews. Part 4 describes development of personnel, covering such topics as training and education, advancement, and performance appraisal. Part 5 addresses the compensation issues of personnel management.

Halper HR, Foster HS (eds): Laboratory Regulation Manual. Rockville, Aspen Publications (updated annually)

Part 10 of Volume III addresses laws concerning clinical laboratory employees. Also of interest might be Part 12 of the same volume dealing with malpractice. The three-volume set is an efficient, complete, and authoritative resource.

Lewis PV: Organizational Communication: The Essence of Effective Management. Columbus, Grid Inc, 1975

This reference is especially useful for considering the communication process in the interview setting. Chapter 11 addresses communication strategies appropriate for planning and conducting pre-employment and counseling interviews.

Metzger N: Personnel Administration in the Health Services Industry. Jamaica, Spectrum Publications, 1979

This book is an excellent administrative overview for personnel management. Chapter 4 has a comprehensive description of the recruitment, screening, and selection process.

McConnell CR: The Effective Health Care Supervisor. Rockville, Aspen Systems, 1982

This book provides a fine description of supervision in the health services industry. Chapter 8, "Interviewing: The Hazardous Hiring Process," provides excellent information on conducting the interview.

Pigors P, Myers CA: Personnel Administration: A Point of View and a Method, 7th ed. New York, McGraw-Hill, 1973

Readers will find this a thought-provoking examination of the ramifications of employee selection and developing human resources with a personnel policy system. The authors provide 19 case illustrations from their experiences, which aid the reader in understanding theoretical concepts.

Strauss G, Sayles LR: Personnel: The Human Problems of Management, 3rd ed. Englewood Cliffs, Prentice-Hall, 1972

Part 5 of this resource deals with manpower and employee development. Chapters 19, 20, and 21 address recruitment and selection, technical training, and minority employment. Readers may also find Chapter 11, "Interviewing: The Fine Art of Listening," to be helpful.

13

Staffing and Scheduling of Laboratory Personnel

Anthony S. Kurec

People don't dislike work ... help them to understand mutual objectives and they'll drive themselves to unbelievable excellence.

Tom Peters[1]

Social, economic, scientific, technologic, and political forces have had significant impact on the clinical laboratory over the years. Human resource management has gained much attention in response to health care reform attempts, penetration of managed care, accommodating changing demographics, and implementation of new technologies.

Because such demands are placed on productivity, efficiency, and cost-containment (the main driving force at this time), and because employees' salaries account for 50% to 70% of most budgets, survival in a highly competitive environment mandates laboratory personnel to be flexible and willing to adapt.[9] To ensure that recruitment, retention, education, and career development of laboratory personnel will be adequate and appropriate to meet the level of expertise required to maintain quality patient care and productivity, the laboratory must have good leadership. Optimal use of personnel is essential to cost-effective management and survival in today's competitive health-care world.

To sustain current laboratory practices and ensure future improvements, long-term, quality employees must be recruited. National vacancy rates have ranged over the past several years from 10% to 19%.[1] The loss of trained, experienced employees is costly. To hire a new technologist may cost $10,000 to $28,000[6,12] when accounting for loss of experience, overtime expenditures, advertising costs, recruiting and interviewing process, morale problems (due to overwork), time spent

training new employees, and administrative actions (eg, orientation, affirmative action, personnel, payroll).

The right people not only possess the appropriate core capabilities, but demonstrate a team-minded spirit and contribute their best to the success of any organization. In such an environment, good leaders need to be sensitive to their employees' needs and concerns. The baby boomer generation has focused more on family values and less on their job. For example, as the number of working mothers rises and as the older segment of the population increases, family care becomes a major concern. Leaders should assist, when appropriate, in resolving work and family conflicts. Through flexibility management, employees are willing to work as a team member, enhancing productivity, maintaining high morale, and being an effective contributor to the overall operation.[26] Moving to this strategy may reduce absenteeism and tardiness, minimize distractions, and otherwise provide a less stressful working environment. Laboratory managers and administrators must develop the skills necessary to take a leadership position. These traits, as outlined in Box 13–1, though not difficult to learn and understand, may be difficult in practice. Thus, in the leadership role, "walking the talk" is the benchmark of success.

RESOURCE MANAGEMENT

By definition, staffing is to provide a group of workers for securing united and cohesive performance in the most effective and cost-efficient way. This process requires short- and long-term planning. Scheduling is staff use: how the staff is organized, how work assignments are planned, and how personnel are used daily to

Box 13•1

Leadership

1. Communication—be open with coworkers.
2. Keep it simple—do not make extra work for yourself or others.
3. Encouragement—Take positive approach, be optimistic, and share information.
4. Praise—Catch them doing something right and praise them.
5. Learn from mistakes—Do not overly criticize or belittle employees; treat each fairly.
6. Knowledge—Develop a solid knowledge base.
7. Patience—Be patient and empathetic.
8. Decisions—Be decisive; have courage to accept responsibility and accountability.
9. Delegation—Don't be afraid to ask for assistance; take the time to teach.
10. Humor—Be serious about your job, but have a sense of humor about yourself.
11. Creativity—Be creative; think outside the "black box."
12. Sensitivity—Be sensitive to employee needs.

accomplish set goals. This involves determining the number and types of positions required and appropriately assigning trained employees to perform these tasks. Work assignments must be designed to meet the needs of the customer, the work flow of the laboratory, or any other issue that could limit effectiveness. Ongoing data acquisition and analysis of workload trends are critical in setting expected productivity levels for the laboratory staff. Laboratory managers and administrators must assess and comprehend the political and economic environments surrounding the laboratory so that appropriate decisions are made. To do this, a clear understanding of purpose and function must be identified (Box 13–2).

To assist in this process, an organization must develop vision and mission statements.[19] A vision statement tells the owners, managers, and employees why the organization exists; an example might be, "The department of pathology assists health-care providers in establishing an accurate diagnosis, prognosis, guidelines in patient management, screening for presence of disease, and monitoring follow-up therapy." A mission statement tells how this will be accomplished: "The Department of Pathology will provide comprehensive, high quality, customer-friendly pathology services in a timely and cost-efficient manner; serve as educator to staff, patients, and community; and sustain and expand research efforts

through state-of-the art technology and advanced procedures." The function and role of the laboratory and how it fits into the overall health-care organization must be clearly defined. Once the purpose of the laboratory has been determined, decisions about efficient use of personnel, facilities, and equipment can be made.

Understanding supply and demand and developing a business plan that sets goals for 1, 5, and 10 years into the future are helpful in anticipating staffing needs. Differences can then be assessed and a plan formulated to recruit and train proficient personnel.

Over the years, the development and refinement of human resources have improved the complex process of people management. Various management styles and practices have evolved through the centuries, from the dogmatic styles of the Egyptians when building the pyramids, the Romans when conquering the "world," and the philosophical discussions by Socrates and Plato,[16] to the quality management and improvement styles (total quality management and continuous quality improvement) of today. In the late 1800s, more scientific approaches were taken, such as Frederick Taylor's suggestion that increased productivity is directly associated with increased financial payment. Henri Fayol set down 14 principles, some of which are seen in practice today (Table 13–1). In 1943, Maslow proposed that individuals are motivated by the Hierarchy of Needs: physiological, safety, social, egotistical, self-fulfillment (in descending order).

The two-factor theory (Herzberg) identifies good feelings associated with content of a job (motivators) and bad feelings associated with job environment (hygiene factors). McGregor presented the idea that employees do not like work and will try to do as little as possible; they are basically lazy, irresponsible, and need constant direction (theory X). However, theory Y takes the opposite approach: Empowered employees will seek and accept responsibilities to meet the goals of the organization. Currently, structure has given way to total quality management and continuous quality im-

Box 13•2

Laboratory's Purpose and Function to Clinicians

1. Confirming or rejecting a diagnosis
2. Providing guidelines in patient management
3. Establishing a prognosis
4. Detecting disease through case finding or screening
5. Monitoring follow-up therapy

Adapted from reference 17.

Table 13-1
Classic Organizational Theory

Principle	Definition
Division of labor	Specialization in task performance
Authority	Formal and personal authority to direct, command, and lead workers
Discipline	Respect for rules and understanding of outcome if not followed
Unity: Command	Report to one "supervisor"
Unity: Direction	Grouping of similar activities under one supervisor
Subordination	Individual interests that do not exceed the goals of the organization
Compensation	Appropriate compensation for services performed
Top-down management	Management from "top down," centralized at the higher levels
Chain of command	Authority and decision making from the "top" and passed down to "subordinates"
Resources	Supplies, materials, and human resources available appropriately
Fairness	Employers fair and equitable in decision making
Security	Employees' position stable and free from unfair management practices
Empowerment	Employees as contributors to the organization
Esprit de corps	Employees as team players

Adapted from Fayol H: General and Industrial Management, Geneva, International Management Institute, 1930

provement concepts, in which management has gone from "top down" to "bottom up."[14,18] Empowered employees are willing to participate in decision making, thus providing total quality at every level during every phase of the procedure, while continually improving at each step. This works toward achieving "zero defects."

FORECASTING STAFFING AND SCHEDULING NEEDS

Forecasting human resource needs is complex. Various techniques have been developed to assist in identifying what is the optimal number of employees to hire at the most economical rate.[30] Overall, these techniques fall under two categories, judgmental forecasting and conventional statistical projections.[32] Judgmental forecasting uses opinions of experts to determine future needs, such as the Delphi technique. This technique is when a group of experts independently prepares statements regarding, in this case, anticipated staffing needs. These statements are reviewed by each member of the group (independently); comments are collected, and the process is repeated until a consensus is obtained.

The nominal grouping technique follows a similar procedure, but it uses a group-review rather than an independent one. Each suggestion is individually prioritized but reported collectively as a group. These brainstorming methods are helpful in identifying and solving organizational problems and staffing concerns. Conventional statistical projections use a mathematical approach, such as simple or linear regressions, productivity ratios, personnel ratios, and time management analyses. Several different systems have been developed for the laboratory using the mathematical approach.

One widely used system was developed by the College of American Pathologists (CAP). The Workload Recording System (WLRS),[10,11] developed in 1969, has been used to assist laboratory managers and hospital administrators in evaluating and making decisions in laboratory operations. WLRS accounts for the number of tests performed and time required to perform each. Tests are reported in workload units (1 unit 1 minute) and subsequently used in various calculations of productivity and use. In 1992, CAP discontinued this service, but many laboratories still use the basic concepts of this system.

Productivity monitoring involves the collection and evaluation of variable workload factors (determining standard unit values) within a fixed time standard to establish target use (accounts for constraints or inefficiencies not controllable by the laboratory manager or supervisor), workload volume, and a report format to collate information. This information then may be used to project workload needs so appropriate changes in practices may be made, such as increasing laboratory operating hours, adjusting test priorities, enhancing test menus, or changing testing frequency. Whatever adjustments are made, changes in staffing and scheduling personnel may be required, thus review and prioritization should be performed periodically. Changes must be shared with staff to allow adequate time for employees to understand and adjust to alterations of the daily schedule. Staff not involved in this process at some level may be resistant to changes, resulting in low productivity, poor morale, and possibly high employee turnover rate. The use of mathematical modeling techniques may be useful in predicting these workload variations.

Staffing assessment can then be made appropriately, and a productivity monitoring system can be constructed; therefore, use of laboratory personnel can be maximized.

In 1990, CAP announced the Laboratory Management Index Program (LMIP), which provides a more comprehensive view of how laboratory staffing, supplies, and service costs are used. This form of benchmarking ("A continuous, systematic process for evaluating the products, services, and work processes of organizations that are recognized as representing best practices for the purpose of organizational improvement."[33]) provides comparative indicators for financial and use management. The main difference between WLRS and LMIP is the former is based on the "workload unit (average minutes to complete a test), while the latter is based on a "billable test."

Other systems have been developed that account for all departments within a hospital, allowing standard comparisons to be made.[25] This information assists administrators and managers in addressing particular needs for each department and provides a greater overview of the organization. In the benchmarking process, laboratories are grouped and compared based on certain characteristics, such as number of output units (billable tests), complexity of testing, acuity of patients, techniques (equipment and procedures), and regional variances (Table 13-2). Whatever system is used, accurate, timely, and comprehensive data collection must be readily available, mandating the need for a well-developed laboratory information system (LIS). In the laboratory environment where work flow may be erratic, anecdotal perceptions of appropriate staffing must be avoided. Access to current workload trends is essential in the decision-making process.

Such decisions cannot be made in haste or lightly, thus a combination of judgmental and statistical forecasting may be appropriate to identify staffing needs correctly.

Table 13-3 shows how one may calculate the required number of full-time equivalents (FTEs) to staff a laboratory adequately that generates 1,000,000 workload units per year using the CAP system. In this example, the laboratory (currently working with 10 FTEs) would require 1 to 2 additional FTEs. Based on this information, appropriate discussions would take place to determine what adjustments in scheduling or staffing are required. In Table 13-4, benchmarking techniques are demonstrated.[25,33] Here laboratory X performs 40,000 billable procedures per year with a staff of 10 FTEs (20,124 worked hours per year). This laboratory spends 0.5 worked hours per procedure. These data are compared with other participating institutions with similar characteristics. In this peer group, laboratories Y and Z spend 0.4 and 0.2 worked hours per procedure,

Table 13-2
Measurements of Productivity and Resource Use

Indices	Measurement
Productivity	Billable inpatient test/FTE
	Billable outpatient test/FTE
	Billable outreach test/FTE
	Billable test/worked hour
	Billable test/paid hour
	Total billable tests/FTE Billable
	Total expense/billable test
	Labor expense/billable test
	Consumable expense/billable test
	Billable test/total tests performed
	Depreciation expense/billable test
Use	Inpatient billable test/day
	Inpatient billable test/discharge
	Inpatient billable test/bed
	Inpatient billable test/total billable tests
	Outpatient billable test/total billable tests
Cost effectiveness	Total expense/discharge
	Total expense/patient day
	Direct expenses/billable test
	Reference laboratory expense/billable test
	Total expenses/total billable tests charges
	Cost of blood purchases/billable test
Revenue comparisons	Billing tests/patient discharge
	Billing tests/patient day
	Billing tests/billable test

respectively. Because these laboratories share similar characteristics (such as number of outpatient tests versus inpatient, number of stats, percent of time supervisors spend at bench, level of automation, pneumatic tube system, bar coding), comparisons with some level of certainty may be made. In this example, laboratory Y can complete an equivalent amount of work with 2 fewer FTEs, while laboratory Z can do with 6 less. These data can be used to identify laboratories that appear to be more productive and determine what specific characteristics make them more efficient.

PERSONNEL SELECTION

In the laboratory, service is the product and people the major resource. An essential part of staffing requires the actual selection and development of personnel to fill

Table 13-3
Measurements of Productivity

Term	Definition	Example
Unit value	1 min (60 U/h)	10 FTEs 1,000,000 WLUs/y 1,000,000 WLU/60 u/h = 16,667 CAP h/y
Paid hours	Salaried time (40 h/w × 52 w = 260 paid d (2,080 h) per year	2,080 × 10 FTE = 20,800 h
	Overtime	50 hrs × 10 FTE = 500 h/y
	On call/recall	1,664 h (weekend coverage for evening/night shifts)
	Total paid time	22,964 h
Worked hours	5 d/52 wk = 260 d/y/FTE	2,080 h/FTE/y × 10 FTE − 20,080 h
	15–20 vacation days/FTE	16 d × 10 = 160 d (1,280 h)
	9–12 holiday/personal days/FTE	10 d × 10 = 100 d (800 h)
	6–10 sick days/FTE	8 d × 10 = 80 d (640 h)
	1–2 other/FTE	1.5 d × 10 = 15 d × 120 h
	Average of 31–44 days off per year	Total time off = 355 d (2,840 h)
	actual *worked* days = 216–229 days per year (1,728–1,832 h off/year/FTE)	Total worked hours = 20,124 h/y
Other	Nonworkload activities (average of 20% of total available time)	Accounting, billing, purchasing
		Administrative activities, telephone calls
		Lunch, breaks, meetings
		Quality assurance/control activites = 4,825 h/y
Standby or idle time	Time remaining *after* work loaded and non–work loaded hours are conted	Standby/idle time = 1,409 h/y
	Average of 5%–10% of total worked hours; 4%–9% paid hours	
Paid productivity	$= \dfrac{\text{Total workload units}}{\text{Paid hours}}$	$\dfrac{1,000,000 \text{ WLU}}{22,964 \text{ paid h}} = 43.5$ U/paid h 43.5 units/paid h/60 U/h × 100 = 72.6%
Worked productivity	$= \dfrac{\text{Total workload units}}{\text{Total hours worked}}$	$\dfrac{1,000,000 \text{ WLU}}{20,124 \text{ worked}} = 49.7$ U worked h 49.7 units/worked h/60 units/h × 100 = 82.8%
Available productivity	$= \dfrac{\text{Workload hours} + \text{nonworkload hours}}{\text{Worked hours}} \times 100$	$\dfrac{14,167 \text{ h} + 4,025 \text{ h}}{20,124 \text{ paid h}} \times 100 = 90.4\%$
Total productivity	$= \dfrac{\text{Workload hours} + \text{nonworkload hours}}{\text{Paid hours}} \times 100$	$\dfrac{14,167 \text{ h} + 4,025 \text{ h}}{22,964 \text{ paid h}} \times 100 = 79.2\%$
Target productivity	$= \dfrac{\text{Total available hours/year/FTE} \times 60 \text{ WLU/hour}}{\text{Paid hours/year/FTE}}$	$\dfrac{14,167 \text{ h}/10 \text{ FTE} \times 60 \text{ WLU/h}}{22,964 \text{ paid h}}$ = 37.0 units/h

(continued)

Table 13-3 continued

Term	Definition	Example
FTEs required	$= \dfrac{\text{Total CAP WLU/year}}{\text{Paid hours/year/FTE} \times \text{target productivity}}$	$\dfrac{1,000,000 \text{ WLU}}{22,964/10 \text{ FTE} \times 37.0}$ $= 11.9$ FTEs required
Expectations	—Paid productivity: 36–28 U/paid h (60%–63%)	72.6%
	—Worked productivity: 42–45 U/workd h (70–75%)	82.8%
	—Available productivity: 90%–95%	90.4%
	—Total productivity: 76%–85%	79.2%

the appropriate job titles. A successful laboratory is dependent on good leadership, and good leadership is dependent on the quality and loyalty of employees. The selection process is critical in matching people and their skills with appropriate jobs. Staffing begins with the recruitment process, followed by employee selection, comprehensive orientation and training, and subsequent performance appraisal. Laboratory managers that have retained high performers who produce quality services generally have spent time and forethought in developing a selection process that allows them to hire the right people. Preparing an accurate job description, using well-developed interviewing techniques, checking references, and offering appropriate orientation and training are essential.[39,40] Great emphasis must be placed on the recruiting process, because these initial decisions in personnel selection are often long-term commitments from the employer and employee. The size and complexity of the laboratory organization will determine who is assigned responsibility for recruiting, but most frequently it is the laboratory director, manager, or supervisor. These decisions should be made in conjunction with supervisors, chief technologists, and other senior staff members who may offer significant insight to the recruitment process and should be included as part of the team.

All employees must understand where they are in the organizational structure. Traditionally, a table of

Table 13-4
Benchmarking Productivity

Procedure	Laboratory X (example)
Number of procedures per year	40,000
Number of worked hours per 10 FTEs	20,124
Number of worked hours per procedure	40,000 procedures/20,124 worked h = 0.5
Laboratory Y (peer) highest worked hours per procedure	0.4 worked h per procedure
Laboratory Z (peer) lowest worked hours per procedure	0.2 worked h per procedure
Difference between Laboratory Y (highest) and Laboratory X	(0.5 − 0.4) × 40,000 procedures = 4,000 additional procedures
Difference between Laboratory Z (lowest) and Laboratory X	(0.5 − 0.2) × 40,000 procedures = 12,000 additional procedures
Number of additional FTEs comparing Laboratory Y with X	4,000 procedures/20,124 worked h = 2.0 FTE
Number of additional FTEs comparing Laboratory Z with X	12,000 procedures/20,124 worked h = 6.0 FTE
Number of FTEs required at Laboratory X's current productivity performance	Laboratory X would require two to six additional FTEs to perform the same amount of work compared with highest best performer and lowest best performer.

organization has been used to present structure and chain of command. This table identifies level of authority, direction of communication, and interrelationships among the components of the institution. Some laboratories have shifted from the hierarchical organization to one that is team based.[7] In this structure, top-down management is "flattening."

Team building is an important part of staff development, maintaining job satisfaction, and promoting high morale. Positions designed around the five characteristics listed in Table 13–5 will frequently produce a higher degree of job satisfaction and motivate employees.[27] Teams assembled and granted the appropriate responsibility, authority, and autonomy will be more effective and significantly contribute to the success of the laboratory. As trust and mutual respect are gained among the team participants, communication is openly shared, conflicts and disagreements expressed and resolved, and future goals planned and executed. Team coordinators and facilitators are identified who assist in setting schedules, policies, quality assurance and control guidelines, and day-to-day supervision. A greater sense of cooperation, client focus, and participation of all staff members is realized, thus enhancing morale and productivity within the organization.

Staffing and scheduling procedures should not be static parameters but adaptable to maintain quality services, promote efficiency, and meet employee expectations. Laboratory managers and administrators must respond quickly and effectively to changes in instrumentation, workload trends, test priorities, costs, and regulatory demands. Therefore, staffing and scheduling are important activities that require use of good management techniques and judgment in the review process. Modification of policies and procedures are made as necessary for optimal effectiveness.

CRITERION-BASED JOB DESCRIPTION

To identify and hire quality employees, clear and comprehensive job descriptions have been traditionally used in the selection process. Both employer and potential employees understand the expectations of the job and where they fit in the organizational structure of the team. Team-based organizations tend to use job descriptions to clarify roles of individuals without necessarily listing specific tasks.[34] These roles are focused on the "clients" and their needs rather than a particular section of the laboratory.

While a variety of formats have been used in developing job descriptions, the most basic should include job title, qualifications and worker traits, job duties, responsibilities and accountability, and job relationships (Fig. 13-1). Qualifications and worker traits should reflect the necessary education, training, or experience required.

The Americans With Disabilities Act (Bureau of National Affairs 42 USC 12101; 12111; 1990; 1992; Bureaus of National Affairs, Washington, DC) prohibits employment discrimination against qualified individuals with physical or mental disabilities (impairments that significantly limit one or more major activities: walking, breathing, speaking, hearing, seeing, learning, and performing manual tasks); therefore, qualifications should reflect minimum standards. Individuals seeking specific employment must possess the appropriate skills, experience, and education and be reasonably able to meet any other job-related requirements. They cannot be discriminated against based on perceived inability to do the job. Specific characteristics of the job should be identified, including limitations, such as physical demands ("capable of lifting 50 lb"), and working conditions unique to the position ("working with potentially biohazardous material"). In addition, one may have to identify parts of the job that could be performed by other employees or completed using mechanical or electronic devices, which may otherwise qualify a disabled individual. However, an employer may be exempt if changes create undue hardship related to costs, extensive modifications, or disruption to business.

Job duties include tasks that if not completed, would significantly change the nature of the job. This would outline the knowledge base and skills required to perform the technical, administrative, educational, or research aspects of the position. This may also include what work aids (equipment, including computers,

Table 13-5 Job Enrichment	
Characteristic	Outcome
Task variation	Performing different tasks with various levels of complexity
Job identity	Performing a job from beginning to end, realizing a sense of completion
Job significance	Impact of how "this job" affects or meets the goals of the institution, public, or self
Autonomy	Accountability and responsibility for self and getting the job done
Feedback	Response from coworkers in how well the job has been performed

JOB DESCRIPTION

Name: _____   Date: _____

Title: _____ Line Item #: _____ Salary Grade: _____

Department: _____ Section: _____

Qualifications: Minimum Educational Requirements; Minimum Years of Experience; Other Requirements (license, certification).

Schedule:

> Identify days and hours to be routinely worked. Overtime, shift work, weekends, holidays, and/or on-call responsibilities must also be noted.

Duties: Job Scope and Function: Summarize primary functions of position that are essential. Identify consequences if the function is not performed.

A. General:

> *The employee understands and agrees to the following policies: report to work at scheduled time; perform assigned duties in an acceptable and timely manner; utilize established laboratory safety measures; participate in quality assurance programs and assist in the continuous quality improvement of the department; and maintain patient confidentiality. Failure to comply with accepted policies will lead to counseling, progressive discipline, and possible termination. These activities may be evaluated as: EXCEEDS, MEETS, or FAILS. The following will be considered failure to meet established policies:*
> *1. More than four (4) unscheduled absences per evaluation year (circumstance specific, reviewed by supervisor).*
> *2. Tardiness of more than fifteen (15) minutes per month or consistent tardiness pattern.*
> *3. Violation of any one (1) mandatory safety policies (Universal precautions).*
> *4. Three (3) failures to record or actively participate in quality assurance or improvement activities.*
> *5. A single (1) breach of confidentiality.*
> *6. Three (3) documented accounts associated with poor customer service.*

B. Technical:

What is the complexity and/or difficulty of the work? Training/Orientation: What initial training does the incumbent receive, what guidance is available, and how is work checked?

Give specific examples of what are routine tasks (require little or no interpretive or analytical skills) and non-routine tasks (requiring a specialized knowledge base or ability). The outcome is measured by quality, quantity, cost-appropriateness, or mastery of performance. These tasks are considered ESSENTIAL; any one (1) violation or failure will lead to counseling.

Specimen Procurement/Processing:
The Technologist must be capable of performing general phlebotomies accurately and successfully; correctly accession patient data; and use standard procedures to process patient specimens. If these tasks are not completed in an accurate and timely manner, patient care is compromised.

Performance of Lab Testing:
The Technologist must understand basic hematologic principles and perform routine testing in a timely and accurate fashion.

FIGURE 13–1. Sample job description.

Reporting Lab Tests:
Communication: The Technologist must accurately report patient results in a timely manner. Identify types of communication (verbal, written, electronic, etc.), frequency, and complexity.

Equipment/instrument Responsibilities:
What type of equipment is used and level of complexity?

C. Administrative Responsibilities:

Supervisory:

		Percent of Time
_____	Requires direct supervision	_____ %
_____	Works under general supervision	_____ %
_____	Works independently with consultive direction	_____ %
_____	May provide some supervision	_____ %
_____	Directly supervises others	_____ %

Accountability
___ Performs simple, well-defined duties, no interpretation required.
___ Limited knowledge of Departmental/Institutional policies required.
___ Moderate knowledge of Departmental/Institutional policies required.
___ Extensive knowledge of Departmental/Institutional policies required.

Budget Responsibility
___ Suggests items for purchase
___ Approves expenditures.
___ Develops and prepares budget recommendations.
___ Approves budget recommendations for section.
___ Approves budget recommendations for department.

D. Teaching/Research Responsibilities:

Responsibilities regarding teaching of staff or students, and research endeavors should be identified.

E. Professional Development:

Requirements for participation and/or presentation of continuing education programs are listed in accordance with regulatory or institutional guidelines.

F. Organizational Relationships:

Include incumbent in Departmental organizational chart; note who is the direct supervisor(s), whom the incumbent supervises, and what the level of responsibility is. In team-based organizations, identify direct team associates, other team affiliations, facilitators, and management members. Identify secondary relationships the incumbent would encounter (i.e., clients, admitting office, maintenance, physicians, nursing, industry associates, etc.)

_____   _____

Employee Signature   Date

_____   _____

Supervisor Signature   Date

FIGURE 13–1.   *(continued)*

tools, machines, or any other device that the employee uses in the job) the employee must be able to use. Responsibility and accountability identify the level of leadership, authority, obligation, and liability of each employee. Job relationships list job titles for which the employee is responsible and to whom the employee would report. In addition, a listing of other departments, types of personnel, or institutions and organizations with whom the individual may directly work and the level of interaction (eg, written reports, verbal presentations) sets the scope of interpersonal skills necessary for this position.

Equal opportunity and affirmative action guidelines must be considered when developing job descriptions and during the recruitment process. Governmental regulations (Table 13–6) regarding discrimination based on age, physical or mental disabilities, gender, color, race, religion, or national origin guarantee proper hiring practices, offer appropriate opportunities for under-represented groups, and ensure safety in the workplace.[32] Use of the criterion-based job description provides a general outline and can be helpful in establishing levels of responsibility (based on definitions set by the Board of Registry of the American Society of Clinical Pathologists; Table 13–7). The criterion-based job description defines positions based on knowledge, technical skills, and administrative and teaching respon-

sibilities (level of judgment, authority, or communication skills required) and allows for other specific duties to be added as deemed necessary by laboratory or hospital administration and accrediting services.

The three traditional levels of laboratory employees are technician, technologist, and specialist (chief technologist, supervisor); these levels reflect core competencies that should be present at entry level. They are hierarchical in that each advanced level would include the skills of the preceding. Furthermore, each of these levels is applicable to most sections of the laboratory.[3,4]

More recently, quality practices have influenced how job descriptions may be developed and used. For each job description, five areas can be addressed (Box 13–3).

Job descriptions should not remain static but should be reviewed periodically for each employee by the laboratory manager or supervisor to ensure that each accurately reflects job titles and meets the needs of the laboratory. Staffing depends on volume of work to be handled for specific hours for each day of operation. This includes number of shifts and proposed availability of laboratory services (frequency and test-menu offered) by shift, weekends, and holidays. In most laboratories, training or teaching of staff or students is required. In addition, laboratories should have some level of ongoing research and development to remain current

Table 13-6
Key Regulatory Issues Associated With Hiring Practices

Regulation	Provision
National Labor Relations Act (1935) Wagner Act	Right to organize unions and represent employees equally
Labor–Management Relations Act (1947) Taft-Hartley Law	Outlaws unfair labor practices by unions; prevents closed shops; illegal to strike during national emergencies, bargaining in good faith
Fair Labor Standards Act (1938) FLSA	Provides for minimum wage, overtime, and limits working hours for children
Civil Rights Act (1964; amended 1972)	Prevents discrimination based on color, race, religion, gender, or national origin; established EEOC
Executive Order 11246 (1965; amended 1966, Order 11375)	Prevents discrimination based on color, race, religion, gender, or national origin
Age Discrimination in Employment Act (1967)	Prevents discrimination based on age
Occupational Safety and Health Act (1970)	Provides for a safe working environment
Equal Opportunity Employment Act (1972)	Enhances power of EEOC; adds state and local government employees
Vocational Rehabilitation Act (1973)	Prevents discrimination based on physical or mental disability; initiates affirmative action
Guidelines on Sexual Harassment (1980)	Defines and establishes standards on what constitutes sexual harassment
Clinical Laboratory Improvement Act 1988 CLIA '88	Redefines laboratory regulations that include personnel standards

Table 13-7
Criterion-Based Job Description

Competency	Technician	Technologist	Specialist
Knowledge	Working knowledge of routine tests	Understands technical aspects of tests, underlying scientific principles, biologic facts, familiar with other laboratory services	Has knowledge of advanced scientific principles within the specialty area; applies knowledge; knows the organization
Technical skills	Performs routine test, instrument maintenance, basics of quality control	Performs routine tests, more complicated tests; implements and monitors quality control; introduces and evaluates new procedures and instruments	Performs all tests within the specialty area; able to maintain and troubleshoot equipment; researches, develops, implements, and evaluates new methods, instrumentation, and quality control
Judgment and decision making	Recognizes common technical problems and able to correct them	Initiates independent judgment of technical/procedural problems; participates in and delegates quality control issues, instrument selection, preventive maintenance, safety reagent/equipment purchases	Implements and delegates decisions in laboratory operations; anticipates and shows independent judgment in problem solving; participates in policy making
Communication	Reports lab results, normal ranges, specimen requirements	Generates technical or general information to medical and nonmedical personnel	Communicates applications and validity of laboratory data, laboratory policies and operations, detailed information about specialty areas
Supervision and management	None	Participates in basic management practices, technical and administrative procedures; supervises technicians, aides, clerical personnel	Performs and directs administrative functions over laboratory personnel
Teaching and training	Demonstrates learned skills	Teaches and evaluates basic theory, technical skills, application of tests	Plans, implements, and evaluates educational programs

Data from Board of Registry, American Society of Clinical Pathologists; Professional levels definitions, Laboratory Med 13:312, 1982

and provide more effective and accurate techniques and procedures. These responsibilities require staff participation and must be scheduled into the work day.

Changes in technologies, equipment, administrative policies, state and federal laws, and accreditation procedures should be considered and incorporated into the job description when appropriate. Reviewing job descriptions with employees is critical to ensure that both understand what is the expectation and to set future goals. A well-developed and current job description can often prevent potential administrative or legal problems. The job description is an essential management tool in the staffing process. It is a training guide, identifying what is expected from each employee, and is a basis for the evaluation process.[28]

SCHEDULING

Laboratory organization charts are helpful for identifying structure within the laboratory. Charts may be designed to include staffing, reporting, physical or facility

Box 13•3

Five Areas of Quality Practices in Job Descriptions

1. *Expectations of employment*—fundamental expectations of *all* employees as terms of general employment. These terms may include time and attendance, ethical conduct, confidentiality, safety, and customer service.
2. *Key job areas* are related job functions assigned within the appropriate level of knowledge, education, and expertise (job title).
3. *Essential tasks* are those requiring the highest level of attention and accuracy (such as patient testing).
4. *Critical tasks* are important to completing the job but if performed incorrectly or not at all would have less impact on outcomes (eg, poor communication skills, attitudes, team spirit). These tasks may be evaluated based on performance, such as "meets," "exceeds," or "fails."
5. *Outcome metrics* measure each task in terms of quantity, quality, cost effectiveness, or performance.

plans, or work flow. Procedure lists, methodologies, time specifications, and instrumentation can also be incorporated into the diagrams. Current operations can be clearly depicted and assist in focusing on particular problems, services, or future trends. Staffing can then be adjusted accordingly.

Once the number and types of employees required to perform assigned tasks are identified, appropriate scheduling must then be considered for each shift. Work flow for busy and slow periods needs to be identified and staffed appropriately. The traditional 40-hour workweek of "9 to 5" may no longer be cost-effective or productive when dealing with outreach customers. Alternative staffing and scheduling might improve efficiency of employee productivity and operating costs. Modified procedures and updated instrumentation will improve work flow and productivity.

Other considerations regarding current health-care issues exist. A significant paradigm shift has occurred in how laboratory services are provided. The implementation of prospective reimbursement of hospitals by diagnostic-related groupings (DRGs; classification of 467 major diagnostic categories used to assign patient case types) has resulted in significant changes in how

hospitals are reimbursed for inpatient stays. More recently, health-care reform and managed care (well-organized plans to provide health-care services to participating members at the lowest cost possible) organizations have again changed how hospitals and hospital laboratories use services. These changes have had a direct impact on organization, staffing, and productivity. Third-party insurers and compulsory rate review agencies are demanding a more bottom-line approach to laboratory use. Laboratories are expected to provide quality testing that is convenient, comprehensive (large test menu), and low cost. Outcome measurements (procedures and processes that directly contribute to the consequence of patient management) will be used to evaluate this process. The emphasis has shifted from maintaining high census numbers to decreasing in-patient length of stay (LOS), thus reducing cost. The laboratory's role is to improve turnaround time for procedures. Additionally, tests offered only once or twice a week are often now required to be performed more frequently to enhance discharge procedures. Increased consumer knowledge ("informed consumer") has led to increased scrutiny of all health-care services. Information is readily available regarding the appropriateness, quality, and accessibility, thus allowing patients to take a more proactive role in monitoring individual and general health care.

Physicians have traditionally used extensive testing to establish the correct diagnosis and treatment and subsequently prevent potential medicolegal action. However, demands to reduce health-care costs have brought laboratory use under intense review. Physician review organizations assess patient records to ensure appropriate services, including those provided by the laboratory, are provided. Health maintenance organizations (HMOs) are particularly concerned with identifying unnecessary laboratory costs and frequently contract for a capitated rate (contracted agreement of payment on a per capita basis of a few dollars [or less] per member per month, regardless of services rendered). For laboratories to afford entry into such contracts, cost accounting for each laboratory test must be assessed. Because labor costs are greater than 50% of overall laboratory expenditures, it is critical for laboratory managers to use staff and equipment as efficiently and effectively as possible to remain competitive. Acute care hospitals are moving toward an integrated health-care system by combining all hospital, physician, and other medical services under one plan to cover participating members of the system from "cradle to grave."

Other considerations when staffing a laboratory are nondiagnostic or technical activities. Phlebotomy, reagent preparation, specimen processing, data entry, test result reporting, charting, quality assurance, telephone calls, filing, and billing all consume large quantities of personnel time within the workday and must be considered in planning the work flow.

Support positions, such as phlebotomists, safety officer, quality assurance coordinator, reagent preparation technicians, glassware workers, receptionists, secretaries, word processors, laboratory aides, computer entry clerks, and computer system managers, play a significant role in meeting established goals. Job descriptions of support personnel must include and match the employee with the kind of work to be performed, the level of responsibility to be assumed, and job requirements to be met. Organizational charts may be useful in identifying appropriateness and usefulness of support personnel and what responsibilities may be assigned to them.

A relatively new category is the multiskilled health-care provider (MSHP).[2] As hospitals and hospital laboratories look at reducing costs, downsizing staff, and enhancing productivity rates, the concept of MSHP provides a viable strategy. MSHPs have been effectively used during staffing shortages, enhance the effectiveness of existing staff, and have been used in developing patient-focused teams. Properly trained, MSHPs may reduce turnaround time, minimize patient movement, increase continuity of care, reduce patient length of stay, enhance job satisfaction, and improve employer flexibility.[5] In some hospitals, internal personnel are cross-trained. Studies show that of the hospitals surveyed, 21% to 70% of the respondents indicated current use of MSHPs in their facilities.[23] Box 13–4 lists a variety of responsibilities that cross standard disciplines. How MSHPs are used depends on their level of education and experience. Creation and implementation of this job title requires planning to ensure that appropriate training and education, experience, legal considerations, and ethical issues are addressed.

Many laboratories use a division of labor in which laboratory sections have specifically trained technologists and technicians. Further, each of these sections requires a supervisor(s) and ancillary support personnel. Depending on size of the section, responsibilities of equipment inventory coordinator, equipment repair specialist, quality assurance coordinator, safety officer, business manager, computer specialist, purchasing agent, and educational coordinator would also be needed. Changes in how health-care dollars are spent have forced some laboratories to relook at how they operate. Because labor is the major expense, the number of personnel and how they are used have come under careful scrutiny. Extensive cross-training, use of more generalists, team-based organizations, and implementation of faster, more efficient instrumentation have contributed to greater cost savings. Use of laboratory computers; discrete, bidirectional analyzers with high volume throughput; point-of-care testing (POCT); molecular diagnostics; robotics; and telepathology are

---

Box 13•4

Potential Responsibilities for Multiskilled Health-Care Providers

Electrocardiographs (ECG)
Electroencephalographs (EEG)
Ultrasound and other imaging procedures (MRI, CAT scan)
X-rays
Nuclear medicine scans
Mammograms
Laboratory tests
Point-of-care testing
Laboratory test use
Phlebotomies
Perfusion technology
Vascular access (start IVs; collect donor units)
Administration of blood products to patients
Vital signs
Quality control/assurance for nonlaboratory areas
Infection control
Interpretation/collaboration in drug/antibiotic monitoring
General safety, biohazard/chemical safety plans
Ophthalmic technology

---

technologies that significantly impact staffing. In the past, analytes that required sophisticated instrumentation, complex methodology, or were too costly to perform were frequently sent out to reference laboratories.[20] As technology has improved and instrumentation has become more diversified, tests once considered labor intensive or too complex may now be brought in house. Laboratories that have increased their workload through outsourcing should return to the laboratory those low volume tests once considered too expensive to perform in house. Test menus should be periodically reviewed in conjunction with reference laboratory send outs to ensure they are appropriate and cost effective.

Consolidation

Consolidations, affiliations, alliances, or takeovers are part of re-engineering (right-sizing, downsizing, restructuring), as seen in health care and other industries. Modifications in staffing and scheduling are defined in terms of enhanced productivity and efficiency. Productivity may increase 400% through laboratory re-engineering.[8] Laboratories have responded to increased workloads by asking employees to be more efficient, enhancing test menus, and extending hours of operation. Aggressive marketing has become a common practice for laboratories on the upward move. Laboratories that want to remain competitive must look at alternative ways to grow. As patient LOS decreases and laboratory testing is carefully monitored, it has become necessary to enhance outsourcing and diversify testing menus to increase workload. Physicians' demands for more preadmission testing and prompt access to laboratory test results and the trend toward outpatient management have required laboratories to review their operations seriously. Traditionally, laboratory services have been primarily physician driven but are now exposed to external factors forcing laboratories to be customer focused. Active participation and practicing of "good customer service" should be incorporated into job descriptions and mission statements. Patients, physicians, employees, students, third-party payors, other health-care providers, and industry partners are now viewed as valued and essential customers.

Hospital laboratories are looking at different ways to develop regional network systems. By forming consolidated or cluster laboratories, resources may be shared in a more cost-effective manner. "Bottom-line" management of resources encourages laboratories to promote better use of personnel and individual exper-

tise; eliminate redundancy of equipment purchases, equipment maintenance, support services, and laboratory supplies; and use limited space more effectively. As seen in Figure 13–2, core laboratories service several hospitals within a given area.[35,36] In addition, other health services, such as clinics, nursing homes, physician office laboratories, and school or workplace dispensaries can also be incorporated into this system. Those hospitals (or other health-care facilities) that serve a specific clientele (such as alcohol and drug rehabilitation facility) may require a unique test service (drug and alcohol levels), thus serving as the "reference" laboratory for other members of the network, while continuing to send the routine laboratory work to the core laboratory. As the public takes greater responsibility for their own health care, the availability and number of home testing kits have increased. Individuals using these kits are more likely to seek out a health-care provider who would refer laboratory testing appropriately.

SCHEDULING FOR EFFICIENT SERVICE

The mission statement requires the laboratory to provide high-quality, cost effective, timely, and efficient services. A helpful guide for staffing and scheduling is

PROPOSED INTEGRATED REGIONAL LABORATORY

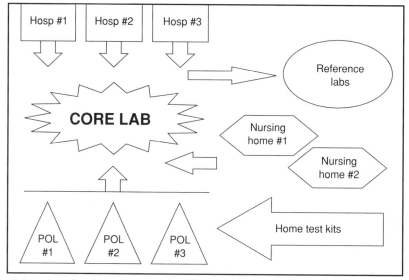

FIGURE 13–2. Schematic diagram of a proposed integrated regional laboratory. (Adapted from Stainer and Root [reference 36])

13–3 is an example of a work flow diagram that may be used to visualize the flow of work. This is particularly helpful when reassigning staff or planning reorganization or rearrangement of the physical facilities. Alterations to the diagram can be easily made, by consolidating similar functions, removing duplication of instrumentation or duties, or identifying underuse and overuse of personnel. Revision might include reassignment of duties or procedures, establishing new priorities, changing the work flow, or rescheduling personnel. Efficiency is further achieved by maintaining continuity and communication.

Factors to Consider When Scheduling Staff

Laboratory Hours

Volume and frequency of specimen procurement dictate the number of personnel per shift to be scheduled. Active marketing and recruiting of non–hospital-based laboratory work increases workload, necessitating a full-time staff for evening and night shifts. Moving some routine "day" work to off-hour shifts may be more efficient. In addition, they may provide equipment maintenance, quality assurance protocols, or assume other duties, thus removing responsibilities from staff during peak hours. As test volume increases and emphasis

---

Box 13•5

Simple Performance Chart

1. ☐ Obtain physician order.
2. ☐ Draw blood.
3. ☐ Receive specimens.
4. ☐ Process and aliquot specimen.
5. ☐ Perform analysis.
6. ☐ Record data.
7. ☐ Report results.
8. ☐ Bill patient.
9. ☐ File data.

---

the performance chart or work flow diagram. Activities within a given operational system are clearly identified as to the current work flow with all steps necessary to reach the desired endpoint presented. Box 13–5 is an example of a simple performance chart that lists all the steps in sequence.

The performance chart can be prepared in as much detail as necessary to identify key operations and how staff is used. This type of listing is not as graphic as a diagram, which can better show the interaction of laboratory areas and employee responsibilities. Figure

Work Flow Diagram for the Laboratory

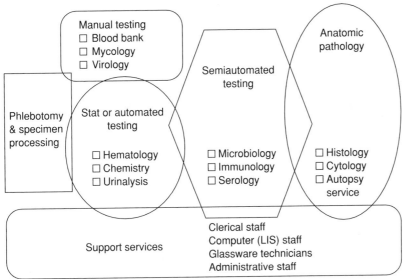

FIGURE 13–3. Flow diagrams are helpful in planning changes in laboratory work flow.

shifts from inpatient to outsourcing, laboratories must consider extending hours of operation, providing better evening and weekend coverage, and improving access to laboratory services.

Laboratories using on-call schedules to cover off hours should carefully review work volumes, trends, and productivity levels to ensure this is cost effective. Improved automation with high throughput, while more expensive initially, requires only a limited number of personnel to be employed during off-shift hours. Alternatives to outright capital equipment purchasing, such as leasing or reagent-rental, should be considered.

Workload Trends

Most laboratories do not maintain a constant workload flow from hour to hour or day to day, resulting in volume peaks and valleys. Monthly fluctuation may also be observed. A review of the previous 12 months of workload will reveal trends that can be used to predict more cost effective and efficient scheduling of personnel as needed. Alternatively, overscheduling of staff may more than accommodate these peak times but result in decreased productivity, short-staffing during off hours, and increased costs. The LIS is helpful in this process. Data should be collected and reviewed often enough to recognize shifts in workload.

Another area to consider is that of stat requests. These requests should be evaluated for frequency, physician use, and appropriateness. Careful collection and review of data can help laboratories become more cost efficient and assist in adequate staffing in a given area, on a given shift, or throughout the laboratory.

Generally, stats interrupt work flow of batch routine procedures, decreasing laboratory efficiency. Where a high percentage of stats exist, inappropriate use of staff may be seen. Careful review of how and when laboratory tests are ordered may require addressing ordering patterns with the medical staff.

Standing orders for laboratory work may include excessive or unnecessary ordering, adding to the cost for inpatient testing (under DRGs). Addressing the need for such a practice with staff physicians and nurses may help reduce costs. The current trend is to reduce inpatient testing and actively pursue non–hospital-based accounts (outsourcing, outreach patient testing). As workload increases and test menus are expanded, esoteric procedures generally sent to reference laboratories may be brought in house, thus instrumentation use and scheduling of personnel may be better optimized.

Performing a test cost analysis helps the manager or administrator know the direct cost of performing any one assay and provides flexibility in negotiating outsourcing contracts. Secondly, as test volume increases, specimen runs are expanded, creating more effective use of reagents, controls, and technician time. Third, support personnel may be optimally employed; specimen processing technicians can spin a full centrifuge carrier; purchasing coordinators can place fewer orders when consumables are bought in larger lots or bulk; and couriers can be fully used in specimen pickup and so forth. Outsourcing may come from physician offices and physician office laboratories (POLs), community clinics, other hospital laboratories, and college or workplace dispensaries.

Personnel Benefits

Nationwide, up to 10% of the work force is absent from work each day. Some of these absences, such as vacation, business leave, and compensatory time, can be predicted and controlled. Other absences owing to illness or other personal reasons are not and may result in understaffing at critical or peak times. To compensate, overstaffing may result when predictable absences are not effectively managed or controlled or when employees take excessive advantage of sick and personal leaves. Monitoring of both is strongly encouraged. Unscheduled absenteeism is costly (Box 13–6) and frequently, if not addressed promptly, results in increased personnel turnover, morale problems, and poor-quality work.

Physical Design

The clinical laboratory has undergone changes in instrumentation, methodologies, workload demands, regulatory mandates, safety issues, and reorganizational endeavors. In some laboratories, the physical design does not effectively meet the needs of fast turnaround times and does not contribute to the efficiency of operations. Historically, as laboratories grew in size and testing became more sophisticated, specialization or subsections of the laboratory appeared (eg, radioimmunoassay [RIA], virology, hematopathology, electron microscopy), creating physical separations or compartmentalization. Today, high-tech methodologies and instrumentation have served as a bridge between various sections. Training is more focused, and the need for specialty training in manual or labor-intensive methods is less common; instrumentation used in chemistry is used in immunology (immunoinstrumentation); molecular diagnostic techniques (molecular probes/polymerase chain reaction) are applicable to many specialty areas; and similar methods are consolidated (eg, electrophoresis for abnormal hemoglobins, serum protein electrophoresis [SPEP]).

The open-laboratory concept has decentralized laboratory sections by removing walls to use space, facilities, personnel, and equipment better. Such consolidation measures will impact on staffing numbers, use,

Box 13•6

Simplified Cost Estimate of Unscheduled Absenteeism

1. Yearly absenteeism rate (%) =

$$\frac{\text{Total \# days absent for all workers}}{\text{Total \# workers} \times 260 \text{ d/worker/y}} \times 100$$

$$\frac{80 \text{ sick d/y}}{10 \text{ workers} \times 260 \text{ d/worker/y}} \times 100 = 3.1\%$$

80 sick d/y $\times$ 8 h/d = 640 sick h/y

2. Paid sick leave is averaged per occupational class and weighted according to use; 53% of absent days were taken by clerical staff, 45% by technologists, and 2% by the supervisor. This calculates to a weighted average salary of $12.63/h.

	Average Hourly Rate	Percent Absenteeism	Weighted Hourly Wage
Clerical	$ 9.60	53%	$ 5.77
Technologists	$14.40	45%	$ 6.48
Supervisor	$19.23	2%	$ 0.38
Total			$12.63

3. Benefits/employee = 25% of weighted hourly salary

Weighted hourly wage = $12.63
Benefits = 25% $\times$ $12.63 = $ 3.16
Total cost/h = $15.79

4. Estimate of cost paid to sick leave

$15.79/h $\times$ 640 sick h/y = $10,106/y paid for no productivity

and overall operational costs. Figure 13–3 shows how a laboratory may "blend" sections so work flow is smooth and efficiency achieved.

In the modern laboratory, the focus will be on how robotics and informatics (see below) are to be integrated in improving efficiency. In one model, automated, semiautomated, and manual laboratory tests are performed in zones, circulating around specimen processing.[24] Functional characteristics of each laboratory section must be considered and planned for appropriately, consolidating when possible. Modular furniture provides maximum use of horizontal and vertical space. Flexibility and portability are added values in meeting the ever-changing laboratory environment. In addition, engineering controls, such as ergonomically correct seating, table heights, padded edges (eg, wrist pads, elbow pads), or mechanical-assisting devices, should be used to prevent work-related traumas (cumulative trauma disorders).[15] In addition, job rotation, job-site modifications, proper orientation and training, and continuing education of all employees are essential to promote a safe work environment. Phlebotomy areas and patient examination rooms (if appropriate) should be customer friendly and accessible. Specimen processing, patient registration, and the LIS should be close to each other.

Adequate electrical power (including emergency power), temperature control, and ventilation must be in place to ensure an optimal and safe environment for employees and equipment. Spacial requirements in relation to other hospital services must be considered: proximity to emergency department, intensive care units, and operating rooms.

Another approach is the regional integrated laboratory network system.[34,35] This network of health-care facilities offers the opportunity to share resources in a given location (see Fig. 13-2). Most laboratory work would be done in a core laboratory, receiving specimens from regional hospitals, POLs, nursing homes, and other health-care providers. The location of the core laboratory might be at an acute care hospital depending on regional accessibility and needs. Low-volume testing once performed in individual hospitals could be consolidated at the core laboratory, increasing menu volume and decreasing costs. Esoteric testing once sent to reference laboratories may now be of adequate volume to be instituted at the core facility. Reference laboratories would function at a significantly higher level, performing those labor-intensive or complex assays that would not be cost-effective if performed locally.

New Technology

The introduction of automation through enhanced informatics and robotics will move the laboratory to the highest level.[29] The laboratory is a source of information to assist clinicians in better patient management and ensure positive outcome measurements. Informatics is technology driven and directly impacts on how laboratories operate. Instrumentation uses state-of-the art computers to provide highly accurate laboratory measurements, enhanced throughput, bidirectional communication with LIS, and relatively simple methodology. Use of pneumatic tubes, conveyor belt systems, and automated guided vehicles have been shown to enhance delivery of specimens to the laboratory.[24] Robotic technology is now being integrated into laboratory instrumentation.[29] Blood specimens will be identified by bar codes, centrifuged, aliquoted, and analyzed all on one instrument. Additional testing may be performed on a second or third instrument that has been "linked," serving as work stations. As laboratories become more automated, staffing needs could be significantly reduced.

The use of telecommunication in pathology (telepathology) and image transfer using computers, work stations, high-resolution video equipment, and multigigabit-per-second telecommunications will generate digitization and high-speed transmission of images, three-dimensional reconstruction of cell and tissue morphology, and intelligence/neural networks.[13] These systems can provide a communication link to hospitals, clinics, extended care facilities, and other health-care provider offices through real-time, robotic microscopy for consultations and well-care evaluations. They can aid in forensic activities, enhance educational endeavors, promote videoconferencing, and assist in the development of regional health-care facilities.

Development of these regional systems could greatly benefit patient services by increasing access to health-care services, improve medical education, and provide continuity in individual health-care maintenance. For the laboratory, this enhances its ability to consolidate services and staff. POCT (near-patient testing, alternate-site testing, patient-focused testing) is used in a variety of settings, such as the emergency department, operating suites, clinics, HMOs, physician offices, and nursing homes. POCT testing brings laboratory testing to the site of the patient rather than obtaining a specimen and sending it to the laboratory. Real-time measurements of a patient's status may be obtained in a short period, allowing the health-care provider to address acute patient needs. POCT brings laboratory testing to the patient, providing patient-focused care. Up to 80% of all inpatient care can be provided at the patient's bedside.[23] Implementation of POCT requires considerable evaluation and planning to maximize its benefits.[20] Studies have shown that patient-focused care can decrease turn-around time (TAT) for certain procedures, reduce patient LOS by 15% to 20%, and reduce expenses by 8% to 12%.[37]

Other hospitals use satellite laboratories that often require redundancy of personnel and equipment. Cost of such an operation versus convenience must be carefully evaluated. Whether a laboratory supports POCT or satellite laboratories (or both), appropriate staffing for these areas must be planned. Careful cost analyses of how laboratory testing may be provided quickly yet cost effectively must be performed and reviewed periodically with hospital staff.

AVAILABLE RESOURCES

Support (ancillary) personnel are critical to overall laboratory operations. These individuals are phlebotomists, laboratory workers, clerks, data entry operators, volunteers, receptionists, and secretaries. Scheduling efficiency, technical performance, and cost savings are quickly realized when these individuals are integrated into daily operations.

This type of staff use relieves other, more costly technical personnel of many time-consuming, nontechnical tasks. In some instances, it may be appropriate to cross-train clerical staff to perform nontechnical functions. Some clerical functions may be contracted to an outside source that specializes in medical report typing. The cost of such a service is generally less than employing a full-time secretary with benefits.

When scheduling, use of time accruals must be considered. Absences cannot always be predicted or controlled. However, in the case of vacations or compensatory time, the supervisor can limit time taken or set limits on the number of employees taking time off on a given day. Supervisors should encourage employees to use accruals during slack periods when possible. Employees should also be encouraged to take vacation year-round instead of just summer months. Use of time accruals should be identified in departmental guidelines and addressed at the time of orientation so that all employees know the rules. In a similar fashion, staffing must be appropriately planned during state and federal holidays. Empowering employees to decide among themselves who will cover when may be advantageous. Whether it is done on a seniority basis (person employed the longest at the laboratory gets first choice) or strictly by volunteering, an equitable policy must be in place and reviewed at orientation.

Laboratories that provide 24-hour service must also account for evenings, nights, weekends, and holidays. While full-time employees may be scheduled to work these hours, costs in overtime (or other compensatory benefit) make this less desirable. Scheduling staff to work a regular 40-hour shift, Tuesday through Saturday, or Sunday through Thursday, is more cost effective because it avoids overtime and is an example of a cost-avoidance measure. Part-time employees can also be used during these off hours. Another potential resource is volunteers. These individuals can be used to perform well-defined, nontechnical tasks, such as delivering reports, mail, specimens, or other similar activities. Often, college students may be available to work during holiday seasons, summers, and other times as needed and are willing to work at more modest wages. Many colleges have work-study or "co-op" programs where "free" labor is exchanged for gaining experience and college credit. These individuals are often more willing and available to work off hours and can perform a variety of functions requiring minimal technical skills.

Part-time employees can be used to fill in during vacations, maternity leaves, and other absences. In some situations, it may be appropriate and within the power of laboratory management to move employees to exempt status (ie, salaried status). The Federal Labor Standards Act states that employees who work more than 40 hours a week must be paid time and a half. Employees of companies involved in noninterstate commerce, seasonal employees, certain salespeople,

executives, administrators, and professionals are considered exempt from this rule. This may obviate payment of overtime; however, other forms of compensation may be offered and accrued, such as compensatory time (time off).

Use of per diem personnel may offer temporary respite during extended periods of absence. Use of such personnel offers flexibility in scheduling, especially when work trends are erratic. While labor costs on a per-hour basis may be the same as full-time staff, generally, reduced or no benefits are required to be paid (benefits are approximately 25% of base salary). Recruitment may be difficult for such positions; however, former staff that have not returned to service for family or other reasons may consider such temporary employment. Placement agencies exist to provide this service, but there may be no-cost savings.

A valuable and important resource available to management is the rotating generalist. Unanticipated and temporary decreases in work force and increases in workload can be handled quickly and adequately with the least interruption in service when cross-trained generalists are available. For employees, this may be an opportunity to maintain their skills and improve job satisfaction; however, maintaining a high level of

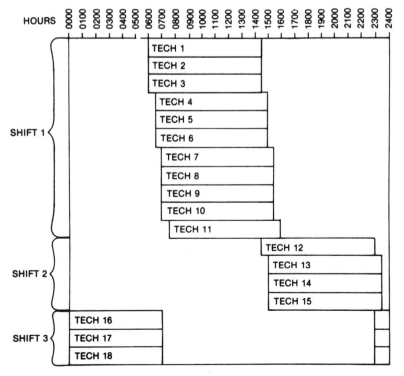

FIGURE 13–4. Staggered shifts. Shifts 1 and 2 are assigned to the chemistry section in 8½-hour shifts with a half-hour lunch period. Shift 3 technologists work all areas of the laboratory, with all three technologies working 8-hour shifts with a starting time of 2300 hours. Staggered starting times enable 1-hour overlap between Shift 3 and Shift 1, allowing Shift 1 technologists time for work list preparation and blood collection. Overlapping hours between 1430 and 1600 allow good work flow from Shift 1 to Shift 2, when the work load is characteristically high. The half-hour overlap between Shift 2 and Shift 3 is usually sufficient for the work flow at that hour; however, if work flow is high, Shift 3 may be assigned a scarring time of 2230 with a half-hour lunch period.

		SUNDAY	MONDAY	TUESDAY	WEDNESDAY	THURSDAY	FRIDAY	SATURDAY
WEEK I	TECH 1		WORK	WORK	WORK			WORK
	2	WORK	WORK			WORK	WORK	
	3	WORK	WORK				WORK	WORK
	4		WORK	WORK	WORK	WORK		
	5			WORK	WORK	WORK	WORK	
	6			WORK	WORK	WORK	WORK	
WEEK II	TECH 1	WORK	WORK			WORK	WORK	
	2			WORK	WORK	WORK	WORK	
	3			WORK	WORK	WORK	WORK	WORK
	4	WORK	WORK				WORK	
	5		WORK	WORK	WORK	WORK		WORK
	6		WORK	WORK	WORK			
WEEK III	TECH 1			WORK	WORK	WORK	WORK	
	2		WORK	WORK	WORK			WORK
	3		WORK	WORK	WORK	WORK		
	4			WORK	WORK	WORK	WORK	
	5	WORK	WORK				WORK	WORK
	6	WORK	WORK			WORK	WORK	
WEEK IV	TECH 1			REPEAT AS ABOVE OR				
	2			REASSIGN LINES AND REPEAT				
	3							
	4							
	5							
	6							

FIGURE 13–5. Schedule for the 10-hour day, 4-day workweek. This schedule is for a microbiology section day shift, with a staff of six technologists.

proficiency may be difficult. Such flexibility is advantageous in effective scheduling and can boost productivity while saving overtime dollars. While generalists offer flexibility, some level of specialization within a section must be preserved to provide continuity, thus the need for specialists. An appropriate balance in "breadth" (generalist) and "depth" (specialist) must be established. How many and where generalists should be stationed will vary based on the needs of each laboratory. Advantages and disadvantages must be carefully evaluated. The need for flexibility in scheduling and cost efficiency versus benefits derived from the expertise and continuity of specialized employees must be reviewed frequently to ensure optimal laboratory operations. Other factors to consider are work volume, test menu offered, and test complexity. In addition, cross-training of ancillary personnel (eg, preparatory technicians, clerical staff) will promote a better understanding of what others do, enhance job satisfaction, and offer significant support to operations during staff down times.

ALTERNATIVE SCHEDULING APPROACHES

Problems that can be encountered with a shift change is the lack of continuity or interruption in service. Staggered work shifts (Fig. 13-4) may offer a better work flow and keep lines of communication open between shifts. A technologist working a split shift from 12:00 PM to 8:00 PM is available for lunch coverage for day-shift technologists and dinner coverage for evening-shift technologists. This provides continuity of services, and the individual is liaison between the shifts. Staff cross-trained to work off hours may be better used and offer flexibility in providing coverage for illnesses, vacations, and other leave periods.[38]

An alternative to routine scheduling is a 10-hour workday in a 4-day workweek (Fig. 13-5). This may be particularly helpful if workload peaks consistently in the morning and again late in the afternoon. This type

of scheduling will decrease overtime but requires commitment from employees. Also, union rules may not allow this practice, and for some, this type of schedule may be too physically tiring or not conducive to personal lifestyle.

A variation of this schedule is 10 consecutive days on (8 h/d) and 4 days off. This type of schedule is helpful for weekend coverage and offers considerable continuity. This also requires a motivated individual willing to

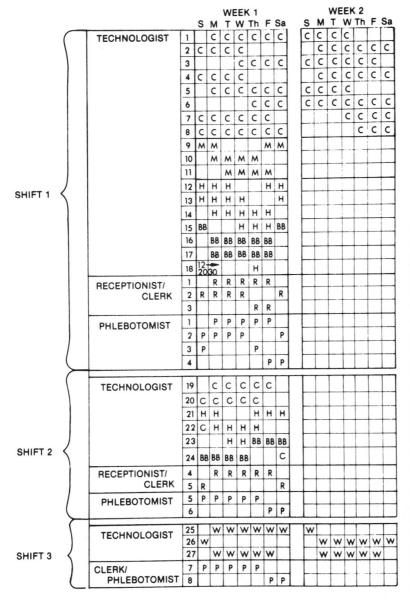

FIGURE 13–6. An example of a clinical laboratory schedule that makes use of innovative scheduling techniques. Technologists 1–11 on Shift 1 are on a 10-days-on/4-days-off schedule with lines assigned on a rotating basis each week. Technologists 12–17 are on a rotating weekend schedule. Technologists 18, part-time, is used in shift-sharing, assigned to the 1200–2030 shift in the blood bank each Sunday. This eliminates the need for additional technologists on both Shift 1 and Shift 2 by providing blood bank coverage during the high work-load periods, primarily preop crossmatches. Part-time employees, used on weekends or during the week, include the receptionists/clerks, the phlebocomists, and the phlebocomist/clerk. Technologists 25 and 26, Shift 3, are on a 7-days-on/7-days-off schedule. They are assigned to a 10-hour shift Monday through Sunday every other week. Two week, 70-hour-schedule pay can be adjusted to 80-hour pay by use of shift differential or by assigning an additional day during the off week.

work 10 consecutive days. Absenteeism in either of the above-mentioned categories can cause serious staffing and productivity problems. An example of a "10/4" schedule is seen in Figure 13–6.[38]

Ordering patterns and test use must be periodically reviewed to ensure proper scheduling of laboratory staff. When peak volumes and stat test orders are routinely seen (especially during the night), prompt review of the situation is essential. Test results required for certain times of the day may be "scheduled" to reduce these peak times. In some facilities, a stat laboratory may be appropriate. If adjustments to time periods cannot be made, additional staff for an early morning shift may be required. By starting a shift 1 or 2 hours before the regular day shift begins, laboratory results are available for morning rounds. The disadvantage is that early shift personnel leave 1 or 2 hours earlier, thus afternoon specimens need to be accounted for, which may necessitate the "10/4" schedule.

Laboratories may take advantage of the open laboratory concept to consolidate instrumentation and personnel for prompt specimen processing and reporting. This eliminates interruptions in routine work flow each time a stat specimen is received. When considering instrumentation purchases, random access and bidirectional (LIS) capabilities should be considered. In some facilities, POCT may be cost effective. Efforts to improve TAT must be monitored and improved on whenever possible. Use of the LIS and broadcast printers, strategic placement of terminals, or use of fax-modems will expedite reporting of laboratory data. Accessibility to patient data contributes to a prompt diagnosis and earlier treatment and allows physicians to discharge patients sooner.

For some highly qualified applicants, full-time employment does not meet their current needs (continuing their education) or lifestyle (family obligations). Job sharing is the policy of allowing two or more employees to occupy one position within a particular job category. This alternative for experienced professionals offers a great value to the laboratory and the employee and should be encouraged. Another alternative is flexitime, which enables employees to perform their job duties during hours they are able to work. In some situations, set work hours are not absolutely necessary for a given position. Job duties, such as reagent preparation, water testing, pipet checking, and inventory control, are not usually restricted to a shift or time. Job descriptions must clearly define all responsibilities, rules, and regulations. Medical technologists who have left the work force for a period of time may be reluctant to resume their careers because of changes in technology. These technologists are a great resource and should not be overlooked as potential contributing employees. Reentry into the profession should be encouraged by offering retraining, with subsequent employment opportunities as they become available on either a full-time or part-time basis.

In summary, selection and placement of employees are continuous processes. Recognizing inter-relationships between the selection process and other human resource functions is essential for effective management. Frequent review of established programs, job descriptions, and workload trends is necessary to make intelligent and accurate decisions in selecting motivated, highly efficient, and loyal employees.

REFERENCES

1. American Society of Clinical Pathologists, 1994 Wage and vacancy study, pp 1–19. Farmington Hills, Market Opinion, 1994.
2. American Society of Clinical Pathologists, Associate Member Section: Laboratory Services and the Multi-skilled Health Care Provider. A Position Paper. Chicago, American Society of Clinical Pathologists, 1994
3. American Society of Clinical Pathologists Board of Registry: The Three Levels of Certification. In Rolen HB (ed): Study Guide for Clinical Laboratory Certification Examinations. Chicago, American Society of Clinical Pathologists Press, 1986
4. American Society of Clinical Pathologists Board of Registry: Professional Levels Definitions. Lab Med 13:312, 1982
5. Bamberg R, Blayney KD: Multiskilled health practitioners: A viable strategy for health-care delivery. Clin Lab Man Rev 7(1):36–42, 1993
6. Bissonette CA: Laboratory employee turnover. Clin Lab Sci 1(5):283, 1988
7. Burdick IM: Implementing work teams in the clinical laboratory. Med Lab Observ 27(1):44–47, 1995
8. Castaneda-Mendez K: Re-engineering: is it right for you? Advance Admin Lab 3(9):16–21, 1994
9. Chruden HJ, Sherman AW Jr: Managing Human Resources. Cincinnati, South-Western Publishing Co, 1984
10. College of American Pathologists: Workload Recording Method and Personnel Management Manual, pp 155–167. Northfield, College of American Pathologists, 1992
11. College of American Pathologists: Workload Recording Method and Personnel Management Manual, pp 169–176. Northfield, College of American Pathologists, 1992
12. Cook JF: Action Alert: A Tool for Laboratory Managers. Chicago, American Society of Clinical Pathologists, 1993
13. Corona R: Telepathology, SUNY Health Science Center Telemedicine Consortium, Syracuse, NY; personal communication, 1994
14. Deming EW: Out of Crisis. Cambridge, MIT, Center for Advanced Engineering Study, 1986
15. Gile TJ: Ergonomics for the laboratory. Clin Lab Man Rev 8(1):5–18 1994
16. Griffin RW: The Development of Management Theory. In Griffin (ed): Management, 2nd ed, pp 34–69. Boston, Houghton Mifflin, 1987
17. Henry JB, Kurec AS: The clinical laboratory: Organization, purposes, and practice. In Henry JB (ed): Clinical Laboratory Diagnosis and Management by Laboratory Methods, 19th ed, pp 3–39. Philadelphia, WB Saunders, 1996

18. Juran J: Juran on Planning for Quality. New York, The Free Press, 1988
19. Kurec AS: The role and functions of the clinical laboratory. In Schofield S, Watters MA, Kurec AS (eds): Guide to Laboratory Management, 2nd ed, pp 1–15. Malvern: CLMA Press, 1995
20. Kurec AS: Implementing point-of care. Clin Lab Sci 6(4): 225–227, 1993
21. Kurec AS: Criteria-based job description. Tech Sample MGM 3:1–4, 1989
22. Maffetone MA, Bielitzki L, Forster C, Hoiberg R: Tools for the Trade, Criteria-Based Management. Rush-Presbyterian-St. Luke's Medical Center: Chicago, IL. Atlanta, Clinical Laboratory Management Association Annual Conference and Exhibition, 1991
23. Makely S: Overview: Multiskilling and the Allied Health Workforce. Washington, DC, Multiskilling and the Allied Health Work Force National Conference, Nov 30–Dec 1, 1994
24. Markin RS: Clinical laboratory automation: Concepts and designs. Sem Diag Pathol 11(4):274–281, 1994
25. Mecon-PeerX: Operational Benchmarking for Managers: Case Study. Syracuse, Workshop, August 9, 1993
26. Michaels B: Flexible management: Strategies for the changing workforce. Clin Lab Man Rev 8(3):246–249, 1994
27. Montebello AR: Teamwork in health care: Opportunities for gains in quality, productivity, and competitive advantage. Clin Lab Manage Rev 8(2):91–110, 1994
28. Nevalainen DE, Berte LM: Training, Verification, and Assessment: Keys to Quality Management. Malvern, Clinical Laboratory Management Association, 1993
29. O'Bryan D: Robotics: A way to link the "islands of automation." Clin Manage Rev 8(5):446–460, 1994
30. Pang CY, Swint JM: Forecasting staffing needs for productivity management in hospital laboratories. J Med Syst 9:365, 1985
31. Schubert E, Gross W, Siderits RH, Deckenbaugh L, He F, Becich MJ: A pathologist-designed imaging system for anatomic pathology signout, teaching, and research. Sem Diag Pathol 11(4):263–273, 1994
32. Schuler RS: Personnel and Human Resource Management, 3rd ed, pp 694–704. St. Paul, West Publishing Co, 1987
33. Spendolini MJ: The Benchmarking Book, pp 1–204. New York, Amacom, 1992
34. Snyder JR: Reengineering the clinical laboratory. Med Lab Observ 27(1):7, 1995
35. Steiner JW, Root JM: Service and value: The decommoditization of laboratory services and impact of managed care. Clin Lab Man Rev 8(3):291–296, 1994.
36. Steiner JW, Root JM: The Decommoditization of Laboratory Services and Impact of Managed Care. Baltimore, Clinical Laboratory Management Association Hot Topic Seminar, Feb 3, 1944
37. Vogel DP: Patient-focused care. Am J Hosp Pharm 50: 2321–2329, 1993
38. Widman J: Using Matrixes to Simplify Scheduling. Med Lab Observ August, 1980.
39. Zinober JW, Maier C: Selecting the best to be the best: How to gain a competitive edge for your organization, Part I. Clin Lab Man Rev 7(6):483–491, 1993
40. Zinober JW, Maier C: Selecting the best to be the best: How to gain a competitive edge for your organization, Part II. Clin Lab Man Rev 8(1):33–42, 1994

BIBLIOGRAPHY

Allred TJ, Steiner L: Alternate-site testing. Consider the analyst. Clin Lab Med 14(3):569–604, 1994
Bureau of National Affairs, 42 USC §12101, Americans with Disabilities Act, 1990
Bureau of National Affairs, 42 USC §12111, Americans with Disabilities Act, 1992
Centers for Disease Control: Recommendations and reports: Guidelines for prevention of transmission of human immunodeficiency virus and hepatitis B virus to health care and public-safety workers. MMWR, 38(S-6), 1989
Cousar JB, Peters TH Jr: Laboratories in patient-centered units. Clin Lab Med 14:525–538, 1994
Dennington SR, Wilkinson DS: CQI in action in the central lab laboratory. Clin Lab Mange Rev 7(6):516–519, 1993
Federal Register, 54, 29CFR 1910; Ergonomic Safety and Health Program Management Guidelines; 1989
Federal Register, 55, 42CFR 493; Clinical Laboratory Improvement Act; 1990
Federal Register, 55, 29CFR 1910; Occupational Exposure to Hazardous Chemicals in Laboratories; 1990
Federal Register 56, CFR 1910.1030; Occupational Exposure to Blood Borne Pathogens, 1992
Federal Register, 57, 42CFR 493; Clinical Laboratory Improvement Act; 1992
Felder RA, Boyd JC, Margrey K, Holman W, Savory J: Robotics in the medical laboratory. Clin Chem 36(9):1534–1543, 1990
Friedman BA: The laboratory information float, time-based competition, and point-of-care testing. Clin Lab Man Rev 8(5): 509–514, 1994
Howanitz PJ, Steindel SJ, Cembrowski GS, et al: Emergency department stat turn-around times. A College of American Pathologists' Q-Probes study for potassium and hemoglobin. Arch Pathol Lab Med 116(2):122–128 1992
Joint Commission on the Accreditation for Healthcare Organizations (JCAHO): Accreditation Manual for Pathology and Laboratory Services, PA 6.4., 1993
Kasten BL, Schrand P, Disney M: Joining the bar code revolution. Med Lab Observ 24:22–27, 1992
Kaufman HW: Specimen pathway analysis aids quality and efficiency. Med Lab Observ 24:33–39, 1992
Koenig AS: Medical Laboratory Planning and Design, pp 1–186. Northfield, College of American Pathologists, 1989
Markin RS: Clinical laboratory automation: A paradigm shift. Clin Lab Man Rev 7:243–251, 1993
Markin RS: A laboratory automation platform: The next robotic step. Med Lab Observ 24:24–28, 1992
Martin BG: Cost containment: Strategies and responsibilities of the laboratory manager. Clinics in Lab Med 5:697, 1985
Martin BG: Change and change makers. Lab Med January: 49–51, 1986
Miller K: How rotation can help boost productivity. Med Lab Observ 19:52, 1987
Woo JH: The advance of technology as a prelude to the laboratory of the twenty-first century. Clin Lab Med 14:459–471, 1994

14

Standards and Appraisals of Laboratory Performance

Jana Wilson Wolfgang • Kenneth E. Wolfgang

Appraisal of performance is part of any human endeavor. After performance of a task, a person will ask himself, "Did I do well?" Similarly, when people pool their efforts under a common leader, the leader may ask whether each person has done his share of the task and whether each performance met the leader's expectations.

In the clinical laboratory, as in other organizations, performance appraisal can play a role in effective management. An appraisal may be formal or informal or both. It may be a vehicle of communication, a basis for promotion or salary decisions, or a means used by managers to change subordinates' behavior.

The benefits of planned, thoughtful appraisals are as great in the laboratory as in nonlaboratory settings. Rapid staff turnover and the special time constraints of the clinical laboratory may seem insurmountable barriers to regular appraisals. On the other hand, the clinical laboratory is uniquely able to deal with the issues associated with performance appraisal. Measurement and its applications are intrinsic to the very processes associated with the laboratory. Issues of reliability and validity are no less critical to the success of a performance appraisal than they are to clinical laboratory testing.

In the following pages, we define some terms associated with performance appraisals and present purposes for which they may be used. We then attempt to distill the essentials of effective appraisal and give examples of the different formats a laboratory manager might consider when planning for this important task.

PERFORMANCE APPRAISALS: DEFINITIONS AND PURPOSES

Some terms applied to periodic assessment of an employee's job performance are employee rating, performance evaluation, merit review, and performance appraisal. The selection of one term over another is usually arbitrary.

Performance appraisal may be defined as a planned, formal, and periodic management activity in which subordinates' on-the-job behavior is evaluated for some purpose. Although the elements of planning, formality, and periodicity are important, the key to this definition is purpose. To function effectively, a performance appraisal should reflect and serve the purpose for which it was designed. Some possible purposes for performance appraisals can be found in Box 14–1.

The most commonly cited reason for evaluating a subordinate is to make salary and promotion decisions.[4,7,10,11,16] In practice, this does not always require direct communication with the subordinate; a manager can, and often does, make such a decision unilaterally. The detrimental effects of such a nonparticipatory action are probably known to many readers from personal experience. The subordinate feels left out of the decision-making process and is often dissatisfied with the results. Some health-care facilities have become so disillusioned with traditional appraisals that they have abolished them altogether.[5]

Another purpose for performance appraisals is to attempt to change a subordinate's behavior. Whether a manager wants to motivate a subordinate who is per-

Box 14•1

Possible Purposes for Performance Appraisals

Salary decisions
Promotion decisions
Behavior modification
Determination of level of competence
Determination of need for training
Communication (obtaining feedback from subordinate)
Evaluation of progress toward or achievement of job objectives
Discussion of interface between subordinate's and organization's goals and how each can be achieved

forming adequately or to bring a below-average performer to an acceptable level, the manager may try to use the performance appraisal to accomplish this goal. If further training is needed to attain an acceptable level of performance, such training would be specified during the evaluation. Attempts to change behavior ordinarily involve face-to-face communication with the subordinate and a more complex performance appraisal system than salary decisions require.

When the primary purpose of a performance appraisal is communication, personal contact between manager and subordinate is essential. The performance appraisal becomes a forum for interactive discussion of the subordinate's responsibilities and how they have been met. Progress toward goals that had been agreed on at the beginning of the period can be examined in light of the actual demands and constraints of the period. Finally, new goals can be set for the future, with the understanding that less formal discussions may take place in the interim before the next performance appraisal.

The various purposes for performance appraisals are not mutually exclusive. However, the purpose or purposes should be clear, both in design and execution, for an evaluation system to function well.

ESSENTIALS OF MEANINGFUL PERFORMANCE APPRAISALS

Without a few critical elements, an appraisal system will not function. These include standards and criteria of performance, communication of these standards and criteria to the subordinate, sufficient frequency of appraisal, and clear communication of appraisal results.

Standards and Criteria

A *standard* can be defined as a measure to which like objects are expected to conform, while a *criterion* is a standard used in forming judgments. For example, a standard for glass cuvettes in the chemistry laboratory might consist of a given internal diameter, such that the cuvette fits into the spectrophotometer. Whether or not the cuvette will go into the spectrophotometer is easily decided; a yes or no answer is possible. In contrast, how readily the cuvette can be removed from the instrument might be a criterion for judging whether the cuvettes are good, bad, or indifferent. To some extent, this is a matter of judgment.

To evaluate performance of a task, both standards and criteria for that performance must exist. This may seem self-evident, but standards and criteria are not always clear. For instance, a new pathologist may be given the responsibility of evaluating the chief technologist without being told what the chief technologist is expected to do. Should the pathologist judge according to the standards of a previous hospital environment? How does the pathologist know what the job of chief technologist entails in the new institution? On the other hand, if the job standards are known, by what criteria should this individual's performance be measured? A good performance in one laboratory might be considered fair somewhere else or excellent at a third institution.

Sources of Standards

Performance standards should be specified for performance to be evaluated meaningfully. One possible source of standards is the job description. Depending on the detail included, this may be a general guideline or a clear understanding of the responsibilities that accompany a given job.

In general, however, job descriptions are short and not very specific. A more exacting set of standards may be derived from a job analysis. In this process, someone who is fulfilling the responsibilities of a job writes down or reports all the different tasks the job includes. Each task may then be broken down into its component skills (task analysis). For example, in the case of a bench-level technologist, a job analysis might show that the technologist runs anticoagulated blood specimens through an automated cell-counting instrument, performs manual differential counts, screens urine specimens using chemical strips, and examines urine sediments. Each of these tasks demands a large number of component skills (eg, use, care, and basic troubleshooting of microscopes and cell counters; recognition of abnormal cells or casts), which could be further subdivided. At the conclusion of the job analysis, a list of tasks and required skills may serve as a set of standards for performance of the job.

A third possible source of standards is mutual consent to specified goals, as found in management by objectives. In this case, the subordinate and manager agree on certain tasks that the subordinate is to perform during the evaluation period. Provided that these standards are clear to both parties, they can provide very useful performance standards.

Performance criteria are more difficult to specify than performance standards. As implied in the definition, criteria are the basis of judgment; they allow performance to be characterized as good, poor, or average. An ideal set of performance criteria would allow 10 different supervisors from 10 clinical laboratories to produce independently exactly the same performance appraisal for one hematology technologist. This is a difficult goal to reach in any situation in which individual judgment is involved.

Performance criteria require clear definitions of what constitutes poor, fair, and excellent performance. If the definition is left to the individual, performance appraisals will be inconsistent from rater to rater and from the same rater at different times. Some reproducibility can be attained through rater training, where managers are taught to use a certain performance appraisal format. However, the validity of a rating system may be increased by providing criteria that are based on observable behaviors.[8] If a criterion gives the rater a clear choice among alternatives A, B, and C, with minimal judgment involved, that criterion is more likely to contribute to a successful performance appraisal.

Communication of Standards and Criteria

Once performance standards and criteria have been specified, the subordinate to be evaluated must be aware of them. Again, this seems obvious, but many laboratory employees have had occasion to ask, "How did I know I was supposed to check the refrigerators every day?" or "Why does my supervisor think my technical skills are average instead of good?" Standards and criteria may be communicated during the initial job orientation session by the manager or personnel department, during the subordinate's first meeting with the manager, or by means of a written document, such as a detailed job description along with the performance appraisal form. In the performance management model, the manager and employee define standards together on an annual basis as part of "performance plan" creation.[15]

Frequency of Evaluation

The frequency with which performance appraisals should take place depends on the purpose they are intended to serve and the efficiency of other means of communication. The most common interval for appraisal is every 12 months; this is usually adequate for salary and promotion decisions. However, formal review of progress toward goals might be required at more frequent intervals, depending on the nature of the job, the subordinate's ability to work independently, and the supervisor's management style. Certainly, if a manager wants to change a subordinate's behavior, regularly scheduled communications must supplement the more formal medium of the performance appraisal.

Communication of Results

A final vital element in effective performance appraisals is communication of the results to the subordinate. These results must be clear and indicate that the purpose of the performance appraisal was fulfilled. Ordinarily, the appraisal will indicate areas for improvement to the subordinate. If these goals are explicit and detailed, they can serve as guides for improvement and as additional criteria against which performance can be measured.

DESIGNING PERFORMANCE APPRAISALS

The structure of a performance appraisal may generally be divided into two areas, the written component and the interview. These areas should complement and reinforce one another in achieving the purpose for which the performance appraisal was designed. Accordingly, a number of formats should be considered during the design process.

Performance Appraisals: The Written Component

Barrett presented a thorough, detailed discussion of designing written performance ratings.[2] As he points out, an employee's on-the-job behavior may be classified and rated in three areas: personality, performance, and product. Evaluation of these areas may involve a variety of formats.

Graphic Scales

The most common method for performance evaluations is probably the use of the *graphic rating scale* (Fig. 14-1). In graphic scales, a quality or characteristic is rated by choosing a point along a horizontal axis. The scale may be discrete (1—2—3—4—5; A—B—C—D—F; excellent—good—fair—poor—unacceptable), or it may be continuous.

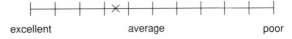

excellent   average   poor

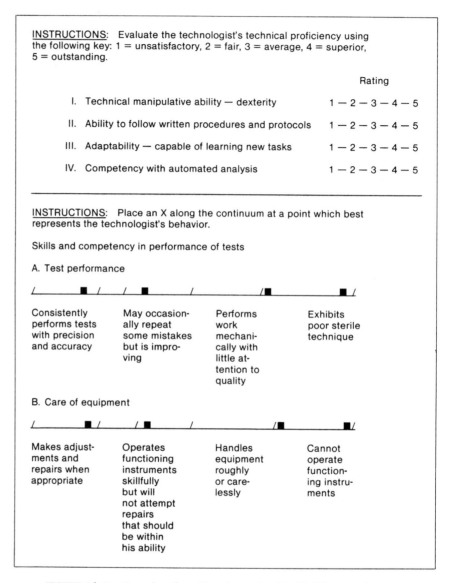

INSTRUCTIONS: Evaluate the technologist's technical proficiency using the following key: 1 = unsatisfactory, 2 = fair, 3 = average, 4 = superior, 5 = outstanding.

Rating

I.   Technical manipulative ability — dexterity   1 — 2 — 3 — 4 — 5

II. Ability to follow written procedures and protocols   1 — 2 — 3 — 4 — 5

III. Adaptability — capable of learning new tasks   1 — 2 — 3 — 4 — 5

IV. Competency with automated analysis   1 — 2 — 3 — 4 — 5

INSTRUCTIONS: Place an X along the continuum at a point which best represents the technologist's behavior.

Skills and competency in performance of tests

A. Test performance

| Consistently performs tests with precision and accuracy | May occasionally repeat some mistakes but is improving | Performs work mechanically with little attention to quality | Exhibits poor sterile technique |

B. Care of equipment

| Makes adjustments and repairs when appropriate | Operates functioning instruments skillfully but will not attempt repairs that should be within his ability | Handles equipment roughly or carelessly | Cannot operate functioning instruments |

FIGURE 14–1. Examples of graphic rating scales. (Modified from Snyder JR, Wilson JC: J Allied Health 9:125–131, 1980 and Lynch BL: Am J Med Tech 43(1):54–63, 1977)

There is usually an uneven number of points on the scale so that a middle or average can be selected. Barrett offers a practical set of guidelines for constructing rating scales.[2] These guidelines can be found in Box 14–2.

Perhaps the most important of these guidelines is to "have raters rate what they observe, not what they infer." Most of the other guidelines help the manager state the behavior being evaluated in an unambiguous manner. Barrett also suggests using between five and nine rating steps to allow the rater to differentiate similar but distinct performances.[2]

An example of a special type of graphic-rating scale is shown in the lower portion of Figure 14–1. This is

Box 14·2

Barrett's Guidelines for Constructing Rating Scales

Express only one thought in a scale.
Use words the rater understands.
Have raters rate what they observe, not what they infer.
Eliminate double negatives.
Express thoughts simply and clearly.
Keep statements internally consistent.
Avoid universals.
Stick to the present.
Avoid vague concepts (eg, honesty).

---

called a *behaviorally anchored rating scale*. It is based on "critical incidents," or actual examples of how people behaved in a given situation. Such critical incidents are gathered and placed along a continuum by groups of judges from the same populations as the raters who will use the rating scale.[1] The technique has been successfully applied to medical technology student evaluation.[8] However, development of behaviorally anchored rating scales requires conscientious input from a group of prospective judges, which may not be feasible in some management situations.

Box 14·3

Sample Checklist Rating Form

Instructions: Circle at least three of the adjectives given below that best describe the technologist's outstanding personal characteristics. The qualities may be desirable or undesirable.

aggressive	flexible	observant
articulate	imaginative	open-minded
careful	immature	punctual
careless	impulsive	pushy
casual	inarticulate	resourceful
cautious	indifferent	responsible
discriminating	inflexible	self-assured
eager	inquisitive	sloppy
efficient	lazy	tenacious
energetic	loud	vigorous
enthusiastic	mature	witty
erratic	meticulous	
excitable	neat	

Checklist

A second common evaluation method is use of the *checklist*. A list of adjectives or descriptive phrases is presented along with instructions for checking those that apply or for circling a prescribed number. A checklist rating form might look like the sample provided in Box 14–3.

According to Barrett, this format is easy to use but rarely distinguishes average from good or poor performers.[2]

Narrative

In combination with other rating methods, the free-written rating or *narrative* is a third common vehicle. The rater may be given explicit directions for writing the narrative or may simply be asked to comment on the adequacy of the subordinate's performance. An example of a narrative evaluation form is provided in Box 14–4.

While easy to construct, this rating method has the dual disadvantages of difficulty in comparing subordinates' ratings and subjective bias.[2]

Ranking

A less common evaluation method is termed *ranking*. Ranking methods have proven neither reliable nor valid experimentally,[2] but they are still used. A group of subordinates who perform similar duties may be *rank-ordered* or assigned a rank in the group according to their

Box 14·4

An Example Narrative Evaluation Form

Instructions: Please give other information that will assist in appraising the technologist. Comment on exceptionally outstanding performance or unsatisfactory ratings and qualities not covered elsewhere. Do not include comments that are only a restatement of the various ratings; specific illustrations are always more helpful than remarks of a general nature. Be concise.

Technical skills
Interpersonal skills
Dependability
Organization
Other

overall performance. Alternatively, subordinates may be compared two at a time (*paired comparison*). In this rating method, ranking occurs on the basis of the number of times a given subordinate is deemed the better performer of a pair. In the very similar *man-to-man comparison*, subordinates are ranked as average, below average, above average, or outstanding on the basis of comparison with *only* those of their peers who are currently performing similar tasks. Last, the *forced distribution* method of ranking subordinates assumes a predetermined distribution of performance. For instance, a rater might be compelled to designate 67% of a group of subordinates as average, with the remaining 33% evenly distributed between above and below average. These four ranking methods share the requirement that subordinates be performing closely similar tasks. They also share the characteristic of subjectivity, because subordinates are usually ranked on the basis of the composite, ill-defined overall performance, rather than on a comparison of performance with present standards.

Forced-Choice Rating

An uncommonly used rating method is the *forced choice*, in which a rater chooses the most applicable of several unrelated descriptions of performance.[2] The choices are purposefully made difficult with the intent of improving the reliability of the rating.

Free-Form

Free-form evaluation methods are in wide use as adjuncts to other methods; they are rarely used as the only evaluation method. One variation of this format not mentioned previously is the *critical incident* performance evaluation. During the evaluation period, the rater observing the subordinate makes written notations of exceptional performance, whether good or bad. For example, if a technologist assumes the responsibilities of the supervisor during the supervisor's absence, the laboratory manager might write that the technologist performed creditably during that period. If the same technologist had a loud argument with the nursing supervisor the following week, this, too, would be noted. These critical incidents and others would be summarized in the written performance evaluation. Among the problems with this rating method is the lack of reference to the day-to-day, noncritical performance that makes up the greatest portion of any person's on-the-job behavior.

Whatever the format used in written appraisals, individual managers will use them to evaluate individual subordinates' behavior. The rater must understand the purpose the appraisal was designed to serve. The appraisal must be flexible enough to allow its use to be adapted to the rater's own management style. Finally, the standards and criteria that underlie the appraisal must allow an objective evaluation of the subordinate.

The Performance Appraisal Interview

For many managers, the interview is the most difficult aspect of the performance appraisal. Some managers avoid the appraisal interview altogether, saying they do not have time or that they have nothing to discuss with the subordinate. Unfortunately, this avoidance of personal interaction denies both the manager and the subordinate a unique opportunity for review, discussion, and planning.

Planning the Interview

The purpose of the appraisal interview is to discuss, modify, or reinforce the written performance appraisal. Therefore, it is important for the manager to plan for the interview carefully. The standards and criteria for the subordinate's job should be close at hand; any written records of performance should be reviewed immediately before the interview. The interview should be scheduled well in advance so that both the subordinate and manager will be prepared. In addition, the interview should be held privately, with no interruptions, so that both can speak freely and without distractions.

Once the interview begins, the interpersonal communication skills of the manager become important. Even when a good relationship exists and a manager and subordinate communicate frequently, the formality of the performance appraisal is likely to make the subordinate (and manager) nervous.

Interview Methods

A number of interview methods have been proposed.[6,9,11,12] Maier, for instance, suggests three basic approaches: the "tell-and-sell" method, the "tell-and-listen" method, and the problem-solving method.[9] In the tell and sell, the manager tells the subordinate the results of the appraisal and tries to talk him into improving on-the-job behavior. This method is advocated for new, young, or timid employees. In the tell-and-listen method, the subordinate has a chance to respond to the manager's observations before returning control of the interview to the manager. In the last method, which is recommended for experienced and mature employees, the subordinate and manager discuss the appraisal as equals. Deficiencies in job performance are considered problems to be solved through joint effort.

Lefton and colleagues have related these ideas to modern management theory and added the concept of the follow-up interview.[6] According to these authors, the performance appraisal is simply the most structured type of feedback along a continuum that also includes ordinary feedback, coaching, and counseling.

Both Scanlan and Swan recommend a results-oriented performance review, emphasizing mutual agreement on standards, criteria, current performance levels, and goals.[11,15] In this type of appraisal, the interview becomes a planning session where both manager and subordinate participate in goal determination.

Although interview methods vary, involving the subordinate in his own appraisal yields improvement in performance. If the manager regards the appraisal interview as an occasion for discussion, preceded by planning and followed up according to a specific timetable, it is most likely to satisfy the needs of both the manager and the subordinate.

Selection or Design of a Performance Appraisal System

Performance appraisal systems are often already in place when a manager assumes responsibility in a new setting. However, a manager may have the opportunity to select an appraisal system, or at least decide how the existing system will be applied. When selecting or designing a written performance evaluation, a manager must consider four factors: (1) the purpose of the appraisal, (2) the work environment, (3) the self-directedness and verbal and analytical skills of the subordinates to be evaluated, and (4) the manager's preferred management style and verbal and analytical skills. Selection of one or more of the written appraisal formats will depend on these factors. For instance, in a busy medical center laboratory, it might not be practical to depend on narrative evaluation alone because of the time and writing skills required. A set of graphic scales, filled out by the shift supervisor and the technologist before the appraisal interview, might be an adequate basis for discussion and planning.

Use of the Personal Computer as a Tool

The personal computer may be a tool after a manager or organization has defined the purpose, measurement standards, and criteria for appraisals. While standard forms have historically been the framework for performance data collection and reporting, they also have been barriers to timely completion. The repetitive task of collecting, transferring, and updating previous employment information sometimes represented a significant time commitment for each appraisal.

With the introduction of the personal computer to the workplace, much of the repetitive aspect of the evaluation process can be eliminated. From scheduling of periodic reviews to criterion linkage to key elements of the employee's position description, efficient use of the computer maintains a high level of management productivity.

Three examples of software programs for performance appraisal are "Employee Appraiser" (3 Lagoon Drive, Suite 340, Redwood City, CA 94065); "Performance Now" (Knowledge Point, 1129 Industrial Ave., Petaluma, CA 94952); and "Workwise Evaluations" (Paradigm Software Development, 2510 Western Ave. #500, Seattle, WA 98121).

Common Evaluation Errors

Managers who have done their homework in designing a performance appraisal instrument still must beware of common evaluation errors, as identified by Feinauer[3]:

- Recent behavior bias: More recent behavior and performance are emphasized to the exclusion of earlier behavior and performance.
- Contrast effect: Performance is compared to that of another employee rather than to an external standard.
- Inconsistent standards: Different evaluators use different standards, so the appraisal process is subject to charges of discrimination.
- Halo effect: One element of the employee's performance dominates the entire evaluation.
- Exclusion of important perspectives: The manager fails to seek input from other supervisors or managers who may have had the opportunity to observe the employee's performance.

PERFORMANCE APPRAISALS IN THE CONTEXT OF PERFORMANCE MANAGEMENT

Performance appraisals do not occur in a vacuum; they are part of the ongoing and variable process of performance management. In the clinical laboratory, application of this concept has been rare. Technical personnel are often promoted on the basis of their technical expertise, not on the basis of managerial skill. Eligibility for positions at higher levels of laboratory management seems to depend on academic or medical degrees, with little regard for the administrative and interpersonal demands of the posts.

The job of any manager is to ensure that the goals of the organization are reached through the people on whom the organization depends. The broad goals of clinical laboratories include accurate and timely laboratory analyses, service to the patient, and service to the physician, with the overriding concern being the welfare of the patient. The people who collect and prepare the specimens and perform the analyses achieve or do not achieve these goals. However, the effort requires teamwork and leadership, which are the responsibility of the laboratory's managers.

Performance management in the clinical laboratory may be perceived as an iterative process involving planning, monitoring, and discussion (Fig. 14-2). Performance appraisal is an integral part of this process.

Goal Setting

In this model, the management process begins with a discussion of the subordinate's responsibilities and goals. For example, consider a hematology technologist for whom a job description was derived earlier. To enter the cycle of the performance management process, let us say that the supervisor of the hematology laboratory undertakes a job analysis with the technologist's help and writes a set of performance standards. The supervisor and the technologist then sit down together and discuss how the standards apply and whether additional ones should be added. Criteria for good performance are discussed and finalized. Finally, the technologist's personal goals—perhaps learning a new technique or attending more professional meetings—are examined and related to the requirements of the job. At the end of this meeting, the technologist and the supervisor leave with a clear understanding and a *written summary* of what the technologist is supposed to do.

Performance Monitoring

The second part of the performance management process is performance monitoring. It is the manager's responsibility to make sure that the subordinate is carrying out his duties. The subordinate's work experience

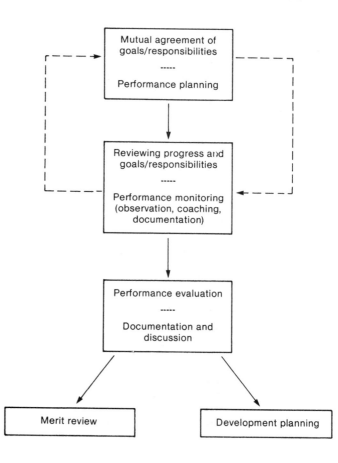

FIGURE 14–2. Clinical laboratory performance management process.

and previous performance will govern how closely he must be observed; a technician with 2 years' experience and an excellent quality-control record might be left to work independently until a question or problem arises, whereas a new phlebotomist might require close supervision and instruction during the first few weeks of work. If a performance problem surfaces, the manager should discuss it with the subordinate as soon as possible so that they may work together to correct it. Such instances should be recorded to facilitate performance appraisal.

Performance Review

When the time arrives for a performance appraisal, the stage is already set. The manager and subordinate can evaluate the subordinate's performance by comparing it with the standards, criteria, and goals agreed on at the beginning of the period. The documentation of performance maintained during the monitoring period is the basis for the appraisal. From this session, new goals can be established. In addition, the appraisal results can be considered when a salary review is undertaken.

In an extremely thorough text, Swan offers eight specific steps for implementing performance appraisal as part of performance management.[15] The first step in this process is to set measurable performance objectives that reflect organizational goals but are specific to the particular job under consideration. The manager and employee create a "performance plan," prioritizing and weighting the objectives and defining clear standards of performance (eg, what constitutes knowledge or behavior that meets, does not meet, or exceeds the expected level). The second step is to observe and document employee performance, giving feedback throughout the period. During the third and subsequent steps, the manager solicits an employee self-evaluation, conducts a discussion of this input, completes the performance appraisal form, reviews it with higher management, and schedules and conducts an appraisal discussion. The discussion and written summary of the discussion become the basis for the next cycle of performance management.

Legal Defensibility

A major advantage to the performance management approach to performance appraisals is legal defensibility. Snyder has clearly conveyed the "legal defense factors" that clinical laboratory managers should consider when assessing their facilities' performance appraisal systems.[13] Appraisals are used for salary adjustments, discipline, and promotions and must be fair; alleged discrim-ination in application has led to court cases under laws such as the Civil Rights Act, the Age Discrimination Act, and the Pregnancy Discrimination Act. Components of the performance management approach, particularly clearly defined standards, feedback, and documentation, are key to defensibility.

PERFORMANCE APPRAISALS AND THE CLINICAL LABORATORY

The potential benefits of a good performance appraisal system may be summarized in terms that are frequently used within the laboratory setting:

A systematic performance management process is *sensitive* to the needs, strengths, and weaknesses of employees and the organization. With this sensitivity, the clinical laboratory manager can expect early detection of problems and personnel development opportunities that otherwise might go unnoticed. Early detection allows corrective action or better use of capabilities.

At the same time, the performance management process is *specific*: Misinformation is avoided by frequent interactions and thorough monitoring. Because misunderstanding of the strengths, needs, or problems of employees leads to errors in decision making, the process increases the effectiveness of the manager.

REFERENCES

1. Anastasi A: Psychological Testing. New York, Macmillan, 1976
2. Barrett R: Performance Rating, pp 33, 46, 47, 52, 54. Chicago, Scientific Research Association, 1966
3. Feinauer D: Making Performance Appraisals a Positive Experience. Clin Lab Manag Rev 4(6):433–438, 1990
4. Fulmer RM: Supervision: Principles of Professional Management. Beverly Hills, Glencoe Press, 1976
5. Gill G, Kendall ER: The Abolishment of Performance Appraisals: Parkview's Story. Joint Commis J Qual Improv 20(12):669–678, 1994
6. Lefton RE, Buzzota VR, Sherberg M, Karraker DL: Effective Motivation Through Performance Appraisal. New York, John Wiley and Sons, 1977
7. Lundberg GD: Managing the Patient-Focused Laboratory. Oradell, Medical Economics, 1975
8. Lynch BL: A behaviorally anchored rating scale for the evaluation of student performance. Am J Med Technol 43: 54–63, 1977
9. Maier NRF: The Appraisal Interview: Three Basic Approaches. La Jolla, University Association, 1976
10. Newell JE: Laboratory Management. Boston, Little, Brown, 1972
11. Scanlan BK: Management 18: A Short Course for Managers. New York, John Wiley and Sons, 1974
12. Smith HP, Brouwer PJ: Performance Appraisal and Human Development. Reading, Addison-Wesley, 1977

13. Snyder JR: Assessing the Legality of Performance Appraisals. Clin Lab Manag Rev 5:483–489, Nov/Dec, 1991
14. Snyder JR, Wilson JC: Evaluation of student performance in the clinical setting using the process skills approach. J Allied Health 9:125–131, 1980
15. Swan WS: How to Do a Superior Performance Appraisal. New York, John Wiley and Sons, 1991
16. Wilcox KR et al: Laboratory management. In Inhorn SL (ed): Quality Assurances Practices for Health Laboratories. Washington, DC, American Public Health Association, 1978

ANNOTATED BIBLIOGRAPHY

Anastasi A: Psychological Testing, 4th ed. New York, Macmillan, 1976

A well-indexed reference text on principles and practice of psychologic testing; addresses issues of validity and reliability of testing, applicable to the development of written performance evaluation.

Barrett RS: Performance Rating. Chicago, Science Research Associates, 1968

An excellent text on a difficult subject. Clearly written and readable, it defines terms, supports conclusions with research and examples, and is eminently reasonable.

Lynch BL: A behaviorally anchored rating scale for the evaluation of student performance. Am J Med Technol 43(1):54–63, 1977

A careful, detailed report of the development of a specific student evaluation tool; an important reference for medical technology educators.

Scanlan BK: Management 18: A Short Course for Managers. In Wiley Professional Development Programs, Business Administration Series. New York, John Wiley and Sons, 1974

A self-instructional text on all aspects of management that is well-organized, concise, and readable. It summarizes management theory and offers examples of practice.

Swan WS: How to Do a Superior Performance Appraisal. New York, John Wiley and Sons, 1991

A complete guide to performance appraisal in the context of performance management. Gives particularly practical guidance for interview techniques, with applicability to management situations beyond the appraisal.

15

Educational Responsibilities of Managers and Supervisors

John R. Snyder • Richard L. Moore II

Change is all around us in the form of threats and opportunities. Flexibility to accommodate, adopt, and adapt to the stimulus of change requires learning. As the business of health care becomes more complex and dynamic and delivery systems become more interconnected, work must become a venue for continual learning. An important extension of the ideas fundamental to total quality management in the laboratory is becoming a learning organization.

What is a "learning organization"? According to Peter M. Senge, principal proponent of the concept, learning organizations are environments in which both managers and employees at all levels "continually expand their capacity to create the results they truly desire; where new and expansive patterns of thinking are nurtured; where collective aspiration is set free; and where people are continually learning to learn together."[22] That is a lofty definition, but embodied in these words are the notion of excitement about learning, a spontaneity of asking "why," a freedom to explore and innovate—all to promote the well-being and mission of the organization. It is possible to become a learning organization because deep down we are all intrinsically inquisitive, natural learners. Consider two times in life when the learning curve is rising dramatically: (1) No one has to teach an infant how to learn and (2) education prepared you for laboratory work.

Learning curves plateau when work becomes routine. Senge's research has identified learning disabilities in organizations: People become their positions, not seeing how their actions affect other positions, or learn from their mistakes because the consequences are felt elsewhere. Organizational hierarchies and levels of authority suggest that someone "at the top" is the grand strategist. New ideas trigger a built-in response from the organization designed to stabilize, thus resisting change.

In *The Fifth Discipline: The Art and Practice of the Learning Organization*, Peter Senge describes five components that converge to innovate a learning organization: systems thinking, personal mastery, mental models, building shared vision, and team learning.[22]

Systems thinking is seeing all of the interrelated effects of our actions and how they will reverberate for years to come. In the clinical laboratory, we are too often caught up in the detailed complexity of what we are doing right now. We need to understand dynamic complexity when the cause and effect of our actions and decisions are distant from each other in time and location.

Personal mastery refers to a special level of proficiency achieved by continually clarifying and deepening one's vision and becoming a lifelong learner. Clinical laboratorians enter practice as well-educated, bright, high-energy scientists. In the absence of the laboratory organization stimulating personal growth, by the time these laboratorians are 30, a few are on the fast track, but most are putting in their time. They've lost the excitement of learning and the sense of mission and commitment to laboratory medicine.

Mental models are ingrained assumptions and generalizations about health-care delivery, the organization, and the role of laboratory medicine. Permission should be granted to think creatively about how things

255

could be different, testing how we view things, and avoiding a "mental prison," denying thoughts about what could be.

Building shared vision fosters genuine commitment if the vision is a common picture of the future, which is translated into movement in a direction. Too often "vision statements" are mistaken for a shared vision that galvanizes an organization, prompting people to excel and learn.

Team learning is also called "thinking together," yielding groups of employees who develop extraordinary capacities for coordinated action. When teams are learning, the collective intelligence of the team exceeds the intelligence of individuals on the team. This results in individual members growing more rapidly than would normally occur by one learner in a vacuum.

Becoming a learning organization is a gradual change process. It requires a redesigning of organizational culture in how people do work and think about work. A learning organization is never finished learning—rather, it is an organization on a path toward fulfilling its mission better.

EDUCATION AND TRAINING IN THE CLINICAL LABORATORY

At one time or another, most technicians, technologists, and pathologists are called on to be teachers.[14,25] Similar to the case made for technical experts to become managers in Chapter 5, these laboratorians are seldom prepared for their teaching role. Teaching responsibilities include a range of activities, from clinical education, in which the manager is asked to help train and supervise medical technology students,[8,15] to orientation of new employees through inservice education[1] and formal continuing education activities for a large peer group.[9]

Current regulations recognize the importance of education and training to the quality performance of laboratory testing. Regulations in the Clinical Laboratory Improvement Amendments of 1988 described in Chapter 2 require that all personnel receive appropriate preservice education and experience, evaluation, and documentation of performance.[21] The Joint Commission on Accreditation of Healthcare Organizations has published a standard for training related to the laboratory environment, facility management, operation, and safety.[5] The College of American Pathologists' inspection checklists contain a variety of training standards.[4] Verification for quality testing performance is addressed in the National Committee for Clinical Laboratory Standards document GP21-A.[16]

This chapter focuses on the need to meet changes occurring in health-care services through acceptance of

educational programming as an overall responsibility of the institution, laboratory management, section supervisors, and the individual laboratorian as a professional within the field of health care. The chapter is divided into sections reviewing some current issues in continuing education; summarizing activities and goals of preservice education, inservice education, and continuing education; listing the strengths and weaknesses of different teaching methodologies; and developing teaching programs.

It is clear that a professional's preparatory formal training in certificate and degree programs is just that—preparatory. The practicing professional is not able to remain abreast of the developments in the field without additional educational activity. To be sure, the laboratorian to a large degree must assume responsibility for continued learning, but it is surely a responsibility of the supervisor to stimulate and provide an environment supportive of learning efforts.

An environment for learning includes a variety of support mechanisms. Among the obvious ones are release time to attend formal education programs, tuition and travel support, and recognition of educational achievement through salary increases and promotions. However, a manager can support and encourage continued learning in other ways (Box 15-1).

One of the most important steps a manager can take to encourage continued learning is the encouragement of professionalism. If the laboratorian identifies himself as a true professional, then he will tend to include educational activities among personal responsibilities. This feeling of professionalism can be enhanced through providing for participation in the activities of the local, state, and national associations and paying dues and membership fees; by encouraging an understanding of issues confronting the profession and assisting laboratorians in becoming involved in resolving professional issues; and by assuming a personal role as supervisor to serve as an advocate for the profession throughout the institution.

An academic program that prepares students to become technologists will involve many different laboratory staff members as teachers, tutors, and clinical supervisors. While there are advantages to such a program through creation of a source of new staff members oriented toward the manner in which the laboratory functions (thereby reducing orientation and familiarization activities), there are also added administrative burdens and budgetary considerations.

LIFELONG LEARNING

In accepting a responsibility for continuing the education of the laboratorian, the manager or supervisor joins a rapidly growing movement generally identified by the

Box 15•1

Ways in Which a Manager Can Support and Encourage Continued Learning

Provision for formal reporting to the other staff members whenever anyone returns from a continuing education course

Formation of study clubs or discussion groups similar to the rounds and conferences commonly attended by physicians in which one person reports on a case or subject of interest

Selection, purchase, and circulation of appropriate journals and newsletters, which provide current relevant information

Provision of funds for staff to select books and reference works for a small laboratory library

Regular rental or free use of audiovisual self-instructional materials, which are available from medical center libraries and biomedical communication centers, regional libraries, pharmaceutical manufacturers, suppliers of laboratory equipment and products, and many of the professional health-related associations

Discussions or informal presentations by other health professionals who are consumers of laboratory services and who can discuss the laboratorian's work in relation to the diagnosis and management of the patient

Box 15•2

Characteristics of Professions Relating to Goals of Lifelong Education

Conceptual characteristics by which the profession establishes a commonly agreed-on function

Performance characteristics, which define the theory and practice of the profession, including mastery of theoretical knowledge, the ability to use that knowledge to solve problems, and the ability to use practical knowledge within the profession

Characteristics of self-enhancement through further individual study

Collective identity characteristics, by which a profession is known to be unique

A system of formal training

Systems for credentialing, which ensure expertise of those in the profession

Existence of a subculture, which includes traditions and language unique to the profession and systems for role definition and recognition

Legal reinforcements, which recognize the activities of the profession with regard to protection of confidences and protection in fulfilling the common functions of the profession

Public acceptance of the field as a profession, which accords a measure of status to its practitioners

A tradition of ethical practice, often formally codified, which sets limits of professional behavior

Penalties available to and enforceable by associations, governments, and agencies that guard against malpractice and incompetence

Relationships with other vocations, which define the role and scope of activity of the professional in relation to allied health occupations

Relationships with users of the service established through the pattern of interactions between professionals and consumers

---

term *lifelong learning*. The concept is based on the idea that the complexity of today's society, the rapid introduction of new technologies, role changes within the many professions, and the interests and desires of the citizenry for greater job satisfaction and more meaningful use of leisure time combine to support learning activities throughout a lifetime, rather than restricting learning to the traditional years of schooling. Continuing professional education identifies the portion of lifelong learning of direct interest to the laboratory supervisor.

Houle speaks to this as he identifies characteristics of professions that can be related to the goals of lifelong education.[11] These he clusters under broad headings (Box 15-2).

All of these characteristics of a profession apply to medical technology and provide opportunities for development of learning activities and responsibilities for the laboratorian. No profession, including laboratory medicine, is static. Indeed, each of these characteristics merely introduces a complex dynamic aspect of the total field that describes ways in which one profession differs from another.

EDUCATIONAL ISSUES

Apart from the issue of a general societal concern for lifelong learning, specific issues are related directly to the education and practice of the laboratorian and other professionals in health care. Among these is the use of educational activity as a criterion for continued licensure, which has grown substantially since New Mexico first required such a step in 1971.[19] Other states soon followed, and today various authors note a wide range of requirements throughout most states. There is no particular pattern as to which states require continuing education for relicensure and for which professionals it is required.

The rationale used in establishing a relicensure requirement for health professionals is a desire to ensure professional competence through continued educational activity. While this assurance is a goal of merit, a direct link between continuing education (or preparatory education) and competence in performance has not been established.

Johnston conducted a year-long study of the relationships among demographic factors, continuing education, and current competence as measured by a career-entry generalist certification examination.[12] Her results showed a positive correlation between continuing education preceding the study and test scores and a negative correlation between years since original career-entry certification and test scores. She concludes that continuing education for continued competence needs an accurate assessment of current knowledge and deficiencies, targeted continuing education activities, and evaluation to determine whether deficiencies have been remedied.

The transfer of cognitive knowledge to performance is difficult, even when the knowledge directly relates to the task to be performed. The relationship between knowledge and performance is even more tenuous when learning activities are only peripherally related, which is the case when a laboratorian attends a course away from the work site. Further, Willoughby, Gammon, and Jonas,[26] among others, in studying competence in physicians and other health professionals, note that although factors such as attitude, peer relations, maturity, and integrity are directly related to competent performance, they are not necessarily related to cognitive knowledge.

Among professionals, there is legitimate concern about the effectiveness of required continuing education for maintenance of competence. However, a man-

ager or supervisor may have some additional concerns. First, there is a budgetary ramification if employees are required to undertake educational activities and therefore need educational support as a possible fringe benefit.[10] Second, the atmosphere (and possibly the value) of the learning experience is potentially different when a large portion of a program audience attends by fiat, rather than by choice. Audience size and attitude clearly affect the learning experience for the participant. Fisher and Britt considered these factors from the perspective of a continuing education provider by identifying preferred formats, schedules, and sites at which to offer programs for practitioners in Florida.[9] They found that attendees preferred lectures and workshops in weekend programs that moved around the state to reduce travel costs to the participants.

To be effective, instruction must be relevant to the laboratorian's work or personal interest. Many institutions have adopted a "just-in-time" approach to inservice and continuing education to seize the "teachable moment." Figure 15-1 shows the relationships between performance-based instructional design and that which an employee must do (ie, task analysis).[17,20]

STAFF DEVELOPMENT

Perhaps the most important teaching role of the manager is in the planned educational activity that results from the performance appraisal conference (see Chapter 14). This educational activity is termed *staff development.* Figure 15-2 illustrates this retraining cycle.[17] Staff development activities are designed to correct deficiencies in current performance and to provide opportunities for employee growth.[2] Many managers fail to provide growth opportunities for their employees, reinforcing the status quo and generating job dissatisfaction for unchallenged laboratorians.

Educational activities that are targeted for staff development involve the manager in the subordinate's career planning.[6] Some laboratory managers feel that they should not take an active part in helping to develop skills that will prepare employees for jobs beyond those within a given laboratory. If a manager risks helping an employee develop his skills beyond the current job, certainly there exists the possibility of the employee leaving to acquire a better position, perhaps with a promotion. However, if the employee is not challenged beyond the routine, the best will leave to find fulfillment elsewhere anyway. This author recalls asking an applicant during a preemployment interview of her career development plans; she said, "I want your job." She was hired—not because her career goals could be soon met in the current position, but because she was ready

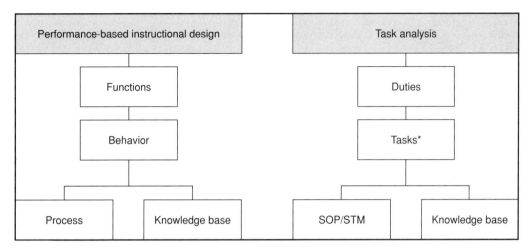

FIGURE 15-1. Performance-based instructional design and task analysis. (SOP, standard operating procedures; STM, standard test method; [1] Modified from Puce [20]; * limited to psychomotor and cognitive behavior) (Nevalainen DE, Berte LM: Training, Verification, and Assessment: Keys to Quality Management, p 5. Malvern, PA: Clinical Laboratory Management Association, 1993; reprinted with permission.)

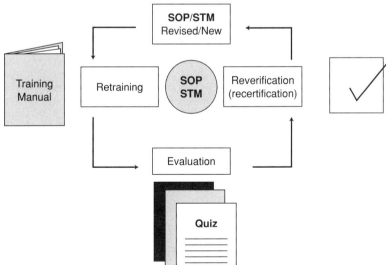

FIGURE 15-2. Retraining cycle. Nevalainen DE, Berte LM: Training, Verification, and Assessment: Keys to Quality Management, p 10. Malvern PA: Clinical Laboratory Management Association, 1993; reprinted with permission.)

for growth and willing to take on educational activities that would make her a more valuable employee than at the time of initial employment. She also welcomed new delegated responsibilities.

Many laboratories are filled with highly qualified bench technologists and have only a few supervisory slots. When considering staff development for clinical laboratorians, beware the trap that the only way to advance is to become a supervisor. Some technologists have no desire to leave their scientific testing role for a position supervising those doing the testing. Unfortunately, too few laboratories have redesigned jobs that allow advancement to positions of "technical specialist," "interdepartmental generalist," or "clinical laboratory practitioner."

Warren has described a staff development program for technologists and technicians who feel their careers have outgrown the growth potential in the laboratory.[24] The program enables movement along technical career development tracks progressing from medical technologist I (MT I) to medical technologist III (MT III). Under the program's guidelines: "(1) A technologist must be able to advance without leaving his or her technical area; (2) the medical center and the employee must make a mutual commitment; and (3) the program must eventually be flexible enough to accommodate all levels of interested laboratorians."[24] Progression from MT I to MT III is based on a mixture of additional education, experience in the institution, and specialty certification. New expanded duties are assigned to match the additional education and experience as one progresses in the career path program.

APPROACHES TO EDUCATIONAL ACTIVITIES

Two areas of educational programming must be explored by the supervisor. These are preservice education and continuing and inservice education. Both are necessary for an efficient laboratory operation.

Preservice Education

One of management's primary responsibilities to the new employee is preservice education. The technologist's first few weeks in a new work environment often are awkward and uneasy. Although the need for additional technical staff generally requires that the new laboratorian function in a technical capacity as soon as possible, the supervisor must ensure that preservice education (or orientation) does not suffer. Too often this critical adjustment period receives too little attention from the responsible superior. Orientation, in fact, is one of management's most overlooked

educational tools. A well-planned and structured preservice education program will ensure that the employee understands his responsibilities, limitations, and expectations initially so as not to hinder full development of performance capabilities. The important components of a preservice program are discussed in the following sections.

Job Description

Although a new employee's duties are discussed during the employment interview, the job description should be thoroughly reviewed at the beginning of the orientation period. The new employee will be more likely to ask questions about the duties and responsibilities of the position, giving the supervisor an opportunity to clarify misunderstandings. The supervisor's frank and open discussion of the job description establishes the foundation for the remainder of the preservice education.

The method of employee evaluation should be related to the job description. A copy of the evaluation form should be reviewed. This discussion about the evaluation and how it reflects the job description will reinforce the specific requirements of the position.

Staff Introduction

An early introduction to the laboratory staff helps develop the effective interpersonal relationships required to build teamwork. Certainly everyone with whom the new employee is to interact directly should be introduced. The size and structure of the laboratory organization will dictate the extent to which staff of other sections should be formally introduced. If the laboratory is small or open in design, all staff may be introduced to foster the "one large family" atmosphere. If, on the other hand, the laboratory has a large staff or is highly departmentalized, the new employee may be introduced only to each section supervisor. In the latter instance, an introduction to everyone at a general staff meeting would be appropriate. The period of individual introductions will include review of the organizational structure and reinforce work relationships for the new employee. In some instances, a personal introduction to the laboratory director may be in order. Attention to this portion of preservice education will enhance the new employee's feelings of belonging in the new environment.

Laboratory Policies and Procedures

Personnel policies and procedures were probably discussed during the initial interview; however, a review of these during the orientation helps to clarify any misunderstandings that might have occurred under the stress of the interview. This responsibility may be retained by the administrative technologist or personnel director or delegated to the section supervisor, depending on who discussed the policies during the interview.

This discussion should include information about the acceptable dress code, appropriate parking areas, security badge requirements, and the mechanism for completing the time sheet or card. Certainly laboratory policy concerning meal times and breaks for the specific work station needs to be addressed, because there is likely to be variation among sections within the laboratory. Coverage of evenings and weekends, call schedules, and vacation and holiday work should be discussed. Economic, educational, and recreational services, such as insurance plans, pensions, continuing and inservice education, athletic or social activities, and health services provided by the institution, should be included. Particular attention should be given to discipline and grievance procedures. Finally, a discussion of the opportunities for promotion and transfer will encourage the employee in self-improvement and productivity in the new laboratory environment.

Specific Laboratory Section

The first three steps in preservice education are oriented toward nonperformance details of the position. After these are sufficiently covered, the attention of the new employee can be focused on the laboratory role. The location of key manuals, reagents, equipment and supplies, and operational manuals and guidelines for instruments in the section where the laboratorian is to work should be explained. The new employee should know the location of particular documents for recording preventive maintenance checks and plotting quality-control data. Appropriate safety equipment both in and near the section should be identified. Outside the immediate working area, the location of certain general-use facilities should be noted, including the sterile preparation area, storeroom, and photocopy equipment.

Finally, the new employee can begin to feel that he has a niche in the laboratory when the area reserved for his personal belongings is pointed out to him. Appropriate stress should be placed on the limits of the institution's responsibility for theft of personal property.

Routine Protocols, Analytical Procedures, and Techniques

A discussion of the routine protocol for daily performance of duties follows orientation in the overall organization and the specific duty station. It is important to note tasks that have priority and tasks that can be completed on a more routine basis. If the section rotates

certain duties and responsibilities among employees, such as ordering supplies or stocking disposables, this also should be explained.

Frequently, a new employee is not informed of criteria that indicate a diversion from the standard operating procedure. By describing these unusual circumstances and explaining why a special protocol is followed, the supervisor will have anticipated and avoided a future problem.

Time must also be allotted for describing the procedures and techniques that the new laboratorian is expected to perform. Initially, all routine and specialized tests should be at least talked through, because certain in-house modifications of test procedures will differ from the individual's previous experience. It is important to emphasize that the methods and procedures established in the laboratory must be followed explicitly. Suggestions for modifying a procedure or technique should be considered by the supervisor. Several days to several weeks usually are required for the new employee to gain sufficient experience to complete all of the procedures and techniques of the section without extra supervision.

One area of preservice education frequently not given sufficient attention is preventive maintenance and troubleshooting problems with the automated equipment the new employee will use. A list of the most commonly occurring problems, noting the cause and outlining a step-by-step approach to resolving each problem, will avoid delays and further orient the employee in unfamiliar equipment. Omission of this important part of orientation inevitably comes back to haunt the supervisor—usually on a weekend or holiday!

Finally, direction regarding the amount of responsibility held in evaluation of quality control and patient data must be given. Approved "panic values" and appropriate actions and the types of test results that require a supervisor's or pathologist's evaluation before a report is issued to the requesting physician should be identified.

Safety Equipment and Procedures

General instructions on the proper use of all laboratory safety equipment is imperative. This may include a demonstration using the fire extinguishers and rolling oneself in a fire blanket and a discussion on the use of safety showers and eyewashes. The new employee should also be made aware of appropriate actions to take in the event of a job-related accident. If appropriate, a written description of the new laboratorian's role in the institution's fire and disaster plan should be provided.

Documentation

A brief summary memorandum of the aspects covered during the preservice education period will reinforce much of the information and provide the documentation necessary to satisfy requirements of the various laboratory accrediting and regulatory agencies.[3] It will also verify the completion of the supervisor's responsibility for employee orientation.

In summary, a well-planned orientation period will help the new employee adapt more readily to the new work environment of the laboratory. The result should be an open channel of communication between the supervisor and the new employee and avoidance of some of the usual misunderstandings associated with the new-job adjustment period. Despite the supervisor's most elaborate orientation approach, however, unscheduled but relevant "orientation" takes place on coffee breaks. Where else can a new employee learn such valuable information as who plans the holiday party, who usually has extra football tickets, and who will take phone messages?

Inservice and Continuing Education

In developing an appropriate postorientation educational program within the organization, the supervisor must first consider program goals. Lauffer indicates that there are two basic orientations or themes on which educational activities are based: improving the capabilities of the laboratorian and improving the manner in which the laboratory functions.[13] Generally, the first of these is called *continuing education* or *staff development*, and the latter is *inservice education*. In reality, however, the distinctions are neither clear nor particularly important. Although the manager will pursue both goals at various times, there must be an awareness of which effort is being pursued at any point.

Improving the capability of the laboratorian can be accomplished in a variety of ways. Attendance at a seminar offered by a hospital or medical center or enrollment in a course at a local university can contribute to individual growth and development. These activities are commonly classified as continuing education in that they are designed to build on previous formal educational experiences. Continuing education rarely provides the initial training required for entering the profession; however, educational activities pursued for enhancing progress within the organization or assuming new functions almost always are considered continuing education. For example, a laboratorian who is promoted to shift supervisor attends a seminar on techniques of supervision; he is attempting to develop a new personal role within the field.

Continuing education, when focusing on improving the capabilities of the laboratorian, is a highly individualistic endeavor, even though one would logically assume that a curriculum could be developed through which all laboratorians could constantly remain current. The fallacy in this attractive idea lies in the variability of employment environments and experiences of the individual after graduation from the initial training program. Individual professional experiences and growth are highly variable. In addition, duties for the laboratorian are likely to vary with work locations.

Because needs, activities, goals, and circumstances of individual practitioners within the field of medical technology vary, care must be given to the selection of continuing education activities. Several questions must be addressed by the professional prior to registering for a seminar.[23] First, can areas of personal need be identified so that the technician will be alert to potential educational opportunities? Examples may include future assumption of new duties that might require review of procedures or mastery of a new technique; the laboratory could be preparing to install new equipment that will require additional knowledge; or the institution could be planning to develop a new health-care service area requiring laboratory support, thereby causing a restructuring of duties.

When the educational goal of the supervisor focuses on the manner in which the laboratory functions, however, educational activity will include a large percentage of the laboratory staff and should be conducted locally. In many cases, no outside consultant will be required, because the educational activity will center on development and implementation of new procedures and techniques. In other cases, the activities might more properly focus on problem-solving steps, such as identification of barriers preventing accomplishment of tasks, motivational sessions that encourage cooperation among staff members, or informational sessions that reiterate policies and procedures. This is the area of inservice education.[1]

A primary concern of the supervisor when focusing on laboratory operation is to ensure that the problem does indeed spring from a lack of training or can be solved through a training activity. A training or educational activity should be held only after it is determined that the lack of performance is not caused by attitudes, lack of motivation, barriers from other departments or personnel, or a lack of resources, such as funding or equipment. Once all of these possible interveners have been examined and discarded, the manager can proceed to the development of an educational activity, taking care that appropriate documentation is prepared for accrediting bodies, such as the Joint Commission on the Accreditation of Healthcare Organizations.[3]

Within the laboratory, target audiences of those

who will participate will vary with the information to be included in the inservice activity. Certain modifications in a department's analytical procedure would be appropriate only for those responsible for performing that particular analysis and for those affected by a change in the procedure. This may involve two separate groups and require separate meetings. Other changes, such as a modification in a personnel benefit policy, may require a session for all staff members. In the case of a technologist experiencing difficulty troubleshooting a certain instrument, perhaps only one participant would be involved in the instructional activity.

There are several approaches to assisting staff members in updating their technical skills within the routine workday. Each of these requires that the supervisor be alert for opportunities to create a learning situation. The College of American Pathologists' Check Sample Program is one such example. By involving everyone in the check sample process, the routine is supplanted by an unusual case. For the highly departmentalized institution, the check sample patient data sheet may provide results from several laboratories to be correlated in defining the intended diagnosis. A subsequent case review is valuable in understanding the pathology behind the check sample findings. This same approach can be used by creating a case study when unusual laboratory results are desired.

Teaching Methodologies

Inservice education is usually a responsibility of laboratory supervisors and managers and requires careful planning and implementation to accomplish the stated goals and objectives. The approaches described here are but a few of the variety available to make inservice more effective for larger groups. The only limitation is one's imagination in creating a learning opportunity as part of the employee's workday.

LECTURE AND DISCUSSION SYMPOSIUM

Most people, when asked to teach, fall back on the dominant technique in American education—the lecture. For presenting new information, the lecture undoubtedly is the most efficient. Because inservice topics are usually of immediate application, the effectiveness of the lecture approach can be greatly enhanced by planning to include time for discussion. Two-way communication (discussion) is more accurate and effective than one-way (lecture only; see Chapter 7). When an inservice topic has several points of view, perhaps two or more speakers may be invited. This becomes a symposium and will increase the perspective of the participants.

PANEL DISCUSSIONS

A panel generally consists of three or four speakers and a moderator. When presenting a change in laboratory protocol, for example, perhaps a panel of supervisors whose sections are affected should briefly describe the change. A moderator would then direct the interaction among panel members and receive and direct the questions from the inservice participants. As in the symposium, the panel is an ideal format for expressing divergent views. Panel members should be carefully selected with attention given to speaking ability, and they should be assigned generally equal amounts of content to present. The responsibility is placed on the moderator to see that timeframes are adhered to and that each panel member is briefed before the session.

PROBLEM-SOLVING SESSION

As noted elsewhere in this text, the commitment to resolution of a problem will be greater if those affected by the problem are involved in solving it. This can become a type of inservice called a *clinic*, in which the speaker is assisted by a panel and the audience in exploring possible solutions to practical problems. When it becomes necessary to modify personnel policies within a department, for example, this approach could be effective. The speaker becomes the leader, relying on the panel for expertise in a judgmental decision area. Even though the content of the discussion may not be totally anticipated, the leader must plan the session to progress through the following stages: (1) defining the problem, (2) stating and ranking the crucial issues, and (3) listing and selecting the best solution.

INTERACTIVE CASE STUDY

Disease correlation with laboratory results and corresponding pathophysiology is best addressed by interactive case study. In this approach, a case is presented in terms of patient history and physical, followed by the laboratory data and a series of questions guiding the audience in a discussion of the case. Several professional journals for clinical laboratory personnel include interactive case studies with appropriate answers and references that may be used.

SIMULATION OR ROLE PLAYING

This approach requires the facilitator to create a representation of reality within which the participants interact. Development of interpersonal relationships, such as dealing with uncooperative patients, is ideally suited for this technique. Of all possible approaches, however, role playing is among the most difficult and requires substantial preparation on the part of the role players to be effective. It may be advantageous to use a prepared "trigger" film or tape, followed by audience discussion, rather than involve participants in acting out the simulated role.

THE PROCESS OF DEVELOPING EDUCATIONAL ACTIVITIES

The process of planning and carrying out effective teaching follows similar steps whether completed in a formal continuing education program or through the efforts of an individual professional who will offer a short seminar for colleagues within the laboratory.[7] In general, these steps are (1) assessing needs, (2) developing objectives, (3) determining content, (4) establishing the teaching method, (5) conducting the activity (teaching), and (6) evaluating the teaching effort.[8] Box 15-3 illustrates one model of training.[7,14] Evaluation logically leads to a reassessment of needs, making the entire process circular and continuous, because in an environment where staff members are involved in inservice activities, each session should identify teaching areas for the next session.[1]

Assessing Needs

Needs assessment is conducted at three levels: institutional, program, and individual. The essential question at each level is, "what shall be taught?"

At the institutional or laboratory level, the process is one of identifying topic areas based on the types of work performed within the laboratory. What are the major tests completed for patient admissions? What comprises the top 10 laboratory orders from outpatient clinic visits? What are the major services provided for inpatients? This analysis of the most common orders for patient–physician support will provide a listing of areas in which programming should be developed. Assessment of current teaching efforts, audit information, physician requests, and comments for information will help to determine appropriate program development priorities.

At the conclusion of this process of identifying subjects, an assessment of information needed for each subject or program must be completed. The first step would be to list the topics to be taught within an inservice program. The unique aspects of the individual program related to the hospital and laboratory should be considered, and priorities of what must be learned on this topic must be set.

The third, and final, level of assessment is that of the individual laboratorian's educational needs as related to the program topic. This analysis of the individual tailors the instruction as much as possible to the individual and to the staff of the laboratory. All of the possible topics that might be included in one program will not be appropriate to every staff member, and some parts may not be appropriate at all. Time also may not be available to cover all desired topics, so the teaching plan must be sequenced to meet areas of greatest deficiency first. A useful strategy often uses an advanced laboratorian as the inservice instructor, thereby creating a tutorial system within the department.

Developing Objectives

The listing of topics that might be taught on any subject provides only a broad guideline. The topics must be refined to summarize actual behaviors that the laboratorian must perform successfully. Some behaviors may be activity based, such as performing a reticulocyte count; some may be knowledge based, such as noting test abnormalities one might expect if a patient were taking a certain medication. The objective is oriented toward the student; that is, the emphasis is on what the student must do rather than on what the teacher will teach.[12] While this may seem to be a subtle distinction, it underlies the philosophy of adult and continuing education.

There are two steps in developing specific objectives for any teaching program. First, a set of standard behaviors for each topic that applies to all students must be listed. These are derived from the topics previously formulated in the needs assessment phase. For the reticulocyte example used earlier, an instructor may list the following behaviors: (1) Prepare a blood–reticulocyte stain mixture; (2) prepare a smear from this mixture for counting; (3) determine the number of reticulocytes/1,000 red cells; and (4) calculate the patient's corrected reticulocyte count.

These activities are then restated as objectives, which contain three elements: the activity or behavior to be performed, the conditions under which the behavior will be performed, and the evaluation criteria that will determine successful performance of the behavior. The acronym ACE serves as a useful reminder of the three elements—activity, condition, evaluation.[18]

The previously mentioned topics could be translated into behavioral objectives:

The student will combine equal amounts of the patient's whole blood and supravital stain in a white cell pipette such that both blood and stain can be mixed in the bulb; smear the blood–stain mixture on a clean glass slide, spreading cells into a monolayer featheredge without accumulation on the edge of the slide; count the number of reticulocytes per 1,000 red cells on two smears with comparative totals of ±5 cells between smears using a light microscope with an oil immersion objective; and, given the hematocrit, calculate the patient's corrected reticulocyte count within ±3 from the known value.

In each of these objectives, the activity to be performed is clear because it is stated in measurable terms; test abnormality expectations will be stated. The condition under which the activity is to be performed is also clear—use of clean slides, use of a light microscope with an oil objective, and calculation from the patient's hematocrit.

The evaluation portion notes the level of competence that must be reached. When unstated, it is understood to be 100%. It could also be stated with ranges of correctness, such as ±5 or 80%. The evaluation criterion provides a signal that teaching has been completed or that additional efforts will be required.

Secondly, the objectives must be sequenced into priority order. The behaviors that are critical would receive the highest priority and be taught to every laboratorian. Less important objectives would be saved for the future or for certain individuals for whom the information is important.

Determining Content

Only the relevant information for the particular objective should be included. While the content should be complete and accurate, the usual tendency to add extra explanatory and background material should be avoided. An overabundance of information that is of marginal importance to the topic may confuse, rather than clarify, understanding.

Once the objective is identified, gather resources that provide information relevant to the topic. Journal articles, texts, manufacturers' publications, and pamphlets and brochures from health associations are all good sources of information. These resources will help clarify objectives; provide clear, concise descriptions, illustrations, and helpful suggestions, such as lists of forms the laboratorian could use; and identify common problems that have been experienced under similar circumstances.

From this information, the actual content of the session, consisting of an outline of the lesson and supplemental notes of drawings, pictures, forms, calendars, and so forth, must be developed. If a particular brochure or article clearly explains one of the teaching points or covers an entire topic, it could be used with little or no modification. In most cases, however, the instructor will want to develop the information to be included using a variety of sources.

Establishing the Teaching Method

The method(s) to be used for teaching the material is developed after the content is determined. The methods available include one-to-one discussion, group meetings, brochures, movies, flip charts, case studies, slide shows, demonstrations, audiotapes and videotapes, and charts. Generally, the use of more than one method is recommended, because a variety of approaches complements the teaching effort. For example, the method to be used should be based on factors such as the time and location available for the teaching; complexity of the information; interfering responsibilities of the clinician, which would affect consistent in-person teaching; type of behavior to be learned; and preference and comfort of the clinician in the teaching situation. A review of the teaching approaches discussed earlier in this chapter will note the strengths and weaknesses of each approach.

The distinction between student-oriented planning and teacher-oriented planning becomes clear when thinking through the teaching methodology. The instructor who has focused on teacher strategies, that is, *what he will do,* will be less flexible in changing approaches when the student does not progress quickly. The instructor who focuses on *what the student must do,* however, generally is open to attempting a variety of activities to help the student successfully accomplish the goal.

Conducting the Activity (Teaching)

Once the objectives are set, lessons planned, and resources and supplemental materials gathered, attention can be given to the actual implementation of the program. Consideration of several factors by the supervisor will enhance the acceptance of the program by the laboratory staff.

First, the supervisor must ensure a positive attitude toward participation, particularly in inservice activities. In-house activities could be seen as conflicting with "real" job duties if insufficient emphasis has been given to helping the staff understand the need for inservice education. Too many meetings will cause resistance, and too few will reduce acceptance of educational activities as an overall part of the laboratory environment.

Second, activities that are attended by staff members and taught by a senior laboratorian on the staff could develop into a social meeting or a gripe session if the goals are not clearly stated or the seriousness of the activity is underemphasized. The use of a committee in the planning process may increase commitment among staff members, and guest speakers may help to reduce side activity during the teaching session.

Third, the supervisor should give careful thought to teaching in the inservice program. For some staff members, the acceptance of the supervisor as a supportive teacher, rather than as a "boss," may be difficult, and this may adversely affect his teaching effectiveness. If the supervisor teaches only sessions with subjects such as policies and procedures, however, he may establish an atmosphere of authoritarianism. Establishing a balance may be difficult but must be considered.

Evaluating the Teaching Effort

There are three types of evaluation to employee student, teacher, and environment. Student evaluation attempts to determine the gains in knowledge resulting from the activity. This evaluation may be formal or informal but must be based on the objectives developed for the instruction. It is not suggested that a paper and pencil test be used, because tests often cause anxiety in adults and negatively affect performance, regardless of the student's knowledge. The test should be as realistic as possible, so actual demonstrations of procedures, case-study discussions, and similar approaches are recommended.

Evaluation of the teacher will help the instructor to improve his approach in the future. Reporting the results to the instructor should be done in a positive, supportive manner.

Evaluation of the teaching environment will reveal distractions and problems, which, if not corrected, may affect the success of future sessions. Statements about interruptions to call technologists back to the laboratory, too much dropping in and out by the supervisor, and the absence of other staff members are all clues for future planning.

REFERENCES

1. Adams CD: Guidelines for in-service programs. Lab Med 16:561–563, 1985
2. Biddle AM: A strategic plan for staff development. MLO 17(1):62–66, 1985
3. Cabonor RP, DeNofa JR: Design and administration of a continuing education policy. Am J Med Technol 47: 715–722, 1981
4. CAP inspection checklists. Northfield, IL, College of American Pathologists, 1996
5. Comprehensive accreditation manual for pathology and clinical laboratory services. Oakbrook Terrace, IL, Joint Commission on Accreditation of Healthcare Organizations, 1996
6. Cross L: Career management development—A system that gets results. Training and Development Journal 37(2): 54–63, 1983
7. Dick W, Carey L: The Systematic Design of Instruction, 4th ed. Glenview, IL, Addison-Wesley Educational Publishers, 1996
8. Ehrmeyer SS, Ehrmeyer GC: A five-step approach to bench teaching. J Med Technol 1:573–577, 1984
9. Fisher F, Britt MS: An assessment of continuing education needs for clinical laboratory personnel. Lab Med 18: 110–114, 1987
10. Garcia LS: A cost containment checklist. MLO 17(4): 67–73, 1985
11. Houle CO: Continuing Learning in the Professions, pp 34–75. San Francisco, Jossey-Bass, 1980
12. Johnston VF: A study of the relationships among demographic factors, continuing education and continued competence. J Med Technol 2:779–785, 1985
13. Lauffer A: The Practice of Continuing Education in the Human Services, p 16. New York, McGraw-Hill, 1977
14. Madura AZ: Instructional design in the laboratory. Lab Med 27: 503–505, 1996
15. Morgenstern F: Clinical teaching: On-the-job training or planned method of instruction? Lab Management 16(1): 52–54, 1978
16. National Committee for Clinical Laboratory Standards (NCCLS): Training verification for laboratory personnel. Approved guideline. NCCLS document GP21-A. Wayne, PA, NCCLS, 1995
17. Nevalainen DE, Berte LM: Training, verification and assessment: Keys to quality management. Malvern, PA, Clinical Laboratory Management Association, 1993
18. Objectives. In Development and Evaluation of Audiovisual Instructional Materials. Atlanta, Educational Training and Consultation Branch, National Medical Audiovisual Center, September 1, 1976
19. Phillips LE: The status of mandatory continuing education for the professions. Presented to the National University Exten-

sion Association, Division of Continuing Education for the Professions, March 21, 1977

20. Pucel DJ: Performance-based Instructional Design. New York, McGraw-Hill, 1989

21. Regulations in implementing the clinical laboratory improvement amendments of 1988 (CLIA). Federal Register 57:180–7181, February 28, 1992

22. Senge PM: The Fifth Discipline: The Art and Practice of the Learning Organization. New York, Doubleday/Currency, 1990

23. Stroul NA, Schuman G: Action planning for workshops. Training and Development Journal 37(7):41–42, 1983

24. Warren J: Building a career ladder for the upward climb. MLO 15(1):72–82, 1983

25. Warshaw M, Welch JL: Guidelines for teaching in the laboratory setting. MLO 15(6):85–87, 1983

26. Willoughby TL, Gammon LC, Jonas HS: Correlates of clinical performance during medical school. J Med Ed 54:453–459, 1979

16

Labor Relations and the Clinical Laboratory

Walton H. Sharp

BACKGROUND

The term *labor relations* encompasses the interactions between an employer, or institution, and a representative of the employees, normally referred to as a *union,* a *labor organization,* or an *employee association.* Labor relations is a subset of the broader discipline of industrial relations, which is concerned with all aspects of the functioning of labor markets and the employer–employee relationship. The purpose of this chapter is to introduce to the laboratory supervisor the study of labor relations and its integral parts and processes: law, collective bargaining, and contract administration.

There are several reasons for laboratory supervisors to understand more fully the labor relations process. First, some 19 million people belong to some form of labor organization in the United States. Second, the passage of the 1974 Health Care Amendments to the National Labor Relations Act provided approximately 1.5 million employees of nonprofit voluntary health-care institutions the opportunity to have union representation. Third, it is proposed here that the laboratory supervisor can be more effective as a part of the management team by understanding the dynamics of the labor relations process.

There is no single encompassing law governing labor relations in the United States. Rather, there are three identifiable legal frameworks: (1) the Civil Service Reform Act, which has jurisdiction over the federal sector; (2) state labor laws, which deal with states and their political subdivisions; and (3) the National Labor Relations Act, which addresses labor relations in the private sector, including profit and nonprofit voluntary health-care institutions (Fig. 16-1).[9] Each of these systems, in turn, must be viewed as dynamic, rather than static, because of changes in the laws themselves, changes in

the regulations, decisions of agencies charged with the administration of the laws, and decisions of the federal and state courts.

LABOR LAW AND THE PUBLIC EMPLOYEE

The National Labor Relations Act exempts the federal government and states and their political subdivisions from the coverage of the Act.[10] Employees of health-care institutions operated by units of government are therefore not protected by the National Labor Relations Act. This is also true of most health-care institutions operated by a taxing authority, such as a hospital district.

Federal Employees

Employees of the federal government did not have a legal right to engage in collective bargaining until 1962, when President Kennedy issued Executive Order 10988. This executive order contained several major inadequacies. First, recognition of a union was based on the proportion of employees in a bargaining unit represented by the union. Second, the number of items about which a union could bargain with the agency was limited. Third, the procedures for resolving contractual disputes between labor and management were a part of the statutory framework of the executive order, were cumbersome, and did not provide for a true independent arbiter of the dispute.

In 1970, President Nixon corrected some of these deficiencies in Executive Order 11491. This executive order created a three-member Federal Labor Relations Council to administer the executive order and to take

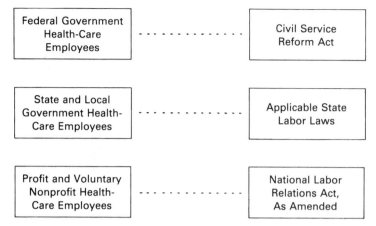

FIGURE 16–1.   Appropriate labor law coverage for health-care institutions and employees.

the leadership role in federal-sector labor relations. The authority to determine union eligibility and to determine the bargaining unit to be represented by the union was placed with the Secretary of Labor. The responsibility for settling disputes arising from contract negotiations was granted to a Federal Services Impasses Panel. Additionally, federal employees were prohibited from striking, picketing, or engaging in a work slow-down or any form of work stoppage, which simply continued the established policy of the federal government.

In 1978, the Congress put federal government labor relations into law through the passage of the Civil Service Reform Act.[4] The Act established the Federal Labor Relations Authority (FLRA) as the agency charged with the responsibility for administration of federal-sector labor relations. The FLRA is composed of three members appointed by the President of the United States, not more than two of whom may be members of the same political party. The scope and functions of the FLRA are similar to the scope and functions of the National Labor Relations Board (NLRB), the agency charged with administration of the National Labor Relations Act, which governs labor–management relations of the private economy. The FLRA determines an appropriate employee unit for purposes of collective bargaining, conducts elections for union representation and certifies the results, hears complaints of unfair labor practices, determines whether bargaining is conducted in good faith, and determines whether certain issues are subject to negotiations between the union and the agency of government. The Civil Service Reform Act also provided for a general counsel to the FLRA, who is appointed by the president. The duties of this office are essentially to file, investigate, and prosecute unfair labor-practice charges, making the duties of the office similar to those of the Office of the General Counsel of the NLRB.

The Civil Service Reform Act also established a Merit Systems Protection Board (MSPB), which is composed of three presidential appointees, no more than two of whom may be from the same political party. The MSPB reviews, on petition by an employee, an adverse action taken by an agency against an employee of the agency. An adverse action may be defined as discipline that involves a removal, a suspension of more than 14 days, a reduction in grade, a reduction in pay, or a furlough of 30 days or less.

Employee complaints that allege discrimination on the basis of race, color, religion, sex, age, marital status, or political affiliation may be processed through the grievance procedure of the labor–agency contract, through arbitration, and then to either the FLRA or to the Equal Employment Opportunity Commission (EEOC). Cases that allege adverse action and discrimination, termed "mixed cases," may be processed through a negotiated grievance procedure, to arbitration, or to the MSPB, the FLRA, or the EEOC. In the event that the findings and decisions of the EEOC and the MSPB disagree, a special panel is convened to resolve the dispute. Finally, the affected employee may appeal to either a United States district court or a United States court of appeals.

After the execution of Executive Order 10988 in the federal sector, states began to enact legislation that granted the employees of state, county, and municipal agencies the right to unionize and to engage in collective bargaining. To date, 36 states grant public employees such rights, although many of these state laws prohibit strikes and limit bargaining issues to those of hours and working conditions. In general, the state laws are not as comprehensive as federal public-sector labor law or the labor laws that govern the private economy.

LABOR LAW AND THE PRIVATE-SECTOR EMPLOYEE

The National Labor Relations Act

In 1935, the Congress of the United States passed the National Labor Relations Act, also referred to as the *Wagner Act.* In doing so, Congress exercised its constitutional authority to govern interstate commerce. Prior to 1967, health-care institutions operated for profit were deemed not to be sufficiently engaged in interstate commerce to be subject to the Act's jurisdiction. This was based on the view of the NLRB that there was not a sufficient flow of patients crossing state lines to receive health care to warrant the inclusion of health-care institutions operated for profit under the Act's jurisdiction. However, in two cases that were heard by the NLRB in 1967, the Board turned its attention to the dollar volume of supplies and equipment that crosses state lines to effectuate a new policy that health-care institutions operated for profit would be subject to the Act's coverage.[3] The Board established a dollar-volume jurisdiction yardstick to determine whether the provisions of the Act should be applied to health-care institutions operated for profit. Hospitals that have annual receipts in excess of $250,000 and nursing homes that have receipts of $100,000 are now subject to the Act's coverage. The Board applied the same yardstick to voluntary nonprofit health-care institutions after the passage of the 1974 Health Care Amendments (discussed later in this chapter) to the National Labor Relations Act.

The Act also established the NLRB as the agency to carry out and oversee the provisions of the Act.[15] As originally established, the board was composed of three members, appointed by the President of the United States, subject to the confirmation of the Senate, who served a specified term of office. The board was also empowered to establish regional and field offices as necessary to carry out the purposes of the Act.

The board has three primary functions: (1) to determine an appropriate bargaining unit when employees seek union representation, (2) to conduct elections for union representation, and (3) to investigate charges of unfair labor practices. These are discussed more fully in the section of this chapter dealing with unions.

Labor–Management Relations Act (Taft–Hartley)

In 1947, Congress amended the National Labor Relations Act and placed additional requirements of labor–management relations into effect with the passage of the Labor–Management Relations Act. Also known as the *Taft–Hartley Act,* the new legislation contained five titles, the first of which amended the National Labor Relations Act. A more detailed discussion of Title I and the amendments follows a brief discussion of Titles II through V.

Title II of the Taft–Hartley Act is concerned with the prevention of work stoppages, especially those that could affect an entire industry and thus threaten the national welfare. In this regard, Congress established the Federal Mediation and Conciliation Service (FMCS) to assist labor and management in resolving impasses in contract negotiations. FMCS is not empowered to make decisions but must use its knowledge and persuasion in attempts to assist labor and management to reach an amicable settlement. Other provisions of Title II outline procedures by which the President of the United States can obtain a federal court injunction when a strike or a threatened strike endangers the national welfare. Under this provision, workers can be compelled to return to work or prohibited from striking for a period of 80 days while attempts are made to settle the dispute between labor and management. Prior to the end of the 80-day period, workers are afforded an opportunity to vote to accept or reject the employer's last offer in a secret-ballot election.

Title III provides that suits to enforce labor–management contracts be brought in a federal district court. This provision is important in the enforcement of grievance–arbitration machinery contained in the majority of union–management contracts.

Title IV established a labor–management commission to study labor–management relations in the United States and to report its findings.

Title V, in Section 502, gives workers a right to refuse to work under abnormally dangerous conditions of employment without such a work stoppage being considered a strike.

Title I made the most substantial changes in the National Labor Relations Act. It increased the size of the NLRB from three to five members and established the Office of the General Counsel of the NLRB. The responsibilities were divided so that the Office of the General Counsel would supervise the regional and field office staffs and the investigation and prosecution of unfair labor practice charges, while the Board itself would adjudicate cases brought before it.

Title I also amended Sections 7 and 8 of the National Labor Relations Act. Section 7 grants employees of employers subject to the Act the right to form, join, or assist in the formation of a labor organization; to bargain through representatives of their own choosing; and to engage in other protected, concerted activities for the purposes of collective bargaining and other mutual aid and protection. Section 8 of the National Labor Relations Act (Box 16–1) outlines a series of employer unfair labor practices that violate employee rights.

An employee or a labor organization has 6 months from the date of the employer's alleged unfair labor practice to file a charge with the Board. (In Section 10, the Act empowers the Board to prevent unfair labor

---

Box 16·1

Employee Unfair Labor Practices as Outlined in Section 8 of the National Labor Relations Act

Interfering, restraining, or coercing employees in the exercise of their rights guaranteed in Section 7

Dominating or interfering with the formation or administration of a labor organization

Discriminating against employees in hiring or promotions because of membership in a labor organization

Discharging or otherwise discriminating against an employee because the employee filed an unfair labor practice charge or gave testimony in a board-conducted hearing

Refusing to bargain with the representative of the employees

---

practices and to require remedial action, including reinstatement of illegally discharged workers, with or without back pay, if the unfair labor practice charge is upheld.)

Section 7 is applicable to union-organizing campaigns and to situations in the absence of a union in which employees band together for purposes of mutual aid and protection. For example, an employer was found guilty of an unfair labor practice for discharging two employees on a construction site who refused to work while it was raining. The employees argued that the work would be dangerous while it was raining and stated that they would resume working when the rain stopped. The supervisor fired the employees, and they, in turn, filed an unfair labor practice charge with the Board. The Board upheld the charge because the employees were engaged in protected, concerted activities for their mutual aid and protection as guaranteed in Section 7; it ordered the employees reinstated with back pay.[2] A union did not represent the employees on the job site. Thus, contrary to popular belief, employees of institutions subject to the National Labor Relations Act enjoy the protection of the Act regardless of the question of unionization.

Taft–Hartley amended Section 7 to grant employees the right to refrain from unionization. Section 8 was also amended to include union unfair labor practices (Box 16–2).

The Taft–Hartley amendments also provide a definition of professional employees in Section 2(12) and in Section 9(b), give professional employees the right to

be represented separately for purposes of unionization, rather than being included in a bargaining unit with other employees. In Section 2(2), the federal government, states and their political subdivisions, and voluntary nonprofit health-care institutions are excluded from the coverage of the Act, although the latter's exclusion was removed with passage of the 1974 Health Care Amendments. Section 14(a) provides that employers are not obliged to recognize nor to bargain with a unit of supervisory employees. Section 14(b) allows individual states to enact laws prohibiting compulsory union membership. These laws are known as *right-to-work* laws and are discussed more fully later in this chapter.

The Labor–Management Reporting and Disclosure Act

Enacted in 1959, The Labor–Management Reporting and Disclosure Act was primarily concerned with the internal affairs of unions, although it did contain some amendments to the National Labor Relations Act. Primarily, the amendments modified Section 8. Unions could not picket for more than 30 days for the purpose of obtaining recognition from an employer, and contract clauses that allow union members to refuse to work with nonunion goods were prohibited.

The 1974 Health Care Amendments

Prior to the enactment of Public Law 93-360 in 1974, the nation's nonprofit health-care institutions were excluded from the coverage of the National Labor Rela-

---

Box 16·2

Union Unfair Labor Practices as Ammended by the Labor Management Relations Act (Taff–Harties)

Restraining or coercing employees in the exercise of their rights guaranteed in Section 7

Refusing to bargain collectively with an employer

Charging excessive or discriminatory union initiation fees and dues

Causing or attempting to cause an employer to pay for services not performed

Engaging in various kinds of secondary boycott activity, which involves striking or placing other economic pressure on an employer, to force it to cease doing business with another employer

---

Box 16·3

1974 Health Care Practitioners That Relate to a Health-Care Setting

1. In initial contract bargaining, a 30-day written notice of the existence of a labor dispute must be given to the other party involved in the negotiation, to the Federal Mediation and Conciliation Service (FMCS, an agency of the federal government), and to any appropriate state agency (such as a state labor relations board) before the party serving the notice may engage in a legal strike, in the case of the union, or a lock out of the employees, in the case of the healthcare institution.[11]
2. A written notice of the union's intent to strike or picket the healthcare institution must be served to a responsible official of the institution and to the FMCS at least 10 days prior to the commencement of such activity of the strike for picketing to be legal.[12]
   The general counsel of the NLRB, in an advisory memorandum, determined that these two sections should be read in tandem, based on the legislative history of the Act.[13] Thus, in initial bargaining, 40 days must elapse after the notice of the existence of a labor dispute has been communicated to the appropriate parties before a union may legally strike or picket. An employee who violates these provisions loses the protections against employer discipline afforded employees by the National Labor Relations Act.
3. In private healthcare settings in which a union–management contract is in effect, a party seeking to terminate or modify the existing contract must serve a written notice of the existence of a labor dispute to the other party at least 90 days before a legal work stoppage can take place and must notify the FMCS and any appropriate state agency at least 60 days prior to the commencement of a work stoppage.[11]
4. Union and management are *required* to participate in negotiation meetings requested by the FMCS.[14]
5. The director of the FMCS is empowered to appoint a board of inquiry in the event that a strike or lockout or a threatened strike or lockout will interrupt the delivery of healthcare services for an entire locality or geographic area. The board of inquiry is to be appointed within 15 days of the receipt of the notice of a labor dispute by the FMCS, and the board of inquiry is to issue a nonbinding report of the facts of the dispute and the positions of the respective parties to the director of the FMCS within 15 days.[14]

---

tions Act. In Section 2(2) of the National Labor Relations Act, these institutions were excluded from the definition of employers subject to the Act, along with the federal government and states and their political subdivisions. In essence, one of the primary features of the 1974 Health Care Amendments was to amend Section 2(2) so that nonprofit health-care institutions were not contained in the grouping of employers excluded from the coverage of the Act. Several other features of the 1974 Health Care Amendments (Box 16–3) are unique to a health-care setting.

Effective August 1, 1979, the FMCS issued new regulations, which afford labor and management jointly an opportunity to nominate people for a board of inquiry if the nominations are received by the FMCS before the notice of the existence of a dispute is served.[5] The FMCS will also defer to a privately agreed on fact-finding procedure established by labor and management and will decline to appoint a board of inquiry if it meets any of the criteria listed in Box 16–4.

The overriding concern of the Congress in passing these amendments was to ensure the continuity of pa-

tient care. Thus, the "ally doctrine" does not apply if a hospital accepts patients transferred from a hospital that is being struck. Under any other circumstances, the acceptance of work normally performed by the striking employees of a struck employer by a neutral employer makes the neutral employer an "ally" of the struck employer. The neutral or "ally" employer may then be legally picketed by the striking employees of another employer.

UNIONS

Why Do Workers Join?

Unless belonging to a union is part of a family tradition, most workers probably know very little about a union and the process of unionization. What, then, is the catalyst that propels employees to seek unionization? There is no single explanation of the dynamics of unionization. This section outlines some of the factors that may cause employees to seek unionization.[21]

Box 16•4

Criteria Necessary for the Federal Mediation and Conciliation Service (FMCS) to Decline to Appoint a Board of Inquiry

a. The fact-finding procedure is automatically invoked at a specified time
b. The fact-finding procedure provides a permanent method of selecting the impartial fact-finding person or board
c. The fact-finding procedure provides that strikes or lockouts will not occur except by mutual agreement prior to, during, and for 7 days after the completion of the fact-finding procedure
d. The person or board conducting the fact-finding procedure makes a written report to labor and management containing the findings and recommendations for setting the dispute and submits a copy to the FMCS.

The FMCS will also decline to appoint a board of inquiry if labor and management have agreed to an interest-arbitration procedure and the procedure meets the following conditions:

e. Except by mutual agreement, the procedure must provide that a work stoppage will not ensue and conditions of employment will not change during the contract negotiations and the time during which the interest arbitration is conducted
f. The award of the interest arbitrator or arbitration panel is final and binding on both parties
g. The procedure contains a fixed method for selecting the interest arbitrator or arbitration panel
h. The procedure provides that the award of the interest arbitrator or arbitration panel must be in writing

Personal Factors

A sense of dissatisfaction with elements of the job and the employing institution often is a stimulus for unionization, especially if the employee perceives that attempts to eliminate dissatisfactions through existing organizational channels would be fruitless. Pay, quality of supervision, the level of fringe benefits, general working conditions in the laboratory, the organization's

rules and policies and the perceived fairness of their administration and enforcement, and the pattern of interpersonal interactions in the laboratory may lead to dissatisfaction. Employees make a number of comparisons based on these variables. First, they compare them in light of their own perceived competence and self-image, and they compare the levels of each of the variables that they perceive they need or deserve and the levels of each that they actually receive. They also compare the levels of these variables that they receive with the levels received by other medical technologists in the laboratory and with other occupational groups in the workplace. They also compare the levels of these benefits with medical technologists employed in other health-care institutions and with other occupational groups in the community.

The perceptions of the individuals, while important, do not lead directly to unionization. Unless the individual perceives or knows that other medical technologists share some of the same concerns, the individual acting alone will probably not attempt to seek union representation and may actually leave the organization. However, as employees interact with each other on and off the job, the sharing of perceived similar dissatisfactions begins to build a critical mass of similarly held beliefs and opinions.[1] Once the critical mass is developed, a group that develops its own norms, values, and sanctions is established. If the group perceives that its dissatisfactions cannot be remedied through existing organizational channels, it may seek outside assistance. It is easy for this group to become the union's internal organizing committee, because this group establishes the norms of behavior for its members and the sanctions against nonmembers.

The Image of the Union

Even though all the necessary ingredients of individual and group attitudes may seem to be present for a successful union-organizing campaign, this does not ensure that the organizing campaign will result in unionization. An important ingredient is the image of the union that seeks to represent the employees, both its general image as a union and its specific image as an effective representative of medical technologists as professionals.

It would be difficult for a traditional blue-collar union to be perceived as an effective representative of what are essentially white-collar professionals. Medical technologists might very well question whether such a union would understand the professional issues that confront the occupational group. On the other hand, a union that has traditionally represented white-collar professionals might be perceived as acceptable, especially if it demonstrates an understanding and knowledge of the professional concerns of medical technologists and if it demonstrates that such concerns can be successfully negotiated with the employer through collective bargaining.

A union perceived as being corrupt and engaging in questionable practices might also be perceived as unacceptable to medical technologists, whereas a union that does not have such a history of adverse publicity might be considered more acceptable.

Although this short discussion by no means includes all the factors that lead to unionization and is not supported by empirical evidence, it does attempt to make the supervisor aware of some of the factors that enter into the decision of employees to seek unionization. The view that medical technologists have of their supervisor is important. The supervisor is one of them, although at the same time, a management representative of the employing institution. If the supervisor is perceived by his employees as effectively representing their personal and professional interests, there will probably not be an effort to unionize. If the supervisor is perceived as representing the employing institution to the detriment of the personal and professional interests of the medical technologists, the supervisor may be perceived as ineffective, and a more effective representative, a union, may be sought.

The Bargaining Unit

If employees seek to be represented by a union for purposes of collective bargaining, usually they will not be voluntarily recognized by the employer. The union must therefore resort to the procedures promulgated by the NLRB to obtain an election for union representation.[6] Suppose the employees of a nonunion employer want to be represented by a union. The union will ask them to sign *authorization cards,* which state that the employee wants to be represented for purposes of collective bargaining by the union named on the cards. From the occupational groups the union seeks to represent, the union must have 30% of the employees sign authorization cards before the board will honor a petition for a union-representation election. In its petition, the union must specify the occupational groups it seeks to represent. This is the start of defining an appropriate *bargaining unit,* the occupational groups of employees the union seeks to represent. The bargaining unit is important because it determines the people who will be eligible to vote in a union-representation election and the people who will be covered by the labor–management contract should the union be successful in winning the election and in negotiating an agreement with the employer.

Regardless of the union's proposed bargaining unit, the final responsibility for determining an appropriate bargaining unit lies with the NLRB.[16] An employer may also challenge the appropriateness of a bargaining unit in a hearing conducted by the board. The employer may want the bargaining unit expanded to include occupational groups perceived not to be in favor of unionization. The main factors considered by the board, other than the pleadings of labor and management, are (1) the history of collective bargaining in the industry and the occupational groups represented; (2) the community of interest among employees, such as common pay plans, interdependent work, and common supervision; and (3) the desires of the employees.[8] After the determination of an appropriate bargaining unit, the board conducts a secret-ballot election among the employees in the bargaining unit. The union must obtain a majority of the votes cast to carry the election and to be certified as the exclusive representative of the employees for purposes of collective bargaining.

It is important in health-care settings to understand that there may be multiple appropriate bargaining units in an employing institution. Congress, in the deliberations that led to the passage of the Act, recognized that a large number of different occupational groups are employed in health-care institutions and that many of these groups have their own professional membership organizations. The Congress, therefore, stated that the board should avoid a proliferation of bargaining units in health-care settings. In general, the board will allow up to six different bargaining units (Box 16–5) in a health-care institution.[7]

However, that the board allows up to six bargaining units in health-care institutions does not mean that the board is required to acknowledge six individual bargaining units. In one instance, the board merged registered nurses and other professional employees into a single bargaining unit.

Once the bargaining unit is determined, the NLRB schedules an election. The election is held at a place and

---

Box 16•5

Six Bargaining Units in a Health-Care Setting

1. Physicians
2. Registered nurses
3. Other professional employees
4. Technical employees
5. Service and maintenance employees
6. Business office clerical employees

time to afford maximum participation by the affected employees in voting for or against union representation. Only employees who are in the bargaining unit are eligible to vote. Notices will be posted at the employer's place of business, usually on bulletin boards, informing employees of the occupational groups in the bargaining unit and the date, time, and place of the election. The election is by secret ballot, and the union must have a majority of the votes cast to win and be certified by the NLRB as the bargaining representative. If the employer carries the election, another election cannot be held in that bargaining unit for 12 months.

If the union carries the election, then the issue of whether or not compulsory union membership will be required of members of the bargaining unit must be decided, according to a number of factors. First, the National Labor Relations Act, as amended by Taft–Hartley in Section 8(a)(3), states that nothing in the law prohibits an employer and a labor organization from negotiating a contract clause that requires union membership, provided that a minimum period of 30 days has elapsed since the employee was hired or the contract clause has been put into effect. Thus, in the first instance, a contract clause that requires union membership is a subject of negotiations, as is the length of the probationary period before an individual is required to join the union. This arrangement is known as a *union-shop clause*. Whether the union is able to obtain such a clause in the contract depends on the strength of the union (the percentage of the employees in the bargaining unit who have voluntarily joined the union) and the union's willingness to strike over the issue.

Although federal labor law does not prohibit such contract clauses, Section 14(b) of the Taft–Hartley amendments allows an individual state or United States territory to enact legislation that prohibits the enforcement of a compulsory union membership contract clause. These right-to-work laws have been enacted in more than 20 states. Thus, in these states, union membership is strictly voluntary. As a result, the bargaining unit is composed of union members and people who refrain from union membership. However, the contract negotiated by the union, in all other respects, applies to the bargaining unit, and both union and nonunion members are subject to its terms and provisions. A union is prohibited from negotiating contract clauses that discriminate against nonunion members of the bargaining unit and must provide representation for nonunion members of the bargaining unit in grievance and arbitration hearings. The reason is that the union, by virtue of winning an election to represent employees for collective bargaining, is certified as the representative of the bargaining unit under Section 9(a) of the National Labor Relations Act.

Because of the prohibitions against compulsory union membership and the realization that nonunion members of a bargaining unit benefit from union representation, some states, especially as part of their state labor relations laws for public employees, enable a union to collect some specified portion of the monthly union dues from nonunion members of the bargaining unit. These are alternately called *agency-shop* or *fair-share laws;* the amount of the monthly financial contribution required from nonunion members of the bargaining unit varies among the states.

As part of the 1974 Health Care Amendments to the National Labor Relations Act, the Congress, in Section 19, stated that people included in bargaining units in voluntary nonprofit health-care institutions who had religious objections to joining or financially contributing to a union would not be required to do so, even if a compulsory membership clause was contained in the collective-bargaining agreement. Rather, these people may contribute the equivalent of the monthly union dues to a nonreligious, nonprofit charitable organization. More recently, the Congress enacted legislation that extended this right to employees of institutions other than voluntary nonprofit health-care institutions. However, in this case, the union is allowed to seek reimbursement for expenses incurred in representing such employees in collective bargaining or contract administration. On December 29, 1980, President Jimmy Carter signed a bill that extended the coverage of Section 19 to all workers.[19]

Bargaining Units for Medical Technologists

Prior to April 28, 1995, the status of clinical laboratorians as either technical or professional employees for purposes of an appropriate collective bargaining unit varied on a case-by-case basis.[18] On that date, however, the NLRB issued a decision declaring medical technologists as *professional employees.* By statute, professional employees and nonprofessional employees cannot belong to the same bargaining unit unless requested by the majority of professional employees. Consequently, medical technologists and other laboratorians have often been grouped with a technical employee bargaining unit.

The NLRB's 1995 deliberations considered the work of medical technologists in light of the strict criteria of a professional employee as defined by the National Labor Relations Act (20 USC 152 (12) 1988). A professional employee is engaged in work (1) that is predominantly intellectual and varied in character, (2) involving the consistent exercise of discretion and judgment in its performance, (3) of such character that the output produced cannot be standardized in relation to a given period of time, and (4) requiring knowledge of an advanced type in a field of science or learning.

The NLRB's decision considered the "totality of duties" of medical technologists.[18] Therefore, while some testing is automated and some procedures not complex, "the degree of intellectual analysis and the consistent exercise of independent judgment and discretion applies to all tests." Moreover, the NLRB recognized other standard responsibilities of medical technologists, such as laboratory operations management, process/methodology development, and quality control, as consistent with a finding of professional status.

The Collective-Bargaining Process

Collective bargaining is characterized by negotiations between the union and the employer in an attempt to establish the wages, hours of work, and other terms and conditions of employment in a contract for a specified time period. Through negotiations, labor and management make known their respective interests. The National Labor Relations Act, as amended, requires the parties to meet at reasonable times and bargain in good faith concerning wages, hours, and other conditions of employment.[17] However, the law does not require that the parties reach an agreement.

Some items of interest to either of the parties are considered to be mandatory subjects of bargaining, meaning that labor or management cannot seek to establish them unilaterally, and neither of the parties can refuse to discuss them. Examples of such items are wages, pensions, fringe benefits, vacations, holidays, work rules, the definition of bargaining-unit work, seniority, promotions, transfers, safety and health provisions, a procedure for the discussion of grievances, the arbitration of unresolved disputes, performance appraisals, and others. If either one of the parties expresses an interest in these issues, the other party is obligated to discuss them, although the two may not be able to reach an agreement.

Although collective bargaining negotiations have historically been characterized by an adversarial relationship between labor and management, some issues are of concern to both parties. For example, there is interest by labor, management, and the government in increasing productivity. Much interest is being expressed in newer labor–management techniques, such as quality circles, which are used in Japan. As a result, some United States companies and unions have begun to experiment with similar concepts. If they are successful, they will eventually permeate all industrial sectors of the economy, including health-care institutions.

The following areas of interest, by no means an inclusive listing of the items contained in all collective-bargaining agreements, provide an overview of the basic elements of a collective-bargaining agreement. Questions are also raised that must be considered by the laboratory supervisor. Finally, there are examples of how some of these issues are being addressed in some existing labor–management agreements.

Wages

Wages are a critical component of the labor–management negotiation. They are of concern to the laboratory supervisor and to the institution, because they represent a cost that to some degree must be controlled. They are also of concern to the union, because they are a benefit to its members. The credibility of the union is enhanced if it can negotiate an increase that is perceived by members to be more than management would grant voluntarily.

Wages include direct pay and a variety of fringe benefits, which are all costs to the employer. Fringe benefits include such items as pensions, health insurance, disability insurance, and premium pay for overtime and shift differentials. The laboratory supervisor must be concerned with these costs because they become part of the laboratory budget. However, the laboratory must do more than simply attempt to control these costs. The supervisor must assess the impact that wages and fringe benefits will have on the retention of present employees and the recruitment of future employees. To accomplish this, the supervisor must be aware of the wage structure of other laboratories and health-care institutions in the geographical area. Today it is not uncommon for the laboratory supervisor to be required to know the pay structure of alternative occupations open to medical technologists with comparable skills or with minimal additional knowledge or training.

Primarily to retain present staff and to recruit qualified medical technologists competitively, the laboratory supervisor must have direct communication with the management personnel responsible for negotiating with the union. The cost of retaining employees must be evaluated against its alternative—employee turnover and the costs of seeking replacements. There are costs associated with advertising open positions, with using supervisory time to interview applicants, and with the administrative overhead of adding new employees to the payroll. If employee turnover requires that other medical technologists work overtime, then premium pay for the hours of overtime should be taken into account. If this resulting overtime occurs too frequently or the duration of each occurrence is long, there will be a cost associated with declining employee morale. Thus, the laboratory supervisor's role is not simply one of controlling costs. By necessity, it must include a realistic assessment of the impact of the institution's ability to retain and attract qualified employees.

Hours of Work

Hours of work, which are normally discussed in negotiations between labor and management, are also important to the laboratory supervisor because of the impact they have on staffing patterns. The supervisor, after all, is responsible for planning, organizing, and directing the accomplishment of work. Most employees will want to work a 40-hour week. The supervisor must consider how long each shift will be, on what day the workweek will begin, whether the workweek will begin on the same day for everyone, whether there will be overlapping shifts to cover peak loads in hospital admissions, whether weekends will be covered by part-time employees or by staggered workweeks of full-time employees, and a number of other issues. These schedules must, in turn, be coordinated with other departments in health-care institutions.

At present, the laboratory supervisor must to some extent consider the desires of employees. The supervisor may have to introduce some variation of flextime, such as 4-days-on/4-days-off or 7-days-on/7-days-off. In this event, the length of the daily shift must be extended, which may entail some amount of premium pay and should concern the supervisor from the standpoint of employee fatigue.

Working Conditions

Working conditions also encompass a wide variety of issues. For example, if the laboratory is large enough and has sufficient volume, will it be departmentalized, and if so, will employees be allowed to rotate among departments to reduce boredom? Will present employees be given preference over outside applicants for openings? Will employees be given the opportunity to transfer to openings on another shift? How will a determination be made if two qualified employees request a shift transfer to a single open position? How much latitude will employees be given to trade with one another? How will promotional opportunities be determined? These questions may be raised during contract negotiations.

Another aspect of working conditions is paid vacations and holidays. To some degree, this will be determined by the policy makers in higher management. However, the laboratory manager should discuss these issues and their impact on the management of the laboratory with higher management. The supervisor should

also have some knowledge of the practices of other laboratories and health-care institutions in the area.

The laboratory supervisor may realize that many of the same issues must be confronted whether or not a union represents the employees. The difference is that if a union is involved, these issues will be subject to negotiations between labor and management, rather than unilaterally determined by the supervisor. Once they are incorporated in the labor–management agreement, these issues cannot be unilaterally changed by management.

Although it is not common, some contracts enable either of the parties to reopen negotiations on any portion or section of the contract by giving the other party a notice of such intent. If this is to be allowed, there is usually a specific clause in the contract that states this right and the amount of advance notice that must be given. Another means of accomplishing the change of a contract clause during the life of a contract is to amend the contract with a letter of agreement concerning a specific issue. Again, however, both labor and management must agree to such a procedure in addition to the content of the change. This second method has appeared in the current economic climate when companies ask employees to forego a scheduled wage increase or to take actual reductions in pay to help the company remain solvent and competitive. In the final analysis, whether such procedures for change are to be included in the contract or are to be accomplished through a letter of agreement depends on whether labor and management prefer to institute procedures for change or would rather invoke them only when confronted with a crisis.

Contract Administration

The most conscientious labor and management negotiators cannot write a perfect contract. The contract must be worded so that it can be applied in a variety of situations. The negotiations cannot possibly envision all the problems that may arise during the life of the contract. Different people will interpret the contract differently. For instance, it is not uncommon for a contract to contain a clause on promotion that gives the promotion to the senior employee (in terms of length of employment) who bids on the job, provided the senior employee is reasonably qualified. The first issue, seniority, may be resolved by consulting employment records. The second issue, being reasonably qualified, is not so easily resolved. A union might interpret it to mean having skill and ability. Management may interpret it to mean having efficiency and dependability in addition to skill and ability. Thus, management may want to deny a promotion to someone because of a record of tardiness and absenteeism. The union may argue that management should handle absenteeism and tardiness through its rules and disciplinary procedures and not through the denial of a promotion. Issues such as this are normally resolved through a formal procedure in which an individual employee may allege that management has violated the labor–management agreement. This process is referred to as *contract administration* and is composed of a grievance procedure that includes arbitration as the terminal step. The purpose of such a procedure is to provide a mechanism for resolving day-to-day differences between labor and management without the union's having to resort to a work stoppage. In most labor–management contracts, the union surrenders its right to strike during the life of the contract in return for a grievance procedure and arbitration.

The grievance procedure is a series of steps or meetings through which an employee's complaint may move in an attempt to resolve it. The initial step of a grievance procedure is normally a verbal discussion of the complaint between the employee and the supervisor with or without a representative of the union being present. The union representative at this step is normally called the *union steward* and is the union's counterpart to the first-line supervisor. Whether or not the union representative is present depends on the wishes of the employee. Under the National Labor Relations Act, the employee has a right to representation by the union, and the union has the obligation to represent all employees in the defined bargaining unit if requested to do so.

Contracts usually specify a given time period, from the date of the action by management that is alleged to violate the contract, within which the allegation must be brought to the attention of management. The length of this period is subject to negotiations and is sometimes as long as 45 days. Regardless of the merits of the employee's complaint, this first step is important in having the employee verbalize the dissatisfaction. Equally important is the manner in which the employee's immediate supervisor conducts this meeting. Even though the allegation may involve the immediate supervisor, the supervisor must listen to the complaint as a member of management and must not be personally offended by the employee's complaint. The supervisor may be uncertain whether the complaint has merit or may need time to investigate the complaint further, but the contract usually allows a given number of days before which the management representative must answer the complaint. This time should be used by the supervisor to discuss the complaint with higher level supervision or with the personnel department. Because management has the responsibility of ensuring that policies and rules are applied consistently and fairly throughout the organization, the supervisor should not hesitate to con-

sult with other levels of management. If the grievance is denied, the union will satisfy itself that the employee's complaint has no merit before it will decide not to appeal the grievance. The contract normally specifies a period of time within which the union may appeal a grievance.

Managers are sometimes perplexed that a union will defend an employee when it seems obvious to management that an employee should be disciplined or discharged. This is a result of the manager's failure to understand the moral and legal role of the union as a representative of the employee. In many instances, the union may be aware of the employee's violation of a rule or policy. The union may also have cautioned the employee that continued infractions of the rules and policies of the institution might result in discipline or discharge. The union, by filing a grievance, may simply want to review management's decision process to ensure that management has applied its rules, policies, and discipline fairly and consistently; that management has followed its own policies in carrying out the discipline; and that the discipline is not more harsh than the offense. The union may object to the strength of the discipline or the manner in which management applied its rules and policies, rather than whether or not the employee should have been disciplined. If it did not challenge management in this manner, the union would be perceived by its own members as not properly representing them. It would also violate its legal duty to represent fairly the employees in the bargaining unit. Supervisors should understand that this is one of the legitimate roles of the union and expect that the union will challenge many of management's decisions.

To continue with the grievance procedure, labor and management negotiate several steps or meetings during which their respective representatives will attempt to resolve the grievance. Each step is characterized by time limits for the union's appeal of the grievance and for management's response after the grievance has been discussed. Each step is also characterized by the addition of higher levels of decision makers by labor and management. For example, the final step of the grievance procedure prior to arbitration might involve the hospital administrator in addition to the personnel manager, the laboratory supervisor, and the first-line supervisor for management. The union might be represented by a representative of the national union, the local union president, the grievance committee chairman, the union steward, and the employee.

What if a resolution is not reached during these meetings? The majority of union–management contracts provide that the union may appeal to arbitration. *Arbitration* is the process whereby an impartial third party is selected to hear the facts pertaining to the dispute and each party's position and then render a final and binding decision. The arbitrator is jointly selected by labor and management and is knowledgeable about labor–management contracts and labor–management relations. There are some full-time arbitrators, but most are fully employed elsewhere. Many arbitrators are practicing attorneys, professors of law or industrial relations, or former employees of agencies of government involved in the labor-relations process.

Two important aspects of the arbitration process should be mentioned. First, if the contract provides for the arbitration of all disputes that arise during the life of the contract, the federal courts will enforce arbitration; that is, if the contract contains an arbitration clause for all disputes and the union appeals a grievance to arbitration, management cannot refuse arbitration simply because it views the employee's complaint as frivolous. To avoid arbitration, management would have to show that the issue is not covered by the language of the contract. The decision of whether or not the dispute is subject to arbitration is the province of the arbitrator. The arbitrator will decide the merits of the grievance, and the award will be final and binding.[20]

One final word on contract administration can be offered. The supervisor must work within the framework of institutional policy for the handling of grievances. The institution may elect to allow supervisors to evaluate and settle employee complaints, or it may choose to centralize this function in the personnel division to ensure uniformity. The supervisor should be aware of the institution's policy.

Management's Rights

Almost all labor–management contracts have a *management's rights clause*. It may range from a brief paragraph to several pages in length. Essentially, a management's rights clause states that management has the sole right and prerogative to make decisions unilaterally concerning the operation of the institution except as it may be limited by the labor–management agreement. These rights usually include, among others, the right to hire, fire, suspend, and discharge for just cause; the right to temporarily assign, promote, or discharge employees according to the needs of the business; and the right to determine the methods of work. The right to suspend and discharge employees for just cause is vitally important, because a union will many times challenge a suspension or discharge for lack of just cause. An employee who has been improperly terminated may be reinstated to the former position by an arbitrator. The arbitrator may also direct remedial action, such as full pay for all time lost and restoration of all benefits that resulted from an improper discharge.

Because of the length of time required to process a grievance to arbitration, which exposes the institution to greater remedial legal liability, some contracts now provide for an expedited grievance procedure for cases that involve discharge and lengthy suspensions. The accused employee is suspended for a short period subject to discharge at the end of that time. The union is notified of the institution's action. If the employee believes that management's action is improper, the employee may file a grievance, and a meeting with all the parties involved is scheduled during the period of suspension and prior to the employee's termination. At this meeting, management will consider the employee's and the union's arguments that the suspension or discharge is unwarranted. This meeting provides an immediate, high-level management review of the discharge and speeds the invocation of arbitration by the union, thereby reducing the institution's potential liability should the arbitrator judge management's action to have been improper.

REFERENCES

1. Antony J: Management and Machiavelli. New York, Bantam Books, 1968
2. Brown & Root, Inc., 246 NLRB 132 (1979)
3. Butte Medical Properties, 168 NLRB 266 (1967) and University Nursing Homes, Inc., 168 NLRB 53 (1967)
4. Civil Service Reform Act, 95 Stat. 454
5. FMCS Services in Health Care Industry Labor Disputes. Code of Federal Regulations, Vol 29, Part 1420
6. McGuiness KC: How to Take a Case before the National Labor Relations Board. Washington, DC, Bureau of National Affairs, 1976
7. Morales G: Unit appropriateness in health care institutions. Labor Law J March, 174–179, 1979
8. Morris CJ (ed): The Developing Labor Law: The Board, The Courts and the National Labor Relations Act. Washington, DC, Bureau of National Affairs, 1971
9. National Labor Relations Act, 49 Stat. 449, as amended by Public Law No. 101, 80th Cong., 1st sess., 1947; Public Law No. 257, 86th Cong., 1st sess., 1959; and Public Law No. 360, 93rd Cong., 2d sess., 1974. Hereinafter referred to the NLRA
10. NLRA, Sec. 2(2)
11. NLRA, Sec. 8(d)(A), 8(d)(B), 8(d)(C)
12. NLRA, Sec. 8(g)
13. NLRA: Guidelines issued by the General Counsel of the National Labor Relations Board for use of board regional offices in unfair labor practice cases arising under the 1974 nonprofit hospital amendments to the Taft–Hartley Act pp 343–365. In Labor Relations Yearbook. Washington, DC, Bureau of National Affairs, 1974
14. NLRA, Sec. 213
15. NLRA, Sec. 3
16. NLRA, Sec. 9(b) and 9(c)
17. NLRA, Sec. 8(d)
18. Parks DG, Altman JP, Lavelle LA: Who are professional employees? Lab Med 26:503–506, 1995

19. Public Law No. 96-593
20. Textile Workers v. Lincoln Mills, 353 U.S. 448 (1957); United Steelworkers of America v. Warrior and Gulf Navigation Co., 363 U.S. 574 (1960); United Steelworkers of America v. Enterprise Wheel and Car Corp., 363 U.S. 593 (1960); United Steelworkers of America v. American Mfg. Co., 363 U.S. 564 (1960)
21. van de Vall M: Labor Organizations: A Macro- and Micro-Sociological Analysis on a Comparative Basis. London, Cambridge University Press, 1970

ANNOTATED BIBLIOGRAPHY

Elkowi F, Elkowi E: How Arbitration Works. Washington, The Bureau of National Affairs Inc., n.d.
> Written by practicing arbitrators, this volume is an invaluable aid to supervisors in understanding the rulings of arbitrators on various issues covered by labor–management agreements. It should assist supervisors in evaluating grievances brought forward by employees.

Fein M: Motivation for work. In Dubin R (ed): Handbook of Work, Organization and Society, pp 465–530. Chicago, Rand McNally & Company, 1976
> Primarily concerned with the effect of payment systems on motivation, this reference nevertheless contains a description of the function of a union in representing employees. It offers a different view of the nature of motivation and a description of the experiences of companions using different payment systems.

Grievance Guide. Washington, DC, The Bureau of National Affairs Inc., n.d.
> A synthesis of rulings of arbitrators on various elements of labor–management contracts. A valuable aid to supervisors because of the policy statements that introduce each topic.

> Updated periodically, it should be of assistance to supervisors in evaluating employee grievances.

Miller RU: Hospitals. In Somers GG (ed): Collective Bargaining: Contemporary American Experience, pp 375–434. Madison, Industrial Relations Research Association, 1980
> This resource includes a good description of the development of unions in the health-care industry. It also includes a description of the unions active in organizing health-care personnel and the history of their involvement.

Morris CR (ed): The Developing Labor Law: The Board, The Courts and the National Labor Relations Act. Washington, DC, The Bureau of National Affairs, Inc., 1971
> This is possibly the most comprehensive work available on the legal aspects of labor–management relations. Updated by annual supplements, the volumes synthesize the major legal developments in labor–management relations. The reader, therefore, should be prepared to research case reports to comprehend fully the rulings of the National Labor Relations Board and the courts.

Sovereign KL, Bognanno M: Positive contract administration. In Yoder D, Heneman HG (eds): Employee and Labor Relations, Vol III, pp 7.145–7.182. ASPA Handbook of Personnel and Industrial Relations. Washington, DC, The Bureau of National Affairs Inc., 1976
> This resource provides a comprehensive discussion of grievances and the role of the union and managerial personnel. It includes a "how-to" section for first-line supervisors. Many of the prescriptions offered apply to employer–employee relations with or without a union.

Tannenbaum AS: Unions. In March JG (ed): Handbook of Organizations, pp 710–763. Chicago, Rand McNally & Company, 1965
> An overview of the structure and functioning of unions, this reference provides a description of internal union processes, which filter into the relationship between management and the union.

Part

IV

Essentials of Effective Laboratory Operation

Clinical Laboratory Design and Refurbishment

Page Pennell C. Painter

Clinical laboratories are integral and necessary components of health-care delivery, the total cost of which is being rapidly forced downward by competitive pressures. To remain viable, clinical laboratories are redefining their mission, reorganizing, restructuring, and generally reinventing themselves to meet the changing needs of their respective institutions. Redesign of all or part of the clinical laboratory is often required to gain the necessary increases in overall fiscal and operational efficiency.

Arriving at an optimal design for a clinical laboratory space requires a thorough understanding of what is to be done in the space and how it might be done, from a near-term and long-term perspective, and planning accordingly. One of the biggest changes in the philosophy of clinical laboratory design today is the realization that multifaceted change, and the ability to fluidly respond to unforeseen change, must be at the foundation of the laboratory design. Elimination of impediments to improved efficiency, whether due to

structural or organizational walls, is widely recognized as an essential component of modern laboratory design and management. This chapter provides a guide to assist in the thought processes that should be used when designing an entire laboratory or a component of the laboratory. A hypothetical Hopeful Hospital laboratory project has been used to show how concepts can be specifically applied.

STARTING THE DESIGN PROCESS: PUTTING IDEAS ON PAPER

Define the Laboratory's Mission With Goals and Limitations

Before beginning the formal laboratory designing process, there should be general discussion meetings to define the laboratory's mission in as much detail as possible. The importance of this step cannot be

283

Box 17•1

Sample Laboratory Goals and Limitations (GOLIMS)

HOPEFUL HOSPITAL

500-bed acute care full-service community hospital. Active outpatient and referral laboratory operations account for 40% of clinical laboratory volume.

GOLIMs

Goals: Laboratory is to provide adequate on-site clinical laboratory services to support institutional needs and create a laboratory that continually optimizes cost effectiveness of all operations.

Limitations: Want current overall operational costs cut by 30% within 3 years. Administration at Hopeful is telling laboratory management that they want all laboratory testing to be of clinically acceptable quality, but they expect that where (in-house versus sending-out) and how (methodology) testing is done to be continually reviewed to optimize cost effectiveness.

follows in the laboratory design process (space size, location, electrical service, heat and air conditioning, cabinetry type) can be directly traceable back to the program statement, as shown in Box 17–3 for the hypothetical merging of chemistry and hematology into a new chematology laboratory at Hopeful Hospital.

Think of the program statement as a "goal specification" document in which you tell the architect or laboratory planner exactly what you are going to do in a given space (general equipment size and current needs from which heat loads can be estimated), how strongly an area must relate to other areas (eg, adjoining, adjacent, remote) and other requested specifics. If a design philosophy has been developed that addresses such items as whether the design will use an open laboratory concept and type of casework to use, these might also appear in the program statement. At the same time the program statements are being developed for each specific area, the summary program statement should be continuously updated to show the proximity relationship of each major space. Laboratory management and administration will have to fine tune the individual program statements so that the final program statements fit the size of overall space available and the budget.

overemphasized. It is particularly important that laboratory management and the institution's administration agree on what the goals and limitations (GOLIMs) will be so that the necessary support can be counted on when enabling operational requests are made to administration (Box 17–1).

Once the GOLIMs have been established, the laboratory operational staff should meet until a plan on how to attain the GOLIMs has been developed (Box 17–2). Everyone needs to be "on board" because historical turf boundaries and structural walls may need to be modified.

Space Considerations and Allocation

Who gets how much space and where that space will be located are critical and frequently organizationally sensitive areas. However, if everyone has been involved with development of the laboratory's GOLIMs plans, the allocation of space should be a more technical rather than political exercise. The document that defines space size and use is called the program statement. The program statement is the laboratory staff's opportunity to tell the planners and architects what space they want and where they want it. Virtually everything that

Box 17•2

Sample Plan to Attain Laboratory GOLIMs

HOPEFUL HOSPITAL

GOLIMs will be attained by:

1. Appropriate use of automation
2. Elimination of organizational and structural barriers to efficiency improvement
3. Reduction of personnel through attrition
4. Merging of substantial portions of chemistry and hematology into a chematology area where technologists would be cross-trained to operate both chemistry and hematology automated analyzers.
5. Connect the laboratory general receiving and stat testing areas to the hospital pneumatic tube system
6. Redesign of the laboratory to eliminate permanent structural barriers to efficiency everywhere possible, the defining of work areas by modular easily reconfigurable casework, movement of synergistic laboratory areas closer together, and use of automation to reduce workstations

Box 17·3

Area-Specific Program Statement

Area number:	2 (Two)	Net sq ft requested:	1,142
Name of area:	Chematology	Max people in area:	10
Laboratory design:	Open lab concept	Furnishings:	Reconfigurable modular

PROXIMITY INFORMATION:

Area	Name	Proximity
1	Receiving	Adjoining
3	Special chemistry	Adjoining
4	Special hematology	Adjoining
5	Chem office	Adjacent
6	Hemo office	Adjacent
7	Blood bank	Adjacent
8	Microbiology	Not critical
9	Micro office	Not critical
10	Immunology	Not critical
11	Main lab office	Keep separated
12	Lab lounge	Keep separated

DESCRIPTION OF AREA USE:

This is the main chemistry and hematology automated analysis area for the department. All testing services in this area must remain in continuous operation because nearly every test performed must be available on a stat basis. Chemistry testing done here includes all automated chemistry profiles, blood gases, whole blood stat chemistry panels, osmolality, therapeutic drugs, drugs of abuse, cardiac markers, and pregnancy tests. Hematology testing includes automated complete blood count, manual differential, automated urinalysis, coagulation testing.

EQUIPMENT:

Name	Number	Size	Volts/AMPs
Chemistry profiler	2	36 × 60 in	206/20
Immunoassay analyzer	2	36 × 60 in	206/20
CBC analyzer	2	36 × 60 in	206/20
Urinalysis analyzer	1	36 × 60 in	206/20
Coagulation inst	2	36 × 48 in	120/10
Blood gas analyzer	4	24 × 24 in	120/10
Whole blood analyzer	2	12 × 24 in	120/10
Osmometer	1	12 × 24 in	120/10
Slide stainer	1	12 × 24 in	120/10
Refrigerators	7	36 × 36 in	120/10
Freezers	5	36 × 48 in	120/10
Printers	6	36 × 48 in	120/10
Computer terminals	14	12 × 12 in	120/10
Label printers	3	12 × 12 in	120/10

SPECIAL ISSUES:

A pneumatic tube portal needs to be installed in this area because stat testing from surgery and other selected areas may need to be sent directly to this area for testing. Furnishings and all utilities (electrical/water) need to be flexible in this area to facilitate reorganization of the space as changes in technology and service dictate.

How Much Space You Need

Unless told otherwise by the architect or planner, when considering space requirements, the space being discussed is net square feet of surface floor space. A surface raised 30 inches above the floor is at sit-down desk height, while a 36-inch high surface is a stand-up work surface height, but the work surfaces all directly translate to the floor surface space beneath them. Consequently, a 36 × 36-inch refrigerator occupies 1,296 sq inches or 9 sq ft (1,296 sq inches ÷ 144 inches ÷ sq ft = 9 sq ft) of floor surface space.

Space Requirement Estimation

Because of the dramatic changes that have occurred in laboratory technology and functional organization during the last decade, most published "rule of thumb" guidelines for estimating clinical laboratory space needs are no longer appropriate. A more defensible yet easy to assemble approach is to use the "space equivalent unit totaling" (SEUT, pronounced See-UT) method. Using the SEUT approach, it is possible to estimate how much minimum total net space (TNS) in square feet is required for the tasks envisioned in that space. As shown in Figure 17–1, TNS is calculated in stepwise fashion. To the TNS total is added the sum of square feet of all floor mounted items, such as chemistry profilers, refrigerators, freezers, and shelving. This TNS does not include the square feet of miscellaneous space (MS) needed for aisles to move between work areas or the square feet occupied by all chase/support components of cabinetry. This MS figure can run between 10% and 30% of the TNS. The TNS-adjusted is then the TNS multiplied by the MS%. If the laboratory has fixed structural walls, the sum of the square feet occupied by walls must accounted for in the gross space required. An example of a space requirement estimation using SEUT is provided in Box 17–4.

Minimum Space Requirements

The minimum amount of space for a clinical laboratory depends on many variables. Arguably, the two most important space-dictating variables are the number of people that will be working in the space and the number of instruments, analyzers, and miscellaneous equipment in the space. The previous SEUT method gives the most reliable and defensible estimate when the required variables are known. The GP18-P document from the National Committee on Clinical Laboratory Standards gives some preliminary recommendations for laboratory minimums as noted in Table 17–1 that can be useful in arriving at aisle width and overall space estimates.

The 1,142 sq ft requested in the program statement for Hopeful Hospital's chematology laboratory falls be-tween the minimum and recommended levels given the 10 full-time employees expected to work in that area. There is also about 400 sq ft of analysis equipment and 720 sq ft allocated for clear bench to work surface for a ratio of 1.8 or almost double the recommended level. This higher ratio would be appropriate if the chematology area must support a good number of manual tests, like high-density lipoprotein cholesterol, that require clear bench surface to do the work, and a good deal of clerical work must be done in the laboratory area.

Space Efficiency: Gross Versus Net Space

When reviewing laboratory plans with architects and planners, there should be a clear understanding about whether the space square footage discussed is gross or net space. Utility chases, support beams, elevators, and corridors can dramatically reduce the amount of usable space from the gross space available, effectively lowering space efficiency. If the architect says a space has a 76.9% efficiency, then the net square feet of space needed should be multiplied by 1.3 (100 ÷ 76.9) to get the gross space needed before construction begins. At Hopeful Hospital, the chematology's TNS-adjusted of 1,142 sq ft would have to start with about 1,484 sq ft of gross space if the laboratory design had a 76.9% efficiency. The TNS and TNS-adjusted space estimates are net usable space estimates.

Laboratory Layout

Once the amount of space needed for the laboratory has been determined, the next step is to decide how the functional areas of the laboratory should be physically located or laid out. The laboratory's layout may need to go through several iterations until sample flow and personnel movement to and through the laboratory and overall layout are optimal for efficient current and future use of resources. The first layouts are best done as free-hand sketches without regard to size using bubble diagrams, circles drawn with strengths of relationships shown by thickness of lines between the circles of space. Architects use a thin transparent paper called TRASH, aptly named because so much ends up in the trash. TRASH comes on a roll, is inexpensive, and will be invaluable throughout the laboratory design process. Block diagrams can then be constructed showing approximate location of the various laboratory parts within the space allocated by administration. The final size of each block will be that approved by administration in the program statement.

Three Defining Issues of Laboratory Design Philosophy

A design philosophy needs to be developed early in the process to provide guidance on at least three issues. First, there must be a decision about whether it is going

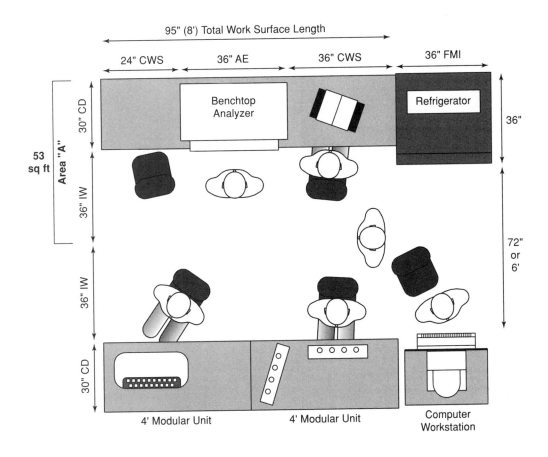

FIGURE 17–1.   The SEUT method of determining the minimum space required.

to be a mostly "open lab" design with work areas defined by casework or a traditional "walled lab" with work areas defined by walls. Second, a decision needs to be made about whether casework will be of the easily reconfigurable modular type or the fixed modular or millwork type. Third, the way utilities, such as deionized water, hot and cold potable water, and electrical service, are going to be supplied to the casework needs

to be decided. These three philosophy issues should be considered in the order given because the first items help define optimal options for the next issue to be resolved. Deciding that the laboratory must have walls around each laboratory work area dramatically impacts many issues like work flow patterns through the laboratory, the amount of functional space available, and even the number of personnel needed as indicated in Figure

Box 17•4

Sample Space Requirement Estimation Using SEUT

Name	Number	W × L	FMI	BTE sq ft
L (in)				
Chem profiler	2	36 × 60 in	30	
Immunoassay analyzer	2	36 × 60 in	30	
CBC analyzer	2	36 × 60 in		120
Urinalysis anal.	1	36 × 60 in	15	
Coagulation inst	2	36 × 48 in		96
Blood gas anal.	4	24 × 24 in		96
Whole blood analyzer	2	12 × 24 in		48
Osmometer	1	12 × 24 in		24
Slide stainer	1	12 × 24 in		24
Refrigerators	7	36 × 36 in	63	
Freezers	5	36 × 36 in	45	
Printers	6	36 × 36 in	54	
Computer terminals	14	12 × 12 in		156
Label printers	3	12 × 12 in		36
Pneumatic tube portal	1	36 × 48 in		48
Shelving	2	24 × 48 in		96
File cabinets	2	24 × 48 in		96
Sum			237	840

Table 17-1
Laboratory Minimums[1]

	Minimum	Recommended
Aisle width between casework units	5 ft	5–6 ft
Aisle width between casework and wall	4 ft	5 ft
Chair vertical adjustment range	5 in	6 in
Knee clearance under sit-down work area	27 in	28 in
Drawer load support at full open position	100 lb	100 lb
Temperature variation	± 10°C	± 5°C
Humidity variation	30%–70%	35%–55%
Air exchanges per hour	6	12–16

From NCCLS Document GP18-P, 1997

17–2. A sample laboratory design philosophy can be found in Box 17–5.

Physical Layout of Laboratory–Working Plans

A complete set of architectural plans will show placement of electrical, plumbing, lighting, and casework layout on separate drawings in sufficient detail to show exactly what is to be constructed. Laboratory staff should be involved in every phase of developing the layout. When considering various layout options, there is absolutely no substitute for firsthand experience. Even the best three-dimensional computer layout programs that allow you to walk in and look around a proposed laboratory on your computer monitor cannot convey the sense you get actually being in a laboratory, seeing where equipment placement causes problems and how people move through the space. A video of laboratories with layouts of interest might help in narrowing the options.

Unit Concept in Laboratory Design

One way to develop a laboratory layout is to view it as a series of units that can be moved around and "built up" to the scale desired. Units might include different

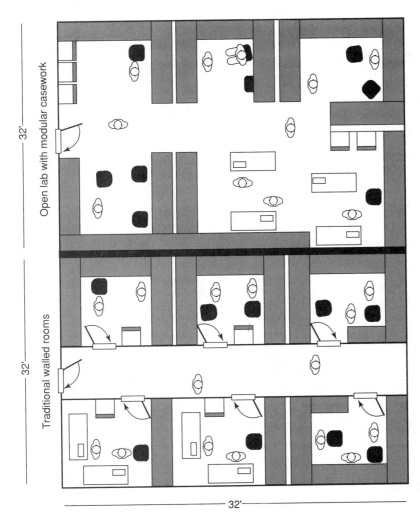

FIGURE 17–2. Two different lab layouts of a 1,024 sqft space.

sets of work station configurations as noted in Figure 17–3. Using such a system helps ensure that each of the units, which have been carefully scrutinized for individual functionality, will be functional when combined. Then the task becomes creating ways to connect the units together with walking paths (aisles and corridors).

Optimal laboratory configuration requires some time spent moving pieces around. Architectural computer-aided design programs facilitate the construction and movement of all elements of design (casework, appliances, equipment, offices, and walls) around a space until an optimal design is attained. Much the same thing can be done by cutting out the size of all the key design elements from properly scaled paper (eg, eight squares to the inch where each square equals 1 in) and moving them around a drawing of the space allocated

done on the same paper. Once completed, the "pasted up" layout could be given to the architects to guide them in constructing their initial layout drawings.

Casework

The benches and cabinetry used in laboratories are collectively termed casework. The two basic types are easily reconfigurable modular and relatively more difficult to reconfigure fixed casework. Before selecting casework, firsthand inspection of various options is required to verify construction, functionality, and appearance concerns. No matter how good something looks, if drawers do not open when loaded and counters sag under weight it will not be functional. If at all possible, casework should be placed over finished flooring to

Box 17·5

Sample Laboratory Design Philosophy

(Issue 1)   Hopeful Hospital has decided the new clinical laboratory will be of the open design. Walls will be eliminated from all technical work areas where possible. Only the lounge, conference room, and officers will have walls.

(Issue 2)   Easily reconfigurable modular casework will be used throughout the technical work areas. Work areas will be defined by the casework. Most casework will have overhead storage.

(Issue 3)   Utilities will be supplied through chases in the support structures holding the modular casework. Utilities (deionized water, potable hot/cold water, and drain pipes) will be routed through all peripheral walls so that casework support chases can be moved along the walls as needed with the assurance that these utilities are available to be attached. Electrical service is routed overhead and dropped either down walls to supply the modular casework cases or through columns as needed for more open room installations.

facilitate rearrangement of casework to new configurations.

Modular casework has components, such as under-counter storage cabinets and drawers assembled as units, that can be lifted from the support structure and interchanged with other modular units to change the configuration. Modular casework typically comes in 48-in lengths. Usually the term modular is used to denote easily reconfigurable casework. However, some modular casework is best considered as fixed because once it is installed, considerable effort is required to extract and reconfigure it. At a minimum, the casework should be able to have the height from the floor easily adjusted and components (eg, 48-in under-counter units) easily interchanged. With modular casework, the counter top often becomes the greatest deterrent to flexibility, so top lengths and construction should be given careful consideration. Counter depths of 30 inches seem to be most functional because 24 inches is too narrow for some bench top analyzers and a 36-inch width can make reaching overhead cabinets difficult.

Fixed casework is almost universally used for home kitchen cabinetry and is consequently the most familiar type of casework to most people. Fixed casework comes in a wider variety of dimensions, colors, and styles than does modular casework. Spans of cabinetry are constructed by combining various fixed units. Special fabrication of fixed casework for units or whole laboratories, especially using plastic laminate over particle board, is still relatively common in some areas.

Moveable casework is becoming increasingly important to support large free-standing analyzers and work surfaces that need to be frequently relocated. This type of casework is especially useful when access to

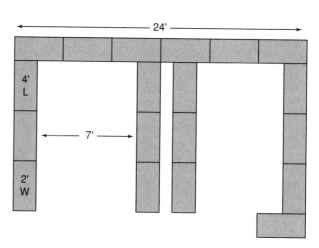

FIGURE 17–3. Modular casework: Build up of two work-areas using 2″ × 4″ units.

the back of a bench top analyzer is required. Some moveable casework designs can support in excess of 500 lb on a 36 × 48-inch top and permit the height adjustment.

Seating in the laboratory should stress comfort and functionality. All seating should have height and back adjustment capability to permit people of different heights to sit comfortably. Seat coverings should resist soiling and be able to be cleaned and disinfected. Cloth fabrics are fine for office seating but may not be functional in the technical work areas.

Computer workstations and other areas where video display terminals (VDT) and keyboards are used require some special considerations and planning. Reflections on VDT screens cause eye fatigue and can contribute to operator entry and review errors. VDTs should be mounted so the viewing height and angle can be adjusted by each individual. Keyboards need to have height and angle adjustments to help minimize wrist fatigue and injury.

UTILITY SERVICES

Services required in all laboratories include electrical, plumbing, and heat and air conditioning. Vacuum and gas may be needed in some areas. How these services are supplied can have a major impact on the flexibility and overall design options available to the laboratory planner. Consequently, every effort should be made to design these systems with change in mind. One way that this can be done is to put all plumbing, such as hot and cold potable water lines, deionized water lines, drain lines, vacuum lines, and gas lines, along all peripheral walls. With such an arrangement, access to these services can be acquired by simply moving casework to a wall, opening an access panel, and routing the services through the casework chases to adjoining casework where specific services are required. The "open lab" in Figure 17–3 could function with such a wall-supplied service system with the exception of the four analyzers, which would require services to be supplied from the ceiling.

Electrical

Clinical laboratories require a large amount of total electrical service per square foot of space. Four or more different types of power may be needed, including general, conditioned, uninterruptable, and uninterruptable or emergency power. General service power is typically supplied to circuit panels feeding the various laboratory outlets as approximately 110V/20A and 208V/20A from step-down transformers in the facility. To supply the stable and clean power required by modern laboratory equipment, it is often necessary to feed the general power into a power conditioner before it gets to the circuit panel or between the panel and the analyzer needing the power. If the analyzer cannot unexpectedly lose power when general power fails, then an uninterruptable power supply (UPS), which also conditions the power fed through it, will be needed to feed a whole circuit panel or between the panel and the analyzer. Because UPS systems typically supply enough power for only a few minutes of operation, the UPS must be attached to generator-supplied emergency power if continuous long-term operation is required when the general power electrical service to the facility fails. Analyzer requirements for dedicated lines, where one outlet is supplied by one circuit breaker, have become a common way for manufacturers to ensure that something else, like a refrigerator or freezer, will not cause erratic power to their equipment. The proliferation of dedicated lines means more circuit panels with more breakers per panel need to be allocated to the laboratory. Electrical power is supplied to work areas either through chases in casework or dropped from the ceiling in posts that serve as utility chases.

Plumbing

Hot and cold potable water is easily routed to work areas either through the walls or dropped from the ceiling. Getting waste water away though drain lines can be more difficult because flow depends on gravity. As a rule, drain lines must have ¼-inch drop per foot to drain properly. This means that a sink usually cannot be located more than 20 ft from the drain it will feed, an important consideration for casework placement. Drains in the floor out in the working laboratory area should be avoided as much as possible because their placement tends to limit layout flexibility. If a large open floor space requires drains some distance from the walls, then several drains should be placed and capped during laboratory construction so there will be several optional locations in the future. There is usually no difficulty in getting gas and vacuum to work areas because they can be fed from the ceiling if necessary. Conditioned water, such as deionized, should be routed on a continuous recirculating system, and dead ends where bacterial contamination could accumulate should be eliminated.

Heating and Air Conditioning

Heat generated by people and equipment in laboratories must be removed through adequate air flow and additional cooled air. Sizing and configuring air handling systems for laboratories require specialized expertise. However, because everything in laboratories generates heat, the biggest problem through most of the year is excess heat. Heating systems are built into chemistry and immunoassay analyzers to keep reaction area temperatures in the 30° to 370°C range. Unfortunately, no provision is made for cooling analyzer reaction areas if the room exceeds the specified reaction area temperature. Humidity is another aspect of laboratory environment that must be maintained within relatively narrow tolerances. If humidity is too low, static electricity causes electrical problems; if it is too high, it can partially reconstitute and destroy tableted reagents and harm electrical circuits.

Lighting

Most laboratory lighting will be supplied by fluorescent ceiling and under-cabinet task lights. The laboratory's lighting needs should be discussed with the architect to make sure adequate illumination is provided for all tasks. The general rule in lighting is that the more prolonged and exacting the task, the greater the illumination in footcandles required. For example, prolonged exacting work on small objects typically would need 500 to 1,000 footcandles of illumination, while other laboratory work might need only 50 to 200 footcandles. This range of illumination needs can be accommodated by supplying individualized output task lighting where needed while using fluorescent overhead lighting for general work tasks. Shadows on work areas can be reduced by orienting ceiling lighting at 90 degrees to the workstations.

Sample Transport Systems

Movement of collected samples to the laboratory over long distances can be accomplished by using a pneumatic tube or track bucket system, sometimes in combination. Most laboratories use a 4-inch diameter tube system with controllers designed to control carrier acceleration and deceleration between tube portals. If one or both of these transport systems are envisioned, the architect will need to plan additional ceiling clearance for their placement. The portals for sending and receiving carriers are about 4 ft across and 2 ft deep. Track type transport systems also exist for transport of individual specimens within the laboratory between sample preparation areas, analyzers, and workstations. Each transport system has its own configuration requirements that will have to be incorporated into the laboratory design.

REFERENCES

1. Painter PC: Laboratory Design Guidelines. National Committee on Clinical Laboratory Standards, GP18-P, 1997
2. Barker JH, Blank CH, Steere NV (eds): Designing a Laboratory. Washington, DC, American Public Health Association, 1989
3. Koenig AS: Medical Laboratory Planning and Design. Chicago, College of American Pathologists, 1989

18

Process Control and Method Evaluation

John A. Lott

PROCESS CONTROL IN THE CLINICAL LABORATORY

Process control (PC) in the clinical laboratory encompasses each step of the chain of events from the preparation of the patient and collection of the specimen to the delivery of the result to the clinician. Every action in the chain of events must be scrutinized to ensure that optimal patient care is achieved. It is clearly not enough to monitor only within-laboratory analytic performance. Many aspects of laboratory policies, procedures, and habits have now been codified in the revised Clinical Laboratory Improvement Act (CLIA) of 1967; the final regulations were promulgated on March 14, 1990, and implemented on January 1, 1991.[1] The rules that apply to PC and method evaluation are described here. This chapter contains a detailed discussion of the CLIA 1988 regulations.[2]

Monitoring the analytic performance of the laboratory is really PC rather than quality control. The quality of the tests is determined largely by the inherent properties of the equipment and materials over which we usually have little or no control. For example, if an antibody we are using for digoxin has some cross-reactivity with digitoxin, we really have no control over this except looking for a different antibody with better specificity. However, we can control the process by which the results are produced, and this activity includes reviewing and controlling the analytic functions of the laboratory. PC includes the interlinked items listed in Box 18–1.

Training and Experience of Laboratory Personnel

The article, "Laboratory Personnel: The Most Important Aspect of Quality Control," speaks to this point.[3] It is possible to have consistently good laboratory performance with well-motivated and trained personnel. A well-educated and experienced staff is the most important asset that a laboratory has. Laboratory personnel must have the necessary technical skills; more important, they must have good judgment. Judgment is acquired and cannot be taught. Good judgment includes the list defined in Box 18–2.

Within-Laboratory Process Control

The increasing sophistication of medicine has placed greater demands on clinical laboratories for reliable analyses. More sensitive and specific laboratory tests have simplified diagnostic medicine and provided signals of diseases earlier in their course.

Process-control programs provide a mechanism by which the analytic performance of clinical laboratories may be evaluated, documented, and improved. A process-control program should contain at least the elements listed in Box 18–3.

The Reference Sample Method of Process Control

The reference sample method is the most efficient and widely used system of PC in clinical laboratories. Controls that mimic patient specimens are analyzed repeatedly within and between days. The reference sample method can be used for evaluation of laboratory performance based on the repeatability of the results and the proximity of the results to the presumed true values. In addition, it can monitor interlaboratory variability when identical specimens or sets of specimens are sent to a group of laboratories.

Commercially Available Controls

Purchased controls have the advantage of convenience. They cannot be used uncritically; criteria for selection must include qualitative characteristics, concentration, stability, cost, and matrix effects. Commercially avail-

293

Box 18•1

Interlinked Items Included in Process Control

- Training and experience of technical and clerical laboratory personnel
- Level of supervision of the clinical laboratory
- Training and experience of phlebotomists
- Patient preparation before acquiring specimens
- Collection, preservation, transportation, and handling of specimens
- Storage of specimens if analysis is delayed
- Time between collection and reporting (ie, the turnaround time)
- Instrument maintenance and checks on instrument functions
- Quality of reagents, kits, and analytical materials; quality of standards and control materials
- Thorough evaluation of any new methods and procedures, including comparison with current methods, linearity checks, preparation of suitable reference ranges, and so on
- Quality and cleanliness of the laboratory environment, equipment, and materials
- Adequacy of procedure manuals, within-laboratory policy manuals, and instructions
- Adequacy of controls and reference specimens in verifying levels of analytical performance
- Assessment of analytical variability by an adequate reference specimen method
- Participation in external quality control surveys
- Policy on extreme values for patients (ie, "panic values")
- Optimum result reporting and delivery, including electronic reporting
- Correctness of reference ("normal") ranges stratified by age and gender when possible
- Interpretive reporting for certain tests
- Record keeping of patients' data
- Long-term storage of patients' and control data and timely retrieval of same
- Laboratory computerization and integration with hospital's computer; access to the hospital database for medical record information, pharmacy, dietary, radiology, and other functions that help the laboratory personnel interpret findings
- Ongoing continuing education of entire professional staff
- A published laboratory guide for users of the laboratory that includes services, policies, reference ranges, telephone numbers, locations of services, and so on
- Well-established safety procedures

Box 18•2

Pieces to Good Judgment

- Recognizing that the specimens are from patients and that erroneous laboratory data can have unpleasant and sometimes serious consequences for the patient, such as unnecessary diagnostic procedures, extra days in the hospital and the attendant costs, mistaken or missed diagnoses, and so forth
- Being able to communicate to the other providers of health care in a professional and helpful way to further patient care
- Identifying and correcting lapses in laboratory performance, such as mistaken values
- Alerting physicians at once when extremely abnormal results are observed in the laboratory and identifying a possible life-threatening situation
- Having a willingness to provide extra effort and time when the situation demands it with ill patients and unusual cases
- Recognizing the need to keep professionally alert and informed on new developments in the field

Box 18•3

Process Control Program

- The precision of the method over the entire dynamic range of normal and abnormal results is known.
- Control materials are used that mimic patients' specimens as closely as possible.
- Simple statistical calculations are made on the control results to give means, standard deviations (SD), and coefficients of variation (CV) of all analytical procedures.
- Control charts (e.g., Levey–Jennings [L–J] charts or similar) are prepared, kept up to date, and are easily retrieved. The control charts contain "warning limits" and "action limits" to assist the technical staff in decision making.
- The limits on the control charts are largely defined in a pragmatic way and with a view toward medical needs and the regulatory environment. Limits based on the statistics of past performance are used appropriately, recognizing that contemporary equipment is better, and strict

- ± 2 SD limits (ie, the 1_{2s} rule) are no longer applicable to all situations.
- Continuous monitoring of analytical performance is carried out by introducing fictitious patient specimens into the laboratory in addition to the control specimens known to the analysts.
- The entire laboratory staff is responsible for the entry of process-control data onto suitable record forms or into a computerized process-control system.
- Certain individuals are responsible for collation of data, for preparing L–J charts, for long-term record keeping, and for record storage and retrieval.
- The corrective actions in "out-of-control" situations are defined, and the role of the various levels of laboratory personnel in correcting such problems is clearly delineated.
- Individuals who have problems performing a given procedure are identified for retraining.

able controls must be certified to be free of hepatitis antigens so that they are safer to use than, for example, pooled serum from the laboratory.

QUALITATIVE CHARACTERISTICS OF PROCESS CONTROL MATERIALS

As closely as possible, PC materials must mimic patient specimens, whether they are whole blood, plasma, serum, urine, body fluids, or other patient-derived materials. A basic assumption of all PC specimens is that the repeatability and accuracy obtained with control materials is the same as that obtained with patients' specimens. If this assumption is correct, the laboratory has an estimate of how well it is performing analyses of patients' specimens. Often, nonhuman PC materials must be used. For example, because of the difficulty in obtaining enzymes from human tissues, animal enzymes are commonly used to fortify control sera. Porcine heart creatine kinase (CK) resembles human skeletal muscle CK[4]; however, calf intestinal alkaline phosphatase (ALP), a common source of ALP, is different from ALP derived from human liver.[5] For some tests, like blood gases, it is nearly impossible to mimic patients' materials, so artificial materials must be used that may not respond like patients' specimens in cases of

analytical failures. For ammonia, ammonium sulfate solutions are commonly used as controls, because serum proteins, even when lyophilized, slowly break down and release ammonia. The disadvantage of ammonium sulfate is that problems with the assay reagent (eg, if it is contaminated with urease) will show increased values owing to this interferant, but the control results will be unaffected.

Lyophilization tends to denature proteins; for example, albumin exhibits changed dye-binding characteristics after lyophilization. Liquid controls containing ethylene glycol are unsuitable for analytic systems using dialysis[6] and dry-film chemistries[7]; however, they are convenient and may be less costly than lyophilized controls because there is less waste. Another advantage is better reproducibility of their target values; the variable associated with reconstitution is absent.

CONCENTRATIONS OF ANALYTES IN CONTROLS

Control sera should have concentrations or activities based largely on medical needs. Methods should be monitored at decision points. Some tests have more than one decision point. For example, hemoglobin, leukocyte count, serum glucose, iron, protein, pH, PCO_2, calcium, digoxin, cortisol, alkaline phosphatase, potassium, magnesium, and most drugs have more than one value where therapeutic, diagnostic, or management decisions are made. Controls should be available with concentrations close to decision values. Other tests, such as creatinine, aspartate aminotransferase, and lactate dehydrogenase (LD), generally have only one decision region. Here, fewer controls are needed. Bilirubin has decision points for newborns that are different from those for adults, and the PC needs are more complex.

Most methods in clinical chemistry are designed to cover a wide dynamic range of concentrations. If possible, controls should be used to monitor the stability of the dynamic range or when a loss in precision has occurred at medically important or decision values.

INTERRELATED CONCENTRATIONS IN CONTROLS

Commercially prepared PC materials that are prepared in sets of two or three should have the concentrations of analytes present in known interrelationships. If the concentrations of the common analytes are present in known ratios, then additional information is obtained in their analysis. For example, a set of controls could have glucose concentrations of 50, 100, 200, and 400 mg/dL. The instrument's response would be graphed versus the expected concentrations to prepare the "operational line" for glucose (see the section on accuracy of controls). Much more PC information is available from an operational line than from repetitive analyses of concentration-unrelated controls.[8]

ACCURACY OF CONTROLS

The true concentration of an analyte in a control is not known; however, good estimates of the true value may be available. A few analytes, such as calcium[9] and glucose[10], have definitive methods, typically gas chromatography-mass spectrometry. Reference methods are one tier below definitive methods, but they have stringent requirements and can yield excellent estimates of the true value. Reference methods have undergone extensive scrutiny; their bias, variability, source of interferences, and so forth, are known. Nearly all the other common analytes have well-established field methods of tested reliability. Control materials should have only one concentration for most analytes. The pressure of the marketplace has created a preposterous situation for some manufacturers of control sera. Ciba Corning Diagnostics Corp. (Irvine, California, 92714), for example, lists 32 unique results for cholesterol for its "lipids" control product; the listed cholesterol values range from 285 to 427 mg/dL, a spread of 142 mg/dL, or 50% of the lower value. The mean and standard deviation (SD) calculated by use of these results are 340 mg/dL and

30.7 mg/dL, respectively. What is the true value? "Matrix effects" could be invoked, but they would hardly explain this huge range of values. Laboratories want to be "in control" for their method, yet they miss the much more serious problem of a substantial bias from the true value.

A major problem with some tests are matrix effects (ie, the analyte in an artificial or modified base material does not act like the same analyte in fresh serum).[11-13] Despite these difficulties, some dry-film methods (eg, Vitros) that show distinct matrix effects can be calibrated with commercially available materials to provide reliable and accurate results on patients' specimens.[14]

Reference methods or candidate reference methods are now available for the analytes listed in Table 18–1.[15] They provide a source of "truth" for many assays and can be used to judge the analytical bias of field methods (ie, those in routine use in clinical laboratories).

Frequency of Analysis of Control Sera

How often should patients' specimens be interspersed with control materials? The frequency of analysis of controls is dictated largely by the variability of the test and what is acceptable drift. The definition of drift in turn describes a batch of specimens. With this gestalt, some drift is acceptable; during the analysis of a batch of specimens, controls are analyzed, along with the speci-

Table 18-1
Methods and Materials Credentialed by the Council of the National Reference System for the Clinical Laboratory[56]

Credentialed Methods and Materials (Date of Action)

Glucose (1988)
Aspartate aminotransferase (1988)
Cholesterol (1988)
Alanine aminotransferase (1988)
Protein, total (1993)
Bilirubin (1988)

Proposed Methods and Materials

Na (1988)
K (1988)
Ca (1989)
Cl (1988)
Urea nitrogen (1988)
Creatine kinase (1993)
Gamma-glutamyl transferase (1993)

mens in the batch. Acceptable drift can be defined as 1 SD of the method during a period of stable performance. For example, if 1 SD of a method for serum glucose is 2 mg/dL at 100 mg/dL, a drift of the mean of the control values from 98 to 100 mg/dL could be disregarded.

On a practical basis, a batch is 5 to 10 specimens for methods using an ion-specific electrode, flame photometry, or atomic absorption measurements; it is 15 to 20 specimens for spectrophotometry, blood cell counters, or many multichannel chemistry instruments. Some instruments, like the Vitros 750XR, are stable, and the analyses of as few as one or two controls in an 8-hour day suffices.

The CLIA regulations require that the laboratory design, document, and implement a PC program.[1] A great deal of latitude is given to the laboratory in the above; the important issue is that the laboratory not violate its own rules. At least two controls at different concentrations must be analyzed at least once a day when the test is performed. These minimal requirements are adequate with highly stable equipment and reagents; most laboratories will opt to assay PC specimens more often than this.

Determination of Laboratory Variation

Levey–Jennings Charts

The most widely used system of PC uses the reference sample system.[16] Here, PC specimens are analyzed singly or in replicate on each day specimens are assayed, and the mean and SD are calculated. Two equations can be used to calculate the SD. The first is as follows:

$$SD = [Sum (Value\ i - Mean)^2/(n - 1)]^{1/2}$$

(Value i − Mean) is the deviation of the ith value from the mean, and n is the number of values. The square root of the entire term is the SD. Alternately, the second equation is as follows:

$$SD = [n(Sum\ value\ i^2) - (Sum\ value\ i)^2/n(n - 1)]^{1/2}$$

(Sum value i^2) is the sum of the squares of the values. (Sum value i)^2 is the sum of the values squared, and n has the same meaning as previously. The second equation is more convenient to use with computers and is used with all hand calculators that have the SD function. With equation 2, the individual points need not be stored by the computer.

When new process-control materials are introduced, it is necessary to establish the acceptable SD. This can only be done when the method has good sta-

bility and the values are not drifting up or down as determined with an established control material. The SD is determined during periods of "good performance" when there are few outliers, the procedure is well controlled, and adequate data have been collected. In general, for small sets of data, as the number of data points (n) increases, the SD increases. Ideally, the number of data points should be large, perhaps 400. For practical purposes, the SD can be calculated if 30 to 50 values are available. With a small sample, the SD may have to be revised as additional data are collected. The data must have a reasonably gaussian distribution. Levey–Jennings (L–J) charts assume the baseline data are gaussian.

There are two schools of thought on the use of L–J charts. The traditional and still most widely used method is performance based; the criteria for future performance are set by experience when the method, instrument, reagents, and so on were "stable." The second school uses some arbitrary limits to define quality based on medical needs or what is required to pass external proficiency surveys. Performance-based criteria are the most popular at present. The difficulty, as discussed below, is the decreasing SD of most methods as better analytical systems have become available.

Use of Levey–Jennings Charts

Stable Performance

A typical L–J chart is shown in Figure 18–1. Two control results are graphed each day on separate charts, and the data for 1 month are displayed. Results outside of ± 2 SD are termed warning limits, and those outside of ± 3 SD are designated action limits. If the mean and SD of the control were established during a period of stability and if the procedure remained stable, new PC data could be used for judging current performance. If the results follow a gaussian pattern, 68.3% of the values will fall within ± 1 SD, 95.5% will fall within ± 2 SD, and 99.7% will fall within ± 3 SD. One in 20 results should be expected to fall outside of ± 2 SD, and only 3 per 1,000 should fall outside of ± 3 SD. Values outside of ± 3 SD should always be questioned, because they are so rare and usually point out unacceptable analytic variability. If a small sample is used to establish the SD, more outliers will occur over time.

Allen and coworkers found that if the control was known to the analyst, the SDs were generally smaller than when the controls were "blind," that is, disguised as a patient specimen.[17] If generally true, the implication of this finding is that the actual performance on patients' specimens is worse than what is determined with PC schemes.

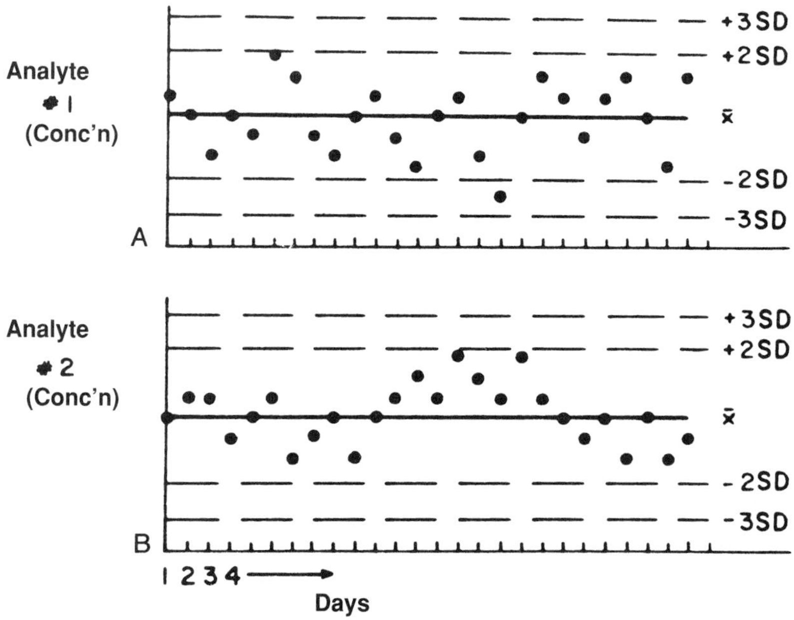

FIGURE 18–1. A Levey-Jennings chart showing the distributions of quality control data using traditional ± 2 SD limits that show day-to-day variability. (*A*) The data are randomly distributed between the limits. (*B*) Over a short period, the data are clustered well within the designated limits; however, small shifts occur from time to time, causing the points to vary between the designated limits. (From Grannis GF, Caragher TE: Quality-control programs in clinical chemistry. CRC Crit Rev Clin Lab Sci 7:327, 1977)

Dispersion or Contraction

A change in precision causes increased dispersion or contraction of the spread of the data. Increased dispersion is shown in Figure 18–2; there is a host of reasons for worsening precision, which is usually apparent from an L–J chart. Some causes are more or new individuals performing tests, inattention to critical steps of procedure, unstable line voltage, greater variability in pipeting specimens or reagents, failures of the instrument, deterioration of the reagents, and so forth.

Trends

Trends in PC data are shown in Figure 18–2. Trends are commonly caused by a gradual deterioration in standards, reagents, instrument condition, and so forth. L–J charts are excellent for detecting trends. A trend is always a signal for remedial action and is generally apparent when at least 10 consecutive values are above or below the mean.

Shifts

Shifts, as shown in Figure 18–2, are commonly caused by the introduction of new lots of standards or reagents and usually with method changes. Shifts caused by a remedy of an unsatisfactory situation are unavoidable and at times desirable. Small trends or shifts within acceptable limits are not a problem.

With many contemporary instruments, for example, the Coulter Stacker, Beckman CX7, Johnson & Johnson Vitros 750XR, and others, the L–J chart often shows tight clusters of data and shifts when new lots of reagent or calibrators are introduced. The analytic range, including the shifts, may be narrow; shifts of this nature are generally unimportant, particularly if they are < 1 SD.

Long-Term Data Records

L–J charts show long-term trends well. In Figure 18-3, monthly coefficients of variation (CVs) are shown for glucose data from the clinical chemistry laboratory of The Ohio State University Hospitals covering a period of nearly 30 years. Each of the data points is the mean of 100 or more values at concentrations of approximately 250 to 300 mg/dL. With improving technology, the CVs have become narrower. This must be considered when setting PC limits; better technology does not necessarily require tighter PC limits. From 1967 to late 1974, the Technicon AutoAnalyzer (Technicon Corporation, Tarrytown, NY, 10591) ferricyanide method was used; monthly CVs were in the 5% to 6% range with occasional months where the CV was close to 9%. Between late 1974 and late 1979, glucose was analyzed on the Technicon SMA-6 with a glucose oxidase method[18]; the precision improved, and the CVs were typically near 4%. In June of 1981, we started using the

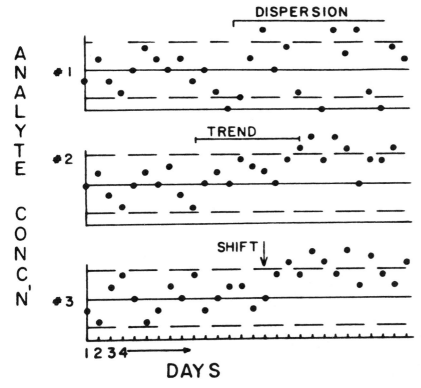

FIGURE 18–2. Examples of three types of changes in quality control data. Chart #1 illustrates dispersion of data characterized by an increased frequency of both high and low outliers. A frequent cause of such dispersion is loss of precision of an automatic dispenser. Chart #2 illustrates an upward trend in the data. Over a period of days, the determined values drift progressively from the prior mean value. Trends are commonly caused by deterioration of instrumental components and by changes in analytic standards. Chart #3 illustrates an abrupt shift in the data to a new mean value. Shifts are commonly caused by changes in analytic systems, such as replacement of components or use of a different lot of standards or reagents. (From Grannis F, Caragher TE: Quality-control programs in clinical chemistry. CRC Crit Rev Clin Lab Sci 7:327, 1977)

Beckman Astra-8 (Beckman Instruments, Fullerton, CA, 92634) and a glucose oxidase-oxygen electrode method and observed a further improvement in precision. CVs are now in the 2% region, that is, a fourfold improvement in precision over the time period shown in Figure 18-3A. From 1985 to the present, we have been using the Vitros 700XR instrument (Johnson & Johnson Clinical Diagnostics, Rochester, NY, 14650), which has provided excellent precision.

Similar long-term data for serum cholesterol are shown in Figure 18-3B. Each point represents the mean of 25 to 30 values at concentrations of 250 to 300 mg/dL. A manual ferric chloride-H_2SO_4 method was used from 1967 to late 1977. CVs averaged 4% to 5%; however, some months showed considerably greater variability. Since late 1977 to about 1985, a cholesterol oxidase method was used on the Abbott ABA-100 Analyzer (Abbott Laboratories, North Chicago, IL, 60064). The precision of this automated enzymatic method is clearly better than that of the manual procedure. The Vitros 700XR, in use since 1985, has further improved precision.

How can the laboratory be certain that long-term stability of the assays is maintained? One tool is to use patients' data; the presumption is that if enough patients

are tested and the data are displayed as a histogram, then a characteristic of the histogram can be used to monitor long-term stability of a test. Another assumption is that there are no shifts in the population with time.

We developed such a method for the long-term (years) monitoring of chemistry tests' stability using results from patients.[19] For each test, histograms of at least 200 to approximately 2,000 data points were obtained on a bimonthly basis, and the median and means were determined from the unmodified data. In about 4 years of data, we found that the medians are extremely stable for most tests, and observed shifts in the medians could all be explained by expected or unexpected events in the laboratory. The means were less useful owing to shifts caused by extreme outliers, especially for enzymes in serum. We recommend the use of medians of patients' data under defined conditions for monitoring the long-term stability of certain clinical chemistry tests. The technique lacks the requisite sensitivity for day-to-day PC and should not be used for that purpose, but it is ideal for identifying gradual shifts occurring over long (years) periods of time.

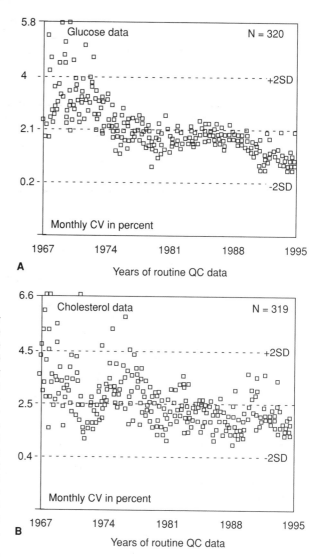

FIGURE 18–3. (*A*) Long-term quality control data for serum glucose obtained in the clinical laboratories of The Ohio State University Hospitals. The monthly mean CVs are shown for controls with glucose concentration between 250 mg/dl and 300 mg/dl. There is a clear trend toward better performance between 1967 and 1995 owing largely to the abandoning of poor methods and establishment of very precise methods such as those obtained with the Vitros instruments. Data are here from the end of 1967 to the first month of 1995. Points shown above the upper horizontal line had values > 5.8. (*B*) Long-term quality control data for serum cholesterol. The monthly mean CVs are shown for controls with cholesterol concentrations between 260 mg/dl and 320 mg/dl. There is distinct improvement in precision over the 29-year period owing largely to the introduction of improved equipment. Data are here from the end of 1967 to the first month of 1995. Points shown above the upper horizontal line had values > 6.6.

Application of Shewhart Control Rules

Westgard described a series of control rules for use in the clinical laboratory to judge if data are acceptable.[20] Certain managerial decisions must be made before the Westgard system can be implemented: A decision is needed on how many controls are to be analyzed with each batch of specimens or per 24-hour period, what the desirable error detection rate is, and what the acceptable false rejection rate of otherwise acceptable data is. The most important decision is determining an acceptable SD for the method.

Development of the Model

The number of control specimens analyzed per batch and the laboratory-determined acceptable SD determine the probability of detecting error (P_{ed}) and the probability of false rejection (P_{fr}) of acceptable data. The CLIA regulations empower laboratories to define acceptable SD limits and their control scheme. Two extremes are easily imagined: Several controls are analyzed with every batch, and the acceptable SD limits are narrow. The (P_{ed}) will be close to one; however, P_{fr} will be unacceptably large. Conversely, with few controls and wide acceptable SD limits, P_{ed} and P_{fr} will be low; many untoward situations will be missed. Clearly, a middle ground is needed. P_{ed} and P_{fr} are defined as follows:

$$P_{ed} = (\text{Proper rejection})/(\text{Proper rejection} + \text{False acceptance})$$

$$R_{fr} = (\text{False rejection})/(\text{False rejection} + \text{Proper acceptance})$$

Westgard has defined the predictive value of a PC scheme to accept data or to reject them as being erroneous. Also described are the theoretical bases of the Shewhart multirule system.[21-24]

Application of the Shewhart Model

Two controls at different concentrations are analyzed with each batch of specimens, and the results are recorded on L–J charts. It is assumed the SD limits are appropriate as described previously. A decision for acceptance or rejection of a batch of results is based on the set of rules defined in Box 18–4.

A violation of the 1_{3S} or R_{4S} control rules generally indicates random error. Violations of the 2_{2S}, 4_{1S}, or 10_X rules indicate systematic error; however, violation of the 1_{3S} rule also points to a large systematic error. The

---

Box 18·4

Factors Used to Decide Acceptance or Rejection of the Shewhart Model

- 1_{2S} rule: The run is rejected when either of two control results are outside the ± 2 SD limits from the mean value.
- 1_{3S} rule: The run is considered out of control when one of the control results exceeds the ± 3 SD limits.
- 2_{2S} rule: The run is rejected when both controls exceed their mean value + 2 SD or the mean − 2 SD limits.
- R_{4S} rule: The run is rejected when one control result exceeds a mean value + 2 SD limit, and the other exceeds the mean − 2 SD limit or when the range of a group of controls exceeds 4 SD.
- 4_{1S} rule: The run is rejected when four consecutive control results exceed the mean + 1 SD or the mean − 1 SD.
- 10_X rule: The run is rejected when the last 10 consecutive control results fall on the same side of the mean.

---

multirule Shewhart procedure could be used with manual calculations; a computer makes the implementation more efficient.

Flow Diagram of Multirule Shewhart Procedure

A flow diagram applying the previous model is shown in Figure 18–4.[20] Analysis of control data with a computer is straightforward, using a proper algorithm based on the flow diagram. The mean and SD of the control must be well established before this procedure can be applied.

The ability of L–J charts or the Shewhart multirule method to detect increasing dispersion, shifts, trends, and so forth depends on the SD of the method. If the procedure has a broad acceptable range, then small increases in imprecision, shifts, or trends will probably be lost in the overall scatter of the data. Amador showed that sudden new biases had to be 1.5 times the SD before they became obvious.[25] Imprecise methods tend to lull the analyst into a false sense of confidence; shifts, trends, and the like occur, but the method remains "in control."

L–J chart limits cannot be based solely on statistical criteria developed during periods of "good performance." Grannis and Caragher recommended that the allowable limits of error be based on ± 2.2 SD found during an "extended period of good performance."[26] They also recommended that the limits undergo periodic review and be "revised downwards whenever possible." When the laboratory was showing better performance, they recommended that the allowable limits (eg, ± 2.2 SD) should be narrowed.

These recommendations must be revised in terms of current technology, medical needs, and the regulatory environment. If only statistical criteria are used, such as ± 2.2 SD, a preposterous situation can develop. Highly precise methods will, by definition, have small limits; outliers, deemed medically unimportant, will create unnecessary concern, reanalysis, wasted resources, and so forth. Less precise methods will have broader PC limits; an outlier of the same magnitude as above will be inside the acceptable limits in such methods. In general, with narrower ± 2 SD limits, there will be more frequent outliers.

The relationship between outlier and PC limits is given in Figure 18–5. Assume that a small sample is taken from a large population of values; for example, ± 2 SD is calculated from 10 replicate determinations of a control and found to be 0.5 U. The true SD for the entire population is 1 U; that is, the sample has grossly underestimated the true SD of the population. This procedure is now put into routine use, and the acceptable

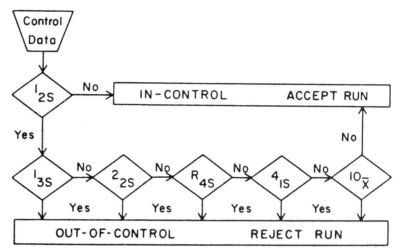

FIGURE 18–4. Logic diagram for applying a series of control rules in the multirule Shewhart procedure. Some laboratories use this approach, although most are using simple rules, such as 1_{2s} and 1_{3s}, to determine the acceptability of results. (From Westgard JO, Barry PL, Hunt MR: A multi-rule Shewhart chart for quality control in clinical chemistry. Clin Chem (27:493, 1981)

PC limits ($\pm$ 2 SD) are set at $\pm$ 1 U. During the early application of the method, the laboratorians quickly find that many of the analyses of the same control yield values outside of the acceptable limits; nearly 32% of the results are "out of control."

The causes of the above are that an inadequate sampling of the population (ie, too few replicates) were used to establish the PC limits; further, the limits are

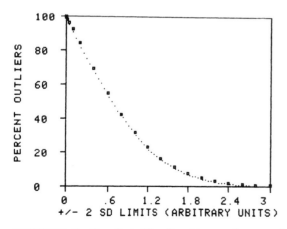

FIGURE 18–5. The effect of the allowable control range and the percent of outliers. As the allowed range is narrowed, there is a sharp increase in the number of outliers. If the allowable limits are set too close together, the consequence is unnecessary reanalyses of specimens, with no gain for the patient or laboratory.

much too narrow. In the above example, the true $\pm$ 2 SD limits were from $-$ 2 to $+$ 2 U; smaller limits will yield many more outliers, as is shown in Figure 18–5. Sometimes even with a large sample, the limits are set to an unrealistically small value, particularly with newer and more precise technology. Some suggested remedies follow.

PC limits can be viewed from another perspective. In 1967, our CV for glucose was quite large (see Fig. 18-3A); better equipment in the period to the present gave us decreasing CVs. With performance-based PC, do you tighten the acceptable limits with each decrease in the CV owing to better technology? The answer is clearly no; in fact, L–J charts could be constructed using medical needs or regulatory criteria so that with very precise methods, outliers would be rare. This then leads to the second school of thinking for PC, that is, PC limits based on medical needs or some other process than the typical Shewhart rules. Many laboratories are moving away from performance-based limits to medical needs-determined or regulation-driven PC limits.

ALLOWABLE ERROR IN THE MEDICAL NEEDS CONTEXT

Defining Allowable Error

Allowable error means there is an acceptable deviation of the determined value from the true value. Bias can be estimated by repetitive analysis of specimens with a known content of analyte. Matrix effects are assumed to be absent. Unfortunately, most of the time the true value or a good estimate of the true value is not known. Total error includes bias, which we assume is known, and random analytic variation. This is better stated as "What is allowable analytic variation?" Barnett used expert clinicians and users of clinical laboratory data to define acceptable error[27]; his approach has been updated and extended.[28-30] Barnett's method is reasonable, and the analytic requirements were linked to the clinical setting. In general, the medically useful precision limits were broader than those based on the current state-of-the-art analytic precision.

Other criteria that have been suggested are Tonk's rule, or one fourth of the reference range or ± 10%, whichever is smaller.[31] Cotlove and coworkers suggested that the "tolerable" analytic variability was 50% of the total biologic variation[32]; the latter is defined as a combination of interpersonal and intrapersonal variability.[33]

Glick[34] recommended that the random error be no greater than 20% of the population-based reference or therapeutic range or no greater than 60% of the medical decision range. For glucose, typical population limits are 65 to 115 mg/dL; 20% of this range is 10 mg/dL. At 120 mg/dL glucose, the medical decision range could be ± 20 mg/dL; 60% of the decision range would be 12 mg/dL. Lindberg and Watson used a "loss to society" approach of a false diagnosis owing to laboratory error[35]; improvements in laboratory precision result in less loss to society. They concluded that there is no simple answer as to what is medically acceptable imprecision. The circumstances under which the test is used dictate what is acceptable.

Effect of Changing Precision on Predictive Value

Allowable error can be calculated for a specific test and purpose with the use of one of three models described by Harris.[36] The first model deals with population screening to detect a biochemical abnormality. The effect of a change in precision on the predictive value of an abnormal test result is calculated; a subjective decision remains as to what loss is acceptable in the predictive value of a result. In population screening studies, the precision needs are less stringent; the within-laboratory variability is small compared with interindividual variability for most tests.

In the second case, Harris examines the effect of improved precision (the reverse is also possible) on the ability to detect abnormal values in a single person. Sharp decision boundaries are defined where the results are abnormal, and estimates are made whether a new

value is truly outside these limits. In the last case, Harris examines the effects of changes in precision on the ability to detect short- or long-term trends of an analyte in one person. Within-person short-term monitoring is the most demanding situation for the laboratory; the greatest precision is required. For example, in a patient being treated for possible acute rejection following renal transplantation, changes in the serum creatinine of as little as 0.2 mg/dL become important.[37] A serum creatinine increase of this magnitude in a renal transplant recipient can result in changes in clinical management. Another example is a patient with a possible problem with internal bleeding. Here changes of 0.3 to 0.5 g/dL in hemoglobin become important, and the laboratory must be as precise as possible. As described by Campbell and Owen,[38] Glick,[35] and Harris,[37] the allowable limit of error should be determined by the diagnostic application and certain other factors, as described below. There is no single acceptable analytic error for any test.

Table 18–2 shows acceptable imprecision for a variety of tests, according to several authors. Notice that the issue of accuracy has not been addressed. Some of the values in Table 18–2 are reasonable target values for CVs in population studies. Skendzel and Barnett[28] based their recommended limits on responses obtained from clinicians. Fraser developed analytical goals based on the biological variation in healthy people.[39] This is a useful device, has a theoretical basis, and could be implemented. For some analytes (eg, albumin, Ca, glucose, LD isoenzymes, total protein, Na, Mg, Cl, creatinine), all at the upper reference limit, the CV goals are unattainable, and the effort to devise analytical methods to meet these goals may not be feasible. Fraser's goals are unreasonably tight, and they do not serve medical needs but rather would foster unnecessary repetition of acceptable test results.

The 40% of CLIA limits is a pragmatic approach based on setting laboratory criteria so that external proficiency challenges are passed nearly all the time.

Cost to Society of Missed Diagnoses

Allowable error will always have a subjective component. What costs to society are acceptable? With overlapping populations, false-positive and false-negative results are inevitable. The key issues are where the decision point or cutoff value is defined and the allowance for analytic variability at this decision point.

Lindberg and Watson described the diagnosis of acute appendicitis as a test case.[36] It is desirable to have

Table 18-2
Acceptable Laboratory Test Imprecision Stated as Percent Coefficient of Variation

Test	Concentration or Activity	Tonks[31]	Harris[36]	Skendzel[28]	Barnett[27]	Fraser[39]*	CLIA[1]†
Acid phosphatase		10				4.5	
Albumin	3.5 g/dL		3.9		7.1	1.4	4.0
ALT						13.6	8.0
Amylase	100 U/L	10				3.7	12
ALP						3.4	12
AST	30 U/L			26		7.2	8.0
Bicarbonate	25 mmol/L		4.2			2.3	
Bilirubin	1 mg/dL			23	20	11.3	20
Bilirubin	20 mg/dL			5	7.5		7.0
Calcium	11 mg/dL	3.0	1.7	5	2.3	0.9	4.0
Chloride	90 mmol/L				2.2		2.0
Chloride	110 mmol/L	2.0	1.4		1.8	0.7	2.0
Cholesterol	250 mg/dL	5.0	6.4	12	8.0	2.7	4.0
CK						20.7	12
CK-MB						15.6	24
Creatinine	1.0 mg/dL	5.0		17		2.2	6.0
GGT						7.4	
Globulin	3.5 g/dL				7.1		
Glucose	100 mg/dL	5.0	5.6	11	5.0	2.2	4.8
HDL-Cholesterol						4.0	12
Hemoglobin	11 g/dL				4.8		
IgG						1.9	
IgM						2.3	
Iron	150 mg/dL			17	26.6	15.9	8.0
LD_1						1.1	12
LD_2						1.7	12
LD_3						1.4	12
LD_4						3.0	12
LD_5						4.0	12
LD, total	200 U/L		9.0			3.9	8.0
Lipase	100 U/L	10				6.5	
Mg	2 mmol/L		1.6			1.1	10.0
pH, arterial	7.4	2.0					0.02
Phosphorus	4.5 mg/dL	5.0	7.5	14	5.6	4.0	
PCO_2	30 mm						3.0
PCO_2	60 mm						3.0
PO_2	40 mm	10					10
PO_2	80 mm	10					10

(continued)

Table 18-2
continued

Test	Concentration or Activity	Tonks[31]	Harris[36]	Skendzel[28]	Barnett[27]	Fraser[39]*	CLIA[1]†
Potassium	3.0 mmol/L			5	8.3	2.4	8.0
Potassium	6.0 mmol/L	4.4	5.0		4.2		4.0
Protein	7.0 g/dL	3.5	2.8		4.3	1.4	4.8
Sodium	130 mmol/L	2.0		2.7	1.5	0.3	1.8
Sodium	150 mmol/L				1.3		1.6
Triglycerides	130 mg/dL			16		11.5	10
Thyroxine	6 μg/dL			17.2		3.4	
Urea	27 mg/dL	6.0	11.9	19	7.4	6.3	3.6
Uric acid	6 mg/dL		10.1	7.3	8.3	4.2	7.0

* Concentrations not stated.
† 40% of allowed CLIA value.

a few false-negative results; a false-negative result carries greater weight than a false-positive result. Operating on a few patients with a normal appendix is acceptable because the cost to society of a missed diagnosis leading to a ruptured appendix, peritonitis, and so forth is much greater. The relative weights of false-positive and false-negative errors are subjective, but where is the line to be drawn?

An example in which the laboratory plays a large role is in the diagnosis of neonatal hypothyroidism. A false-negative diagnosis carries a much greater cost than a false-positive one; a large number of false-positive results are an acceptable cost. If we assume that the test for thyroxine (T_4) is the primary screening test, then the decision point to identify "abnormal" newborns is set to allow for considerable analytic variation. The test must be as sensitive as possible at the cost of specificity. The hypothyroid and euthyroid neonates will have overlapping T_4 values; the cutoff point should be set to include all the hypothyroid cases plus 4 SD of the analytic variation. If a T_4 value of 4 μg/dL includes all hypothyroid cases and the SD of the method is 0.5 μg/dL, then the decision point is 6 μg/dL. Infants with a T_4 value below 6 μg/dL receive further testing.

The last example is a hospitalized patient who is known to have diabetes mellitus. If the laboratory variability is so great that the high glucose result is incorrectly reported as normal, then the test result is falsely negative. The cost to society of the false-negative result is probably minimal because of the likelihood of further testing. The costs of a false-positive and a false-negative result appear to be the same.

Variables Affecting Allowable Error

Degree of Overlap

In instances of greatly overlapping population of well and sick, less laboratory imprecision is acceptable than in nonoverlapping cases. A change in precision in a test for patients in the overlap region has much more effect on the predictive value of a positive test (PV[+]) as compared with the same test with a value at a decision point for nonoverlapping populations.

Disease Prevalence

In overlapping populations, disease prevalence is a major factor in determining PV(+) (Table 18–3). The PV(+) may be such that the test is not worth doing regardless of the analytic variability. Watson and Tang showed that serum acid phosphatase had no value as a screening test for prostatic cancer.[40] The PV(+) was low because of the considerable overlap and low prevalence. Obviously, a PV(+) of 50% or less is no better than a guess.

Biologic Variability

The data in Table 18–3 assume an overlap of 3% of the well and sick.[41] A decrease in precision has its greatest effect on PV(+) for tests that have a small interpersonal

Table 18-3
Effect of Prevalence and Change in Precision on PV (+)[41]*

Test	C_B*	$C'C_A/C_A$†	PV (+)†	PV (+)‡	PV (+)§
Prevalence			**50%**	**10%**	**1%**
Any	29%	1.0	97.7	82.5	30.0
Calcium	0.6%	1.9	87.1	42.9	6.4
Glucose	9.6%	1.5	97.6	81.9	29.1
Urea nitrogen	16.8%	2.3	97.1	78.8	25.3

* Predictive value of a positive test.
† Percent interpersonal variability.
‡ Ratio of "poor" (C'_A) to "good" (C_A) precision of listed tests.
§ Predictive value of a positive test at indicated prevalence.

biologic variability (C_B). Calcium has a C_B of about 1%. It shows the most rapid decline in PV(+) with a decreasing prevalence. For glucose and urea nitrogen, which have much larger C_B values, the PV(+) at 10% prevalence is nearly twice that of calcium.

Summary of Discussion of Medically Acceptable Error

Medically acceptable error is a subjective value. However, certain circumstances require highly precise laboratory values, or a large number of false-positive results is acceptable:

- The overlap between the well and sick populations is small. An example is a borderline increase of serum gastrin in a patient with suspected Zollinger-Ellison syndrome. A decision must be made regarding further testing. False-positive results are acceptable because of the serious consequences of missing a treatable case.
- The prevalence of disease is low. An example is neonatal hypothyroidism. Screening tests must be both sensitive and precise, and one must accept a significant number of false-positive results.
- The within-person biologic variability is small. Renal transplant patients, if they are stable, show only small changes in serum creatinine. A precise test is needed to detect an upward trend in the serum creatinine.[37]

ALLOWED ERROR BASED ON CLIA RULES

One of the CLIA mandates is that five proficiency testing (PT) challenges must be analyzed every quarter. Failing to meet the CLIA allowed limits for the same test in two

or three consecutive PT challenges can result in severe regulatory consequences called "adverse actions." Missing two or more tests in a single challenge of five specimens is also a bad mark. The punitive details are described elsewhere,[1] and they include stopping the performance of the test that failed the PT challenges, stopping all testing in a section of the laboratory, and even closing the laboratory. With this gestalt, it is natural for laboratorians to seek ways of passing the PT challenges.

CLIA Challenges

The tests for which CLIA limits have been defined are given in Table 18–4. The laboratory must return results on PT challenges that are within the allowed limits; results outside of these limits are PT failures. The allowed limits are fairly broad; however, for a laboratory to pass PT challenges consistently, the bias of a test from the presumed true value must be small, and the intralaboratory imprecision must be substantially less than the allowed CLIA limits. Ehrmeyer and coworkers[42] performed computer simulations to determine the chances of failing a "two-of-five event" (ie, having two or more failures for a specified test in a five-test challenge). Figure 18–6 shows the likelihood of failing, given the imprecision of the laboratory relative to the allowed limits and zero bias. The X-axis is set to the percent of the allowed limits (100% is the allowed limit); to pass consistently, the internal CV of the laboratory must then be a fraction of this. With no bias and a CV of between 30% and 40%, the chances of failing are small. Ehrmeyer and coworkers[42] recommended that a laboratory set as a goal that the maximum imprecision not exceed 33% of the allowed CLIA value. Using 40% of the allowed

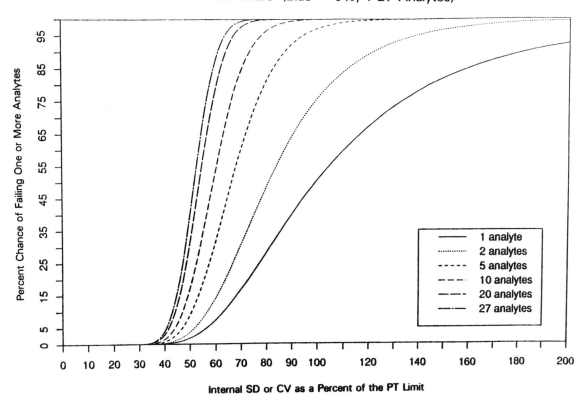

FIGURE 18–6. Chance of failing a CLIA PT challenge (score < 80%) based on the variability of the laboratory relative to the allowed CLIA limits. If the variability of the laboratory is <40% of the allowed limits, the chances of failing are small. (From Ehrmeyer SS, Laessig RH, Leinweber JE, Oryall FF: 1990 Medicare/CLIA final rules for proficiency testing: Minimal intra-laboratory performance characteristics (CV and bias) needed to pass. Clin Chem 36: 1736, 1990)

Table 18-4
Setting Process Control Limits for Routine Testing Based on CLIA Allowances

Test	CLIA Allowance, $\pm^1$	Decision Concentration	Fraser's goal, 1 SD[39]*	OSU Performance, 1 SD	CLIA-Allowed Error, Concentration	40% of CLIA Allowance	Shewhart Rule for Accepting Results
Albumin	10%	3.5 g/dL	0.049 g/dL	0.06 g/dL	0.35 g/dL	0.35×0.4 = 0.14 g/dL	0.14/0.06 = 2.3. Use $1_{2.3s}$ rule
Alkaline phosphatase	30%	150 U/L	5.1 U/L	1.7 U/L	45 U/L	18 U/L	1_{10s}
ALT	20%	80 U/L	10.9 U/L	3.2 U/L	16 U/L	6.4 U/L	1_{2s}
Amylase	30%	100 U/L	3.7 U/L	3.3 U/L	30 U/L	12 U/L	$1_{3.6s}$
AST	20%	80 U/L	5.8 U/L	3.5 U/L	16 U/L	6.4 U/L	1_{2s}
Bilirubin (1)	20% or 0.4 mg	1.5 mg/dL	0.17 mg/dL	0.07 mg/dL	0.4 mg/dL	0.16 mg/dL	$1_{2.3s}$
Bilirubin (2)	20% or 0.4 mg	20 mg/dL	ND†	0.48 mg/dL	4 mg/dL	1.6 mg/dL	$1_{5.3s}$
Calcium (1)	1.0 mg/dL	8.5 mg/dL	0.08 mg/dL	0.07 mg/dL	1.0 mg/dL	0.4 mg/dL	$1_{5.7s}$
Calcium (2)	1.0 mg/dL	11.0 mg/dL	0.10 mg/dL	0.10 mg/dL	1.0 mg/dL	0.4 mg/dL	1_{4s}
Chloride (1)	5%	90 mmol/L	0.63 mmol/L	1.0 mmol/L	4.5 mmol/L	1.8 mmol/L	1_{2s}
Chloride (2)	5%	110 mmol/L	0.77 mmol/L	1.0 mmol/L	5.5 mmol/L	2.2 mmol/L	$1_{2.2s}$
Cholesterol	10%	240 mg/dL	6.5 mg/dL	3.4 mg/dL	24 mg/dL	9.6 mg/dL	$1_{2.8s}$
CK	30%	200 U/L	41.1 U/L	4.9 U/L	60 U/L	24 U/L	$1_{4.9s}$
CK-MB	$\pm$ 3 SD	5 U/L	0.78 U/L	0.55 U/L	3 U/L (?)	1.2 U/L	$1_{2.2s}$

Creatinine (1)	0.3 mg/dL or 15%	1.0 mg/dL	0.022 mg/dL	0.02 mg/dL	0.30 mg/dL	0.12 mg/dL	1_{6s}
Creatinine (2)	0.3 mg/dL or 15%	4.0 mg/dL	0.088 mg/dL	0.08 mg/dL	0.6 mg/dL	0.24 mg/dL	1_{3s}
Glucose (1)	6 mg/dL or 10%	50 mg/dL	1.1 mg/dL	0.82 mg/dL	6.0 mg/dL	2.4 mg/dL	$1_{3.9s}$
Glucose (2)	6 mg/dL or 10%	120 mg/dL	2.64 mg/dL	1.2 mg/dL	12.0 mg/dL	4.8 mg/dL	1_{4s}
HDL-Cholesterol	30%	35 mg/dL	1.4 mg/dL	1.2 mg/dL	10.5 mg/dL	4.2 mg/dL	$1_{3.5s}$
Iron	20%	150 µg/dL	24 µg/dL	1.5 µg/L	30 µg/dL	12 µg/dL	1_{8s}
LD	20%	1,000 U/L	39 U/L	20 U/L	200 U/L	80 U/L	1_{4s}
Magnesium	25%	2.0 mg/dL	0.022 mg/dL	0.05 mg/dL	0.5 mg/dL	0.2 mg/dL	1_{4s}
PCO$_2$ (1)	5 mm or 8%	30 mm	0.72 mm	0.92 mm	5 mm	2 mm	$1_{2.2s}$
PCO$_2$ (2)	5 mm or 8%	60 mm	1.44 mm	1.43 mm	5 mm	2 mm	1_{2s}
pH	0.040 U	7.40 U	0.14 U (?)	0.004 U	0.04 U	0.016 U	1_{4s}
PO$_2$ (1)	± 3 SD	40 mm	ND	1.20 mm	10 mm (?)	4 mm	$1_{3.3s}$
PO$_2$ (2)	± 3 SD	80 mm	ND	1.34 mm	10 mm (?)	4 mm	1_{3s}
Potassium (1)	0.5 mmol/L	3.0 mmol/L	0.072 mmol/L	0.07 mmol/L	0.5 mmol/L	0.2 mmol/L	$1_{2.9s}$
Potassium (2)	0.5 mmol/L	6.0 mmol/L	0.14 mmol/L	0.09 mmol/L	0.5 mmol/L	0.2 mmol/L	$1_{2.2s}$
Protein, total	10%	8.0 g/dL	0.11 g/dL	0.09 g/dL	0.8 g/dL	0.32 g/dL	$1_{3.6s}$
Sodium (1)	4 mmol/L	130 mmol/L	0.39 mmol/L	1.2 mmol/L	4 mmol/L	1.6 mmol/L	1_{2s}
Sodium (2)	4 mmol/L	150 mmol/L	0.45 mmol/L	1.4 mmol/L	4 mmol/L	1.6 mmol/L	1_{2s}
Triglycerides	25%	250 mg/dL	29 mg/dL	1.2 mg/dL	63 mg/dL	25.2 mg/dL	1_{10s}
Urea N	2 mg/dL or 9%	30 mg/dL	1.9 mg/dL	0.5 mg/dL	2.7 mg/dL	1.08 mg/dL	$1_{2.2s}$
Uric acid	17%	8 mg/dL	0.34 mg/dL	0.1 mg/dL	1.4 mg/dL	0.56 mg/dL	$1_{5.6s}$

* Values in this column are calculated from Fraser's Table 1. Fraser goal = (his % CV X decision concn.)/100.

† Ehrmeyer[42] recommended using 33% of the allowed CLIA limit rather than 40% as shown here. You may want to use their stricter limits.

‡ No data given.

CLIA limits gives quite similar results. For example, the allowed CLIA limit for albumin is ± 10%. Thus, for a specimen with 3.5 g/dL albumin, the CLIA allowed error is 0.35 g/dL, and 40% of this is 0.14 g/dL as the allowed error to pass PT most of the time. Now look at our laboratory's performance of this test in Table 18–4. The SD for albumin is 0.06 g/dL, and the laboratory can safely use the $1_{2.3s}$ rule as its primary guide for result acceptance (ie, the action limits are ± 0.14 g/dL). Fractional SD allowances are permitted, and the 1_{2s} rule is too restrictive with contemporary stable and precise instruments. Not surprisingly, as the number of tests in a PT challenge increases, so do the chances of failing (Fig. 18-6).

Effect of Bias

When bias is introduced (Figs. 18-7 and 18-8), the chances of failure increase with the magnitude of the bias. The chance of failing does not increase linearly with bias, rather an increase in bias from 0% to 20% of the allowed CLIA limit has a much smaller effect than when going from a bias of 20% to 50% of the allowed CLIA PT limit.

Some common-sense rules for increasing the chances of passing a CLIA PT challenge are defined in Box 18–5.

If the bias is 50% of the allowed CLIA limit, then the chances of failing are quite significant. In most labo-

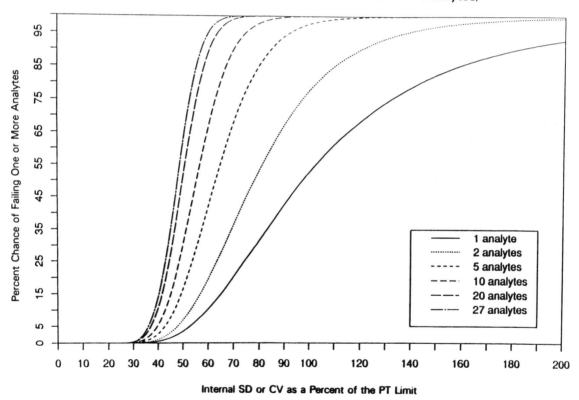

FIGURE 18–7. Chance of failing a CLIA PT challenge (score < 80%) based on the variability of the laboratory relative to the allowed CLIA limits. A bias of 20% of the allowed CLIA variability has been added to the previous figure. Note the shift of the curves to the left. With added bias, the chances of failing a challenge are greater. (From Ehrmeyer SS, Laessig RH, Leinweber JE, Oryall FF: 1990 Medicare/CLIA final rules for proficiency testing: Minimum intra-laboratory performance characteristics (CV and bias) needed to pass. Clin Chem 36:1736, 1990)

1 PT Event Failure (Bias = 50%, 1-27 Analytes)

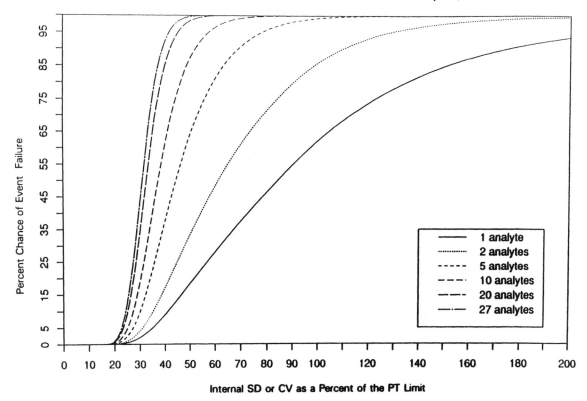

FIGURE 18–8. Chance of failing a CLIA PT challenge (score < 80%) based on the variability of the laboratory relative to the allowed CLIA limits. A bias of 50% of the allowed CLIA variability has been added to the previous figure. Note the still greater shift of the curves to the left. With added bias, the chances of failing a challenge are greater. (From Ehrmeyer SS, Laessig RH, Leinweber JE, Oryall FF: 1990 Medicare/CLIA final rules for proficiency testing: Minimum intra-laboratory performance characteristics (CV and bias) needed to pass. Clin Chem 36:1736, 1990)

ratories today, imprecision is not the problem but bias is. Sample problems illustrating the application of CLIA rules to PC issues are given in Appendix 18–1.

INTERLABORATORY SURVEYS

Interlaboratory proficiency surveys, or laboratory improvement programs (a better term), provide PC and management information for participants. Because a large cohort of laboratories analyze the same material, group mean values can be determined that are generally excellent estimates of the true value. From survey data, a participating laboratory can determine whether its val-

ues are biased relative to those of peer laboratories using the same method or whether the laboratory's variability is generally larger than that of the peer group.

Most surveys report the methods being used, precision data, and how many participants are using a particular method. This provides management information; laboratories should abandon obsolete methods or those that give results that are consistently different from the consensus mean. Finally, surveys provide information on the state-of-the-art of common analyses and can provide the basis for goal setting or improvements in methodology. Based on survey data, improved performance in the determination of serum calcium, creatinine, and thyroxin was recommended in a symposium on analytic

---

Box 18·5

Common-Sense Rules for the CLIA PT Challenge

1. Because bias rather than imprecision is the main reason why laboratories fail PT, perform preventive maintenance on your instrument, check that all performance indicators are within specifications, and run calibrators and controls to assess any bias or other problems. If the internal PC data are acceptable, then the PT challenges can be analyzed.
2. Check for recent trends in the data. If there are any, then fix the problem first.
3. Designate a key operator to assay the PT challenges to avoid the mistakes of the inexperienced. Have the same person complete the questionnaires.
4. Do not hesitate to replicate PT challenges that are outside of your dynamic test range if this is a normal and documented practice in your laboratory.
5. Assay PT challenges along with controls and patients' specimens. Reject all results if PC indicates an out-of-control situation.

---

goals.[43] Target values for improvement are shown in Figure 18–9; calcium and creatinine are analytes that require further attention to improve precision.

Professional, Private, Commercial, and Governmental Organizations Providing Surveys

The groups providing external proficiency surveys in clinical chemistry are shown in Appendix 18–2. The largest survey by far is that of the College of American Pathologists (CAP, Table 18–5) and is the most compre-

hensive evaluation of the common and unusual tests performed in clinical laboratories. The American Association of Bioanalysts also provides surveys with a broad menu of tests.

Government Agencies Providing Surveys

Several state health departments and regulatory agencies provide surveys. Prominent among these are the programs in Wisconsin, New York, and New Jersey (see Appendix 18–2).

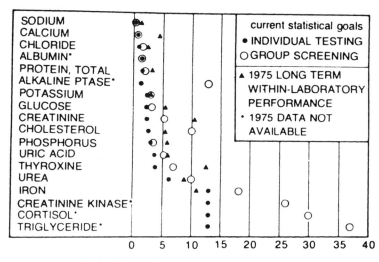

FIGURE 18–9. Some analytical goals for clinical analytes. For some tests (e.g., urea), analytical goals have been met. For others (e.g., thyroxine and creatinine) more work is needed to improve analytical precision. (From Aspen Conference on Analytical Goals: College of American Pathologists, Skokie, IL, p. 5, 1976)

Table 18-5
Data from CAP 1994 C-C Comprehensive Chemistry Survey

Analyte	Method	No. of Labs*	C-11 Mean	C-11 %CV	No. of Labs*	C-15 Mean	C-15 %CV
Albumin	All	5,928	2.71	8.8	5,899	4.48	7.1
	Automated BCG	3,490	2.62	9.8	3,476	4.33	7.0
Bilirubin, total	All	6,077	1.18	11.0	5,994	2.50	7.2
	Diazo-dyphylline coupling	1,411	1.18	8.0	1,400	2.45	5.3
Calcium	All	6,181	10.58	2.8	6,187	11.01	3.4
	Arsenazo III dye	2,910	10.64	2.7	2,923	11.23	3.0
Creatinine	All	6,704	1.26	9.4	6,646	2.77	6.0
	Enzymatic	1,437	1.20	3.6	1,431	2.86	3.0
Glucose	All	6,894	292.9	3.2	6,843	152.8	2.9
	Glucose oxidase colorimetric	1,546	285.2	1.9	1,547	151.7	2.5
Potassium	All	6,636	2.82	3.0	6,674	4.89	2.5
	ISE, direct	2,644	2.86	3.1	2,645	4.96	2.5
Urea N	All	6,733	18.4	7.7	6,720	31.3	6.7
	Urease quinolinium dye	1,457	16.4	3.8	1,454	28.3	3.3
Cholesterol	All	5,878	162.8	5.1	5,840	233.8	4.8
	Enzymatic	5,778	162.8	5.1	5,739	233.7	4.8

* Number of participants in the survey.
† Challenge number.

Commercial Surveys

Manufacturers of control materials have provided proficiency surveys. Because the availability of these programs changes frequently, laboratories should discuss their needs with manufacturers' representatives.

RESOLVING ANALYTICAL ERRORS WITH INTERRELATED SPECIMENS

When an out-of-control situation arises in the laboratory, it is often difficult to identify the problem as having to do with instrumentation, reagents, or inappropriate standardization. The use of interrelated specimens in a constant, pooled human-serum matrix can often resolve the problem. The advantages of these materials are several: Only the analytes of interest vary from specimen to specimen. The concentrations of protein, other analytes, and possible interferants are constant. They are prepared from pooled serum; therefore, they mimic patient specimens closely. Reference-grade materials can be used as the supplement for some analytes. With careful weighing, the concentration added to the pool can be calculated. More than one analyte can be checked at a time. If an enzyme is being investigated, the supplement can contain a simple analyte, such as NaCl, in addition to the enzyme. If on analysis for Na^+ or Cl^-, the expected linear relationships are obtained, then the specimens were prepared correctly. If the enzyme results are unsatisfactory, the problem lies not with the specimens, but with the method, instrument, or some other factor.

Interrelated specimens (Appendix 18–3) can be used in any laboratory for resolving an analytic problem. The supplementing material need not be highly purified; crude organ extracts can be used successfully for enzyme tests. For simple analytes like Na^+, Cl^-, glucose, and uric acid, pure materials should be used, because they will permit a calculation of the expected delta values as described in the appendix.

Operational Lines

The analytic results for tests fall on an operational line, that is, a plot of found (Y) versus expected (X) analytic values.[8] Typical operational lines are shown in Figure 18–10, which can be of great help in diagnosing analytic problems. Ideally, the operational line should have a slope of 1.00 and an intercept of zero.

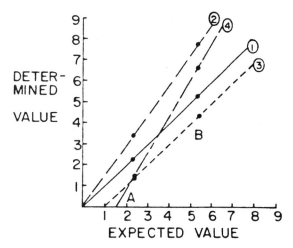

FIGURE 18–10. Illustration of some possible operational lines. When determined values are compared to expected values, the results should ideally agree and fall along line 1. Actual results may fall along lines 2, 3, 4, depending on the standard curve used for the determination. The data illustrate typical "operational lines" for analytical procedures. The operational lines can indicate specific kinds of method mis-standardization. See Table 18–6 for analyses of the operational lines. (From Grannis GF, Gruemer H-D, Lott JA, et al: Proficiency evaluation of clinical chemistry laboratories. Clin Chem 18:222, 1972)

Preparation of Operational Lines

How are operational lines determined? A simple procedure is to analyze CAP survey serum or other serum-based material of known content at the same time that calibrating materials are being used by the laboratory. CAP survey serum has been analyzed by thousands of laboratories. The values can be assumed to be correct or are an excellent estimate of the true values. Some examples of CAP data from the 1994 Comprehensive Chemistry Survey are given in Table 18–5. Results for the well-accepted methods are shown and the mean of all results. The means are extremely close, supporting the premise that extreme outliers become unimportant when the cohort is large.

A plot of the results from the known material (Y) versus the calibrators (X) used in the laboratory produces the operational line. Grannis showed that laboratories produced the expected relationships of interrelated survey specimens, suggesting that the mean values of all laboratories are excellent estimates of the true values. For serum calcium, the mean survey results by atomic absorption agreed with the values determined by the National Bureau of Standards using an

exacting method.[44] Assuming the survey specimens have not deteriorated, they are the most widely available materials that mimic patient specimens and for which an excellent estimate of the true value of the concentrations of the common analytes is available.

Analysis of Operational Lines

The types of operational lines in Figure 18–10 are summarized in Table 18–6. Line 1 is the ideal case of perfect agreement. For line 2, all values are too high by a proportional amount because the standards are less concentrated than believed. The mirror image about line 1 could be imagined; that is, all values are too low by a proportional amount because of standards that are more concentrated than believed. Line 4 occurs in an interesting way with instruments using single-point calibration if the baseline is misset.[45] Only results at the calibration point, or close to it, will be correct. If the baseline is set at 95% T, rather than 100% T, then all results below the standard will be too high, and all results above the standard will be too low. The error is not proportional to concentration but is related to it in a complex way as shown in the following equations:

$$\% \text{ Error} = [(A_{observed} - A_{correct})/A_{correct})] \times 100$$

$$\% \text{ Error} = Ab[1 - Cu/Cs)/As(Cu/Cs)] \times 100$$

where Ab is the absorbance setting of the baseline. As is the absorbance of the standard, Cs is the concentration of the standard, and Cu is the concentration of the unknown.

The absorbance of the standard plays a role; the worst errors occur with specimens that are less concentrated than the standard and with a standard having a low absorbance.[45]

LABORATORY MISTAKES

Defining Blunders

A mistake, or blunder, as distinct from analytic error, can result in grossly incorrect results leaving the laboratory. Much attention has been given to improving precision. The worst culprit—mistakes—deserves more attention in the laboratory. Typically, physicians are more aware of laboratory mistakes than the laboratory staff.

Blunder Detection

Grannis and coworkers estimated the mistake rate in a clinical chemistry laboratory based on suspect values coming to the PC section.[8] Mistakes were confirmed

Table 18-6
Analysis of Operational Lines From Figure 18-10

Line No.	Possible Problem(s)	Constant Bias	Proportional Bias
1	None	No	No
2	Standards less concentrated than believed: incorrect preparation, dilution, decomposition, and so forth	No	Yes
3	Inappropriate blank, all values too low by a fixed amount	Yes	No
4	Use of single-point calibration and inappropriate baseline; could also be combination of 2 and 3 above	Yes	Yes
5	Nonlinear response: loss of analytic sensitivity (line not shown)	No	?

before they were counted, and the rate was 3.5% for the laboratory and 0.2% for the PC section. Northam estimated errors from a proficiency survey[46]: 13% of the outliers were more than 10 SD from the mean, 22% were between 5 and 10 SDs, and 65% were between 3.2 and 5 SDs from the mean. A 5-SD error for sodium was 11 mmol/L. Some of the worst laboratories had a blunder rate of 10%.

In the CAP Enzyme Survey, specimen mix-ups are readily detected, because the results from a set of specimens within a mailing must be in a known sequence of increasing or decreasing values. Lott and coworkers estimated the blunder rate in the CAP Enzyme Survey at 4.1%; the mistakes probably occurred because of specimen mix-ups.[47]

Types of Mistakes

Grannis and coworkers provided a complete list of typical blunders.[8] The most serious blunders were mislabeling and misplacing specimens in an analyzer tray. The latter error can affect all of the specimens in the tray. Other types of mistakes were chart-reading errors, calculation errors, errors due to inappropriate reagents or faulty standards, errors due to neglect, unrecognized instrument problems, and mentally calculated results.

Reducing Laboratory Mistakes

Is a 3% to 4% mistake rate the irreducible minimum? For a clinical laboratory performing 6 million tests a year, this means 240,000 mistakes a year, or 657 a day! On the basis of our observations and those of Northam,

it is suggested that the procedures in Box 18–6 be implemented to reduce blunders.

EVALUATION OF NEW METHODS

Selection of a new method for any test in a clinical laboratory is a vital aspect for maintaining high-quality laboratory testing. Discussed here are primarily procedures that give a numeric result; however, some of the concepts are applicable to qualitative methods. The reasons for establishing a new test fall into two categories: (1) the test is new to the laboratory, or (2) the new test replaces an existing method.

Old methods are replaced for a host of reasons: the old procedure may be obsolete (eg, glucose by neocuproine); it may have poor clinical sensitivity or specificity (eg, the thymol turbidity test); it requires too large a specimen (eg, the Technicon SMAC); it has poor accuracy (eg, the titan yellow method for magnesium); it has poor precision (eg, the olive oil emulsion method for serum lipase); the reagents are poisonous or carcinogenic (eg, the NaCN–urea method for uric acid or the use of o-toluidine or benzidine). Many other reasons can be given for abandoning older procedures.

Before a new method is chosen, considerations of convenience, cost, and so forth, should be made. In Table 18–7 is a checklist of the most important factors that should be evaluated before a new procedure is implemented in the laboratory: patient-related factors, laboratory and associated personnel issues, and costs.

Method Comparison Studies

Clinical laboratorians are typically conservative. They want some assurance that the results of tests they are reporting are "correct." A new or replacement test can

Box 18•6

Suggested Procedures to Reduce Blunders

- The laboratory has a computerized information system for test requisitioning, accessioning, interfacing of equipment, reporting, log generation, inquiry, test requisitioning, and so forth.
- Primary tube sampling, where the instrument sips out of the bar-coded blood collection tube, is possible for most tests.
- Orders for laboratory studies are entered at the nursing station directly into a host or laboratory computer. The orders are transmitted automatically to the laboratory.
- Phlebotomists carry a portable computer or label maker and downloads orders periodically to their computer through telephone jacks or other means.
- The phlebotomist wands the patient's bar-coded wrist band. This identifies the patient, the computer determines if an active order exists for this patient, and the device makes a bar-coded label at the bedside.
- The bar-coded specimen (primary tube) is sampled directly in the laboratory on the analytical instrument; transfer tubes, "take-off" tubes, and the like are never used in the laboratory. The bar code on the tube identifies the specimen to the instrument. Only computer-generated log sheets are used.
- Manual pipeting is not done, and dilutions are never made. When the instrument encounters an out-of-range specimen, the instrument automatically makes a dilution and reanalyzes the specimen.
- Reagents are labeled with machine-readable tags; the instrument checks the validity of the reagent vessel and its expected contents, keeps a perpetual inventory, and warns the operator of a low-reagent situation.
- Real-time feedback of out-of-control results for proficiency specimens is available through the computer system.
- The number of steps or procedures between receipt of the specimen (or its collection) and delivery of the report are kept to an absolute minimum.
- Manual calculations are never performed, and hand-held calculators are forbidden. Only laboratory computer-controlled calculations are performed with suitable safeguards in the computer program.
- Real-time checks of today's patient results against previous results are made to identify impossible or erroneous values.[48]
- Multivariate computer checks are made of single results and sets of results for flagging impossible values or unlikely data, for example, high calcium and high phosphorus levels, low sodium and high chloride levels, and so on.[49]
- The laboratory staff is well trained and highly motivated to provide the best laboratory services possible. They can quickly identify unlikely results or unusual situations.[3]
- Pre-employment testing is performed to identify individuals who are likely to make transcription errors and similar mistakes.
- The automated equipment has an elaborate system of self-diagnostic steps and internal checks to detect malfunctions.

be judged for correctness only with considerable difficulty. A utopian and essentially impossible procedure is to compare the new and old methods with many specimens from patients with a great variety of disorders, the same receiving a long list of drugs, and patients of all ages and of both genders, including newborns and children. Furthermore, the new test is compared with the contemporary "gold standard" if possible. The latter may be extremely cumbersome and costly to carry out (eg, isotope dilution-mass spectrometry). In the real world, some compromises must be made. Nevertheless, a logical and cost-effective evaluation is possible.

Selection of a Reference Method

The most difficult aspect of method evaluation is judging accuracy. Absolute accuracy is unknowable; however, in some instances, good estimates of truth are possible. A few tests have been investigated in great detail, and reference methods or candidate reference methods exist that give excellent estimates of the true value if the details of the methods are adhered to with great care. They are listed in Table 18–1 as "Credentialed" or "Proposed" methods or materials. At the other extreme are tests for nearly all proteins (eg, immunoglobu-

Table 18-7
Checklist to Consider Before Implementing New Methods

Patient-Related Factors

Clinical sensitivity and specificity of test
Volume of specimen required
Difficulty in obtaining specimen
Reference ranges

Laboratory Personnel Issues

Accuracy and precision of method
Complexity of test or instrument, time to learn procedure
Dynamic or reportable range of test; linearity
Safety: presence of carcinogens, poisons, radionuclides
Throughput/automation, turnaround time
Freedom from interferences (ie, drugs, metabolites, other)
Convenience for one or many tests
Performed by all personnel on any shift
Analytical sensitivity and specificity

Costs

Costs of materials, instrument, service, utilities, personnel, maintenance contracts, and so on
Increase or decrease of costs in implementing new test
Costs of training laboratory staff
Disposal costs

lins); many hormones; trace elements, such as Al and Cr; coagulation factors; and other minor metabolites where there is extreme disagreement among various methods and no reference methods exist.

Comparison Studies

Assume that a reference method or a well-accepted procedure exists that will serve as the anchor or comparative protocol for the new method. The reference method need not be a "routine" method; that is, it could be one that is used only for comparison purposes. Required are patients' specimens that cover the dynamic range of the test. Preferably, the specimens should come from the well and sick and should include most or all of the clinical cases for which the test is designed. Three groups of patients that should always be included are babies, patients with end-stage renal disease, and pregnant individuals. The reason for this is that these patients often harbor unusual metabolites or unusual concentrations of known metabolites. If no test interferences are found with these groups, the test is probably generally free from interferences. The specimens are

analyzed by the new and reference procedures, preferably in duplicate, and graphed.

Typical X–Y charts are shown in Figure 18–11.[50] Here the reference titration method for serum lipase is compared to three candidate methods. Graphing the data is always necessary. Statistical evaluation, as discussed below, is necessary but insufficient. Graphs will reveal the degree of dispersion, disagreement, nonlinearity, gross errors, and slope or intercept errors. Some of these factors will not be apparent from the usual statistical calculations.

Statistical Tests of Comparison Data

Westgard and Hunt[51] evaluated the commonly performed statistical tests. The statistics with the greatest information content are the slope and intercept of the least-squares regression line and the SD of the scatter (in the Y direction), that is, Sy•x. The student-paired t test and the correlation coefficient contain little information or are impossible to evaluate (Table 18–8).

Slope of the Line

A sample regression plot is shown in Figure 18–12. The slope of the line is a measure of proportional bias. Assuming that there are no gross outliers, a slope greater than 1 means the Y values are generally higher. A slope of 1.11 means the Y values are on average 11% higher than the X values.

Intercept of the Line

The equation for the line in Figure 18–12 is Y = 1.11 X + 12. The method has a constant bias, and all Y values are at least 12 U higher than the X values.

Table 18-8
Value of Statistical Tests in Method-Comparison Studies

Statistical Test	Type of Error Detected		
	Random	Constant	Proportional
Slope of line	No	No	Yes
Y intercept of line	No	Yes	No
Sy·X	Yes	No	No
Correlation coefficient	Yes	No	No

Westgard JO, Barry PL, Hunt MR: A multi-rule Shewhart chart for quality control in clinical chemistry. Clin Chem 27:493, 1981

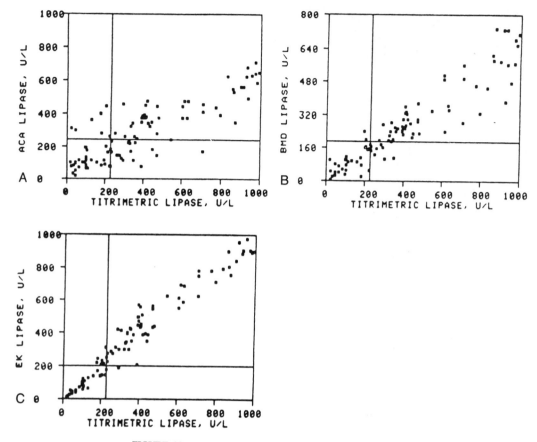

FIGURE 18–11. Correlation plots for serum lipase determinations. The same method is shown on the X-axis in all cases. The scatter about the line decreases from *A* to *B* to *C* and is reflected in the Sy·x statistic: for *A*, it is 201; for *B* it is 192; and for *C* it is 164. The horizontal and vertical lines within the figures are the upper reference limits of the two methods in each case. (From Lott JA, Patel ST, Sawhney AK, Kazmierczak SC, Love JE, Jr: Assays of serum lipase: Analytical and clinical considerations. Clin Chem, 32:1290, 1986)

Standard Error, Sy·x

The best-fit line to the paired data is shown in Figure 18–12. Vertical bars could be drawn to indicate the deviation of each point from the line in the Y direction. The mean bar length is proportional to the Sy·x statistic, and it is a measure of the scatter about the line. If all the points fit exactly in the line, Sy·x would be zero.

Correlation Coefficient (r)

This statistic is frequently quoted but poorly understood. An r value close to 1 does not mean agreement, only that the values go up and down in tandem. It is possible to have a huge proportional or constant bias and still have a near-perfect r. In Figure 18–12, r is 0.9967; however, the two methods really show poor agreement. A value of 50 by the "X" method corresponds to a value of 68 by the "Y" method.

Caragher and Grannis showed graphically that the r value is highly dependent on the distribution of the data: If a few outliers on the 45-degree line are added to a random cluster of data about the line, the r value increases dramatically.[52] In short, the r statistic is inappropriate and uninterpretable for the typical method comparison data being generated in clinical laboratories.

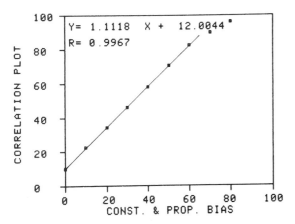

FIGURE 18–12. A sample correlation plot obtained during a method-comparison study. The regression equation, Y = mX + b, is shown at the top. There is a proportional bias (m) of about 11% and a constant bias (b) of 12 units. Note that the r value is very close to 1 despite the large proportional and large constant bias and a loss of linearity above about 80 units.

CLIA REQUIREMENTS FOR NEW METHODS

The CLIA requirements must be fulfilled before a new method can be implemented in the laboratory. The requirements are described elsewhere[1] and are summarized here.

Estimates of Accuracy

The laboratory must verify accuracy that can be performed by comparing patients' results with an accepted method, assaying materials with known values, or assaying sera from interlaboratory surveys. Determinations of accuracy are difficult. At best, an estimate can be made. To judge accuracy, a gold standard method must be available. A material that mimics patients' specimens closely and contains a known quantity of the analyte under study is also helpful. In Table 18–9 are techniques that have been used to estimate accuracy, how good these methods are, and how difficult it is to carry out the indicated study.

Estimates of Precision

Measuring the precision of a new method is straightforward. Control materials at two or more concentrations, preferably near decision points, are analyzed at least 10 times on each of 10 successive days. The within-day and between-day SDs are calculated, and L–J charts can be prepared and analyzed as described previously.

Analytical Sensitivity

Analytical sensitivity is confirmed by preparing dilutions of controls, standards, or specimens and determining the lowest concentration that can be determined reliably. Zero concentration is meaningless, and values that are smaller than the SD of the method also have no meaning.

Analytical Specificity

Analytical specificity can come from the manufacturer; however, checking for the effect of hemolysis, lipemia, and icterus is good laboratory practice. The study of potential interferants, if properly done, is generally elaborate.[18,53] The number of drugs in common use is huge, and seriously ill individuals typically receive 8 to 12 different drugs. An interference study should include the effects of lipemia, icterus, and hemolysis. Lipemia should be due to endogenous hypertriglyceridemia and not added Intralipid (Kabi Pharmacia, Clayton, NC, 60015), milk, or cream. Also, bilirubin should be added from patients' specimens. Adding bilirubin from an alkaline solution does not represent the endogenous form. A study of drugs should include the 20 or so most frequently prescribed agents; obviously, all drugs cannot be examined. A recovery study should be performed with the technique of interrelated specimens, as described previously. Ideally, adding the analyte to the blood or serum specimen should not change the endogenous matrix.

Table 18-9
Judging the Accuracy of a New Method

Approach	Value	Difficulty in Performing
Comparison with "definitive method"	Best	Extremely difficult
Comparison with "reference method"	Excellent	Difficult
Analysis of specimens with known values	Good	Easy
Comparison to routine method	Fair or poor	Easy
Recovery studies	Fair	Easy

Reportable Range of a Method

The reportable or dynamic range of a method is determined by analyzing a range of calibrators to define the upper and lower limits of the method. Generally, the reportable range includes the dynamic range where the instrument produces a linear response as the concentration is increased or decreased. The reportable range defines where dilutions must be made.

Reference Ranges

Finally, reference ranges must be established. Manufacturers' values can be used, or the laboratory can analyze specimens from 10 to 20 individuals in good health. Although this meets CLIA requirements, analysis of 10 to 20 specimens does not provide a reliable or usable reference range. Generally, at least 200 specimens from individuals in good health should be analyzed.[54]

Judging the Acceptability of a Method

The procedure described in Appendix 18–4 as a case study follows the approach of Westgard and coworkers.[55] Before this can be used, one must know the medically acceptable error or maximum error from the true value; an estimate of the true value must also be available.

REFERENCES

1. Health Care Financing Administration, Medicare, Medicaid and CLIA Programs; Revision of the clinical laboratory regulations for the Medicare, Medicaid, and Clinical Laboratory Improvement Act of 1967 programs; proposed rule. Fed Regist 53:29590, 1988
2. Passey R: Laboratory regulations: CLIA 1967. In Snyder JR, Wilkinson DS (eds): Management in Laboratory Medicine, 3rd ed, Philadelphia, J.B. Lippincott, 1995
3. Lott JA: Laboratory personnel: The most important aspect of quality control. Med Instrument 8:22, 1974
4. Lott JA, Wenger WC, Massion CG, et al: Inter-laboratory survey of enzyme analyses: IV. Human versus porcine tissue as source of creatine kinase for survey serum. Am J Clin Pathol 78:626, 1982
5. O'Donnell NJ, Lott JA: Intra-laboratory survey of alkaline phosphatase methods. Am J Clin Pathol 76:567, 1981
6. Pope WT, Caragher TE, Grannis GF: An evaluation of ethylene glycol-based liquid specimens for use in quality control. Clin Chem 25:413, 1979
7. Curme HG, et al: Multilayer film elements for clinical analysis. Clin Chem 24:1335, 1978
8. Grannis GF, Gruemer H-D, Lott JA, et al: Proficiency evaluation of clinical chemistry laboratories. Clin Chem 18:222, 1972
9. Cali JP, Mandel J, Moore L, et al: A referee method for the determination of calcium in serum. NBS Spec. Publ. 260-36, US Dept. of Commerce, National Bureau of Standards. Cat. No. C13.10:260. Washington, DC, US Government Printing Office, 1972
10. Neese JW, Duncan P, Bayse D, et al: Development and evaluation of a hexokinase/glucose-6 phosphate dehydrogenase procedure for use as a national glucose reference method. HEW Publication No. (CDC) 778830, Atlanta, Centers for Disease Control, 1976
11. Naito HK, Kwak Y-S, Hartfield JL, et al: Matrix effects on proficiency testing materials. Arch Pathol Lab Med 117:345, 1993
12. Eckfeldt JH, Copeland KR: Accuracy verification and identification of matrix effects. Arch Pathol Lab Med 117:381, 1993
13. Ross JW, Myers GL, Gilmore BF, et al: Matrix effects and the accuracy of cholesterol analysis. Arch Pathol Lab Med 117:393, 1993
14. Lasky FD: Achieving accuracy for routine clinical chemistry methods by using patient specimen correlations to assign calibrator values. Arch Pathol Lab Med 117:412, 1993
15. Lott JA, Bowers GN Jr: College of American Pathologists Conference XXIII on matrix effects and accuracy assessment in clinical chemistry. Arch Pathol Lab Med 117:433, 1993
16. Levey S, Jennings EF: The use of control charts in the clinical laboratory. Am J Clin Pathol 20:1059, 1950
17. Allen JR, Earp R, Farrell EC Jr, et al: Analytical bias in a quality control scheme. Clin Chem 15:1039, 1969
18. Lott JA, Turner K: Evaluation of Trinder's glucose oxidase method for measuring glucose in serum and urine. Clin Chem 21:1754, 1975
19. Lott JA, Smith DA, Mitchell LC, Moeschberger ML: Use of medians and "average of normals" of patients' data for the assessment of long-term analytical stability, Clin Chem 42:888, 1996
20. Westgard JO, Barry PL, Hunt MR: A multi-rule Shewhart chart for quality control in clinical chemistry. Clin Chem 27:493, 1981
21. Westgard JO: An internal quality control system for the assessment of quality and the assurance of test rules. Scand J Clin Lab Invest 44:315, 1984
22. Westgard JO, Falk H, Groth T: Influence of a between-run component of variation, choice of control limits, and shape of error distribution on the performance characteristics of rules for internal quality control. Clin Chem 25:394, 1979
23. Westgard JO, Groth T: Power functions for statistical control rules. Clin Chem 25:863, 1979
24. Westgard JO, Groth T, DeVerdier CH: Principles of developing improved quality control procedures. Scand J Clin Invest 44(Suppl 172):19, 1984
25. Amador E: Quality control by the reference sample method. Am J Clin Pathol 50:360, 1968
26. Grannis GF, Caragher TE: Quality-control programs in clinical chemistry. CRC Crit Rev Clin Lab Sci 7:327, 1977
27. Barnett RN: Medical significance of laboratory results. Am J Clin Pathol 50:671, 1968
28. Skendzel LP, Barnett RN, Platt R: Medically useful criteria for analytic performance of laboratory tests. Am J Clin Pathol 83:200, 1985

29. Lott JA, Manning NR, Kyler MK: Proficiency testing in a medical-needs context. Clin Chem 35:347–354, 1989

30. Lott JA, Surufka N, Massion CG: Proficiency testing of serum enzymes based on medical-needs criteria. Arch Pathol Lab Med 115:11, 1991

31. Tonks DB: A study of the accuracy and precision of clinical chemistry determinations in 170 Canadian laboratories. Clin Chem 9:217, 1963

32. Cotlove E, Harris EK, Williams GZ: Biological and analytic components of variation in long-term studies of serum constituents in normal subjects: III. Physiological and medical implications. Clin Chem 16:1028, 1970

33. Harris EK, Kanofsky P, Shakarji G, et al: Biological and analytical components of variation in long-term studies of serum constituents in normal subjects: II. Estimating biological components of variation. Clin Chem 16:1022, 1970

34. Glick JH: Expression of random analytical error as a percentage of the range of clinical interest. Clin Chem 22:475, 1976

35. Lindberg DAB, Watson FR: Imprecision of laboratory determinations and diagnostic accuracy: Theoretical considerations. Meth Inform Med 13:151, 1974

36. Harris EK: Statistical principles underlying analytic goal-setting in clinical chemistry. Am J Clin Pathol 72:374, 1979

37. Lott JA, Hebert LA, Baer SG: Use of computer graphics to assess trends in glomerular filtration rate (GFR) from sequential serum creatinine values. J Med Tech 1:361, 1984

38. Campbell DG, Owen JA: Clinical laboratory error in perspective. Clin Biochem 1:3, 1968

39. Fraser CG: The application of theoretical goals based on biological variation data in proficiency testing. Arch Pathol Lab Med 112,4, 1988

40. Watson RA, Tang DB: The predictive value of prostatic acid phosphatase as a screening test for prostatic cancer. N Engl J Med 303:497, 1980

41. Lott JA, Abbott LB, Koch DD: An evaluation of the DuPont aca IV: Does it meet medical needs? Clin Chem 31:281, 1985

42. Ehrmeyer SS, Laessig RH, Leinweber JE, Oryall FF: 1990 Medicare/CLIA final rules for proficiency testing: Minimum intra-laboratory performance characteristics (CV and bias) needed to pass. Clin Chem 36:1736, 1990

43. Aspen Conference on Analytical Goals, p 5. College of American Pathologists, Skokie, IL, 1976

44. Grannis GF: Studies of the reliability of constituent target values established in a large inter-laboratory survey. Clin Chem 22:1027, 1976

45. Lott JA: Hazards of incorrect use of the calibration wheel and single-point calibration. Lab Med 8:25, 1977

46. Northam BE: Whither automation? Ann Clin Biochem 18:189, 1981

47. Lott JA, O'Donnell NJ, Grannis GF: Inter-laboratory survey of enzyme analyses III. Does College of American Pathologists' Survey Serum mimic clinical specimens? Am J Clin Pathol 76:554, 1981

48. Ladenson JH: Patients as their own controls: Use of the computer to identify "laboratory error." Clin Chem 21:1648, 1976

49. Lindberg DAB, Vanpeenen HS, Couch RD: Patterns in clinical chemistry. Am J Clin Pathol 44:315, 1965

50. Lott JA, Patel ST, Sawhney AK, Kazmierczak SC, Love JE Jr: Assays of serum lipase: Analytical and clinical considerations. Clin Chem 32:1290, 1986

51. Westgard JO, Hunt MR: Use and interpretation of common statistical tests in method-comparison studies. Clin Chem 19:49, 1973

52. Caragher TE, Grannis GF: Design of quality-control specimens for use with a small multi-channel analyzer. Clin Chem 23:2011, 1977

53. Lott JA, Stephan VA, Pritchard KA Jr: Evaluation of the Coomassie Brilliant Blue G-250 method for urinary protein. Clin Chem 29:1046, 1983

54. Lott JA, Mitchell LS, Moeschberger ML, Sutherland DE: Estimation of reference ranges: How many subjects are needed? Clin Chem 38:648, 1992

55. Westgard JO, Carey RN, Wold S: Criteria for judging precision and accuracy in method development and evaluation. Clin Chem 20:825, 1974

56. National Committee for Clinical Laboratory Standards (NCCLS), 771 E. Lancaster Avenue, Villanova, PA 19085. 610-525-2435.

57. Physician Office Laboratory News, February 1995

ACKNOWLEDGEMENTS

I wish to thank Bernadette L. Thornton for her help in the many tasks of the Proficiency Testing Laboratory and for her extensive help in collecting the process control statistics.

APPENDIX 18–1 PROBLEMS IN PROCESS CONTROL (PC) AND PROFICIENCY TESTING (PT)

Summary of problems:

1. Definition of performance and PC limits
2. Setting PC limits
3. Achieving agreement of two (or more) analyzers
4. Controlling and testing for bias
5. Frequency of analysis of PC materials
6. Checking for shifts in the mean with a change in reagents
7. Establishing mean values for PC materials
8. Checking for stability of patient's values with a change in reagents
9. Change in appearance of Levey–Jennings (L–J) charts
10. Bias and random error: their impact on passing CLIA challenges
11. The "problem" tests that require more attention

Examples:

1. What is the difference between performance and PC limits?
   - Performance limits are those calculated from results obtained on an instrument. The standard deviation (SD) is calculated in the usual way from a set of values. PC limits are defined as limits used in routine use that meet 40% of the allowed CLIA

criteria or medical needs, whichever is more appropriate. Performance and PC limits are *not* the same.

2. The personnel in a laboratory want to set PC limits for glucose. Their current routine performance with a mainframe instrument is $+/- 1.2$ mg/dL (1 SD) at 120 mg/dL (6.66 mmol/L). For glucose, the CLIA-allowed error limits are $+/- 6$ mg/dL or $+/- 10\%$, whichever is greater. What upper limit (UL) and lower limit (LL) should they set to ensure meeting medical needs and to pass CLIA challenges consistently?

   - Use 40% of the allowed CLIA limits (= 10%) here. At a glucose concentration of 120 mg/dL, this is 120 mg/dL $\times$ 0.10 $\times$ 0.40 = 4.8 mg/dL. This value is 4 SDs, therefore, they use a 1_{4s} rule for the PC charts and routine assays. All values falling outside of $+/- 4.8$ mg/dL from the mean are considered to be out of control. The bias in this laboratory is very close to zero as determined with the method described below in question 4.

   What about the same PC QC limits for their high-concentration glucose control (ie, 300 mg/dL [16.7 mmol/L]) 1 SD at 300 mg/dL is 3 mg/dL.

   - Use the same 40% of the allowed CLIA limits; 40% of the CLIA allowance is 300 mg/dL $\times$ 0.10 $\times$ 0.40 = 12 mg/dL. The laboratory elects to use the 1_{4s} rule, and their PC charts are constructed accordingly. Any value outside of 300 $\pm$ 12 mg/dL is out of control.

3. A laboratory with two mainframe analyzers attempts always to have the two instruments agree on all tests. The same cholesterol control shows a long-term mean of 303 mg/dL (7.77 mmol/L) on instrument A and 305 mg/dL (7.90 mmol/L) on instrument B. Both instruments A and B consistently produce data with 1 SD of 4.0 mg/dL at 300 mg/dL. From a conservative perspective, should either instrument A or B be recalibrated?

   - 1 SD for either instrument is 4.0 mg/dL. Because the instruments agree within 2 mg/dL that is less than 1 SD (performance limits), no recalibration is needed at this time. If the two instruments consistently do not differ by more than 1 SD, no recalibration is required.

4. Prior to assaying CLIA challenges, a laboratory wants to be certain that their bias is as low as possible. What are some ways of checking for bias?

   - a. Assay calibrators at least five times as unknowns and average the results. The mean should be < 1 SD (performance limits) from the labeled and presumed correct value.
   - b. Assay CAP or other well-assayed survey serum, and compare your value with the expected or published value. The mean should

be < 1 SD (performance limits) from the labeled value.
   - c. Assay any other fluid that has established values and does not exhibit matrix effects on the instrument, and follow the protocol above.

5. How often should I assay PC materials on my instrument?

   - The general recommendation is that two different controls should be assayed at least once per 24 hours, which meets CLIA standards. We ask our staff to assay the controls at the beginning of their shift to ensure themselves that the patients' results are in control.

6. When we shifted to another lot of the same generation of Vitros slides, our glucose mean, determined on 30 replicates over a 1-week period, shifted from 100 to 101 mg/dL. Should we recalibrate our instrument with the lot change?

   - For glucose at 100 mg/dL, the laboratory's 1 SD performance limit is 1.0 mg/dL. Because the shift is = 1 SD, the instrument is not recalibrated.

7. How can we establish the mean of an unassayed control fluid?

   - The mean can be established with good reliability if at least five replicates are analyzed per day over a 7-day period. The 1 SD for the values must not exceed the 1 SD (performance) limits, established during periods of "good" or "stable" performance. There must be no slide lot changes nor recent adjustments of any kind of the instrument.

8. If I start using a new generation of slides, how can I be sure that my results on patients do not shift?

   - A simple approach is to reassay at least 20 patients' specimens before and after the generation change. Determine the mean bias, which should be < 1 SD (performance limits).

9. With the new definition of PC with UL and LL, my L–J charts look different than in the past; the values are clustered together near the mean; there are very few values near the UL or LL and no values outside of UL or LL. I'm not used to the way my charts look, and the CAP inspector questioned the appearance of our L–J charts, particularly for some tests like LD for which I'm using a 1_{4s} rule.

   - Yes, the PC QC charts look different than they did in the past; it is the expected result because performance is better. With good documentation of how you derived your limits and sign-off by your director, there should be no question of the validity of your approach. Complete documentation is critical according to CLIA regulations. A signed document stating your policies from your lead technologist, director, or department head should serve this purpose.

10. In the assay for total protein with a mean value of 8.0 g/dL, we had a bias of 0.3 g/dL and a perfor-

mance SD of 0.4 g/dL. What is the likelihood that we will fail a CLIA challenge?[42]

- The CLIA allowance for total protein is 10% of the value; for a specimen with a TP of 8.0 g/dL, 10% is 0.8 g/dL. On the chart from Ehrmeyer and co-workers,[42] the horizontal line for a 0.3 g/dL bias (40% of CLIA allowance) and the vertical line for a SD of 0.4 g/dL random error (50% of CLIA allowance) cross at an approximately 3% chance of failing the CLIA challenge. If the bias is reduced to zero, the chance of failing drops to about 1.5%.

11. What are the "problem" tests where we have the greatest likelihood of failing a CLIA challenge?
- These tests are evident from the Table 18–4 where you must use the most restrictive PC limits (ie, the 1_{2s} rule). The tests are ALT, AST, Cl, PCO_2, and Na. Here, the SD for even excellent performance is close to 40% of the CLIA limit. The CLIA limits for ALT and AST are too tight ($\pm$ 20%), and it is illogical that for the other enzyme tests, a $\pm$ 30% allowance is given.

* Note that the Vitros is used as the example instrument. The principles here apply to other clinical analyzers as well.

APPENDIX 18–2 PROFICIENCY TESTING PROVIDERS[57]

Accutest
P.O. Box 999
Westford, MA 01886-0031
(800) 356-6788

American Academy of Family Physicians
8880 Ward Parkway
Kansas City, MO 64114-2797
(800) 274-2237

American Academy of Pediatrics
P.O. Box 927
Elk Grove Village, IL 60009-0927
(800) 433-9016

American Association of Bioanalysts
205 West Levee Street
Brownsville, TX 78520-5596
(800) 234-5315

American Osteopathic Association
142 East Ontario Street
Chicago, IL 60611
(800) 621-1773

American Proficiency Institute
121 East Front Street, Suite 201
Traverse City, MI 49684
(800) 333-0958

American Society of Internal Medicine
Medical Laboratory Evaluation
2011 Pennsylvania Ave. NW #800
Washington, DC 20006-1808
(800) 338-2746

American Thoracic Society
1740 Broadway
New York, NY 10019-4374
(212) 315-7400

California Thoracic Society
202 Fashion Lane #219
Tustin, CA 92680
(714) 730-1944

College of American Pathologists
325 Wankegan Road
Northfield, IL 60093-2750
(800) 323-4040

Idaho Bureau of Laboratories
2220 Old Penitentiary Road
Boise, Idaho 83712
(208) 334-2235

New Jersey Department of Health
CN 360
Trenton, NJ 08625-0360
(609) 530-6172

New York State Department of Health
Nelson Rockefeller Empire State Plaza
P.O. Box 509
Albany, NY 12201-0509
(518) 474-8739

Ohio Department of Health
1571 Perry Street
P.O. Box 2568
Columbus, OH 43216-2568
(614) 466-2278

Pacific Biometrics Research Foundation
1100 Eastlake Avenue East
Seattle, WA 98109
(206) 233-9151

Pennsylvania Department of Health
Bureau of Laboratories
P.O. Box 500
Exton, PA 19341-0500
(215) 363-8500

Puerto Rico Department of Health
Laboratory Services Program
Building A
Call Box 70184
San Juan, PR 00936
(809) 764-6945

Solomon Park Research Institute
12815 N.E. 124th Street
Kirkland, WA 98034
(206) 821-7005

Wisconsin State Laboratory of Hygiene
465 Henry Mall
Madison, WI 53706-1578
(800) 462-5261

APPENDIX 18-3 USE OF INTERRELATED SPECIMENS TO RESOLVE ANALYTICAL PROBLEMS

In the example here, uric acid is used as the test analyte being investigated. Creatinine has been added to the supplement to permit checking if the specimens have been prepared properly.

Preparation of Interrelated Specimens With Uric Acid Supplement

Using universal precautions, pool about 60 mL of fresh patients' sera. Use only clean, nonturbid, nonhemolyzed, nonicteric sera. Strain through gauze for the removal of small fibrin clots. This is the base pool. Prepare the uric acid supplementing solution, and prepare on the day of use; do not add formaldehyde if a uricase method is being used. The recipe is:

Uric acid (reagent grade or equivalent): 100 mg
    (weigh to nearest 0.1 mg)
Creatinine: 100 mg (weigh to nearest 0.1 mg)
Lithium carbonate: 100 mg
Distilled H_2O, enough to make 100 mL of solution

Dissolve the Li_2CO_3 in 80 mL H_2O, add the uric acid and creatinine, dissolve, and bring to 100 mL in a volumetric flask with distilled water. Prepare two pools as follows:

Pool A: 25-mL base pool + 2 mL supplement (1 mg uric acid + 1 mg creatinine/mL)
Pool B: 25-mL base pool + 2 mL 154 mmol/l NaCl (saline)

Note: The concentration of the uric acid in the supplement is about 10 to 20 times normal, and the volume of the supplement used is about 5% to 10% of the total volume of Pool A. The volume of the supplement is kept low to prevent excessive dilution of the base pool matrix.

Prepare interrelated specimens as shown in Table 18-10.

Note that the matrix of the interrelated specimens is constant, and the difference in uric acid and creatinine concentration, that is, the delta concentration between adjacent specimens, is constant, assuming that the specimens have been prepared properly.

Table 18-10
Interrelated Specimen Example

Specimen number	1	2	3	4	5	6
Parts or volumes of Pool A	0	1	2	3	4	5
Parts or volumes of Pool B	5	4	3	2	1	0
Total volume or parts	5	5	5	5	5	5

Analysis

Analyze the specimens for uric acid and creatinine. If an independent method is available for uric acid, use it also for the six interrelated specimens.

Calculations

The values determined by analysis for samples 1 to 6 are used in the calculations. Incorrect values for uric acid as determined by analysis do not render the method useless; the data are still usable, although of lesser value.

Calculate the expected values as follows:

Pool A concn. = [25 (concn. base pool) + 2 (concn. in supplement)]/27
Pool B concn. = [25 (concn. base pool) + 0]/27
For Specimen 1, the concentrations are the same as in Pool A.
Specimen 2 = [80 (Pool A concn.) + 20 (Pool B concn.)]/100
Specimen 3 = [60 (Pool A concn.) + 40 (Pool B concn.)]/100

and so on. The delta values are simply the difference in concentration of uric acid or creatinine of adjacent specimens, that is:

Delta 1 for uric acid = uric acid found in Specimen 1 − uric acid found in Specimen 2.
Delta 2 for uric acid = uric acid found in Specimen 2 − uric acid found in Specimen 3 and so on.

Data Analysis

If the deltas for the control analyte, creatinine, are very similar, and the found values are very close to the expected values, then the specimens were properly prepared. If the deltas for the test analyte, uric acid, are

- highly variable, the method has poor precision.
- increasing with increasing concentration of uric acid, the method has a positive proportional bias.
- decreasing with increasing concentration of uric acid, the method has a negative proportional bias.

Also, if a plot of found concentration of uric acid versus percent pool A in the specimens is not straight, then the response is nonlinear, or there is a loss of linearity at higher concentrations.

APPENDIX 18±4

A Case Study of Method Acceptability
Work through the problem below; the answers follow. A new uric acid test method is to be evaluated. The test method uses uricase coupled to an insoluble matrix plus an electrode that determines oxygen consumption as in the following reaction:

$$\text{Uric acid} + 2\,H_2O + O_2$$

$$\uparrow \text{allantoin} + CO_2 + H_2O_2$$

The reference method also uses the above reaction but with a colorimetric end-point. The reference method is considered to be reliable and is believed to give accurate results.

Data

1. The medically acceptable error over the analytic range of 3.0 to 12 mg/DL is ± 10% (CV). Thus, at 5.0 mg/dL, the allowable error is ± 0.5 mg/dL.
2. A control serum analyzed 34 times over 1 month with the test method gives a mean 5.2 ± 0.14 (SD) mg/dL.

3. Linear regression analysis of the test method with the reference method on 50 patient specimens gives:

$$Y\,(\text{ref}) = mx(\text{test}) + b$$

where m is the slope, and b is the intercept on the Y axis.

$$Y = 1.02 \times + 0.10$$

4. At 5.0 mg/dL for test, the reference method gives $Y = 1.02\,(5.0) + 0.10 = 5.3$ mg/dL. Thus, the test method has a proportional error of 2% (slope of 1.02) and a constant error of 0.10 mg/dL (intercept of 0.10).
5. Is the test method acceptable? (Answers are below.)

a. Random error (RE)
   RE = 2 × SD = _____ mg/dL. (Use the SD determined from the control.)

The random error is acceptable/not acceptable (circle) because it is less than/greater than the allowable error of 0.5 mg/dL.

b. Systematic error (SE)
   SE = Found − Correct value
   5.20 − 5.0 = _____ mg/dL

The systematic error is acceptable/not acceptable (circle) because it is less than/greater than allowable error of 0.5 mg/dL.

c. Total error (TE) = RE + SE
   TE = _____ mg/dl + _____ mg/dL.

The total error is acceptable/not acceptable (circle) because it is less than/greater than allowable error of 0.5 mg/dL.

Answers:
a. RE = 0.28, acceptable, less than
b. SE = 0.20, acceptable, less than
c. TE = 0.48, acceptable, less than

19

Computers and Laboratory Information Systems

John R. Svirbely • Jack W. Smith, Jr. • Carl Speicher

Clinical laboratories perform the laboratory tests requested by physicians. They must generate the right data on the right person and deliver it to a locatable place within a medically useful period of time. Many kinds of tests are performed, several of which must be available 24 hours a day. This results in a considerable flow of information into, through, and out of the laboratory.

The collection and communication of information by the clinical laboratories may be viewed simplistically as two separate processing cycles (Fig. 19-1), one being an extralaboratory communication cycle and the other an intralaboratory analysis cycle. The extralaboratory cycle consists of afferent and efferent limbs. The afferent limb involves test ordering, specimen collection, and its delivery, while the efferent limb consists of report generation and delivery to the physician. The intralaboratory cycle involves accessioning test requests and patient specimens, dividing the specimens into aliquots, delivering them to the appropriate workstation, performing the test, and generating the result report. The organization of an institution and its laboratory profoundly affects the information flow so that, in practice, numerous subcycles arise for failure in handling and troubleshooting situations.

Computers were introduced into clinical laboratories during the 1960s to aid in the information-processing task. Today, computers are extensively distributed and integrated within the clinical laboratory. They serve an essential role in information processing and are expected to have an increasingly larger role in the future. This chapter is an overview of how the modern laboratory information system (LIS) uses computers for efficient information management. We first discuss the problems encountered in information processing before the advent of computers. We then cover the "clas-

sic" roles for computers in the laboratory and the newer roles computers have today. Finally, we discuss how to select and install an LIS.

PROBLEMS IN INFORMATION HANDLING PRIOR TO COMPUTERIZATION

Manual information systems can function adequately when the workload is limited in volume, the timeliness of the results is unimportant, and a level of tolerance to error exists. However, for the last 3 decades, there has been a relatively constant rate of increase in the number of tests performed annually, with a greater need for urgency in reporting results for which any degree of error is unacceptable.

By the late 1950s, laboratories were already finding themselves unable to handle the constantly rising workload. Most test procedures in the clinical laboratories at that time were done individually, by hand. In addition, much of the clerical work associated with the tests was done by the same technologist who was performing the test. For each test, several stages were involved in information handling, each of which could delay processing or result in an error. Particularly troublesome were specimen misidentification, transcription errors, illegible handwriting, and misplaced reports.

There was hope that the introduction of automated analytic instruments would solve some of these problems. However, because data could be generated in large amounts rapidly, the capacity of the data-interpretive processes within the laboratory was easily overwhelmed. Rather than simplifying the situation, test automation contributed to further decompensation. The emergence of automated information processing was necessitated.

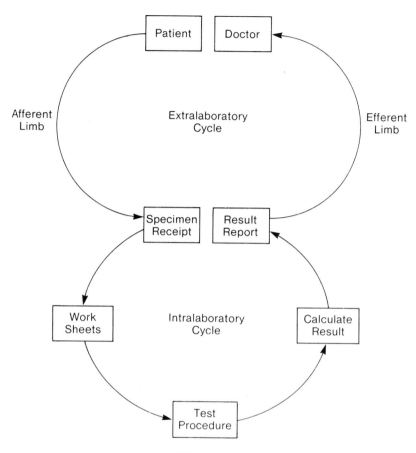

FIGURE 19–1. The laboratory information cycles.

OVERVIEW OF COMPUTER SYSTEMS

A computer alone does not constitute an LIS. An LIS consists of computer hardware, software, data, and personnel.

Computer hardware consists of the actual computer machinery. The central processing unit (CPU) is where the principal computer operations are performed. Data being sent to or received from the CPU are stored in random access memory, which is fast but typically of a finite size (measured in bytes, where one megabyte is 1 million bytes). Larger amounts of data require slower storage devices, such as magnetic disks, magnetic tapes, and optical disks; these media permit more "permanent" storage of information.

Users can directly access computers by means of terminals, such as the cathode ray tube, or microcomputers running terminal emulation software. These devices may be directly connected to the computer if nearby or may make use of modulating-demodulating devices (modems) if remote from the computer. Information stored in the computer is output on printers, which range in their capabilities in speed and output quality.

Computers can be connected to each other over communication networks, which use sophisticated protocols for exchange of information. Laboratory instruments, which usually contain their own microprocessors, can directly exchange data with the LIS computer by means of instrument "interfaces." These interfaces may be one way from the instrument to the LIS (unidirectional) or may allow downloading of patient demographics from the LIS to the instrument with uploading of results to the LIS (bidirectional).

Software consists of the commands by which the hardware is controlled and directed. Computers operate by means of a binary code (0, or off; 1, or on); however, the actual language used by the machine (machine code) is both difficult and time-consuming for people to use. This has necessitated development of high-level languages, such as FORTRAN or UNIX, which are easier for programmers to use, but whose commands must be translated by the computer into the machine code that it understands. The operating system is the software that allocates system resources among the different processes running simultaneously. Software packages, such as an LIS, consist of a number (often very large) of specialized programs written in high- or low-level languages to implement certain desired functions. The functional implementation of the LIS is discussed in the next section.

Data are the actual information the computer uses or generates in its computations. Data may be acquired by direct manual entry but more often is input over instrument interfaces. This information can be stored on various kinds of hardware devices, the choice of which depends on how much data must be stored, how fast it must be retrieved, how often it will be accessed, and how long it needs to be available. Because patient information is confidential and may be sensitive, special provisions for data security are required, as are discussed in the next section.

Specially trained personnel are required for optimal computer system operation. The system manager is the director for the computer system; he interfaces with hospital administrators, allocates resources, and directs projects. Programmers develop and maintain software programs. System analysts interface between system users and programmers to design the applications that will be implemented by the programmers. Operators are the people who perform the actual support functions for the computer system (printer maintenance, report generation, data backup to or retrieval from storage media).

THE FUNDAMENTAL FUNCTIONS OF THE LABORATORY INFORMATION SYSTEM

An LIS must be capable of performing many different functions. We describe these in relation to their location in the laboratory information cycles, as shown in Figure 19–1.

The Laboratory Information System and the Extralaboratory Cycle—Afferent Limb

The afferent limb of the extralaboratory information cycle involves test ordering and the delivery of necessary specimens to the laboratory. Test ordering minimally requires completion of a test requisition form (paper or computer based) with sufficient information to identify the patient uniquely (full name and a unique identification number), indication of the type of determinations required, and indication of the person to whom the results should be reported. After a test is ordered, specimens should be correctly collected, labeled, and then transported to the laboratory.

The most important problem in this cycle involves specimen and patient identification. No completely reliable, generally accepted, and cost effective system for specimen and patient identification is available. Patient identification systems using bar codes are becoming more widespread but are expensive and require cooperation between different hospital departments. In most laboratories, patient identification still requires that the specimen collection personnel either read the patient's identification bracelet or ask the patient his or her name and birthdate.

In other ways, however, the LIS can simplify the afferent limb for the laboratory. By referring to centralized patient demographic (admission-discharge-transfer, or ADT) information, the LIS can update patient status and location on an ongoing basis. This permits accurate collection of specimens and reporting of results, with a minimum of delays and errors. Much of the information required to complete a test requisition can be automatically retrieved from this source.

Communication links between patient care units and the laboratory computer greatly improve the test-ordering process, in comparison with older manual methods. The ability of patient care units to order tests and obtain results by such links improves handling of information transfer, particularly in emergency situations.

For nonemergency situations, the LIS can use requisition data to prepare collection lists for specimen collection personnel; such lists permit more efficient specimen collection and result in fewer collection errors. By synchronizing specimen collection times throughout an institution, maximum advantage can be taken of economies of scale in high throughput laboratory instrumentation, with resources adjusted for peak periods of demand. This can provide a cost-effective and acceptable turnaround time for the majority of test requests. New hand-held devices allow phlebotomists to document collection times and specimen information while on the patient units; this information can be uploaded into the LIS on return to the laboratory.

The Intralaboratory Cycle

Clerical Functions

Within the laboratory, many clerical duties are associated with performing tests. First, test requests must be tabulated and arrangements made for specimen collection. When a specimen is received in the laboratory, it is recorded and assigned a unique identifier (accessioned). The specimen is then divided into appropriate aliquots, which are distributed with worksheets to the different analytic workstations. After tests are performed and the results verified, reports are generated in a useful format and delivered to the appropriate physician offices and patient locations. Finally, any inquiries concerning pending or incomplete procedures must be answered, whereas completed reports must be placed in archival storage in a retrievable manner.

Reduction in clerical errors and improvement in efficiency were some of the first improvements noted with the introduction of computers into the laboratory. The LIS can integrate the accessioning process, generate worksheets, and data collection. An essential feature is the ability to maintain a tracking log for each test request, which contains the data entered on that request at each stage of processing. This record maintains the connection of the specimen to the patient, permits interim status inquiries, and is needed for data interpretation. Later we further discuss the role of the LIS in reporting results.

Data Acquisition and Manipulation for Quantitative Tests

Laboratories can be roughly divided into two kinds based on the general nature of the results that they generate. One kind generates data that are primarily numeric and are the result of quantitative analyses. The second kind generates primarily descriptive results, which are expressed in varying amounts of text. Examples of the first kind are the chemistry and hematology laboratories; examples of the second are the microbiology and surgical pathology laboratories. The success of computers in data handling has varied because of this essential difference in the type of data generated.

Some of the earliest uses of computers in the laboratory involved their use for data acquisition from laboratory instruments. The advent of semiautomated and then fully automated instruments, which were capable of performing multiple analyses on a single specimen, made the ability to collect and store the increased amount of data in a similarly automated way desirable. This eliminated human error and time delays associated with data collection and entry. The first attempts at data acquisition used off-line input with mark-sense or punched cards and some human coding of instrument outputs. Subsequent instruments produced output on a machine-readable medium that could later be fed into a computer. Later, direct instrument–computer interfaces, for which the computer used the analog output from instruments to obtain digitalized results, were used for data input. The earliest success with this direct interface was achieved with the AutoAnalyzer (Technicon

Corporation), the IL flame photometer, and the Coulter blood cell analyzer. Once data were stored in the computer, it was a simple matter to perform data manipulation, with curve interpolation, statistical calculation, or other mathematic functions being used to generate analyte results directly from raw data. The combination of automated analyses and automated data handling allowed development of powerful instruments that permit a very high volume of testing to be performed.

Let us examine more closely how the typical online instrument interface transmits data in real time through a direct hardware connection without human intervention. In the AutoAnalyzer (Fig. 19-2), the transmittance of light through a solution is measured by an electronic detector, which generates a voltage. The peak value of this voltage is directly proportional to the amount of the analyte being measured, with the proportionality factor determined by testing a series of standard solutions of known concentration and generating a working curve. To determine the analyte value, a computer must digitalize the voltage over time (analog-to-digital conversion). The peak value may then be found by making use of various peak detection algorithms that make use of curvature parameters, such as slope changes or derivatives of the input. This value is then interpolated to a working curve for obtaining a result, which may be subjected to further calculations for a final determination of the actual analyte value. The data acquisition computer must have a list of how to associate each peak with a specimen type and the analyte being measured. This is traditionally accomplished by the input of "loading" lists that specify the identity of each sample as "patient specimen," "test standard," or "quality assurance sample." In this way, the online interface can convert data in a raw form (varying voltage) to a digital analyte value, which can be stored.

The data acquisition interface was originally achieved in the central laboratory computer. However, developments in computer interfacing have taken it out of the central computer and placed it directly in the instrument. Many automated instruments now come equipped with preprocessors that convert the raw data generated by the instrument into data results, which are output in a uniform digital format. Indeed, other aspects of data handling can now be achieved locally in the instruments themselves.

A computer may be used as a process controller for the mechanical operation of the instruments and for data handling. In 1970 the first computer-controlled laboratory instrument, the Automated Clinical Analyzer (ACA, DuPont), was made available. It incorporated a hard-wired computer to control instrument function and calculate results from raw data and output results for direct reporting. Size and price reductions have hastened the incorporation of computers into laboratory

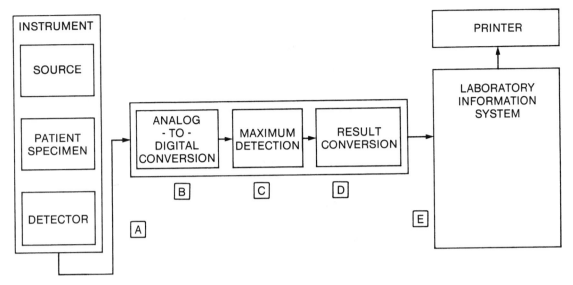

FIGURE 19–2. Data acquisition from an analytical instrument. Data from an online instrument are processed in the following steps:

A. Instrument output

B. Analog-to-digital conversion

C. Maximum (peak) detection

D. Result calculation (converting test data to an analyte value). The amount of a substance can be determined by interpolating the slope of its reactivity curve to a working curve made by testing standard solutions of known activity.

E. Storage of result in the central LIS

The intermediate processing steps (B–D) involved in converting instrument output were initially located in the central LIS computer, but now they are usually located in the instruments themselves.

instruments to control instrumentation components, acquire and process data, and format instrumental output. Since then, the trend is toward highly automated, intelligent, stand-alone instrument systems with dedicated processing and control computers.

Data Acquisition and Manipulation in Descriptive Domains

Computerization has been slower and more difficult in laboratory divisions like microbiology and the anatomic pathology services, where data are non-numeric and often visually oriented. This has not been due to a lack of effort, because the advantages of computerized information processing in these domains were appreciated early. However, certain features of the domains have limited development of computerized systems. Specimens analyzed in these laboratories may undergo many nonautomated processing and interpretive steps; these may take varying periods of time—days, weeks, even

months—to complete. In addition, their reports may make use of a nonstandard terminology and use variable amounts of natural language text ("free text") in nonstandard formats, all of which are unpredictable at the time of specimen receipt. These factors make data storage and retrieval more difficult than for the quantitative domains, where the results are more constrained and predictable.

Specimen tracking through the laboratory, which ensures that appropriate information is associated with the specimen at each stage of processing, is often a problem for computerized systems handling descriptive domains. Because no standard terminology has emerged to describe all of the steps involved, the LIS vendors may adopt an idiosyncratic terminology or format for describing specimen-processing status. This may force a laboratory to make compromises between making extensive changes in the LIS system to match its operation and making changes in a laboratory's internal procedures to match the system.

Generation of reports and retrieval of information contained within are major problems for these areas. Word processing, combined with coded text retrieval, has been used in such laboratory areas. Recently, computer systems have been introduced that provide for voice recognition, whereby dictation can be converted directly to transcribed reports. While offering great promise in the future, these may require either a constrained vocabulary or involve extensive training of the computer to recognize specific users.

The development of standardized coding schemes, such as systematized nomenclature of medicine (SNOMED), have partially resolved some of the problems with nonstandard terminology. These coding schemes provide a way to index and retrieve specimens numerically on the basis of descriptors, such as anatomic location, diagnosis, or cause. Although widely used, this approach suffers from the general problems of any controlled vocabulary indexing scheme, where the text being indexed may be subject to multiple interpretations or for which the indexers may not be exact. This is especially true when a laboratory modifies index terms to meet its own particular operation. Another approach to the terminology problem entails free text entry, with indexing based on the use of all uncommon words (key words in context).

Data Storage and Retrieval

Today, the wide range in choices to store information has greatly reduced storage and retrieval problems. The best option for a specific laboratory requires consideration of the constraints in cost, use, and space. Peripheral storage devices, such as magnetic discs, offer more rapid retrieval at a higher cost. Many laboratories use these modalities for short-term or frequently queried domains. Many laboratories still rely on paper records or magnetic tapes for long-term storage; however, this practice often is plagued by storage problems and inefficient retrieval. The availability of other media, such as microfiche and more recently, optical discs, offers useful yet economic alternatives.

Descriptive domains are problematic for memory storage and result retrieval because of the following: (1) The amount of text required to report a case is unpredictable at the time of specimen receipt. (2) A relatively long and variable period is required for specimen processing (24 hours or more in anatomic pathology, 24 hours to 3 or more weeks in microbiology). (3) The steps in specimen processing can vary considerably and unpredictably, depending on interpretations made at various stages of specimen processing. For example, a sputum Gram stain and smear showing no organisms and salivary contamination may not be processed further, whereas one showing white cells and a uniform

collection of gram-negative organisms will be cultured on a variety of media, with each separate isolate tested for antibiotic sensitivities. The LIS must be capable of handling these complex storage requirements.

Although the length of time that records must be stored varies for each laboratory, there has been a tendency toward longer periods of storage. Records must be retained for specified periods as stipulated by the regulatory agencies. Stored data can be used for purposes such as replacing lost reports or noting patient trends over long periods of time. Many laboratories, particularly at larger teaching institutions, use records for educational and research purposes. Most laboratories store their reports for at least 1 year; exceptions include blood banks, which must keep blood product records for 5 years, and anatomic pathology services, which often keep their records indefinitely.

It is important to guarantee the confidentiality and security of patient data because of the economic, social, and legal consequences of access by unauthorized people. The conflict to be resolved is between the need for ease of access dictated by the demands of medical practice and the need to limit access by security measures. Most LISs offer several different levels of protection through the use of passwords and access-limited accounts. In addition, users may be distinguished by what functions they can use in their interaction with the LIS. Typically, physicians have "read-only" access, laboratory technologists have "read and write" access, and supervisory personnel have full privileges to alter key files.

Quality Control Functions

Quality control is an essential concern of any laboratory. Its purpose is to monitor the quality of work produced by the laboratory and ensure that high standards in practice are followed. Quality control involves several different functions with the common goal of permitting better laboratory service. Examination of quality control records is an important part of laboratory accreditation, while statistics based on quality control data permit comparison in the proficiency of different laboratories. The LIS can help by storing the various records required and by statistical analysis of control samples.

Repetitive analysis of standard samples with known composition is a standard quality control activity and is done for two reasons. Results obtained on control samples included within a particular analytic procedure permit the technologist to verify that the data generated during that examination are valid. Statistical analysis of control sample data over longer periods can be used for evaluation of the laboratory's accuracy and precision and can detect trends in data due to problems in instruments or reagents.

In addition to the statistical reports on control materials, a variety of reports that summarize those patient results showing a feature of interest are reviewed daily by the laboratory supervisory personnel. The "delta" check is a consistency check that involves the review of test results that exhibit a statistically significant difference from previous analyses performed on the same patient. If a reasonable explanation for this difference cannot be found in the patient's medical condition, then review of other samples analyzed at the same time is performed. This may result in detection of sample mixups, contamination, or reagent problems that otherwise might not be evident. Other reports may include all tests with critical ("panic") values, with long stat turnaround times, or that were cancelled. An LIS allows problem documentation (people called, resolution) to be stored directly with the order, which allows for efficient retrieval of this information at a later date.

Finally, all the equipment and most of the utilities in the laboratory need to be monitored and maintained, with the service records required for inspections. Time and personnel must be scheduled for some tasks daily and for others periodically throughout the year. Reagents must be assayed to verify that they are properly prepared and labeled. These and other records are handled much better and with more accuracy in a computerized LIS than by manual systems.

The Extralaboratory Cycle

Reporting Along the Efferent Loop

Once analysis is complete, the results need to be delivered to the ordering physician. Reports need to be a concise, readable, chronologic representation of information if they are to be interpretable. The LIS can generate standard report forms and present the same information in alternative representations that may be more useful in a given situation. Interim reports permit delivery of information about test results as they become available, rather than delaying the report for completion of all the requested testing. Cumulative reports summarize all the information on a patient over a given period of time, with information arranged by related data items. Physician reports summarize the data on all of the patients of a particular physician. Ward or service reports similarly can be useful, especially if they list the work still to be performed.

Delivery of laboratory reports is often among the greatest problems faced by laboratory directors. Verbal reports are subject to misinterpretation or incomplete data transferral, and manual report delivery can result in a significant percentage of lost or misplaced reports. As an alternative to these report delivery methods, various transmission devices for communication with the laboratory have been used, particularly to key areas such as the emergency room and intensive care units. While pneumatic tube delivery to selected stations has advantages over manual transmission, it is also restricted, inflexible, and expensive. The use of telecommunications between the laboratory and the end-user has greatly improved the ability of laboratories to deliver results rapidly and accurately. Fax modules are available for most computer systems, allowing direct facsimile transmission of results from terminals.

Due to the increases in the type and amount of data being generated, it is becoming less acceptable simply to report test result data. One of the most important developments in laboratory medicine has been the interpretive reporting of test results, which is an attempt to transform data into relevant information pertinent to patient care. Several workers have presented schemes for interpreting laboratory data with computers. One method has been the implementation of computer-assisted strategies to aid clinical decision making and highlight important information on recurring patterns and associations of laboratory measurements. Simple attempts in this direction have been made in the past by (1) marking abnormal results, providing reference values adjacent to test results, and grouping data by system or organs; (2) displaying data in more informative ways; (3) calculating ratios or indexes automatically when the required information is available; (4) generating diagnostic possibilities based on patterns of test results; (5) making interpretive comments; (6) suggesting additional studies or performing additional studies automatically; and (7) providing reminders when certain clinical situations occur.

Others have attempted to discover relationships in data that are useful for clinical problem solving, using various forms of analysis, such as multivariate analysis, numeric taxonomy, and discriminant functions. However, surveys of interpretive reporting in clinical pathology indicate that although there a wide variety of interpretive reports is currently in use, few are integrated directly into the LIS. To work effectively, the LIS will need to incorporate data retrieval with computer-based decision aids for interpretive reporting.

CURRENT AND FUTURE REQUIREMENTS FOR LABORATORY INFORMATION SYSTEMS

Modern clinical laboratories must be cost effective, which requires greater efficiency at all stages of management. Moreover, providing clinicians with laboratory results in formats that aid decision making can improve patient care. Because many departments in the health-care system need to share information and are computerized, there is an increasing need for networking the hospital computers, resulting in highly distributed computer systems.

Cost Effectiveness

In the past, most hospital laboratories were revenue-generating operations. Today, because of changes in reimbursement legislation, laboratories will eventually become cost centers and must face the conflict between the need to reduce total operating costs and the need to meet the continuing rise in demand for services. It will be an economic necessity that automation, miniaturization, systemization, and computerized information handling in laboratories continue to evolve. There are at least three major ways that the LIS can help contain costs.

First, because personnel costs for wages and benefits represent a significant proportion of any laboratory budget, LIS functions that result in savings in labor will be beneficial. The LIS has proven cost effective in the performance of numerous clerical functions, such as data collection and report preparation. The demand for bar coding on automated instruments to reduce body substance exposure and to provide positive specimen identification has resulted in the widespread use of such codes in the laboratory, increasing the potential to automate other clerical and specimen handling functions. It is envisioned that the laboratory of the future will be fully automated with minimal personnel, using robots for most functions.

Second, an LIS can contribute to the decentralization of the clinical laboratories, a process that will result in a significant reduction in transportation time and costs (while possibly increasing technical error). In the past, it was desirable to maintain centralized laboratories, because large automated analyzers were expensive and needed to be operated by highly trained individuals. Newer instruments can perform an increasing number of measurements on smaller samples, and their cost and complexity of operation are decreasing. These instruments use built-in microcomputers, which control operation and provide digital outputs of fully processed data for direct display or transmission to other computers. With the increasing availability of such instruments, physical dispersion of laboratory testing to points of patient care is likely, especially when there is high laboratory usage and demand for fast turnaround times. However, this should not be done with attention to the details of good laboratory practice; issues that must be resolved are responsibilities for quality control, equipment maintenance, user competency training, and capture of the results into the medical record.

Finally, the LIS can reduce laboratory testing costs by reducing the number of tests performed. More extensive networking of LISs, with creation of regional data banks and long-term storage, would reduce the amount of duplicate testing performed on patients, particularly those transferred between care facilities. By automatic ordering of additional laboratory tests based on symptoms, diagnoses, or screening test results, it is possible to reduce replicate testing and to shorten patient hospital stays.

Management Support Functions

Careful management of clinical laboratories is required for efficient operation. This requires access to accurate and diverse information from a variety of sources. Many of the tasks required are amenable to information-processing techniques.

Operations management is a very important function, particularly in large laboratories that provide continuous operation throughout the week. To perform this task intelligently, one must perform workload and work flow analyses. These studies permit each procedure to be reviewed as to the number of times that it was performed, who performed it, and to what extent usage patterns may be changing. This information allows for optimizing productivity in the laboratory. The Laboratory Management Improvement Program of the College of American Pathologists (CAP) can assist in providing a quantitative measure of performance in each area of the laboratory and compare productivity with other institutions. This program requires access to extensive and specific information, all of which can be best achieved through the LIS. Changes in personnel or resource allocation can be made based on analysis of these values. In addition, computers can monitor parameters such as laboratory turnaround time or usage volume (Fig. 19-3) to maintain efficient service or to troubleshoot problems.

With increased emphasis on quality assurance and improvement, valuable information on employee performance and productivity can be retrieved from the LIS. This has become increasingly important as technologists are required to rotate through several different sections of the laboratory, rather than staying in one area or on one shift. The LIS can also retain records on employee training and competency testing.

Fiscal control is another management activity. Budgets for personnel and purchase of capital equipment or reagents need to be calculated. The billing for the testing performed must be recorded and collected. The LIS significantly reduces errors and decreases the time involved in billing when compared with manual systems. At the same time, it increases the recovery of

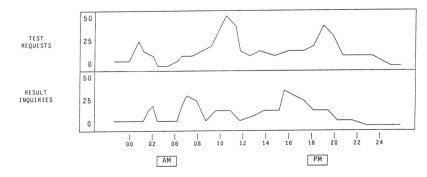

FIGURE 19–3. Assistance for making management decisions. The LIS computer can be used to monitor test ordering and test result inquiry patterns. This information can be used to determine staffing for periods of more critical need. In this example, maximum staffing for logging test results should be planned to cover the hours of 1 A.M. and 7 P.M.

charges and permits a greater flexibility in test ordering by allowing tests to be ordered in different combinations. Changes to the health-care marketplace have introduced new problems to be overcome, as restrictions placed by insurance carriers and health maintenance organizations have created a complex maze affecting patients based on their status as outpatients, emergency department clients, ambulatory surgery patients, or inpatients. Medicaid and Medicare constantly update their reimbursements, placing restrictions on charges for panels or individual tests. Without the precise numbers provided by the LIS, coping with these demands is overwhelming.

Inventory control poses a significant problem in certain laboratories. The blood bank needs to maintain careful inventory of all available blood products, not only within the blood bank itself, but also at satellite storage sites, such as in the operating suite. Microbiology and molecular pathology laboratories may similarly maintain large inventories of frozen organisms or cells. Database capabilities in the LIS can greatly simplify the paperwork entailed in such data storage situations.

Managers must ensure that the laboratories meet licensure requirements and regulations, which have been increasing since the passage of the Clinical Laboratories Improvement Acts of 1967 and 1988. Currently, several agencies inspect and certify clinical laboratories, notably the Joint Committee for Accreditation of Hospitals and the CAP. In addition, some laboratory divisions are inspected by specialty organizations, such as the American Association of Blood Banks and the Nuclear Regulatory Commission. Government agencies, such as the Occupational Safety and Health Administration, inspect laboratories to ensure that they are in compliance with safety regulations. These groups all set certain standards for test performance, personnel, and the laboratory work environment. By maintaining records and manuals, the LIS can greatly simplify the clerical labor involved in preparing for laboratory inspections. Even the LIS is not exempt from scrutiny, with the Food and

Drug Administration viewing health-care computer systems as medical devices requiring validation and testing.

Finally, the LIS can improve communications within the laboratory and with outside departments through electronic mail and bulletin boards. This is especially important for exchanging information between shifts and for contacting part-time employees. Because receipt of messages can be documented within the computer, uncertainty in the communication links can be removed as a concern.

Decision Support Aids

In the future, computers will be increasingly used to assist physicians in ordering and interpreting laboratory test data. Not only is the sheer volume of laboratory testing already beyond the capacity of humans to assimilate it, but the knowledge required to use it effectively is vast and constantly increasing. The combination of these factors has caused clinicians to underuse or misinterpret a large proportion of the laboratory data from their patients. The following has been shown:

1. A high percentage of significantly abnormal laboratory results have no measurable effect on physician decisions.
2. A significant disparity exists between the criteria that physicians use to determine whether a laboratory measurement has changed and the analytic limitations for detecting such a change, based on the underlying methodology.
3. Laboratory use differs significantly between physicians managing patients with similar diagnoses.

Recent studies have supported the thesis that current laboratory use is less than ideal and suggest that it is often inappropriate and excessive.

Improvements in the capabilities of the LIS for data retrieval and manipulation can be used to make patient data more interpretable. The benefits of being able to interpret a patient's results in reference to precisely defined populations matched to the patient's personal characteristics or to the patient's prior data have long been appreciated. By being able to store and collate large amounts of information, the LIS can provide a greater ability to define the normal and abnormal values for the body's chemical constituents. Correction of patient results for the influence of drugs and physiologic abnormalities will become possible through altering or rejecting affected test data. The development of information systems databanks in such areas as the causes of specific laboratory abnormalities will allow retrieval of relatively inaccessible information. Information services from the laboratory, such as on-line assistance for test interpretation, should become commonplace.

The decision models used in the past have paralleled the mathematic models most popular in computer-assisted diagnostic systems: Baye's theorem, decision analysis, algorithms, or sequential branching strategies. Knowledge-based LIS decision support modules incorporating the techniques of artificial intelligence are just beginning to emerge. We expect that knowledge-based expert systems will increasingly be incorporated into the LIS. Expert systems technology has been applied in a limited way to some laboratory interpretation tasks already and reached sufficient maturity to be incorporated in commercial products. For example, the EXPERT language has been used for construction of a series of decision-making models for endocrinology, serum protein analysis, and interpretation of a select number of enzyme tests. Several of these modules are now available as add-ons for a commercially available serum protein electrophoresis instrument.

Distributed Computing Systems

In the past, the LIS was designed to run on a single, stand-alone minicomputer, which handled all of the information system functions for the entire laboratory. This choice was dictated by the available computer technology. However, for efficient laboratory operation, more flexible computational abilities and communication links between the individual laboratory divisions are required. Laboratory divisions need to exchange data with other hospital services outside of the laboratory (Table 19–1). The needs for communication to acquire and disseminate data are compatible with the use of distributed computing through a community of networked computers located within and outside of the actual laboratory.

Each member of the network provides one or more functions to the other members, which reduces the need for duplicate storage and the attendant problems of version control. The hospital information system, which itself may be a network of computers, usually maintains patient demographics, ADT information, and long-term patient data collation and billing; it exchanges this information with the departmental and patient care information systems. The main laboratory computer can act as a gateway and server to the microcomputers and workstations within the laboratories, providing more extensive database, communication, and printing services. The minicomputers and

Table 19-1 Some Examples of the Communication Exchanges Between Laboratory Divisions and Different Hospital Departments		
Hospital Division	Laboratory	Information
Emergency room, intensive care unit, operating room, wards	Blood bank	Blood product usage
	Chemistry	Chemical analyses
	Hematology	Blood indices
	Microbiology	Culture results
	Surgical pathology	Tissue diagnoses
Monitoring services (eg, epidemiology, tumor registry)	Morobiology	Bacterial lactasis
	Surgical pathology	Tumor diagnoses
Support Services (eg, pharmacy, sterile supply)	Chemistry	Drug levels
		Drug adverse effects
	Microbiology	Sterility checks
		Drug susceptibility

workstations dispersed in the divisional laboratories will locally process data and transmit it to the LIS for further processing, merging with patient data and rendering of interpretations, prior to transmission to the other information systems.

The introduction of powerful, specialized image analyzing workstations has revolutionized previously undercomputerized, labor-intensive descriptive domains, such cytogenetics and surgical pathology. Image storage, manipulation, and transmission are significant problems for imaging systems due to the large size and complexity of the files involved. These functionalities can be handled by photograph archiving and communication systems. Connecting such systems for distributed access over networks has been hampered by the need for high speed and capacity in the data networks and by the scarcity of high-resolution display stations.

Just as demand has driven the need for information exchange within the hospital, there is increasing demand for exchanging information with others outside of the hospital. Major developments in telecommunications have made feasible connections with physician offices and, through cellular communications and mobile computing, with the physician directly. While the high-speed data links required for telemedicine are available in only a few areas, such facilities are expected to be commonplace in a few years. Widespread accessibility to the Internet has made access to national databases feasible from the smallest institution.

Despite the opportunities offered by such advances, several problems have arisen. The medical record has become highly fragmented between the hospital, physician offices, clinics, and insurance-dictated referral laboratories. Despite the government's proposal for a unified electronic medical record, this is likely to be many years away and extremely expensive to maintain. Fortunately, standards for data transmission and exchange have been under development for many years by the American Society of Testing and Materials. However, the demand to provide for data security and confidentiality while having the information readily accessible by qualified practitioners is likely to be problematic for some time.

ACQUIRING AN LIS

Before selecting an LIS, the following questions must be answered:

1. Is computerization really necessary?
2. What needs to be computerized and to what extent? Will the system need to interface with other computer systems, either internal or external to the laboratory?

3. What resources, particularly how much money, are available? How will this affect where the computer is located relative to the laboratory, and who will control its operation?
4. Should system development be done in-house or by an outside vendor?
5. What guidelines are to be used for evaluating and selecting from among the different options available?
6. How will the the system installation be done?

Necessity of Computerization

Before computerization is decided on as a solution to a problem, it is first necessary to decide exactly what problems are to be addressed and what benefits are to be achieved by computerization. Simply putting something on a computer may not make a problem any more solvable or easy to handle, because many problems are not optimally handled by computer. A systems analysis should therefore be performed to define the problems to be considered for computerization and to help in deciding what options are available for their solution (Box 19–1).

A comparison of the expected cost for an LIS versus its potential benefits is fundamental in determining the need for computerization. The potential benefits of an LIS can be great, as shown. However, the cost of most systems is also great, because it includes not only the expense of the system but also personnel and supply costs. Many laboratory directors and health-care administrators have expressed dissatisfaction at the economic impact of computers in laboratory medicine, citing the

---

Box 19•1

Some Benefits of a Computerized Laboratory Information System

Decrease in turnaround time
Decrease in clerical errors and loss of results
Decrease in boring and tedious jobs
Flexibility in report formats and interpretations
Increased accuracy in patient and research data retrieval
Increased accuracy in billing information
Increased accuracy in quality control data and inventory records
Increased efficiency and productivity of technologists
Optimalization of work flow and organization

failure to see any drop in laboratory expenses since the introduction of their use. However, evaluation of the direct and indirect economic impacts of an LIS does not support this view. The direct economic impact of such systems includes decreased data handling expenses, greater personnel productivity, and greater control over finances, particularly with regard to recoverable charges. The indirect economic impact includes improved patient care and improved laboratory morale. When evaluating the economic impact of an information system, one must examine factors that affect laboratory expenses (inflation, billing practices of the institution) and reevaluate managerial decisions that may be resulting in a failure to use the system optimally.

Extent of Computerization

Key factors in determining the choice of an LIS are the size of the laboratory, the size of the hospital in which the laboratory is located, and whether the entire laboratory or only some of its divisions are to be computerized. In general, options for a small laboratory in a small hospital are more extensive than for a large laboratory in a large teaching hospital.

For most laboratories, a single integrated computer system is preferable to several systems from different vendors, where the problems increase exponentially with the number of systems involved. An integrated system is easier to manage and involves less duplication in personnel training, fewer supply and storage problems, simpler data exchanges, and better data integration. Even if multiple systems can be brought up successfully, inevitable changes or upgrades in software or hardware can be simply devastating for the support staff due to unforeseen repercussions through the systems.

The need to network with other computers is a significant decision that can place constraints on subsequent decisions and may restrict choices to only a few vendors with the necessary expertise. With hospitals consolidating services or merging, the need for different LISs to exchange information effectively is becoming increasingly important.

Available Resources

Based on the goals, sufficient resources must be available. Requirements for a computer system include those listed in Box 19–2.

If any of these requirements is inadequate, it is better to reevaluate goals than to proceed with computerization.

Often it is more cost-effective to have several departmental information systems maintained centrally

---

Box 19·2

Requirements for a Computer System

A proper environment
Proper support personnel
Proper training of laboratory personnel
An adequate budget
Support from the administration

---

within the hospital. While offering many advantages, this approach can also introduce problems if the hospital administration maintains tight control without involving the departments in the decision-making process.

In-House Versus Vendor System Development

An LIS may be developed either through in-house ("do-it-yourself") programming or by purchase from a commercial software vendor of a "turnkey" system. In-house LIS development typically uses personnel and hardware of an already existing hospital computer system. Although this approach would seem to be effective use of available computer resources, many of these systems have failed. This is because of the difficulty of the task and the need to maintain software for long periods by people familiar with the unique features of the system. Moreover, much of the work required is needless duplication of efforts already done by others.

The majority of laboratories use vendor-developed commercial systems, specifically designed for use in the clinical laboratory. These turnkey systems derive their name from the theory that one can purchase an entire computer system, have it installed, and begin operation by simply "turning the key." There are several advantages to this approach of LIS development. The extremely high cost involved in the development of a computer system is distributed among the many users, as is the cost of software maintenance and updating. Groups of system users can solve common problems, advise the vendor about the needs for improvements in programs, and develop new computer programs. However, several potential problems can occur if a turnkey system is purchased (Box 19–3). Most of these problems are well known, so the hazards can be minimized. For example, most vendors offer more flexibility in system function through the use of modular programs and of table-driven system definitions.

Some Hazards of Vendor Systems

Restriction in computer hardware choices to
those dictated by the vendor
A loss of flexibility in laboratory operations
The expense to modify and maintain changes
Dependence on the vendor's commercial
viability

Evaluation and Selection

The choice of an LIS from among the alternative systems requires a careful evaluation of the systems, with comparison of the laboratory's information processing needs with the functions provided by the different systems available.

This process has been greatly simplified by independent evaluations, which exhaustively compare the features of the commercial systems. The CAP (through its newsletter *CAP Today*) maintains information on computer systems. The Department of Pathology at the University of Michigan has provided particularly valuable resources over the years, through its annual Laboratory Information System Symposium at the University of Michigan and its recently introduced service LIS-FAX (1-800-4-LISFAX) for accessing system descriptions.

Evaluation of each prospective vendor-provided system should include the points provided in Box 19-4.

Based on the results of these investigations, a request for proposal is sent to vendors who seem to meet the needs of the institution. This is an exhaustive process, not only in its generation, but also in the evaluation of the responses, with the need to clarify what is provided by the vendor for each level of support. Before any contract is signed, it must be carefully reviewed by legal counsel to ensure that recourse is available if problems arise.

In general, it is advisable to avoid using a system that integrates the hardware of several manufacturers and to avoid being the first laboratory to use a new computer system (or to implement a major software change). It is particularly important that the hardware specifications be as generous as possible; vendors often will undersize the computer to keep the price low, while users are unforgiving of a slow or unresponsive system.

Installation

The installation of the LIS can be a long and tedious process, even for a small system. Thus, sufficient resources must be allocated for this critical operation.

One person should be given authority to manage the installation. This position requires great tact and diplomacy, with the ability to balance the desire for control versus the need for user input. This person will typically serve as the system manager after the installation is complete. He or she will often have assistants, who may be temporarily assigned from another laboratory section for this project.

Before and during the installation, sufficiently detailed diagrams of the instrument, terminal, and communication layout are essential. This not only allows concrete planning, but also is useful for new user orientation. Later, when changes are made to the system, such diagrams can significantly reduce the confusion pursuant.

Careful documentation of the installation process is essential, particularly in the blood bank, where system validation is required for accreditation. Records should include orientation of users, demonstration of competency, and descriptions of problems encountered ("bugs"). While time consuming and often neglected, such documentation can be extremely useful if unexpected failures occur.

Prospective Vendor-Provided System Evaluations

Interviewing other users of the laboratory
information system (LIS), especially those with
laboratories and hospitals similar in size to
one's own hospital
Visiting one or more sites where the LIS is
installed (site visit)
Having an on-site demonstration of the system
Validating the compatibility of the proposed
system and its ability to be integrated with
existing computers at the institution
Asking what other hospital information systems
the company is developing that might
adversely compete with support for the LIS
Checking on the economic viability of the
vendor and the stability of the programming
support staff.

BIBLIOGRAPHY

Aller RD, Elevitch FR: The ABCs of LIS—Computerizing Your Laboratory Information System. Chicago, ASCP Press, 1989

Friedman BA, Mitchell W: Integrating information from decentralized laboratory testing sites. Am J Clin Pathol 99:637–642, 1993

Furfine CS: The FDA's policy on the regulation of computerized medical devices. MD Computing 9:97–100, 1992

Griesser G, Jardel JP et al (eds): Data Protection in Health Information Systems. New York, North Holland, 1983

Speicher CE, Smith JW: Choosing Effective Laboratory Tests. Philadelphia, WB Saunders, 1983

Statland BE, Burke WP, Galen RS: Quantitative Approaches Used in Evaluating Laboratory Measurements and Other Clinical Data. Philadelphia, WB Saunders, 1979

20

Concepts of Preventive Maintenance for Laboratory Instrumentation[*]

John S. Davis

The establishment and documentation of preventive maintenance programs have become responsibilities of pathologists, clinical chemists, and medical technologists as a result of requirements by accrediting agencies. Preventive maintenance should also be considered from a practical point of view. A patient's treatment is often dependent on quick turnaround time for critical laboratory tests, so any type of equipment malfunction could potentially affect patient care. When an instrument malfunctions, it is expensive for a laboratory to maintain backup equipment or send tests to another laboratory. Benefits of a preventive maintenance program are summarized in Box 20–1.[5]

The purpose of a preventive maintenance program is to ensure that equipment operates properly and safely. Yapit describes a comprehensive system of preventive maintenance, including instrument manuals, troubleshooting specialists, and breakdown/repair documentation resulting in a 54% reduction in downtime.[13] This can be accomplished by checking critical operating characteristics of an instrument and performing the recommended maintenance on a scheduled basis. Preventive maintenance can be divided into two categories: function verification, which includes checks and tests to ensure that an instrument is working properly and is

correctly calibrated, and maintenance, which includes replacement, adjustment, or repair to prolong the life of an instrument and prevent mechanical malfunctions.[7] A preventive maintenance program contains the following:

Accrediting agency requirements
Instrument selection and implementation
Documentation
Performance responsibility of personnel

ACCREDITING AGENCY REQUIREMENTS

Accreditation by both the Joint Commission on Accreditation of Healthcare Organizations (JCAHO) and College of American Pathologists (CAP) requires preventive maintenance programs.

The JCAHO outlines general guidelines requiring a system of periodic maintenance, inspection, and performance testing for all equipment and instruments with appropriate documentation (Box 20–2).[4]

The CAP requires a detailed program of preventive maintenance with documentation and provides the laboratory with a checklist of requirements that must be met on inspection.[3] This checklist covers instrument operating characteristics, interval of inspection and maintenance, tolerance limits, and documentation. Meeting requirements for accreditation is not a major

---

[*] This chapter is revised from the second edition chapter authorized by Judith Thompson and Peggy Prinz Luebbert.

341

Box 20•1

Benefits of a Preventive Maintenance Program

- Improved product quality
- Greater operator safety
- Fewer interruptions of production
- Decreased employee idle time
- Lower repair costs
- Avoidance of premature replacement
- Reduction of standby ("backup") equipment
- Identification of high maintenance costs
- Better spare parts control

---

task if a laboratory establishes a preventive maintenance program following these guidelines and maintains documentation on a routine basis.[4]

The guidance and questions in Box 20–3 are from the CAP Inspections Form, and they describe instrument maintenance quality probes.

INSTRUMENT SELECTION AND IMPLEMENTATION

Preventive maintenance programs begin by selecting instruments that will operative effectively for a reasonable period of time. The routine operation of the instrument should be considered. Is it an instrument that will be used by many people and operated 24 hours a day, or is it a highly specialized instrument that will be used infrequently? Before purchasing an instrument, inquiries should be made at laboratories using similar equipment regarding the performance record of their particular instrument and the quality of service provided by the manufacturer.

When the decision has been made to purchase an instrument, specific items should be outlined in the purchase contract. These should include installation of the instrument, training of personnel, and an evaluation period (generally 30 to 60 days) during which the instrument can be returned at no cost if it does not meet expected performance.

As soon as an instrument is delivered and installed, it should be evaluated. Before the evaluation, it is important to define specific operating characteristics with tolerable limits or performance for acceptance. The manufacturer's operation manual is a good reference source, as are publications on laboratory instrumentation. These publications list function checks needed and frequency of performance.[1,12] After the instrument has been evaluated and has met the criteria for accep-

tance using method evaluation, it can be implemented for routine use. At this time, a preventive maintenance program for the instrument should be initiated. The operating parameters and tolerance limits that have been defined in the initial evaluation can be incorporated into the program.

For some instruments, commercial service is required as part of the routine preventive maintenance program. For example, cleaning the objectives and oiling and aligning a microscope require skill and should not be attempted by an untrained person. Also, analytical balances should be cleaned and calibrated annually by a qualified service agent. Service contracts can be purchased for more sophisticated instruments and may include routine calibration and maintenance. When considering a service contract, one should note whether parts, labor, travel, emergency service, and calibration are covered. Also, the availability of competent in-house service personnel should be considered.

An important aspect of implementing a new instrument into routine use is training of personnel.[10] This can be accomplished in several ways. The company representative who installs an instrument generally will give basic instructions on use and care. Often the manufacturer holds an instrument training program at its applications laboratory for technologists. The training session and expenses can be included as part of the initial purchase agreement. In-house continuing education sessions are an effective way of informing groups of technologists about the underlying principles and operation of the instrument and preventive maintenance procedures. An obvious source of instruction, but one that is frequently overlooked, is the operation manual provided with the instrument. It contains basic operating instructions, maintenance, and a troubleshooting guide. The operation manual and warranty should always be kept in a convenient location near the instrument.

When an instrument has been carefully chosen, its operating characteristics evaluated, its operators well trained, and preventive maintenance regularly performed, it should perform well for its expected lifetime.

The key to a good preventive maintenance program is organization. This includes developing protocols for function check limits and routine maintenance for each instrument, performing these checks at scheduled intervals, and carefully documenting this information and any repair work or service done to the instrument.[2] It is important for these records to be complete and kept up to date.

Organization of a program begins with a careful inventory of all equipment and instrumentation. This inventory can be in the form of a card file, notebook, or computer listing. It should include the following information for each item of equipment: name of instru-

Box 20·2

General Guidelines of the Joint Commission on Accreditation of Healthcare Organizations

EC.1.6: A management plan addresses laboratory equipment.

INTENT OF EC.1.6

A management plan describes how the laboratory will establish and maintain a laboratory equipment management program to promote safe and effective use of laboratory equipment. The plan provides processes for the following:

a. Selecting and acquiring equipment
b. Establishing criteria for identifying, evaluating, and taking inventory of laboratory equipment to be included in the management program before the equipment is used; these criteria address the following:
   • Equipment function
   • Risks associated with use
   • Maintenance requirements
   • Equipment incident history
c. Assessing equipment use through inspection, testing, and maintenance, including the following:
   • Preventive maintenance, periodic inspection, and performance testing of equipment and instruments
   • Evaluation of analytical measuring equipment and instruments with respect to all critical operating characteristics
   • Evaluation of automated volumetric equipment
   • Test performance and instrument operation within the temperature and humidity ranges required for proper performance
   • Documentation for the monitoring of temperature-controlled spaces and equipment
d. Monitoring and acting on equipment hazard notices and recalls
e. Monitoring and reporting incidents in which a medical device is connected with the death, serious injury, or serious illnesses of any individual, as required by the Safe Medical Devices Act of 1990
f. Investigating equipment problems, failures, and user errors
g. Providing an orientation and education program addressing laboratory equipment management

h. Setting performance standards for personnel laboratory equipment management knowledge and skill
i. Conducting an annual evaluation of the laboratory equipment management plan.

A historical record is maintained for each instrument or piece of equipment in the laboratory. Detailed records identifying daily, weekly, or monthly performance testing and function checks are retained for at least 2 years. Records of major repairs, parts replacement, and annual maintenance are retained for the life of the instrument or equipment.

EXAMPLES OF EVIDENCE OF IMPLEMENTATION FOR EC.1.6

1. The following promote safe and reliable equipment functioning:
   • Execution of performance testing, function checks, preventive maintenance, and calibration or calibration verification of each piece of equipment
   • Written descriptions of each equipment testing and maintenance phase with detailed instructions and defined intervals
   • Documentation of the maintenance performance testing, calibration, and calibration verification as defined in the written instructions. Protocols defining performance testing, maintenance, and calibration are at least as stringent as manufacturer's guidelines, if available. If the manufacturer has not defined suggested guidelines, recommendations found in current literature for this similar equipment should be used.
   Testing, maintenance, and calibration frequency are related to the laboratory's use of the equipment or instrument and to its documentation history of performance.
2. In the laboratory, the daily, weekly, and monthly performance testing is performed by the laboratorian. Major repairs and annual maintenance are performed by the biomedical personnel or the manufacturer.

Reprinted with permission from JCAHO. Comprehensive accreditation manual for pathology and clinical laboratory services, 1996.

Box 20•3

College of American Pathologists' Guidance and Questions

Questions in this section apply to *all* instruments in the general/automated chemistry section. The procedures and schedules for instrument maintenance must be as thorough and as frequent as specified by the manufacturer.

Is there a schedule or system *available at the instrument* for the regular checking or the critical operating characteristics for all instruments in use?

Note: This must include, but is not limited to, electronic, mechanical, and operational checks. The procedure and schedule must be as thorough and as frequent as specified by the manufacturer.

Are there documented instructions for instrument check system (ie, manufacturer's manual or system prepared by the laboratory)?

Are function checks documented *by the technical operator* and readily available to detect trends or malfunctions?

Are tolerance limits for acceptable function documented for specific instruments wherever appropriate?

Are instructions provided for minor troubleshooting and repairs of instruments (such as manufacturer's service manual)?

Are records maintained *at or near* each instrument to document all repairs and service procedure?

Are *recent* instrument maintenance, service, and repair records (or copies) promptly available to, and usable by, all technical staff operating the equipment on all shifts?

Note: The investigation of method failure begins with the bench technologist. Instrument records are essential to such investigations. Off-site storage, such as with centralized medical maintenance or computer files, is not precluded if the inspector is satisfied that prompt retrieval exists.

Reprinted with permission from CAP. Commission on Laboratory Accreditation Inspection Checklist, 1994.

---

ment, manufacturer, model number, serial number, inventory number, purchase date and price, service representative, and service phone numbers. It also may be helpful to include a list of spare parts with part description number, price, and vendor (Fig. 20–1). A copy of the list of spare parts should also be filed with the inventory control department of the laboratory.

After all equipment has been itemized, an outline of function checks and routine maintenance must be developed for each instrument (Table 20–1). The instrument operation manual contains a list of necessary function checks, a maintenance protocol, and a troubleshooting guide. If the operation manual has been misplaced, it can be replaced by contacting the manufacturer's headquarters. Other sources of information are also available.[1,12]

After the function checks and routine maintenance requirements have been outlined, a written protocol should be developed. This should include performance criteria and concise, step-by-step instructions covering each item in the outline. Performance criteria for each function check can be obtained from the operation manual or other reference sources.[7,12] Also, information from an in-house evaluation of the instrument can be

used. This written protocol should also include a brief troubleshooting guide or referral to the troubleshooting guide in the operation manual. A typical written maintenance protocol for wavelength calibration check, using the holmium oxide filter from the Chemetrics Spectro-Standard set, can be seen in Box 20–4.

A system of charts and records should also be de-

Table 20-1
Spectropbotometer Maintenance Outline

Function Verification

1. Check linearity with National Bureau of Standards standard weekly.
2. Check wavelength calibration montly.
3. Check for stray light monthly.

Routine Maintenance

1. Check cuvette well weekly.
2. Dust optical surfaces weekly.
3. Check exciter lamp monthly.
4. Check silica gel monthly

INVENTORY RECORD CARD

Name of Instrument:_____
Laboratory Location:_____
Model Number:_____
Serial Number:_____
Inventory Number:_____
Manufacturer:_____
Purchase Date:_____
Purchase Price:_____
Service Representative:_____
Service Phone Number:_____

(back side)

SPARE PARTS

Description	Order Number	Price	Vendor

FIGURE 20–1.   Inventory record card (5 × 7 in).

Box 20•4

A Typical Written Maintenance Protocol for Wavelength Calibration Check

1. Turn operation switch on, tungsten lamp on, filter to appropriate setting for wavelength being checked, lamp selector to visible, sensitivity to high.
2. Read instructions included with Chemetrics Standard set on handling of filters.
3. Place holmium oxide filter in cell holder of spectrophotometer.
4. Set wavelength on spectrophotometer at 536 nm.
5. Turn operation switch to meter. Adjust transmittance to approximately 50% T.
6. Slowly change the wavelength on either side of the selected value until a minimum % T value is obtained. (Do final rotating of knob in clockwise direction to eliminate backlash error.)
7. Wavelength of minimum % T should correspond to specific holmium oxide value within the tolerances specified by the spectrophotometer manufacturer (± 0.5 nm). If adjustment is required, see operation manual.

veloped. Each laboratory can devise charts that best suit its needs. A good chart should include a title, date, results of a function check, comments, and a place for the technologist's and reviewer's initials. It is also helpful to include the established performance limits so that the technologist can immediately see whether the day's reading is acceptable. The chart should be simple, well-organized, and permit easy and rapid review of equipment function (Fig. 20–2).

A maintenance schedule should be established and incorporated into the routine work flow. Many different types of reminder techniques have been developed.[8,11] Specific tasks may be assigned to a work unit or person, and a reminder system of calendars, charts, and file cards can be developed (Fig. 20–3). Provision should also be made for doing critical function checks and maintenance on weekends and during the evening and night shift. The checklists, charts, and written protocols should be kept on the bench next to the instrument so that the technologist has easy access to them.

A troubleshooting log for each instrument must be maintained. The following should be included: problem, action taken, comments, date, and technologist's

initials (Fig. 20–4). When the service representative repairs the instrument, this information can be obtained from the customer's copy of the service report.

It may be beneficial to incorporate external interlaboratory survey programs into the preventive maintenance program.[6] The CAP conducts an instrument survey program, which can be used for comparison of instrument performance with established standards and other laboratories. Check samples are provided for spectrophotometers, analytical balances, and pH meters. Each participating laboratory receives a summary of all data obtained for the check sample and educational material outlining procedures for calibration and performance validation.

PERFORMANCE RESPONSIBILITY

Responsibility and accountability for a preventive maintenance program begin with the technologist at the bench. Before attempting to use an instrument, the technologist must learn the operation of the instrument, its performance capabilities, preventive maintenance protocol, documentation, and simple troubleshooting. This is accomplished by on-the-job training, continuing education seminars, manufacturer's training programs, and reading the operation manual provided with the instrument. The technologist performs the daily function verification and routine maintenance for the instrument. Each time an instrument reading is taken, it should be compared with established performance criteria. If the reading exceeds these limits, the technologist should perform simple troubleshooting to restore instrument function or notify the supervisor so that appropriate action can be taken. This should be carefully documented in the troubleshooting log by recording the problems, corrective action, date, and technologist's initials.[9]

The department supervisor is responsible for coordination and review of the preventive maintenance program. The supervisor should designate specific maintenance assignments and provide a schedule with effective reminders for bench technologists. Preventive maintenance should be scheduled during a time when the instrument is not heavily used. These assignments should be given to a specific person or work unit, which provides a system of accountability. The supervisor should review all records on a monthly basis to ensure that the procedures are being followed, identify potential problems, and review corrective action. The supervisor usually initiates all repair work and sees that it is documented.

A full-time or part-time instrumentation technologist can be beneficial. This position can be effective for a small laboratory that does not have access to biomedical

Daily refrigerator/freezer temperatures _____ 19 _____

Room # _____ Refrigerator or freezer # _____

Limits: ± 5°C of assigned temperature _____

Reviewed by _____

Date	Initial	Temperature	Comments	Date	Initial	Temperature	Comments
1				16			
2				17			
3				18			
4				19			
5				20			
6				21			
7				22			
8				23			
9				24			
10				25			
11				26			
12				27			
13				28			
14				29			
15				30			

FIGURE 20–2.   Daily maintenance chart.

engineers or for a large laboratory that has a wide variety of equipment requiring one person to coordinate and maintain the preventive maintenance program. General qualifications for this position include a medical technology background with a special interest in instrumentation and electronics. This person should be responsible for all preventive maintenance and troubleshooting for equipment. He should be able to provide emergency repairs, communicate with the service representative, maintain an inventory of spare parts, supervise the maintenance program, and instruct technologists and students on the care and troubleshooting of laboratory instrumentation. Having an instrumentation technologist coordinate the preventive maintenance

program can result in repair-cost savings and reduction of instrument downtime.

Most large hospitals and institutions have biomedical engineers responsible for general repair and maintenance of all hospital instrumentation. They provide a useful service to the laboratory by repairing common instruments, such as centrifuges and water baths; installing replacement parts; and performing emergency repair. Plant maintenance engineers can provide service for refrigerators and freezers.

Generally, all instrument manufacturers have field service representatives who have been trained to repair their instruments. They provide service on a request basis and initial set-up and testing of a new instrument.

WEEK I			DATE	INITIALS
Clean Mechanical Pipettes				
Clean Heat Sealers				
Check and Clean Balances				
Platelet Quality Control (4 units/month)				
Temp of Incoming Shipment	Source	Temp		
WEEK II				
Clean All Microscopes				
JHH Platelet Culture—Unit #				
Donor Arm Culture—Unit #				
Check and Clean Refrigerated Centrifuges				
Temp of Incoming Shipment	Source	Temp		
WEEK III				
Check Refrigerator & Freezer Alarms				
Temp of Incoming Shipment	Source	Temp		
WEEK IV				
Check FFP and Cryo				
Check Thermometers Against Standard				
Check Heat Blocks and Water Baths				
Check Agglutination Viewing Mirrors				
Check Platelet Rotator				
Temp of Incoming Shipment	Source	Temp		

FIGURE 20–3. Monthly maintenance and quality control chart. (Baldwin M, Barrasso C: The development and operation of an efficient laboratory preventive maintenance program. Am J Med Technol 45:216–218, 1979)

Date:_____
Technologist:_____
Service Representative:_____
Costs:_____
Problem:_____
_____
_____
_____
_____
_____
_____

Action Taken:_____
_____
_____
_____
_____
_____

Comments:_____
_____
_____
_____
_____
_____
_____
_____

FIGURE 20–4.   Trouble shooting log and repair record.

Their services can also be covered by a service contract. When a service representative is called for instrument repair, the laboratory should explain the problem, how it was identified, and what initial repair work has been done. When field service is necessary, the service representative should be prompt, answering the call within 24 hours if the problem is acute and affecting patient care. When the service representative arrives, the laboratory should have someone available to explain the problem and provide necessary assistance. After the repair work has been done, the representative should fill out a field service report, listing the problem, work done, and cost (parts, labor, travel). These services may be covered by a warranty or service contract or paid by individual call. Good communication between the representative and customer is important for good service.

BENEFITS OF PREVENTIVE MAINTENANCE

The preventive maintenance program should be periodically reviewed for the frequency and cost of repairs for each instrument. The program should be analyzed for determining whether (1) a change should be made in preventive maintenance frequency or action criteria;

(2) certain preventive maintenance checks should be discontinued for equipment needing infrequent repair; (3) modification, overhaul, or replacement of equipment is needed because of the increasing costs of the maintenance and repairs; and (4) a service contract is cost effective. A preventive maintenance program is cost effective when repairs and adjustments are made at a convenient time instead of when a breakdown occurs. This decreases the number of outside service calls, lowers repair costs, and decreases equipment downtime. A well-organized preventive maintenance program can provide additional benefits to the laboratory. A good program improves the morale and self-confidence of the technologists by giving them a working knowledge of how to use and take care of instruments. It also reduces the frustration caused by an inefficiently operating instrument. The technologist will have the confidence needed for accurate laboratory results when he knows his instrument is performing at the desired levels of precision and accuracy.

REFERENCES

1. A Guide on Laboratory Administration. Publication VIII, Maintenance. Laboratory Consultation Office, Bureau of Laboratories, Atlanta, Centers for Disease Control and Prevention, 1976

2. Baldwin M, Barrassoz C: The development and operation of an efficient laboratory preventive maintenance program. Am J Med Technol 45:216–218, 1979

3. CAP Inspection Checklists. Northfield, IL, College of American Pathologists, 1996

4. Comprehensive Accreditation Manual for Pathology and Laboratory Services. Oakbrook Terrace, IL, Joint Commission on Accreditation of Healthcare Organizations, 1996

5. Fink JG, Narayanan S: Preventive maintenance and troubleshooting. In Ward KM, Lehmann CA, Leiken AM (eds): Clinical Laboratory Instrumentation and Automation: Principles, Applications, and Selection, pp 415–443. Philadelphia, W.B. Saunders, 1994

6. Hamill RD: Quality control in the laboratory. Clin Toxicol 12(2):213–217, 1978

7. Hamlin WB, Duckworth JK, Gilmer PR, et al: Laboratory Instrumentation Maintenance Manual. Chicago, College of American Pathologists, 1970

8. Jaglinski K: A flexible reminder system for preventative maintenance. MLO 8(5):79–86, 1976

9. Johnson JE: "The machine Isn't working"—a set of diagnostic questions for instrument troubleshooting. MLO 18(8): 77–81, 1986

10. Lee LW (ed): Elementary Principles of Laboratory Instruments, 4th ed, pp 287–289. St Louis, CV Mosby, 1978

11. McDonald CW: Keeping track of preventive maintenance. MLO 12(3):77–84, 1980

12. Ottaviano PJ, DiSalvo AF: Quality Control in the Clinical Laboratory: A Procedural Text, pp 9–16. Baltimore, University Park Press, 1977

13. Yapit MK: Keeping your instruments happy. MLO 15(11): 33–39, 1983

21

Clinical Laboratory Safety and OSHA

Peggy P. Luebbert

One of the most important recent trends in health care is an increasing interest in the safety and well-being of employees. This interest revolves around the desire to decrease risk of infections and other physical and chemical hazards in the workplace.

Increasing awareness of these issues is a direct result of several factors. First is the acquired immunodeficiency syndrome (AIDS) epidemic, which has greatly increased public awareness of the dangers of transmission of blood-borne pathogens. In addition, the emergence of antibiotic-resistant strains of bacteria and the striking rise in the incidence of tuberculosis, foodborne, and skin illnesses have reemphasized the importance of preventing infections at all levels of health care. Similarly, a better understanding of the dangers of certain physical and chemical hazards is vital in reducing the risk of hazard exposure to health-care workers.

The responsibility for laboratory safety resides ultimately with the director of the laboratory. Under United States laws, the employer has a legal duty to provide a safe work environment. Should the employer fail to meet these legal duties or provide less than the acceptable work environment, he or she may be held liable. These standards of care are imposed or defined by laws from various federal, state, and local governing bodies; regulations and guidelines developed and made public by appropriate agencies; standards of conduct or acceptable practices recommended by private and professional organizations; and common law and practices.[19]

For day-to-day operations, a safety officer who is familiar with the laboratory practices and hazards should be appointed among the laboratory staff. The safety officer should be responsible for giving advice and consulting with the laboratory staff, providing orientation and training programs, developing and maintaining policies and procedures, beginning an effective chemical inventory, and documenting all medical records, including a hepatitis B vaccination program and exposures. In hospital laboratories, the safety officer should also consult with and report new information to the hospital's infection control practitioner and safety officer. When appropriate, reports should be made to the hospital's infection control and safety committees and to local and state health departments.

A good safety plan includes an effective incident investigation program.[22] Incident investigation requires that information be collected to reconstruct accurately the accident and determine the underlying reasons for its cause. Once the primary causes of the accident have been determined, preventive measures can be taken. All accidents must be investigated promptly, regardless of their severity. Even incidents that caused no injury or damage should be investigated to trend activities or problems that may lead to more serious consequences in the future.[11] Incidents that do involve injury or personal harm should be documented in an accident report. This report, at a minimum, should include the name of the individual involved; date of report; employee's job classification, age, and sex; date, time, and exact location of incident; description of the incident; nature of injuries; cause of accident; witness testimony; future preventive measures; and necessary follow-up.

REGULATIONS AND ENFORCEMENTS

Many government and private organizations influence the safety and health programs in today's laboratories through their formal recommendations and inspection processes. A few of the most prominent are listed below.

Occupational Safety and Health Act

In 1970, Congress passed the Occupational Safety and Health Act (OSHA) "to assure so far as possible every working man and woman in the Nation safe and healthful working conditions." Under the Act, OSHA was created within the Department of Labor. Among other purposes, OSHA develops mandatory job safety and health general industry standards (Code of Federal Regulations [CFR] 1910) or laws. Many of these standards affect clinical laboratories. This list includes but is not limited to:

1910.38	Emergency and fire precaution plans
1910.95	Occupational noise exposure
1910.101	Compressed gases
1910.134	Respiratory protection
1910.120	Hazardous waste operations and emergency response
1910.157	Portable fire extinguishers
1910.164	Fire detection systems
1910.1048	Formaldehyde
1910.1200	Hazardous communications
1910.1450	Occupational exposure to hazardous chemicals in laboratories
1910.147	Lockout/tagout
1910.1030	Bloodborne pathogens

Each year, the office of federal regulation publishes all current regulations and standards in the CFR, which is available at many libraries and from the Government Printing Office.

To enforce its standards, OSHA is authorized under the Act to conduct workplace inspections. Most clinical facilities are inspected following employee complaints, but OSHA may conduct planned inspections of high-hazard industries. Once in a facility, the compliance officer may inspect all areas if he or she suspects a concern besides the initial complaint. Penalties for failure to follow OSHA standards range from a maximum willful penalty of $70,000 to a serious violation of $700 and $1,000 for record-keeping concerns.

Employers of 11 or more employees must maintain records of occupational injuries and illnesses as they occur. These incidents must be recorded on OSHA's "Log and Summary of Occupational Injuries and Illnesses" (OSHA No. 200) or its equivalent. The summary page of the log must be posted no later than February 1 and must remain in place until May 1 for all employees to see.

Employers are also responsible for keeping employees informed about OSHA and about the various safety and health matters with which they are involved. The OSHA poster (OSHA 2203) that informs employees of their rights and responsibilities must be posted in a prominent spot for all employees to see. Also employees must be told annually of their right to examine any records kept by their employers regarding their exposure to hazardous materials or the results of medical surveillance.

College of American Pathologists

The College of American Pathologists (CAP) is a private organization that provides a peer review accrediting process every 2 years for clinical laboratories. Its inspection process consists of two portions. The first portion (manuals and records) relates to reviews of documents, whereas the second portion (physical inspection of the laboratory) requires direct inspection of the various laboratory areas to observe environmental safety compliance and actual employee practices. Most noncompliances will become phase two deficiencies.

Joint Commission for the Accreditation of Healthcare Organizations

The Joint Commission for the Accreditation of Healthcare Organizations (JCAHO) is also a private organization that on request will inspect laboratories on a 3-year review. JCAHO's safety requirements are listed in the environment of care or the infection control sections of the *Comprehensive Accreditation Manual for Hospitals.* The Environment of Care section is broken down into seven areas of concern: general safety, hazardous chemicals, security, life safety, emergency preparedness, equipment safety, and utilities. This agency is moving toward reviewing processes and outcomes rather than policy and procedure.

Clinical Laboratory Improvement Amendments

The Clinical Laboratory Improvement Amendments (CLIA) of 1988 was enacted to ensure that clinical laboratories accurately test samples of materials derived from the human body. The responsibility for enforcement of this law has been delegated to the Health Care Financing Administration on the state level. CLIA inspectors have included the majority of OSHA's and CAP's safety requirements into their own system of inspections.

INFECTIOUS HAZARDS

Because medical histories and examinations cannot reliably identify the infectivity of body fluids and tissues, precautions should be used when handling any of these substances.[27] The concept of universal precautions was first introduced in 1987 by the Centers for Disease Control and Prevention (CDC) to decrease the occupational risks of blood-borne diseases, such as AIDS and hepatitis B, to health-care workers.[8,9] In 1991, OSHA issued their final standard on occupational exposure to blood-borne pathogens, which mandates the use of Universal

Precautions for protection against blood-borne pathogens. Since then, this concept has evolved to include protection from all pathogens in all body substances. In general, the use of protective measures should now be based on the health-care worker's contact or interaction with body fluids rather than on the patient's diagnosis. This concept originally known as body substance isolation has now been adapted and incorporated into CDC's two-tiered isolation guidelines as Standard Precautions.[16]

According to CDC, the first tier of protection, Standard Precautions, applies to blood, all body fluids, secretions, and excretions regardless of the diagnosis of the patient or whether or not they contain visible blood. They also apply to nonintact skin and mucous membranes. The three transmission-based second-tier precautions, airborne, droplet, and contact, are designed for patients documented or suspected to be infected with highly transmissible or epidemiologic pathogens for which additional precautions are needed.

Airborne precautions are used for patients known or suspected to be infected with microorganisms transmitted by airborne droplet nuclei. The organisms can remain suspended in the air and can be widely dispersed by air currents within a room or over a long distance. Sample organisms include measles, varicella, and tuberculosis.[24] These patients will be placed in specially ventilated private rooms. Employees susceptible to measles or varicella should not enter the room, and all employees should wear respirator protection when entering a possible tuberculosis patient's room.

Droplet precautions should be used in addition to standard precautions when patients are known or suspected to be infected with microorganism transmitted by large particle droplets (pertussis, influenza) that can be generated by the patient during coughing, sneezing, talking, or performing procedures. These patients ideally should also be placed in private rooms but may be cohorted or even share a room with noninfected patients as long as at least 3 ft is placed between the infected patient and the other patients. A mask (not a respirator) should be worn when working within 3 ft of the patient.

Contact precautions should be used when caring for specified patients known or suspected to be infected or colonized with epidemiologic microorganisms that can be transmitted by direct contact. Organisms of concern today include the multidrug-resistant bacteria, *Clostridium difficile, Escherichia coli* 0157:H7, and rotavirus. Contact may include hand or skin contact that occurs when performing patient care activities that require touching the patient's dry skin or indirect contact by touching environmental surfaces or patient care items in the patient's environment. In general, these precautions expand standard precautions from not only using protection when coming in contact with body fluids but also when coming in contact with the body or environment contaminated by the body. Gloves should be worn when entering the room and changed when contaminated or when leaving the room. Hands should be washed with an antimicrobial soap.[17] If substantial contact with the patient or the contaminated environment is expected, clean, nonsterile gowns should be worn. Noncritical patient care items, such as tourniquets, should be dedicated to a specific patient. If use of common equipment or items is unavoidable, then the items should be adequately cleaned and disinfected between patient use.

Protective Measures

In 1991, OSHA issued their final standard on occupational exposure to blood-borne pathogens, which mandates the use of universal precautions for protection against blood-borne pathogens. At the time, OSHA estimated that this rule will protect more than 5.6 million workers and prevent more than 200 deaths and 9,200 blood-borne infections each year. This standard mandates that each laboratory must develop an exposure control plan with control measures specifically suited to the laboratory. These measures include engineering controls, safe work practices, the use of protective equipment, proper waste handling, and a program for free hepatitis B vaccinations.[7,18]

Engineering controls that isolate or remove the hazard of a pathogen are supplied by the employer and are considered the first level of protection by OSHA. It is always better to eliminate or minimize the risk of exposure by using an engineering control than to try to protect oneself from the risk by use of protective equipment. For example, if an employee is popping corks and aerosols are produced, it is better to use an engineering control, such as a splash shield and a safe technique (cover the cork with gauze), than to put on goggles and masks for protection. Examples of engineering controls in the laboratory include those listed in Box 21–1.

Personal protective equipment (PPE) should be used as barriers to protect the employee's skin, clothing, and mucous membranes against contact with all body fluids.[14] Common protective equipment that is provided, maintained, and cleaned by the employer includes gloves, laboratory coats, aprons, face shields, goggles, and cardiopulmonary resuscitation (CPR) masks. This protective equipment must fit properly to provide adequate protection and to avoid the increased risk of exposure. It should not impede the ability to work. The equipment should be conveniently placed in areas where risk is expected and should be worn only when at risk. Gloves should be changed between

---

Box 21·1

Examples of Engineering Controls in the Laboratory

Secondary containers for handling or transporting specimens if the primary container leaks, is contaminated, or is accidentally punctured

Biosafety cabinets available for use when working with infectious aerosols[7]

Splash shields used during activities that entail risk of body fluid splashes into the face

Impervious needle boxes labeled with biohazard symbols placed in strategic positions in the laboratory, patient rooms, and phlebotomy drawing areas for disposal of sharp objects, such as needles, scalpels, and broken pipettes

Automatic pipettes available for use when pipetting potentially infectious body fluids or other fluids that may have been contaminated

Centrifuge caps used to prevent the production of aerosols

Self-sheathing needles used to eliminate risks associated with recapping and disposal of used needles

Safe work practice controls reduce the risk of exposure by performing the activity by the safest technique possible. It is always better to eliminate or minimize the risk by changing a procedure than to try to protect oneself from the risk by use of protective equipment. Some common work practice controls found in the laboratory for protection from body fluids include:

Do not eat, drink, apply cosmetics, or handle contact lenses in laboratories or anywhere that body fluids or other potentially infectious materials are present.[18]

Be aware of hand-to-face contact to avoid inadvertent inoculation of mucous membranes (eye, nose). When caring for coughing patients, ask them to turn away or use a tissue to cover their mouths.

Cover corks or lids, and open them away from oneself when popping open test tubes.

Wash hands with an appropriate antiseptic after every patient contact (including phlebotomy); after removing gloves and other protective wear; after distributing specimens; when visibly contaminated with blood, body fluids, or tissues; before leaving the clinical work area; and periodically during the day when handling and testing body fluids.[17]

Contaminated sharps should be recapped, bent, broken, or removed. If there is no feasible alternative method or mechanism available, sharps may be recapped by using the "scoop" technique or by a mechanical resheating device.

Handle broken contaminated glassware with mechanical means, such as vacuuming or sweeping into a hard-sided receptacle. Tongs may also be used.[27]

---

patients, but laboratory coats can be worn between patients (as in phlebotomy) or between procedures. If obviously contaminated, the equipment should be removed as soon as feasibly possible.[6] Quality assurance monitors should be established to review the use of the protective gear. Employees should review regular updates on their appropriate use.

Gloves are the most common protective clothing worn in the laboratory. Gloves should be worn when hand contact with body fluids or tissue is expected, during all phlebotomy procedures, when handling contaminated items or surfaces, or when cleaning up after a body fluid spill. These gloves should be available in a variety of sizes and should not irritate or sensitize the skin. Allergies to latex have become a serious problem for health-care workers, and employers should be

aware of the symptoms and the alternatives available in gloving materials.[1,2] Gloves should be changed as soon as practical when contaminated. If an employee is working with contaminated gloves, the contaminated material could be transferred by direct contact to doorknobs, keyboards, or telephones, which could then be an indirect source of infection.

The type and characteristics of protective body clothing chosen for protection depend on the task and the degree of exposure anticipated during the task. For example, if an activity rarely entails exposure to body fluids (ie, clerical work), any type of coat or gown can be worn to protect from day-to-day soiling. Disposable or reusable coats, however, that repel fluids should be worn if there is a potential for splashing or spraying of infectious materials. Impervious coats are necessary if soaking of clothes could potentially occur. A variety of fabric types is now available to offer excellent protection in any of these instances.

If facial exposure is a possibility, the eyes, nose, and mouth must all be protected by masks and goggles or chin-length face shields. Pulmonary resuscitation devices for administering CPR procedures should also be available in patient care areas such as outpatient phlebotomy areas.

In areas where laboratory testing of body fluids is performed, specific procedures for maintaining a clean, safe environment must be developed.[13] Low-level disinfection should occur on noncritical surfaces, such as floors, walls, and doorknobs. Quaternary ammonia products, alcohols, and phenolics are considered low-level disinfectants. Intermediate-level disinfection is necessary in noncritical surfaces (ie, laboratory bench counters, tourniquets) that may come in contact routinely with body fluids.[3] These chemicals should have a product label claim for effectiveness against tuberculosis or human immunodeficiency virus or contain 550 ppm of free chlorine, such as in a fresh 1:100 dilution of common household bleach. Bench tops should be disinfected after completion of a procedure, when leaving the work area, at the end of each shift, and when obviously contaminated.

In general, the following waste items should be "rendered noninfectious" according to local regulations: liquid or semiliquid body fluids, contaminated items that would release body fluids if compressed, items that are caked with dried body fluids and are capable of releasing these materials during handling, contaminated sharps, and pathologic and microbiologic wastes. The appropriate disposal containers should be labeled with a biohazard symbol or color coded for identification. If outside contamination of the regulated waste container occurs, it should be placed in a second container that is closable and leakproof.

CHEMICAL SAFETY

In 1983, OSHA introduced the hazard communication standard (right-to-know; CFR 1910.1200) to regulate the use of hazardous materials in the industrial workplace. In 1990, OSHA recognized, however, that the requirements of the right-to-know regulation could not be applied to laboratories and promulgated the occupational exposures to hazardous chemicals in laboratories standard (CFR 1910.1450). This regulation is to be followed by all facilities that use chemicals on a laboratory scale and perform multiple chemical procedures that are not part of a production process. This regulation, commonly known as the hazardous chemical (haz chem) standard, requires the employer to develop, implement, and maintain at the workplace a written, comprehensive hazard communication program that includes provisions for identifying and classifying chemicals, chemical inventories, container labeling, a documented employee-training program, and availability of material safety data sheets (MSDS).

Classification of Chemicals

Many federal agencies have developed methods of classifying hazardous chemicals. OSHA, the Department of Transportation, the Environmental Protection Agency, and the National Fire Protection Association (NFPA) have all developed specific methods of classification based on their areas of interest and concern.

The hazards of handling chemicals in the laboratory are broadly classified by OSHA according to the dangers they present as physical hazards to the environment or health hazards to living tissues (Appendix 21–1). This method of classification is the most commonly used in clinical laboratories.

In the text of NFPA-704, a system for identifying hazardous materials that may present a hazard during a fire has also been used in laboratories. This method was developed to identify hazards with which a firefighter or responder might come in contact. Their warning system includes a diamond-shaped label with the information listed in Box 21–2.

Chemical Inventories

A listing of hazardous chemicals used in the laboratory must be developed and annually reviewed. This list may include the name of the chemical, name and address of manufacture, physical state (liquid, gas, solid), maximum amount of chemical present at one time, storage area, method of disposal, and identification of hazards. An up-to-date copy of this list should be available to emergency personnel in case of a fire, explosion, or any other type of emergency.

Labeling

Manufacturer labels are required to list the name of the chemical, hazards associated with the chemical, and name and address of the manufacturer, importer, or responsible party.

Once a hazardous chemical is transferred to another container, the name of the chemicals and the associated hazards must also be transferred. This information is not required by law if you plan to use the chemical immediately. The label may also contain other information that may be required by other agencies.

Box 21•2

Warning of Hazardous Materials a Firefighter or Responder May Encounter

HEALTH–BLUE

Indicates that the material may directly or indirectly cause permanent or temporary injury due to acute exposure by physical contact, inhalation, or ingestion

4—Deadly
3—Extreme danger
2—Hazardous
1—Slightly hazardous
0—Normal material

FLAMMABILITY–RED

Assesses the relative susceptibility of materials to fire burst, based on the form or condition of the material and its surrounding environment

4—below 70°F
3—Below 100°F
2—Below 20°F
1—Above 200°F
0—Will not burn

REACTIVITY–YELLOW

Advises that the material may be susceptible to explosion, whether through self-reaction or polymerization or by exposure to certain conditions or substances

4—May detonate
3—Shock and heat may detonate
2—Violent chemical change
1—Unstable if heated
0—Stable

SPECIFIC HAZARD–WHITE

Covers special properties and other hazards associated with a particular material; especially useful for emergency response or firefighting teams:

Oxidizer (Ox)
Corrosive (Cor)
Use *no* water
Radiation

Material Safety Data Sheets

All hazardous chemicals present in the laboratory will have an MSDS that has been developed to protect and inform workers on how to handle hazardous materials and how to respond to emergencies. Employees are responsible for knowing and understanding the information on these sheets. The original format contained the eight sections listed in Box 21–3.

A new format for standardizing MSDSs has been developed to improve its readability and use in emergency situations.[10,31] Until all manufacturers change over to the new format, the employee should be familiar with both formats. The new system is formatted into the 16 sections detailed in Box 21–4.

Employee Training Program

The chemical hygiene plan for a laboratory will require that all employees be trained when hired, when new chemicals are introduced, and if conditions for handling the chemicals change. Topics listed in Box 21–5 should be included.

Prevention and Controls

Once existing and potential chemical hazards in the laboratory have been recognized, laboratorians at risk have been identified, and existing control measures have been evaluated, the next step is to assess the need for prevention, control, or PPE.[15] Laboratory policies and procedures should describe the use of appropriate methods of controls, such as engineering and administrative controls, safe work practices, and appropriate PPE.

Box 21•3

Eight Sections of the Original Material Safety Data Sheet

Section I: Chemical identity
Section II: Hazardous ingredients
Section III: Physical and chemical characteristics
Section IV: Fire and explosion hazards
Section V: Reactivity data
Section VI: Health hazards
Section VII: Precautions for safe handling and use
Section VIII: Control measures

Sixteen Sections of New Standardized Material Safety Data Sheets

Section 1: Identification
Section 2: Composition and ingredients
    information
Section 3: Hazards identification
Section 4: First-aid procedures
Section 5: Firefighting procedures
Section 6: Accidental release measures
Section 7: Exposure control (personal protective
    equipment)
Section 8: Handling and storage
Section 9: Physical and chemical properties
Section 10: Stability and reactivity information
Section 11: Toxicologic information
Section 12: Ecologic information
Section 13: Disposal guidelines
Section 14: Transport information
Section 15: Regulatory information and
    considerations
Section 16: Other information

Engineering controls, the preferred method for controlling hazards, use technologic means to isolate or remove chemical hazards from the laboratory workplace. Examples include splash shields, flammable cabinets, covered switches, light fixtures, flammable refrigerators and freezers, and ventilation hoods. Ventilation

Topics for Instruction Under the Chemical Hygiene Plan

The location and labeling of the hazardous
    chemicals in the laboratory
Whereabouts of the written chemical hygiene
    plan and chemical inventories
Use and location of the MSDSs
Physical and health hazards presented by
    chemicals
Proper use and location of engineering controls,
    administrative controls, safe work practices,
    and personal protective equipment

MSDS, Material Safety data Sheets.

hoods not only protect laboratorians from toxic, offensive, or flammable vapors, but also act as a barrier in case of an explosion or chemical spill. The hood should be used whenever operations might result in release of toxic chemical vapors or dust or when working with any appreciably volatile substances with a TLV of less than 50 ppm. These hoods should be evaluated before use to ensure adequate face velocities, which are typically between 60 and 100 lfms. The hood should also be kept closed at all times except when adjustments within the hood are being made. Materials stored in the hood should be kept at a minimum and should not block vents or air flow. The hood should be left on when it is not in active use if toxic substances are stored in it or if it is uncertain whether adequate general laboratory ventilation will be maintained when it is off (Box 21–6).

Safe work practices reduce the likelihood of exposure to occupational chemical hazards by altering the manner in which a task is performed. PPE is specialized clothing or equipment worn by an employee for protection against a hazard.[25] The use of PPE, such as gloves, goggles, aprons, respirators, ear plugs, ear muffs, and boots, is the last resort for reducing or eliminating worker exposure. PPEs typically are used when other engineering and work practice controls are not feasible or until other controls can be implemented. Traditionally, PPE is a supplement to minimize workers' exposure, not a primary source of control.

Workers must be trained in the proper selection, use, and maintenance of employee-supplied PPEs. A physical evaluation also may be required before workers are assigned to areas requiring the use of some PPEs, such as respirators.

Because skin contact is probably the most common chemical exposure in the clinical laboratory, appropriate gloves and long sleeve protective coats, gowns, or jackets can drastically minimize the number and severity of chemical exposures.

Gloves should be worn whenever handling corrosive materials, rough or sharp-edged objects, very hot or very cold materials, or body fluids or whenever protection is needed against accidental exposure to chemicals. Latex gloves can be worn when handling most of the common laboratory chemicals. However, specialty gloves, such as neoprene, polyvinyl chloride, nitril leather, and insulated gloves may be required for handling certain chemicals. For example, aromatic chemicals, such as benzene and chloroform, will attack latex but are more resistant to nitrile gloves. Glove manufacture catalogs will often list the proper glove for specific chemicals.

Laboratory coats or gowns are also necessary protective equipment in a clinical laboratory. They are intended to prevent contact with dirt and minor chemical

---

Box 21·6

Examples of Safe Work Practices

Avoid eating, drinking, smoking, gum chewing, or applying cosmetics or lip balm in areas where
laboratory chemicals are present. Wash hands before conducting these activities.

Avoid storing, handling, or consuming food or beverages in storage areas, refrigerators, glassware, or
utensils that are also used for laboratory operation.

Do not mouth pipette.

Empty containers may still have traces of chemical in them, so treat these containers as contaminated
waste. Do not use them to store any other fluids.

Dispose of chemicals in sealed labeled containers.

Use glassware equipment only for its designed purpose.

Keep the work area clean and uncluttered, with chemicals and equipment properly labeled and stored;
clean up the work area on completion of a procedure or at the end of the shift.

Do not smell or taste chemicals.

Use only chemicals for which the quality of the available ventilation system is appropriate.

Be aware of unsafe conditions, and see that they are corrected when detected.

An exhaust hood should be used whenever appreciable quantities of flammable substances are:
Transferred form one container to another
Allowed to stand in open containers
Heated in open containers
Handled in any hazardous way

All flammable reagents are to be kept in the flammable storage facilities at all times when not in use. Most
experts recommend that no more than one gallon of total flammable fluids by stored on open shelving
in a 100 sq ft room. Up to 2 gallons may be stored in safety cans and safety cabinets for each 100 sq ft.[29]

Any solutions compounded from these reagents should be labeled as flammable.

Flammable substances should be handled only in areas free of ignition sources.

Flammable substances should not be heated by using an open flame. Preferred heat sources include steam
baths, water baths, oil baths, heating mantles, and hot air baths.

When transferring flammable liquids in metal equipment, static generated sparks should be avoided by
bonding and the use of ground strips.

Administrative controls reduce or eliminate a worker's exposure by changing the duration, frequency, or
severity of exposure. For example, if toxic air exposures may exist and cannot be reduced to the
permissible exposure limits through engineering or work practice controls, administrative controls may
be used as an alternative means to reduce laboratorians' exposure. Examples of administrative controls
include rotating employees to jobs free of the specific hazard, adjusting work schedules, and providing
adequate staffing when the work output is increased.

---

splashes or spills. However, when handling larger
amounts of chemicals, disposal impermeable gowns
may be necessary for better protection.

When procedures that involve potential hazards to
the eyes and face are performed, facial protection may
be necessary. Safety glasses with eye shields, goggles,
or face shields are commonly worn. Full face shields
that protect the face and throat should always be worn
when maximum protection from flying particles and
harmful liquids is needed; for full protection in extreme
cases, safety glass should be worn in combination with
the face shields.

Chemical Spills and Releases

All chemical spills should be handled as potential hazards. Many times significant exposures occur before
you actually see or smell the chemical. Therefore, all
employees must always aware of the risk of a spill and
what is normal handling, storage, and disposal of each
chemical. Should a spill or release occur, immediate
action should be taken according to the laboratory's
emergency plan.[23] Chemical spill kits should be available to assist in containing the spills. The kits should
contain absorbent materials, protective clothing, gloves

and goggles, appropriate air purifying respirators (ie, formaldehyde and organic cartridges), and hazardous area warning tape.

In general, employees should be taught the following basic rules for handling the three types of chemical spills: unknown or untrained spill; small, contained spills; and chemical emergencies.

If you are unfamiliar with the released chemical and if you have not been trained in its use and handling or do not recognize the involved chemical, do not attempt to clean up the spill. Secure the area according to your laboratory's plan, and notify your supervisor and other people in the immediate area about the spill. Attend to any people who may have been contaminated. If the spilled material is potentially flammable, turn off ignition and light sources. Avoid breathing vapors of the material. Leave on or establish exhaust ventilation if it is safe to do so. Finally, notify proper authorities in your facility. Do not take further action. Leave the rest to trained personnel.

If you are familiar with the spilled chemical and decide to contain a minor spill yourself, approach the spill with caution. Secure the area as described previously, and do not attempt to handle the spill until you have protected yourself and others around you. If possible, identify the chemical by name brand and manufacturer. Contact your supervisor or your laboratory safety officer to make sure someone else is aware of the spill and will respond quickly to back you up if necessary. No matter how comfortable you are with a chemical, review the MSDS before you proceed. The spill and leak procedure section of these sheets will tell you how to safely absorb, neutralize, or otherwise control the spilled chemical. The special protection data section of the MSDS will explain what protective equipment is recommended in the clean-up process. Once contained, dispose of the chemical as directed by the MSDS or your laboratory's established policy. If you become contaminated with a hazardous chemical during a spill, call for help immediately.

A large uncontrollable chemical spill or release should be considered a chemical emergency if it causes airborne concentrations of toxic chemicals above permissible exposure limits, is life or injury threatening, requires employee evacuation, poses immediate danger to life and health conditions, poses a risk for fire or explosion, or promotes an oxygen-deficient condition. Employees should be trained to identify these conditions and to report them to the appropriate management immediately. The need for evacuation of personnel and resources should be assessed immediately and appropriate measures taken to evacuate effectively. Trained in-house spill teams or community hazardous materials control units should take over all responsibilities for containment and removal of these hazardous chemicals. Many laboratories are developing their own response teams based on OSHA's hazardous waste operations and emergency response standard (CFR 1910.120).[5,26] These specifically trained teams can quickly respond to minimize physical damage or injury to personnel.

Chemical Exposures and First Aid

Chemicals may cause health hazards to the body by either inhalation, ingestion, skin contact, contact with eyes, and injection. The necessary first aid is based on the method of exposure.

Inhalation of toxic vapors, gases, dust, or mists can produce poisoning by absorption through the mucous membrane of the mouth, throat, and lungs. The degree of severity depends on the toxicity of the material and its solubility in tissue fluids and on its concentration and the duration of exposure. Some chemicals, such as benzene, are cumulative poisons that can produce body damage through exposure to small concentrations over a long period. The best way to avoid exposure to toxic aerosolized chemicals is to prevent the escape of such materials into the working atmosphere and to ensure adequate ventilation by the use of exhaust hoods and other local ventilation. Chemicals of unknown toxicity should not be smelled.

Many values have been developed to measure the risk associated with respiratory exposure to a chemical. The most common include those listed in Box 21–7.

Many chemicals used in the laboratory could cause physical harm if ingested. The ingestion hazard is measured by its LD50 rating. An LD50 is defined as the quantity of material that when ingested or applied to the skin in a single dose will cause the death of 50% of the test animals. It is expressed in grams or milligrams per kilogram of body weight. In general, if chemicals are accidentally ingested, the person would be encouraged to drink large amounts of water. The MSDS should be consulted for further first aid and medical follow-up.

Skin contact with hazardous chemicals is the most common route of exposure in the clinical laboratory. The main portals of entry for chemicals is through hair follicles, sebaceous glands, sweat glands, cuts, and abrasions. In the event of skin contact, all contaminated clothing and jewelry should be quickly removed. Chemical spills on leather products, such as watchbands, belts, or shoes, can be quickly absorbed and then held close to the skin. At the time of the contact, the affected areas should be flushed with copious amounts of cold water. Wash off chemicals by using a mild soap and water. Consult the MSDS for further first aid and medical follow-up. Medical attention should be sought if symptoms persist.

Box 21·7

Common Values Developed to Measure the Risk Associated With Respiratory Exposure to a Chemical

PEL: Permissible exposure limit. A PEL is the maximum airborne concentration of a substance regulated by OSHA to which a worker by be exposed. These values are enforced by law. These limits must be interpreted by a trained industrial hygienist based on air sampling methodology, material levels, exposure duration, and individual worker size, sex, age, and body chemistry.

ppm: Parts per million.

REL: Recommended exposure limit. Established by the National Institute for Occupational Safety and Health (NIOSH), REL is the maximum recommended exposure to a chemical or physical agent in the workplace. The REL is intended to prevent adverse health effects for all occupational exposed workers.

TLV: Threshold limit value. A TLV is the airborne concentration of a substance to which nearly all workers can be exposed repeatedly day after day without adverse effect. The American Conference of Government Industrial Hygienists (ACGIH) recommends and publishes these values annually on the basis of the most current scientific interpretations. TLVs are not OSHA standards and are not enforced by law.

TLV-C: Threshold limit value-ceiling. The TLV-C is the airborne concentration of a substance that should not be exceeded—even for an instant—during any part of the working exposure.

TLV-SKIN: Threshold limit value—skin absorption. TLV-SKIN refers to the potential contribution of absorption through the skin—including mucous membranes and eyes—to a worker's overall exposure by airborne or direct contact with a substance.

TLV-STEL: Threshold limit value-short term exposure. The TLV-STEL is the maximum exposure concentration allowed for up to 15 minutes during a maximum of four periods each workday. Each exposure period should be at least 60 minutes after the last period.

TWA: Time-weighted average. The TWA is the average exposure concentration during an 8-hour workday. Exposure for more than 8 hours per day or more than 40 hours per week, even at or below the TLV or PEL, may represent a health hazard. NIOSH recommendations typically include 10 hour TWAs for up to a 40 hour workweek. The TWA for an 8-hour workday is calculated as follows:

$$\frac{\text{sum of [(exposure period)} \times \text{(exposure concentration)] for each exposure period}}{\text{8-hour workday}}$$

For example, formaldehyde exposure in a laboratory might be:

$$\frac{(5 \text{ ppm} \times 2 \text{ hours}) + (1 \text{ ppm} \times 6 \text{ hours})}{\text{8-hour workday}} = \frac{10 + 6}{8} = 2.0 \text{ ppm TWA}$$

Most chemicals in the laboratory are considered minimal eye irritants. However, some chemicals, such as strong acids and bases, are hazardous enough to cause burns and loss of vision. Also, because eyes are very vascular, chemicals are rapidly absorbed through this route. Eye protection, such as safety glasses, goggles, or shields, provide good protection to eyes. In the event of a splash to the eyes, the eyes should be flushed with copious amounts of water for at least 15 minutes, and medical attention should be sought whether or not symptoms persist.

Laboratorians are rarely exposed to chemicals through injection. However, this could occur through cuts or punctures with contaminated glass or sharp metals or needles.

Formaldehyde

In 1992, OSHA's special law for handling formaldehyde promulgated its final rule on the occupational exposure to formaldehyde (cfr 1910.1048). In histology, anatomy, and pathology laboratories, an alcohol-based formaldehyde product, formalin, is often used for preserving tissue and anatomic body parts. Because of its unique nature to be able to become airborne, OSHA felt a spe-

---

Box 21•8

Initial Training for Personnel Who Handle Formalin

A discussion of the contents of this regulation and the contents of the material safety data sheets

A description of the potential health hazards associated with exposure

A description of the signs and symptoms of exposure to formaldehyde

Instructions to report immediately to the employer the development of any adverse signs or symptoms that the employee suspects is attributable to exposure

Description of appropriate engineering and safe work practice controls

The purpose for, proper use of, and limitations of personal protective clothing and equipment

Instructions for the handling of spills, emergencies, and clean-up procedures

---

Box 21•9

OSHA Regulations for Respirators

The use of negative pressure respirators

A quantitative fit test at the time the respirator use begins and annually thereafter

A medical assessment provided at no charge to the employee to be sure that the employee is physically able to wear a respirator

The regularly changing the purifying chemical cartridge in the respirator

---

cific regulation was necessary. This regulation requires a written formaldehyde exposure plan that describes how occupational exposure can be reduced through safe work practices, proper ventilation, the use of PPEs, and periodic monitoring of air samples.

Health hazards that have been associated with formaldehyde use include skin and eye irritation, skin sensitization, and respiratory toxin and carcinogen exposure. Personnel who handle formalin must receive training at the time of initial assignment, whenever a new exposure to the chemical is introduced into the work area, and on an annual basis. This training must be easily accessible and include the materials listed in Box 21–8.

In most clinical laboratories, engineering controls and good work practices keep formaldehyde vapor levels at a safe range. If necessary, personal protective equipment and clothing should be provided at no cost to the employee and usually includes a cover gown or apron, safety goggles or goggles and face shield, and gloves compatible with formaldehyde (nitrile, neoprene, or vinyl). If vapor levels are above the acceptable

level, respirators must be worn. This respirator usage must meet OSHA regulations for respirators (Box 21–9).

Equipment should be repaired or replaced as needed to ensure its effectiveness. If contaminated, it must be safely removed and cleaned or disposed of properly. PPE, contaminated or not, should not be taken home or otherwise removed from the laboratory.

Initial exposure monitoring to formaldehyde should be performed to verify that vapor levels are below allowable levels. If so, then this monitoring only needs to be repeated if there is a change in the volume of the chemical handled, equipment, process, personnel, or control measures that may result in new or additional exposure. Repeat monitoring must also be performed if employees note signs or symptoms of respiratory or dermal conditions associated with formaldehyde overexposure.

If initial monitoring exceeds allowable limits, periodic monitoring must also be performed at least every 6 months until the levels fall below the action level of 0.5 ppm or STEL of 2 ppm for two consecutive sampling periods at least 7 days apart. While levels are high, this area of the laboratory must be labeled with a sign (Box 21–10).

Box 21•10

Formaldehyde Laboratory Monitoring Sign

Danger
Formaldehyde
Irritant and potential cancer hazard
Authorized personnel only

All results of monitoring must be shared with the employee within 15 days of knowledge of results. If acceptable levels of exposure are exceeded, a written plan to reduce the employee's exposure will be given to each exposed employee, which describes the corrective actions being taken to decrease exposure. Also, a medical evaluation must also be conducted to assess for any irritation or sensitization of the skin or eyes, shortness of breath, or abnormal pulmonary function tests.

Procedures to follow in case of an emergency associated with a formaldehyde release have been developed for each laboratory that uses formaldehyde. It is the employee's responsibility to be familiar with these procedures. It is the employer's responsibility to train all employees in their specific duties.

If a spill of appreciable quantity occurs, the area should be vacated immediately unless specific duties have been previously designated. Designated employees should isolate the hazard area and deny entry except for necessary people protected by suitable protective equipment (clothing and respirators) adequate for exposure.

Compressed Liquids and Gases

Liquids or gases compressed into containers for use in the clinical laboratory present a unique concern.[20] These containers represent the potential of chemical and physical hazards. The OSHA standard (CFR 1910.101), based on recommendations in pamphlets developed by the Compressed Gas Association, requires special identification, handling, transportation, and storage of these chemicals. Some effective safe work practices in the laboratory include those listed in Box 21–11.

FIRE (LIFE) SAFETY

Fires and explosions are a constant threat in the clinical laboratory.[28] Frequent causes of fires in this area include carelessness, inattention, lack of knowledge, unattended equipment, and faulty electrical wiring and equipment. Most fire regulations and guidelines are based on recommendations of the NFPA, who update their codes on a regular basis. Copies of these codes may be obtained through a local fire marshall or NFPA itself.

Multiple flammable and combustible chemicals that exist sometimes in large quantities in the laboratory add to the morbidity of a fire. The number and size of these flammable chemical containers should be kept at a minimum and always stored in closed explosion-proof cabinets, refrigerators, or freezers. Chemicals on the working bench should also be limited to those necessary for daily needs. When transferring flammable liquids in metal containers, static-generated sparks are avoided by bonding and the use of ground straps.[29]

The multitude of electrical equipment in a clinical laboratory can also increase the risk of fires.

All spark-causing relays, switches, motors, or hot plates should be eliminated. Only Underwriters Laboratories (UL) equipment should be used. Extension cords must only be used as a temporary measure and must be UL approved as well.

The NFPA has set specific requirements for facilities to minimize damage in case of a true fire.[12] Each laboratory must check with the local fire marshall to be sure that all necessary precautions are in place. In general, an automatic sprinkler system is required for laboratories separated from inpatient areas by a 1-hour construction wall and class C self-closing doors. For facilities with no inpatients that have 2-hour construction and class B self-closing doors, no sprinkler system is required. Also, each room larger than 1,000 sq ft that contains flammables must have at least two lighted exit doors remote from each other, one of which opens directly into a means of egress. Fire detection systems must be in place and fire alarms audible in all parts of the laboratory. Quarterly fire drills must be in place with each employee participating at least annually.

Damage caused by fire can be minimized by knowing the proper steps to take when a fire is discovered. These steps can best be described by the use of the acronym RACE:

R—Rescue
A—Alarm
C—Confine
E—Evacuate

The order in which these steps are used depends on each situation. For example, many small fires can be contained before having to rescue personnel or patients; however, in fires that are out of control, rescue should come first.

R—Rescue Personnel and Patients

When a fire is discovered, rescuing personnel or patients in immediate life-threatening danger is always the top priority. Stop to investigate all unusual odors. If you smell smoke coming from behind a closed door, feel the door with the back of your hand before opening it. If it is hot, do not open it. If it's touchable, open it slowly. If you must enter the scene of a fire to rescue, stay low. Smoke and heat rise to the ceiling.

A—Sound the Alarm

After discovering a fire, alert authorities as soon as possible. IF you must rescue personnel or patients in immediate danger, call out to other staff so that they can

Box 21•11

Effective Safe Work Practices in Laboratories Containing Compressed Liquids and Gases

1. Signs should be conspicuously posted in areas in which flammable compressed gases are stored, identifying the substances and the appropriate precautions.
2. Cylinders should have a permanent legible label that identifies its contents and hazards. Color coding is not a reliable method of identifying because colors may vary from manufacturer to manufacturer.
3. Stored cylinders are secured to a wall or vertical support by means of a strap, chain, or container. Avoid routinely storing cylinders in a cylinder cart. Cylinders should be assigned to a definite area for storage. Segregate full and empty cylinders in their storage area.
4. Keep cylinders protected from excessive temperatures by storing them away from heat sources.
5. Do not store oxygen cylinder and flammable gas cylinders in the same room unless there is adequate separation by distance or fire-resistant partitioning walls.
6. Never use oxygen as a substitute for compressed air.
7. When moving cylinders, use the appropriate-size cart with a chain restraint in place. Do not drag cylinders or carry them in your arms.
8. For cylinders equipped with valve protection caps, keep the cap on cylinders at all times when not in use.
9. Cylinders should never be dropped or rolled in a horizontal position because the cylinder valve might be broken off.
10. Return leaking cylinders to personnel authorized to return as soon as possible to the supplier. Label or tag the tank denoting the problem.
11. Combustible leaking gas tanks should be moved to a well-ventilated, preferably outdoor area away from combustible materials.
12. Never force a post-type valve (brass valve) onto the regulator. Check to be sure the right gas regulator is being used for that specific tank. A pin index safety system is in place to prevent the possibility of accidental substitution of the wrong gas on a yoke-type connection apparatus.
13. If a cylinder protective cap is extremely difficult to remove, do not apply excessive force or pry the cap loose with a bar inserted into the ventilation openings. Attach a label or tag to the cylinder identifying the problem, and return the cylinder to the supplier.
14. Wrenches should not be used on valves equipped with a handwheel. If the valve is faulty, attach a label or tag to the cylinder identifying the problem, and return the cylinder to the supplier.
15. Inspect the overall condition of the regulator on a regular basis for any signs of damage. Report any damage to the inlet fitting and porous filter and the outlet fitting before using.
16. Return any cylinder with a damaged valve or one that shows any signs of contamination to the supplier. If the valve is undamaged, point the outlet away from yourself or any other person, stand to one side, and "crack" open slightly to clear the valve of particulate matter such as dust. Make sure that all smoking and open flame rules are enforced.
17. A face shield and resistant gloves should be worn when handling liquid gases and other cryogenic fluids. Contact with skin should be avoided because even a brief skin contact with a cryogenic liquid may cause thermal burns.

sound the alarm. Review your facility's alarm procedure with your coworkers.

C—Confine the Fire

Laboratory units are divided and separated from the rest of the facility by heavy fire doors. Once the alarm is sounded, these doors will close automatically to keep the fire from spreading. To help confine the fire within your unit, close all doors, windows, and vertical open-

ings, such as laundry chutes or "dumb waiters." Stuffing damp towels underneath doors can help keep smoke out. Shut off oxygen if you are directed to do so.

E—Evacuate

If the fire is out of control and cannot be contained, you must evacuate the area. Initially evacuate beyond the first set of designated fire doors. These doors are developed to give protection for a specific amount of time. If necessary, leave the facility. Establish a predetermined meeting place.

Fire Extinguisher

Most fire extinguishers in today's laboratories are of the multipurpose classification. These ABC extinguishers are recommended for all types of fires, including combustibles, liquids, and electrical fires. OSHA mandates that clinical laboratory employees receive annual training in the use of fire extinguishers. A simple method to remember how to use a fire extinguisher includes the use of the acronym PASS.

P—Pull the Pin

Hold the bottom of the handle of the extinguisher and pull the pin out from the handle.

A—Aim at the Bottom

Stand 8 to 10 feet away from the fire. Aim the nozzle at the bottom of the fire, because the bottom of the flames is actually what is burning.

S—Squeeze the Handle

Squeeze the handle to release the extinguishing agent in short bursts of 5 to 10 seconds.

S—Spray Back and Forth

Spray the extinguishing agent in a back-and-forth sweeping motion at the bottom of the fire to extinguish all burning materials.

ERGONOMICS

From the perspective of employees, ergonomics in a laboratory can be defined as making facilities more user friendly, thereby minimizing risks. The goals for a good program should include improving employee well-being; reducing cumulative trauma disorders (CTDs) and related workers' compensation costs; improving patient service and facility efficiency; improving job satisfaction, morale, and employee relations; and reducing absenteeism and turnover.[4] Elements of a good ergonomics program will include an organized plan with proper training, a job analysis to review all jobs for issues and methods of improvement, a medical management program to identify

and treat employees with symptoms, and a monitoring process that will measure and evaluate the program.[21]

An overall plan should include assigning responsibilities and resources. The coordinator of the ergonomic program should be assigned specific authority and sufficient resources for assigning staff time and employee time off to be involved in the program. This written plan should also identify the organizational structure, outline program goals and objectives, and provide a timetable for achieving them. An ergonomics team may be necessary to identify concerns and to coordinate and implement any changes.[30] This team should consist of qualified, interested employees. Mechanisms should be established to obtain employee input through suggestions or complaints, interviews, formal surveys, or small group discussions.

Training in basic concepts of ergonomics and cumulative trauma should be provided early in the development of an ergonomics program. This information should be pertinent to each group's role in the program. Employees who perform tasks that involve risk factors for CTDs should be provided with information that includes the basic symptoms and how employees should report any problems. Job-specific training may be needed to help employees use smooth and easy work techniques.

Often, the common reason for the failure of ergonomic programs is poor communication among the players. If individuals are not told what is going on, they may assume nothing is happening. Also communication and participation often help pave the way for accepting any changes in jobs that might occur with the implementation of a new program.

Job analysis should begin with a background review to identify ergonomic hazards already present in the laboratory. Begin with a review of existing medical, safety, and insurance records, including the OSHA 200 logs and workers' compensation injury reports for evidence of CTDs. Often, available recorded medical data are not complete. Records are dependent on employee awareness of the need and the importance of the reported problems. Ways of soliciting information from employees could include simple informal discussions or a self-administered questionnaire. A simple one-page anonymous "symptom questionnaire" that asks employees if they experience physical discomfort from their jobs usually by referring to a part of the body and an index of severity can be effective. Also, occupational therapy departments can assist with some easy, quick screening methods to identify employees at risk of such illnesses as carpal tunnel syndrome.

Once you are confident that you have identified all present employees with symptoms, you can calculate annual rates for upper extremity disorders and lower back injuries per 100 full-time workers in each laboratory:

$$\text{Incidence rate} = \frac{\text{(No. of new cases/year)} \times \text{(200,000 work hours) per laboratory}}{\text{No. of hours worked/facility/year}}$$

The second step is a detailed baseline screening survey to identify jobs that put employees at risk of developing CTDs. The survey should be performed with an ergonomic checklist that includes such components as posture, materials handling, and upper extremity factors. The risk factors that should be identified through the survey include those defined in Box 21–12.

Also, review human resources records for jobs that have high turnover, are universally disliked, are lowest on bid lists, and are used as entry-level jobs due to undesirability.

Once knowledgeable to ergonomics concerns, problem areas may be identified by a walk-through of the area.

Problem solving should be prioritized once risks have been recognized. First identify the steps of the job, noting specific risk factors for each step. If necessary, videotape processes to become familiar with each.

Finding ways to improve jobs is the key part of the process. Look at short-term and long-term improvements using concepts of "continuous improvement." Sources to use can include in-house personnel, ergonomics literature, ergonomics consultants, contractors, equipment suppliers, and professional contacts. A good tracking system of job evaluation results, ideas for improvement, planned changes, and overall progress should be incorporated into your safety program. Concerns often noted in the laboratory include those responsible for improper positioning (Box 21–13).

Low-level noise or white noise is often a problem in clinical laboratories due to the large amounts of instrumentation. White noise can result in fatigue, irritation, and headache. To minimize these risks, employees should be required to take breaks and lunches away from the area as much as possible.

Using OSHA's tiered systems of protection, some common protective measures are useful to minimize ergonomic risks in the laboratory:

- *Administrative controls*: rearranging of work flow, rotating of personnel, quality assurance indicators, preventive maintenance programs for equipment, and an effective housekeeping program
- *Engineering controls*: proper chairs and stools, automatic pipettes, antifatigue mats, pencil grips, swivel mounted keyboards, automatic reagent mixing analyzers, touch-controlled video display terminal (VDT) screens, VDT glare screens, document holders at VDTs, easy access fume hoods, hands-free microscopes, tilting binocular head microscopes, swivel mounted microtones, work bench edge cushions, telephone headsets, foot rests, lumbar cushions, and magnifiers
- *Safe work practices*: early detection of signs and symptoms, proper work postures, breaks, and exercises
- *Personnel protective equipment*: possibly wrist or arm supports and back supports (though OSHA is now questioning their effectiveness)

Medical management is a vital element of the overall ergonomic program. Programs should include early recognition, systematic evaluation and referral, conservative treatment and follow-up, integration of health care with ergonomics, and accurate record keeping.

Periodic evaluation of the ergonomic program should also be conducted to review the management of the overall program, injury and illness trends and incident rates, ergonomic job improvement log, and

---

Box 21•12

CTD Risk Factor Survey

Repetitive and prolonged activities
Forceful exertions, usually with the hands
Prolonged static postures
Awkward postures of the upper body, including reaching above the shoulders or behind the back
Continued physical contact with work surfaces, such as contact with edges
Excessive vibration from equipment
Cold temperatures
Inappropriate or inadequate hand equipment
Poor body mechanics, for example, continued bending at the waist, continued lifting from below the knuckles or above the shoulders, or twisting at the waist, especially while lifting
Lifting or moving objects of excessive weight or asymmetric size
Prolonged sitting, especially with poor posture
Lack of adjustable chairs, foot rest, body supports, and work surfaces at work stations
Slippery footing

Box 21·13

Improper Positioning Concerns

WHEN SITTING

Do not hunch shoulders over, always bend forward from the hip.

Incline work surfaces; aim toward "right angle" work surface.

Use a well-defined and adjusted chair.

If heels rise up off the floor when you lean back in chair, use a foot rest.

WHILE SEATED

Allow room between tops of legs and work surfaces.

Work heights should include the following:
26–28 in for typing and light assembly work
28–31 in for writing and reading
31–44 in for precise work

FROM A SEATED POSITION

Keep materials 6–14 in from the front of the work area and no more than 10 in above the work surface.

Sideways reaches should be limited to about 16 in from the center of the body.

Only lift objects less than 10 lb.

Avoid body contact with hard surfaces: tilt boxes/bins toward you or use "holders."

WHILE STANDING

Use a footrest.

Reaches over 20 in and above shoulder height should be avoided. Keep within 10 in for frequent reaches.

Work surfaces heights while standing should be positioned:
Precise work: just above elbow height with forearm support
Light work: just below elbow height—keeping "right angle" working position
Heavy work: no higher than 4–8 in below elbow height

Tilt boxes or bins toward you to avoid body contact.

Use antifatigue floor mats to minimize foot pressure.

---

performance indicators, including employee survey results, compensation costs, turnover, absenteeism, quality, and productivity.

REFERENCES

1. Asa R: Allergens spur hospitals to offer latex-free care. Materials Management June:28–34, 1994
2. Mendyka BE, Clochesy JM, Workman ML: Latex hypersensitivity: An iatrogenic and occupational risk. American Journal of Critical Care 3(3):198–201, 1994
3. Bond WW, Favero MS, Peterson NJ, Gravell CR, Ebert JW, Maynard JE: Survival of hepatitis B virus after drying and storage for one week. Lancet i:550–551, 1981
4. Brzezicki LA: Conquering the causes of cumulative trauma. Advance Administrators of the Laboratory March:20–23, 1994
5. Burt SA: Health facilities not exempt from HAZWOPER. Health Facilities Management October:41–43, 1993
6. Centers for Disease Control and Prevention: Hepatitis B contamination in a clinical laboratory—Colorado. MMWR 29:459–460, 1980
7. Centers for Disease Control and Prevention/National Institutes of Health: Biosafety in microbiological and biomedical laboratories, 3rd ed. HHS Publication No. (CDC)93-8395. U.S. Government Printing Office, Washington, DC, 1993
8. Centers for Disease Control and Prevention: Recommendations for prevention of HIV transmission in health care settings. MMWR 36(2S):1–18, 1987
9. Centers for Disease Control and Prevention: Update: Universal precautions for prevention of transmission of human immunodeficiency virus, hepatitis B virus, and other bloodborne pathogens in health-care settings. MMWR 37:377–388, 1988
10. Chemical Manufacturers Association: Standard for the Preparation Material Safety Data Sheets. Proposed draft submitted to American National Standards Institute (ANSI). February 11, 1993
11. Dienstag JL, Ryan DM: Occupational exposure to hepatitis B virus in hospital personnel: Infection or immunization? Am J Epidemiol 115:26–39, 1982
12. Erickson DS: New life safety code contains key fire changes. Health Facilities Management December:42–45, 1992
13. Favero MS, Bond WW: Chemical Disinfection of medical and surgical materials, pp 617–641. In Block SS (ed): Dis-

infection, Sterilization and Preservation, 4th ed. Philadelphia, Lea & Febiger, 1991

14. Favero MS, Bond WW: Transmission and control of laboratory-acquired hepatitis infection, pp 19–32. In Fleming DO, Richardson JH, Tulis JJ, Vesley D (eds): Laboratory Safety—Principles and Practices, 2nd ed. Washington, DC, ASM Press, 1995

15. Fawcett HH, Wood W: Safety and Accident Prevention in Chemical Operations. New York, Interscience Publishers, 1965

16. Federal Register: Draft Guidelines for Isolation Precautions in Hospitals. U.S. Washington, DC, Government Printing Office, 59(214):55552–55570, 1995

17. Garner JS, Favero MS: Guidelines for handwashing and hospital environmental control. HHS Publication No. 99-1117. Centers for Disease Control, Atlanta, 1985

18. Goreschel DHM, Strain BA: Laboratory safety in clinical microbiology, pp 49–58. In Balows A, Hausler WJ, Hermann KL, Isenberg HD, Shadomy HJ (eds): Manual of Clinical Microbiology, 5th ed. Washington, DC, American Society for Microbiology, 1991

19. Haines H: Safety and compliance: Legal and punitive considerations. In Orynich RE (ed): Policies and Procedures Program Manual. Houston, TX, Health Safe Systems, 1992

20. Hospital Safety Information Service: Care, use and handling of compressed gas cylinders. Scientific Enterprises Sept–Oct:70–73, 1993

21. Joint Commission on Accreditation of Healthcare Organizations: Ergonomics in health care facilities. Plant, technology and safety Management Series No. 2, 1994

22. Kiyosawa KT, Sodeyama E, Tanaka Y, Nakano S, Furuta K, Nishioka RH, Purcell TJ, Alter HJ: Hepatitis C in hospital employee with needlestick injuries. Ann Intern Med 115: 367–369, 1991

23. Landesman LY: Hospital Preparedness for Chemical Accidents Plant, technology and safety management. Series 2: 33–38, 1990

24. Luebbert PP: New TB risk categories. Advance for Administrators of the Laboratory 4(1):39–42, 1995

25. National Research Council: Prudent Practices for Handling Hazardous Chemicals in Laboratories. Washington, DC, National Academy Press, 1981

26. Occupational Safety and Health Administration (OSHA 3114): Hazardous Waste and Emergency Response OSHA Publications Office, Washington, DC, 1992

27. Pike RM: Laboratory-associated infections: Incidence, fatalities, causes and prevention. Annu Rev Microbiol 33: 41–46, 1979

28. Stern A, Ries H, Flynn D, Vance A: Fire safety in the laboratory: Part 1. Laboratory Medicine 24(5):275–277, 1993

29. Stevens AM: How to store and handle flammable, combustible liquids used in hospitals. Health Facilities Management May:20–24, 1992

30. Tapp LM: Establishing an Employee Ergonomics Task Force. Professional Safety (American Society of Safety Engineers) July:26–28, 1994

31. Turk AR: ANSI standardizes material safety data sheets. Health Facilities Management April:36–38, 1993

APPENDIX 21–1 OSHA'S PHYSICAL HAZARDS

Combustible Liquids

Any liquid having a flashpoint at or above 100°F (37.8°C) but below 200°F (93.3°C), except any mixture having components with flash points of 200°F (93.3°C), the total volume of which make up 99% or more of the total volume of the mixture

Compressed Gas

1. A gas or mixture of gases having, in a container, an absolute pressure exceeding 40 psi or 70°F (21.1°C)
2. A gas or mixture of gases having, in a container, an absolute pressure exceeding 104 psi at 130°F (54.4°C), regardless of the pressure at 70°F (21.1°C)

Explosive

A chemical that causes a sudden, almost instantaneous release of pressure, gas, and heat when subjected to sudden shock, pressure, or high temperature

Flammable Gas

A gas that, at ambient temperature and pressure, forms a flammable mixture with air at a concentration of 13% by volume or less or a gas that, at ambient temperature and pressure, forms a range of flammable mixtures with air wider than 12% by volume regardless of the lower limit

Flammable Liquid

Any liquid having a flashpoint below 100°F (37.8°C), except any mixture having components with flashpoints of 100°F (37.8°C) or higher, the total of which make up 99% or more of the total volume of the mixture

Solid Flammable

A solid, other than a blasting agent or explosive, that is liable to cause fire through friction, absorption of moisture, spontaneous chemical change, or retained heat from manufacturing or processing or that can be ignited readily and when ignited burns so vigorously and persistently as to create a serious hazard. A chemical is considered to be a flammable solid if when tested, it ignites and burns with a self-sustained flame at a rate greater than one tenth of an inch per second along its major axis.

Oxidizer

A chemical other than a blasting agent or explosive that initiates or promotes combustion in other materials, thereby causing fire either of itself or through the release of oxygen or other gases

Water Reactive

A chemical that reacts with water to release a gas that is either flammable or presents a health hazard

Pyrophoric

A chemical that will ignite spontaneously in air at a temperature of 130°F (54.4°C) or below

Reactive (Unstable)

A chemical which in a pure state or as produced or transported will vigorously polymerize, decompose, condense, or become selfreactive under conditions of shocks, pressure, or temperature

OSHA's Health Hazards

Chemicals where exposure may produce acute or chronic health effects include:

Carcinogens: Chemicals that have been evaluated by the International Agency for Research on Cancer (IARC) and found to be a carcinogen or potential carcinogen or listed in the Annual Report on Carcinogens published by the National Toxicology Program (NTP) or regulated by OSHA as a carcinogen
Irritants: A chemical that causes a reversible inflammatory effect on living tissue by chemical action at the site of contact
Corrosives: A chemical that causes visible destruction or irreversible alterations in living tissue by chemical action at the site of contact; does not refer to action on inanimate surfaces
Sensitizers: A chemical that causes a substantial proportion of exposed people or animals to develop an allergic reaction in normal tissue after repeated exposure to the chemical

Toxins

Toxin is a term that can be applied to almost any chemical in quantity. In the laboratory, a substance is considered toxic if serious biologic effects may follow inhalation, ingestion, or skin contact with relatively small amounts. Acute toxins are hazardous chemicals that cause adverse effects to target organs after a short period of time following a one-time high exposure to the substance. Chronic toxins include hazardous chemicals causing adverse effects to target organs that develop after a long time following or during repeated contacts with the substance.

The following list illustrates the range of toxic agents but is not all-inclusive:

Hepatotoxins: Chemicals that produce liver damage
Nephrotoxins: Chemicals that produce kidney damage
Neurotoxins: Chemicals that produce their primary toxic effects on the nervous system
Hematopoietic hazards: Agents that act on the blood or hematopoietic system: decrease hemoglobin function; deprive the body tissues of oxygen
Lung hazards: Agents that damage the lung; chemicals that irritate or damage the pulmonary tissue
Reproductive toxins: Chemicals that affect the reproductive capabilities, including chromosomal damage (mutations) and effects on fetuses (teratogenesis)
Skin hazards: Chemicals that affect the dermal layer of the body
Eye hazards: Chemicals that affect the eye or visual capacity

22

Laboratory Regulation, Certification, and Accreditation

Gary B. Clark

FORCES DRIVING REGULATORY CHANGE

Over the past several decades, there has been a steady increase of regulatory control of the entire health-care delivery system, including clinical laboratories. Senhauser attributed this spiraling growth of technocratic oversight to the growing importance of laboratory testing in the increasingly technologic practice of medicine.[1]

Based on economies of scale, any increased volume of testing tends to produce a proportionately higher incidence of production errors and utilization abuse. Thus, it is predictable that legislation and peer review ultimately arrive to ensure the health and safety of the consumer for good reasons.

Actually, an even more complicated combination of socioeconomic forces are stimulating the control of health-care laboratory operations. These determinants include (1) evolving consumer influence, (2) burgeoning managed care, (3) reactive governmental involvement, and (4) supportive peer review.

First, the public is gaining in its appreciation of health-care quality. If not better read professionally, our primary customer, the patient, is certainly aware of the front page news. Consequently, there is continually heightened public understanding of the diagnostic-therapeutic scope and technologic nature of health care, including that of clinical laboratory testing.

Subsequently, there has been growing public concern that some aspects of medical care quality are eroding due to the robotic complexity of modern techno-

logic health care, relentless medicolegal pressures, severe cost-containment measures, and quality management resource constraints. The media occasionally reports shoddy clinical laboratory testing. For example, the publicized hue and cry over faulty Pap smear testing greatly influenced the passage of the Clinical Laboratory Improvement Amendments of 1988 (CLIA '88).

Dennis S. O'Leary, MD, President of the Joint Commission on Accreditation of Healthcare Organizations (JCAHO), has pointed out that public concerns about quality have resulted in a demand for greater accountability by hospitals, physicians, and others involved in providing health-care services, including clinical laboratories.[2] Customer pressures catalyze the complex interactions among federal and state lawmakers, regulators, credentialing agencies, and professional societies.

Managed health care, the second determinant, has become an overwhelming force of change, emerging on the health-care business scene with incredible rapidity. The largest managed health-care corporations have swept away weaker competitors with juggernaut-like efficiency. Under the guise of cost-containment, managed care has eliminated wastefulness that evolved during the more lucrative, resource-rich years of the Burton-Hill Act of 1946. Now, there is a new focus on trimming the size of health-care organizations and altering organizational structures and processes to fit modern management, technologic, and customer satisfaction needs.

Managed care initially concerned itself with minimizing inpatient services. However, the quest for improved outpatient services has become increasingly important. Unfortunately, health-care quality management resources, including those of the laboratory, have remained limited.

Early on managed care was perceived as a rescuer. Some have hoped that managed health care would assist in reducing national health-care costs and budget deficits at the federal and state levels. For example, some state Medicare and Medicaid budgets have been going into the red, and it has been predicted that the federal Medicare/Medicaid programs may be insolvent by 2002.[3] To help alleviate these fiscal problems, various programs have been proposed on Capitol Hill. For example, the federal government has extended waivers to some states, allowing them the right to enroll their Medicare/Medicaid participants into managed care programs. This approach has been received with some enthusiasm: More states have applied for waivers than have received them. However, the program has raised more questions about the efficacy of federal- and state-managed health care.

As time has passed, managed care has been perceived more and more as a villain. Many wonder if managed care is really working to the patient's benefit or if it is dictating medical decisions for financial reasons. Because of the unabated growth of this inappropriate power in the marketplace, there is growing clamor for legislation to regulate the managed health-care industry and other third-party insurers.

How does the clinical laboratory fit into managed care at this time? Regardless of whether health-care management is the rescuer or the villain, laboratories must learn to compete effectively in the modern economic milieu. They need to continue to do what they have been doing all along: increasing overall efficiency by streamlining organization and process, modernizing customer services, and improving customer satisfaction. In current parlance, all of this is known as reengineering, restructuring, and downsizing, which means systematic quality management in a continuous quality improvement environment.[4,5]

Unfortunately, clinical laboratories must do all of this while fighting the encroachment of the market place by point-of-care testing and home testing. Ultimately, they will have to contend with the looming specter of "bottom line" oriented, entrepreneurial approaches, such as competitive bidding.

Clinical laboratory operations as a nationwide industry represented about $39.5 billion in 1995 health-care dollars, as compared with $988 billion in total 1995 health-care costs. Thus, clinical laboratory health-care costs equal about 4% of total national health-care costs.[6]

There is a third determinant of laboratory regulatory control: as the tides of the economy ebb and flow, so fluctuate the government's perceptions and concerns. Most recently, federal and state involvement in health care has become increasingly manifold, particularly in regard to the curbing of costs.

Clearly, mounting regulatory pressures are challenging many resource-constrained facilities. Often, quality-related regulatory activities are encountering reluctant acceptance by various health-care organizations; especially by primary care providers who often have the most limited quality management resources. This has spurred the implementation of less expensive, interim self-inspections at both governmental and peer review levels of laboratory control.

As a fourth determinant of laboratory control, private sector peer review has had an increasingly positive impact on improved health-care quality; however, it has also contributed to burgeoning management costs. Peer review consists of oversight by fellow professionals through inspection and accreditation. In the case of laboratory medicine, it is usually a matter of laboratorians inspecting other laboratorians.

Peer review standards parallel federal-level regulations, translating technocratic rules into operational reality. This dynamic process is aimed at improving health-care quality, including that of the peer review process. Organizational-level quality control and operative-level quality surveillance have offered important approaches for surviving these changes. Examples of clinical laboratory peer review programs include those of the JCAHO, the College of American Pathologists (CAP), and the American Association of Blood Banks (AABB), among many others.

Still other factors confound health-care organizational operations. These include (1) the pernicious role of the health insurance companies in influencing clinical decisions, (2) the revolutionary advances in science and technology that create increased laboratory complexity and health-care cost increases (or greater testing simplicity fit for home use that results in decreased laboratory revenues), and (3) the need for quality management systems that pervade the entire path of organizational work flow.

Laboratories must maintain a balance between the extrinsic demands of consumer concern, managed care, governmental regulation, and peer review versus the intrinsic outcomes of high quality health care. There is a break-even point between those extrinsic demands and the intrinsic outcomes. There can be too much or too little regulatory control, either of which affects patient care quality and the health-care management cost.

The details of specific regulatory requirements and performance standards change from year to year and from locale to locale. Therefore, this chapter addresses only the general principles of regulation and accreditation. The reader should become familiar with local, state, and federal regulations and with the voluntary certification and accreditation requirements that apply to one's own laboratory.

DEFINITIONS

A major source of difficulty in understanding the process of laboratory regulation and accreditation is the imprecise definition of the terminology used in discussing these complex issues. The definitions that follow include terms that address governmental control and assurance and professional peer assurance. These definitions can be somewhat confusing due to overlap between public and private sector usage and popular interpretation of the terms.

Regulation

Regulation is defined as government intervention in an economic market, including the health-care market, to control entry into or change the behavior of participants in that marketplace through the specification of rules for those participants. Governmental regulatory programs evolve through a series of legislative and executive branch steps, often leading to peer-level oversight. Table 22–1 illustrates the typical path of government-based intervention.

Federal and state agencies regulate laboratory operations through various mechanisms, including licensure, certification, and registration. Such governmental oversight includes control of entire organizations or in-

dividuals who participate in the marketplace. Control of organizations is directed at their structure, process, or outcome. Control of individuals is directed at their reviewing past credentials and assessing current competence.

The *Code of Federal Regulations* (CFR) is a systemized classification of final rules published in the *Federal Register* by agencies of the federal government. The Code is divided into 50 titles, which represent the broadest of areas subject to federal regulation. Each title is divided into chapters that bear the name of the issuing agency; each chapter is subdivided into parts and sections covering more specific regulatory areas. For example, the CLIA '88 regulations covering general provisions can be cited by CFR title, chapter, subchapter, part, subpart, and section number as "42 CFR, Part 493, Subpart A, Section 1 through 20."

Licensure

Licensure is the process by which a competent public authority grants permission to an organization or individual to engage in a specific professional practice, occupation, or activity. Requiring a license is the most restrictive form of government regulation of professional practice. Licensure makes it illegal for an unlicensed organization or individual to provide a profes-

---

Table 22-1
Events Leading From Legislative Branch Lawmaking, to Executive Branch Administration, to Peer Organizational Surveillance

Regulatory Event	Example
Federal-level legislative branch passes a bill that is ratified by the President, resulting in statutory law.	Congress enacts Clinical Laboratory Improvement Amendments Act of 1988 (CLIA '88). The President signs Public Law 100-578.
Federal-level executive branch implements the law by directing an administrative agency with statutory authority to design rules of implementation.	Department of Health and Human Services (DHHS) and Health Care Financing Administration (HCFA) formulate CLIA '88 implementation rules, which are published in the Federal Register.
DHHS/HCFA establish regional and state CLIA '88 offices and grant exempt status to individual state governments and deeming authority to peer organizations to implement and enforce federal statutory requirements.	State-level CLIA '88 offices establish state-wide policies for inspection and certification. Exempted states and JCAHO, COLA, CAP, AABB, and other peer organizations incorporate CLIA '88 requirements into their accreditation standards and enforce compliance of all volunteer participants.
Public and private laboratories develop policies and procedures for quality operations and interim assessment in compliance with CLIA regulations and peer review standards.	Ideally, laboratories produce quality clinical testing with reproducible accuracy and precision and demonstrate an unfailing quality surveillance record.

sional service within a scope of practice that is defined by statute.

Licensing is designed to protect the public from inadequate manufacturing practice and incompetent practitioners. These permits include a precise definition of the practice being regulated and the criteria by which competence is measured.

Applicants must demonstrate a minimal degree of competency as determined necessary to ensure public health and safety. These are mandatory requirements, not voluntary.

Organizational Licensure

Health-care facilities obtain licenses from governmental agencies. For example, at the federal level, the Food and Drug Administration (FDA) licenses all blood banks. The granting of such a license is based on a stringent application and inspection process that strives to ensure safety and effectiveness through sound design and good manufacturing practices.

Personnel Licensure

Usually at the state level (including the District of Columbia), a license is required for individual practitioners of various disciplines to engage in lawful practice.

At the state level, licensing boards serve as consumer-advocacy boards. They have two basic functions:

1. Establish entry-level standards that will ensure safe practice.
2. Monitor the continued competence and ethicality of the licensee's practice.

Individual practitioner licensure is usually granted by an appointed board of competent peer authority. The board grants a license on the basis of proof of education and written or oral examination. The license is usually permanent and conditioned on the periodic payment of fees, proof of continuing education, or proof of continued competence. Usually, possession of a medical license from one state will suffice to obtain a license from another by reciprocity. Some states, however, do not recognize reciprocity and insist on an entrance examination. Commonly accepted grounds for revocation of a license include incompetence, commission of a crime (whether or not related to the licensed practice), and moral turpitude.

For example, all physicians (including pathologists), dentists, podiatrists, laboratory-based nurses, and physician assistants are licensed. In addition, the licensing of medical technologists has become more prevalent. In 1937, California was the first state to enact clinical laboratory and technologist licensing legislation.

Since then, others have passed some form of legislation; these states include Florida, Georgia, Hawaii, Louisiana, Montana, Nevada, North Dakota, Rhode Island, Tennessee, and West Virginia; and the territory of Puerto Rico, which requires licensure of nonphysician personnel.[3,7–10]

Most states have enacted clinical laboratory legislation in some form or another. As expected, there are significant pros and cons to state regulation, including licensure. Overall, it does ensure minimal qualifications for essential laboratory personnel.[11]

Certification

Certification is a process by which a federal or state governmental agency or a peer level professional association officially recognizes a laboratory organization or an individual as having met certain predetermined qualifications. As an example of organizational certification by a government agency, the Health Care Financing Administration (HCFA) certifies laboratories for fulfilling the requirements of CLIA '88. One way that this is accomplished is by state-level CLIA agencies under contract by HCFA.

First, the laboratory applies for a certificate at a certain level of testing complexity through the state-level agency to HCFA. After the application is processed and an initial certificate is granted, the laboratory can operate at the granted level of complexity. For laboratories performing moderate and high complexity testing, the provisional certification is eventually followed by a regularly scheduled on-site inspection. Following a successful inspection, the laboratory receives follow-up certification. This is an example of a mandatory certification program.

Certification is also a process by which a state or nongovernmental professional association can grant recognition of competence to individuals who have met certain predetermined qualifications as specified by that agency or association. This form of special recognition began as a voluntary process for those desiring to demonstrate competence and be competitive in the job market. Noncertified individuals can still offer similar services to the public, but they could not advertise themselves as being certified or use a related title in dealing with clients.[12] Box 22–1 lists several laboratory organizations and their certifying programs.

In light of the most recent CLIA '88 legislation, individual certification has changed in its significance. Under these rules, personnel are federally mandated to meet various levels of competence to match specific levels of testing complexity. Statutory law and implementation rules spell out these levels of ability in terms of the knowledge, training, and experience that are re-

Box 22·1

Organizations That Provide Laboratory Registry and Certification in the United States[8,13,14]

American Academy of Microbiology (AAM)
  Diplomate, American Board of Medical
    Laboratory Immunology
  Diplomate, American Board of Medical
    Microbiology
American Board of Bioanalysts (ABB)
  Bioanalyst Clinical Laboratory Director (BCLD)
  Bioanalyst Laboratory Director (BLD)
  Bioanalytical Laboratory Manager (BLM)
  Clinical Laboratory Director (CLD)
  Laboratory Supervisor (LS)
American Board of Pathology
  Diplomate, Anatomic and/or Clinical Pathology
  Special Qualification in Blood Banking and
    Transfusion Medicine
  Special Qualification in Chemical Pathology
  Special Qualification in Cytopathology
  Special Qualification in Dermatopathology (in
    conjunction with the American Board of
    Dermatology)
  Special Qualification in Forensic Pathology
  Special Qualification in Hematology
  Special Qualification in Immunopathology
  Special Qualification in Medical Microscopy
  Special Qualification in Neuropathology
  Special Qualification in Pediatric Pathology
American Board of Clinical Chemistry (ABCC)
  Diplomate, American Board of Clinical Chemistry
American Medical Technologists (AMT)
  Certified Office Laboratory Technician (COLT)
  Medical Laboratory Technician (MLT)
  Medical Technologist (MT)
  Phlebotomy Technician (RPT)
American Society of Clinical Pathologists (ASCP)
  Assistants
    Certified Laboratory Assistants (CLA [ASCP])
  Technicians
    Phlebotomy Technician (PBT [ASCP])
    Histologic Technician (HT [ASCP])
    Medical Laboratory Technician (MLT [ASCP])
  Technologists
    Cytotechnologist (CT [ASCP])
    Medical Technologist (MT [ASCP])
    Technologist in Blood Banking (BB [ASCP])
    Technologist in Chemistry (C [ASCP])
    Technologist in Hematology (H [ASCP])

  Histotechnologist (HTL [ASCP])
  Technologist in Immunology (I [ASCP])
  Technologist in Microbiology (M [ASCP])
  Technologist in Nuclear Medicine (NM [ASCP])[†]
Specialists
  Hemapheresis Practitioner (HP [ASCP])
  Specialist in Blood Banking (SBB [ASCP])
  Specialist in Chemistry (SC [ASCP])
  Specialist in Cytotechnology (SCT [ASCP])
  Specialist in Hematology (SH [ASCP])
  Specialist in Immunology (SI [ASCP])
  Specialist in Microbiology (SM [ASCP])
Diplomates
  Diplomate in Laboratory Management (DLM
    [ASCP])
American Society of Phlebotomy Technicians
  (ASPT)
Department of Health Education and Welfare
  (DHEW)
  Clinical Laboratory Technologist (CLT)[‡]
International Academy of Cytology (IAC)
  Cytotechnologist Member (CM [IAC])
  Cytotechnologist Fellow (CF [IAC])
International Society for Clinical Laboratory
  Technology (ISCLT)
  Physicians Office Laboratory Technician (POLT)
  Registered Laboratory Technician (RLT)
  Registered Medical Technologist (RMT)
National Certification Agency for Medical Laboratory
  Personnel (NCA)
  Clinical Laboratory Scientist Generalist (CLS)
  Clinical Laboratory Phlebotomist (CLP1b)
  Clinical Laboratory Technician (CLT)
  Clinical Laboratory Scientist in Chemistry (CLS/C)
  Clinical Laboratory Scientist in Hematology
    (CLS/H)
  Clinical Laboratory Scientist in
    Immunohematology (CLS/I)
  Clinical Laboratory Scientist/Microbiology (CLS/M)
  Clinical Laboratory Specialist in Cytogenetics
    (CLSp[CG])
  Clinical Laboratory Specialist in Hematology
    (CLSp[H])
  Clinical Laboratory Director (CLDir)
  Clinical Laboratory Supervisor (CLSup)

* Discontinued in 1982; these individuals have been invited to sit for the ASCP technician level examination.
† Discontinued in 1992; this certification was merged with the Nuclear Medicine Certification Board examination.
‡ A federal government certification granted to assure that military personnel were qualified under CLIA '67.

quired. These rules are translated then into terms of laboratory certification levels. The general trend is for federal requirements to be less stringent than those of the professional certifying agencies. This is a balancing process whereby the federal government seeks to ensure that laboratory testing is as universally accessible as possible. At the same time, the professional organizations seek to maintain personnel requirements with skill levels that are technically appropriate.

Registration

Registration is the least restrictive form of governmental regulatory control. On one hand, an organization is required to file with a government agency. For example, medical device manufacturers must register annually with the FDA. On the other hand, an individual is required simply to file name, address, and qualifications with a government agency before practicing a given profession. Such personnel registration is usually practiced at the state level and does not pertain to laboratory personnel at this time.

However, a professional association can provide the administrative mechanism for national registration by preparing standards of performance, developing and administering appropriate examinations, and developing appropriate scoring procedures. Often this form of registration is accompanied by peer level certification and is administered by a board of registry.

Again, this is usually considered a "voluntary" process that is recommended for the individual to be most competitive. Several organizations provide this type of registry surveillance in the United States, as listed in Table 22–2.

The mode of regulatory control by licensure, certification, or registration will vary from jurisdiction to jurisdiction. For example, a given health-care profession might be registered in some states and certified or licensed in others.

PROFESSIONAL PEER LEVEL ASSURANCE

In the private sector, professional organizations often exercise oversight of their constituent organizations and individual members. At the highest national level, the JCAHO wields tremendous peer influence over member health-care organizations through its on-site survey and accreditation program. At the specialty level, organizations such as CAP run on-site and interim inspection and accreditation programs and adjunct surveillance and comparison services, such as proficiency testing and laboratory management improvement. There are also several, more focused organizations, such as the AABB, that inspect and accredit subspecialty laboratories.

Within a health-care facility (eg, a hospital), there are usually two levels of peer review: a higher administrative (total organizational or operational) level and a lower managerial (operative) level. At the hospital-wide administrative level, peer review is rendered in the form of committee-driven quality assessment and improvement (QI) of organizational performance. This form of quality management might be incorporated with utilization and risk management programs. Within the laboratory, peer review can be exercised at the departmental-wide administrative level in the form of committee-driven QI. This is linked with peer review at the intradepartmental, managerial level in the form of operative quality or peer control.[4,5]

Accreditation

Accreditation is the process by which a private, peer-level commission or association evaluates and ensures that a program of professional study or activity in an institution is meeting appropriate standards of organizational performance. The accrediting body usually defines its standards as essential elements of organizational structure, process, and outcome. These include governance, administrative services, medical and other professional staff management, scope and organization of services, personnel management, methods and procedures, instruments and other equipment, supplies, and the physical plant.

Outcome is the chief indicator of laboratory excellence. Thus *patient care* and *employee health and welfare outcomes* should be the laboratory organization's true "bottom line measurement of effectiveness." Still, process and structure are of paramount importance in the long run of resolving quality of performance problems.

Accreditation is usually a voluntary process by which a laboratory elects to be inspected and assisted by professional peers rather than submitting to mandatory external review and control by governmental agencies. Often, however, the professional value of volunteerism has become moot, because accreditation is usually a prerequisite for Medicare/Medicaid reimbursement eligibility. CLIA '88 certifies a laboratory as being accredited if inspected by a deeming status organization such as the JCAHO or CAP.

Unlike licensure, accreditation is not a condition of lawful practice, but is intended to ensure high-quality practice. However, because federal Medicare/Medicaid reimbursement is often predicated on accreditation, the latter has the same effect as licensure.

Credentialing

Credentialing is a broad generic term, defined as the formal recognition of professional or technical competence. Credentialization is the process of reviewing an individual's evidence of education, licensing, certification, registration, malpractice claims, *curriculum vitae,* and other professional documents for the purpose of verifying proof of identity and competence. This process is exercised by any agency or other health-care organization that renders any sort of a professional privilege. For example, a credentials review would be required of an individual (eg, physician) who is applying for some privilege, such as attending a degree-level course of health-care instruction, practicing health-care in a state, or performing diagnostic or therapeutic privileges in a hospital.

FEDERAL REGULATION OF CLINICAL LABORATORIES

As a response to professional studies, tort law, and legislation, standards of health-care practice are established and enforced at the governmental and peer level. A fundamental basis for legislation of health care is the tort law system in the United States. The definition of legal liability for medical negligence has evolved over time. The general, objective standard is "what a reasonable physician, possessed of the same degree of skill and learning, would have done under the same or similar circumstances."[15]

Over the years, the courts have gradually fine-tuned the definition of medical negligence through a body of legal precedence known as tort law. Certain legal tenets have been of some importance, such as *charitable immunity* and *respondeat superior* (ie, "let the master answer or be responsible").

Before the 1900s, civil courts usually looked on hospitals as centers for treatment of the indigent. Consequently, such beneficent health-care facilities were not held liable for malpractice and enjoyed "charitable immunity." More affluent patients who sought medical care from private clinics had the right to legal recourse if there were any adverse result.

In the early 1900s, hospitals became more commercialized, charging patients for their services. As the quality of hospital care improved, more physicians hospitalized their private patients. Inevitably, medical-legal scrutiny began to focus on the quality of hospital health care. In turn, the differences between institutional and health-care provider responsibilities began to be more clearly defined.

At first, only the hospital was held liable for organizational misconduct. Gradually, the tenet of *respondeat superior* guided the legal system toward recognizing the additional liability of the individual practitioners and their subordinates, including those in the clinical laboratory. As a consequence, a large number of medically related court rulings have been found throughout this century. The more salient of these court precedents have engendered government-level health-care legislation.[4,16]

When addressing health-care regulations, it is also helpful to understand the structure and role of the various government agencies that have become involved during the last century. The Biologics Control Act (or so-called Virus-Toxin Act) of 1902 was enacted subsequent to several children dying from diphtheria antitoxin contaminated with *Clostridium tetani* toxin. In joint passage, the Public Health Service Act created the U.S. Public Health Service (PHS) as part of the Department of the Treasury.

In 1905, the Pure Food and Drugs Act was enacted, creating the FDA as part of the Department of Agriculture, initially based in the Department of Agriculture's Bureau of Chemistry. In 1930, the Hygienic Laboratory of the PHS became the National Institute of Health (NIH). In 1945, the NIH issued its first license to a blood bank in Philadelphia. By 1948, the NIH had enlarged to become the National Institutes of Health.

In 1938, the Food, Drug, and Cosmetic Act was enacted, singling out the role of the FDA. In 1940, the FDA, along with the PHS, were placed under the Federal Security Agency. In 1953, the Federal Security Agency became the Department of Health, Education, and Welfare (DHEW). The DHEW has since been reorganized as the Department of Health and Human Services (DHHS). Education was placed under the jurisdiction of the Department of Education, allowing the DHHS to focus more specifically on public health and health-care economics.[17]

Department of Health and Human Services

As illustrated in Figure 22–1, the DHHS consists of (1) the PHS, within which resides the Centers for Disease Control and Prevention (CDC); (2) the FDA, within which reside the Center for Devices and Radiological Health and Center for Biological Evaluation and Research; and (3) the HCFA, within which reside the Health Quality Standards Bureau and the Office of Survey and Certification.[18]

Medicare and Medicaid Regulations

Federal and state governments can mandate standards and inspection programs through their authority to certify and reimburse health-care facilities, including clini-

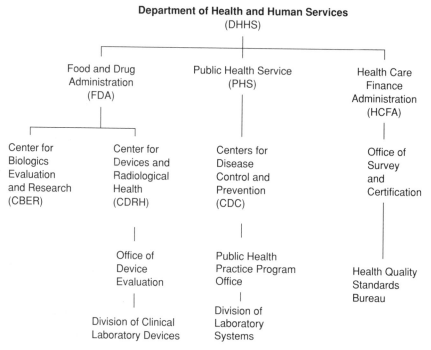

FIGURE 22–1. Structure of the Department of Health and Human Services. (Adapted from CLIA '88 Regulatory Handbook. Abbott Park, IL, Abbott Quality Institute, 1994)

cal laboratories. Such power is derived from the enactment of laws by the various legislative bodies under their duty to protect the public health, safety, and welfare.

Prior to the 1960s, several states (notably California and New York) had begun to legislate health-care reimbursement reform. In 1965, state rules were effectively eclipsed by the federal government's enacting Public Law 89-97. This law created the Medicare and Medicaid programs by amending Titles XVIII and XIX of the Social Security Act of 1939. The Medicare regulatory program awarded *statutory authority* to the Secretary of the DHEW to set standards that ensure the health and safety of Medicare and Medicaid beneficiaries. As a result of these laws, the DHEW developed standards for all clinical laboratories operating in inpatient and outpatient settings, including hospital and independent laboratories (ie, the latter being physically and organizationally separate from a hospital and the patient's attending physician). Physician office laboratories (POLs) were exempt.

To provide enforcement at the peer level, the DHHS appointed the JCAHO to set the specific standards and survey for accreditation. That is, the DHEW granted *deeming authority* to the JCAHO to act in the DHEW's stead and implement the new regulation at the professional level.

A major weakness of the Medicare/Medicaid law was that POLs were exempt from having to meet the standard requirements for reimbursement eligibility. Most of these laboratories were operated by licensed physicians, osteopaths, dentists, or podiatrists who performed laboratory tests or procedures for the treatment of their own patients.

The essential power of Public Law 89-97 to regulate clinical laboratories has rested in its *conditions of participation in the Medicare/Medicaid program.* Under these provisions, a health-care facility, including a subject clinical laboratory, could be barred from receiving reimbursement for services if the conditions were not met.

Following their inception in 1965, the Medicare/Medicaid regulations for hospital-based and independent clinical laboratories eventually addressed standards for personnel, record keeping, management, safety, and internal and external quality control systems, including proficiency testing. Standards for independent laboratories included more detailed personnel standards for the director, technical supervisor, general supervisor, technologist, and technician. Whereas hos-

**Department of Health
and Human Services Departments
Important to the Clinical Laboratory**

- The Food and Drug Administration (FDA),
  which regulates the market entry of clinical
  laboratory instruments, reagents, and systems
  manufactured by the clinical laboratory device
  industry; determines what devices will be sold
  to the public on the open market and how the
  public will use those devices on a day-to-day
  basis. The FDA also regulates production of
  donor blood and its components as a drug and
  biologic, licensing blood bank facilities.
- The Centers for Disease Control and
  Prevention (CDC), which provides technical
  input for the classification of laboratory
  technology and methods according to the
  criteria of the CLIA '88 complexity model
- The Health Care Finance Administration
  (HCFA), which determines CLIA requirements,
  sets performance and facility standards,
  monitors compliance, accredits outside
  organizations to inspect laboratories and
  provide proficiency testing programs, sets
  reimbursement schedules, registers
  laboratories, collects fees, manages federal
  health-care expenditures, and enforces
  regulations

pital laboratories were approved as part of the overall
facility, independent laboratories were approved by
specialty and subspecialty activity (eg, chemistry, radioimmunoassay).

Clinical Laboratory Improvement Act of 1967

Subsequent to the enactment of the Medicare/Medicaid
laboratory standards in 1965, Congress became concerned that significant problems existed in the quality
of services provided to Medicare recipients by clinical
laboratories engaged in interstate commerce. Thus,
Congress resolved to address these problems by passing separate legislation, Clinical Laboratory Improvement Act of 1967 (CLIA '67).

The provisions of CLIA '67 were founded on a geopolitical approach, mandating licensure of only laboratories that were engaged in interstate commerce. The
Act defined such laboratories as those accepting more
than 100 out-of-state specimens during each year in various major testing categories (eg, microbiologic, serologic, hematologic, chemical). Laboratories receiving
fewer than 100 specimens could obtain a letter of exemption on application to the CDC in Atlanta.

As in the case of the Medicare regulations, clinical
office laboratories (ie, POLs) were exempt from this
law. Thus, mainly independent laboratories that were
involved in interstate commerce were prohibited from
operating in that market sphere unless they obtained a
CLIA '67 license issued by the DHEW or by a designee
with deeming authority.

The CLIA '67 technical standards were essentially
the same as those for independent laboratories under
Medicare/Medicaid. However, CLIA '67 was significantly different administratively in that sanctions were
based on licensure, rather than reimbursement. The
newer act also differed in that it regulated on the basis
of laboratory test groupings, rather than the laboratory
as a component of a hospital organization.

The power to license interstate laboratories was
delegated to the PHS through its CDC, which administered the CLIA '67 program until 1976 when the HCFA
assumed that role. Also, licensed laboratories were required to participate successfully in a proficiency testing
program operated by the CDC.

With both Medicare/Medicaid and CLIA '67 in
force, the government found itself administering two
separate regulatory programs for clinical laboratories.
There were overlapping as well as differing requirements. During the following years, there also were complications caused by shifting authority among various
and often rival governmental agencies being charged
with administering the regulations.

The laboratorian experienced genuine frustration
from the sheer complexity of these overlapping regulations. For example, the rules implementing CLIA '67
were published in an entirely different section of the
CFR as those promulgating the laboratory regulations
for Medicare/Medicaid. Considering how the FDA currently regulates blood and blood components both as
biologics and drugs, times really have not changed.

Following the enactment of CLIA '67, the federal
government enacted several laws with significant impact on clinical laboratories. For example, the 1982 Tax
Equity and Fiscal Responsibility Act (ie, TEFRA) placed
hospital laboratories under reimbursement limitations
and changed the basis of pathologist reimbursement,
limiting the latter to a reasonable compensation equivalent (RCE). The Social Security Amendments of 1983
replaced the RCE basis for Part A Medicare reimbursement with a prospective payment system. This system
relied on the diagnostic related grouping (ie, DRG) as
a reimbursement limitation tool.

In 1987, the Omnibus Budget Reconciliation Act (OBRA '87) ruled that POLs performing greater than 5,000 tests per year were under the control of CLIA '67 for Medicaid/Medicare eligibility. However, OBRA '89 rescinded the greater than 5,000 test volume limitation, extending CLIA '67 Medicare/Medicaid interstate commerce eligibility requirements to *all* laboratories—including all POLs—regardless of testing volume. On March 14, 1990, the final rule revising CLIA '67 was published, serving as a transition between the 1967 and 1988 laboratory inprovement laws. Thus, center stage was set for CLIA '88.

Clinical Laboratory Improvement Amendments of 1988

In 1988, the 100th Congress enacted and President Bush signed into law Public Law 100-578, known as CLIA '88. These were amendments to Section 353 of the Public Service Act and Sections 1861 and 1902 of the Social Security Act. This legislation occurred in response to particular public concern about the quality of laboratory testing in POLs and Pap smear laboratories.[19]

CLIA '88 replaced both the Medicare/Medicaid and CLIA '67 regulations for laboratory control with a more unified set of "minimum" standards that apply to almost all clinical laboratory testing of human specimens regardless of location, size, or type of laboratory. On February 28, 1992, the CLIA '88 final rule was published as 42 CFR Part 493 with correcting amendments published later.[20]

42 CFR Part 493 consists of four separate sets of rules that establish (1) laboratory performance standards (HSQ-176), (2) application procedures and user fees (HSQ-177), (3) enforcement or sanction procedures (HSQ-179), and (4) approval of accreditation programs (HSQ-181). The laboratory standards cover the major issues of certification, inspections, personnel qualifications, patient test management, quality control, quality assurance, and proficiency testing.*

This most current of clinical laboratory laws addresses quality management through several new surveillance initiatives as directed by the HCFA. An additional voice of professional expertise for the ongoing interpretation and updating of CLIA '88 is provided by the Clinical Laboratory Improvement Advisory Committee (CLIAC). Although the Secretary of DHHS appoints the committee members, CLIAC is under the administrative control of CDC. This committee provides technical expertise to the HCFA and CDC on CLIA-related issues.

Compared to the geopolitical approach of CLIA '67, CLIA '88 established an equal-protection-under-the-law (or site neutrality) approach to regulating clinical laboratories. Thus, *all* laboratories, including those desiring eligibility for Medicare/Medicaid reimbursement, must be certified every 2 years. This includes all civilian not-for-profit or federal, state, or local government laboratory sites doing limited public health testing. HCFA-appointed state certifying agencies or approved private, nonprofit organizations are considered "deeming" authorities under Section 353 of the Public Health Service Act, as amended by CLIA '88. In turn, 42 CFR Part 493 laboratories are "deemed" to be meeting that law's requirements and are eligible to receive Medicare and Medicaid reimbursement.

The universality or site neutrality of CLIA '88 ensures the inclusion of POLs and all the other intraoffice laboratories originally exempted by the Medicaid/Medicare Act of 1965 and CLIA '67. The concern about a

---

*CLIA '88 amendments are cited as 42 CFR Parts 74, 405, 411, 416, 440, 482, 483, and 488 (including all antecedent laws regarding Medicare/Medicaid and CLIA '67), and Part 493 (which is CLIA '88 specific). These are all archived in the Federal Register, volume 55, pages 9538 to 9610. A portion of CLIA '88 is also cited as an amendment to Part 11 of the Health and Safety Standards, Section 353 of the Public Health Service Act.

Box 22•3

Laboratories Exempt from CLIA '88 Jurisdiction

1. Those subject to rules published and enforced by the Veterans Administration
2. Those subject to rules published and enforced by the Department of Defense for personnel drug surveillance and enforcement purposes*
3. Those licensed by approved state licensure programs
4. Those operated by law enforcement agencies to determine the legal status of individuals for personnel drug surveillance and enforcement purposes*
5. Those performing testing for forensic purposes
6. Those performing in vivo and externally attached patient-dedicated monitoring
7. Those performing research testing, the patient-specific results from which are not reported for clinical use
8. Those performing any other drug testing that is certified by SAMHSA

*Administered by The Substance and Mental Health Services Administration (SAMHSA)

organizations. Currently, the latter group includes the Commission on Office Laboratory Accreditation, JCAHO, CAP, AABB, American Society for Histocompatibility and Immunogenetics, American Osteopathic Association, New York State—and the list continues to grow.[23]

Further in its process of delegating authority, HCFA

laboratory's involvement with interstate commerce is no longer relevant.

The result of this legislation has been the inclusion of many heretofore unregulated laboratories. Prior to 1988, less than 10% of all clinical laboratories were required to meet quality standards (ie, only about 12,000 hospital and independent laboratories were involved). Subsequent to CLIA '88, more than 150,000 laboratories are now regulated. Some laboratories remain exempt from direct CLIA '88 control (Box 22–3).[21]

Also exempted are tests that are FDA cleared devices for home use.[22] Box 22–4 lists general locations of CLIA-certified laboratories and indicates their general prominence.[23,24]

Also fundamental to CLIA '88 is that laboratory regulatory control is based on the *complexity of tests performed* (Box 22–5). This categorization system is based on a stratification of the regulatory requirements according to technical complexity and judged by a variety of selection criteria.

Through a certification process, HCFA manages the approval of laboratories under CLIA '88. There are five types of certificates depending on initial inspection status and level of complexity (Box 22–6). Laboratories in CLIA-exempt states number about 7000 and are issued certificates by the states, themselves.[19,23]

To obtain certification, a laboratory must formally apply to HCFA through (1) a state-level CLIA office, (2) an accrediting agency that has been granted deeming authority by HCFA, or (3) a state certification office that has been awarded CLIA exempt status. Initially, HCFA contracted responsibilities for managing application information and inspecting for compliance to state departments of health; these state-level agencies are organized under the oversight of 10 regional HCFA offices. The list of state-level agencies with deeming authority then expanded to a number of peer review

Box 22•7

Proficiency Testing Programs

Accutest
American Academy of Family Physicians
American Academy of Pediatrics
American Association of Bioanalysts
American Proficiency Institute
American Society of Internal Medicine
American Thoracic Society
California Thoracic Society
College of American Pathologists Surveys
College of American Pathologists EXCEL
Pacific Biometrics Research Foundation
Solomon Park Research Institute
Wisconsin State Laboratory of Hygiene

State/Commonwealth Health Departments
Idaho Bureau of Laboratories
Maryland Division of Laboratory Licensure
New Jersey Department of Health
New York State Department of Health
Ohio Department of Health
Pennsylvania Commonwealth Bureau of
   Laboratories
Puerto Rico Health Department Lab Services

CLIA Watch: which labs fare best, worst on PT? National
Intelligence Report, 1996;10:80

Such an ongoing program should rest on the establishment of performance standards that reflect reasonable and measurable expectations. Actual performance must then be monitored and assessed by an ongoing evaluation process. Performance indicators range from error rates to measurements of value system, affective (attitudinal) behavior, cognitive (technical and analytical) skills, and psychomotor (physical performance) skills. All of these measurements must be made keeping in mind that individual motivation and professional ability operate in a milieu of organizational incentive and inspiration.[25]

In regard to proficiency testing, Box 22–7 lists various proficiency testing programs that are available. A testing site is contacted by its respective accrediting agency for remedial measures if two out of three PT sets are unsatisfactory.

Waived testing is the lowest or simplest level of complexity and includes a limited listing of comparatively simple procedures that meet one of the following three statutory definitions:

1. The test must have been cleared by the FDA for home use; or
2. The test must use methodology that is so simple and accurate as to render the likelihood of erroneous results negligible; or

has recognized certain states as being totally exempt from HCFA's certifying program. These states are allowed to carry on their own CLIA-based laboratory surveillance and award their own certificates of compliance. These states currently include New York (except for POLS), Oregon, and Washington.

A CLIA '88 inspection covers five major areas for compliance founded on an outcome based process: (1) personnel qualifications, including personnel competence assessment; (2) patient test management; (3) quality control; (4) quality assurance; and (5) proficiency testing. Subsequent to inspection, the accreditation agencies notify HCFA of the sites that do and do not comply with the CLIA regulations. The actual inspection process varies depending on whether it is performed by HCFA, a deeming authority or an exempt state. For example, to date, the CAP is still using a process-oriented checklist which is in transition to a more outcome based approach.

Regarding personnel competence, the laboratory director must have an ongoing mechanism to evaluate the effectiveness of his policies and procedures for assessing employee and consultant competence.

Box 22•8

CLIA '88 Waived Tests*

1. Dipstick or tablet reagent urinalysis (nonautomated) for bilirubin, glucose, hemoglobin, ketone, leukocytes, nitrate, pH, protein, specific gravity, and urobilinogen
2. Fecal occult blood
3. Ovulation tests, visual color comparison methods for human luteinizing hormone
4. Urine pregnancy tests, visual color comparison methods
5. Erythrocyte sedimentation rate, nonautomated
6. Hemoglobin-copper sulfate method, nonautomated
7. Blood glucose by devices approved by the FDA for home use
8. Spun microhematocrit
9. Hemoglobin by single analyte with self-contained or component features

Federal Register, 1995;60:47535.
* This list is subject to continual modification.

Box 22·9

Categorization of Moderately Complex and Highly Complex Levels

1. Knowledge required of the laboratorian through education
2. Training and experience required of the laboratorian
3. Reagent material and preparation complexity
4. Procedural or operational step complexity
5. Calibration, quality control, and proficiency testing material complexity and availability
6. Maintenance and trouble shooting complexity
7. Interpretation and judgment required of the laboratorian

A Summary of the Provisions of the Final Rules Implementing the Clinical Laboratory Improvement Amendments of 1988. Washington, DC, American Society of Clinical Pathologists and College of American Pathologists, 1992

---

3. The test must pose no reasonable risk of harm to the patient if the test is performed incorrectly

Box 22–8 lists the tests included in this category. The number of test methods and devices included in the waived category are extremely limited, but it represents about 46% of registered laboratories. It can be expected that this list of waived tests will grow in length and breadth of scope as the health-care industry develops devices suitable to FDA criteria. The general process for granting waived status is under significant revision. The list will eventually contain the above nine items plus those cleared by the FDA for home use and those cleared by the CDC waiver process.

Laboratories operating under the authority of a certificate of waiver are not subject to inspection for certification or recertification. However, they are expected to follow whatever processes for quality control and assurance are explained in manufacturers' instructions. They still must expect to be surveyed randomly if ever a complaint is raised to a CLIA agency.

The next two levels of moderate complexity and high complexity are categorized on the basis of seven test characteristics (Box 22–9).[27]

Moderately complex laboratory tests are manual or include procedures with limited steps and with limited sample or reagent preparation or are automated tests that require minimal operator intervention during testing (Box 22–10). The moderately complex category includes about 75% of the methods and devices currently on hand.[21]

To date, the moderately complex testing category includes the one subcategory of provider-performed microscopy (PPM). Laboratory tests falling under the PPM category require proficiency in the use of the microscope and in identifying cellular elements present in the specimen (Box 22–11). Specific tests included in this PPM subcategory are listed in Box 22–12.

Limited to bright field or phase contrast, PPM is used to recognize the presence or absence of human cellar, bacterial, fungal, or parasitic elements and to differentiate these from artifacts. It is not to be used for definitive identification or enumeration or with any staining. The number of test methods and devices included in the PPM category is also extremely limited, but it represents about 20% of registered laboratories.[28]

A second subcategory of moderately complex test-

Box 22·10

Characteristics of Moderately Complex Laboratory Tests

1. Some basic scientific and technical knowledge is required to perform preanalytical, analytical, or postanalytical phases of the testing.
2. Some basic training and experience are required for preanalytical, analytical, and postanalytical phases of the testing process.
3. Reagents and materials are generally stable and reliable but require some specific storage precautions.
4. Operational steps are not fully automated and require some monitoring, timing, or simple calculations.
5. Calibration materials do not validate the entire analytic process, are vastly different from the specimen matrix, or are supplied by the laboratory as previously assayed patient samples. Proficiency testing materials are in a format other than that of the clinical specimen.
6. Test system troubleshooting requires some independent technical skill decision making or intervention by the analyst.
7. Some interpretation and judgment are required of the analyst before releasing results.

A Summary of Major Provisions of the Final Rules Implementing the Clinical Laboratory Improvement Amendments of 1988. Washington, DC, American Society of Clinical Pathologists and College of American Pathologists, 1992.

Box 22•11

Characteristics of Provider-Performed Microscopy

1. Tests are personally performed during the patient's visit only by licensed physicians (ie, MD or DO), dentists (DDM or DDS), podiatrists, and mid-level practitioners, (ie, nurse practitioners, nurse midwives, and physician assistants).
2. The procedure must be categorized as moderately complex.
3. The primary instrument for performing the test is a microscope.
4. The specimen is labile, or delay in performing the test could compromise the accuracy of the test result.
5. Control materials are not available to monitor the entire testing process.
6. Limited specimen handling is required.

ing, accurate and precise technology tests, has been proposed. Strongly opposed by the clinical laboratory community but supported by clinical practitioners, this subcategory would include a large number of tests that have been heretofore considered to be the simpler, fully automated tests included in the moderately complex grouping. If recognized as a new subcategory, these tests would require less personnel and quality management qualifications, similar to those in the waived testing category. To date, this proposed subcategory has not been written into the CLIA regulations.

Highly complex laboratory tests are manual procedures with multiple steps in sample or reagent processing or multiple steps in the analytical process or are automated procedures requiring significant operator intervention (Box 22–13). The highly complex category includes about 25% of the methods and devices.[21]

For both moderately and highly complex certified laboratories, participation in a proficiency testing program is mandatory for certain, specially listed analytes. In fact, this is a major tool used by HCFA to maintain

Box 22•12

CLIA '88 Provider-Performed Microscopy Procedures*

1. Wet mounts, including preparations of vaginal, cervical, or skin specimens
2. All potassium hydroxide (KOH) preparations
3. Pinworm examinations
4. Fern tests
5. Postcoital direct, qualitative examinations of vaginal or cervical mucous
6. Urine sediment examination
7. Nasal smears for eosinophils
8. Fecal leukocyte examination
9. Semen analysis, limited to presence or absence of sperm and motility

* This list is subject to continual modification.

Box 22•13

Characteristics of Highly Complex Laboratory Tests

1. Specialized scientific and technical knowledge is required to perform preanalytical, analytical, or postanalytical phases of the testing.
2. High level training and experience are required to perform the preanalytical, analytical, and postanalytical phases of the testing process.
3. Reagents and materials are extremely labile and require special handling or preparation to ensure reliability; reagent and material preparation may include manual steps, such as gravimetric or volumetric measurements.
4. Operational steps in the testing process are extensive or complex, requiring manual manipulation and close monitoring or control.
5. Calibration materials, are so labile that quality control or proficiency testing are not available or cannot duplicate any part of the sample matrix.
6. Troubleshooting requires high level decision making and extensive intervention to resolve most problems.
7. Significant independent interpretation and judgment are required to perform preanalytical, analytical or postanalytical processes.

A Summary of Major Provisions of the Final Rules Implementing the Clinical Laboratory Improvement Amendments of 1988. Washington, DC, American Society of Clinical Pathologists and College of American Pathologists, 1992.

Table 22-2
Health Care Financing Administration Comparison of 1994 CLIA '88 Proficiency Testing Failures Comparing Physician Office Laboratories (POLs) and Other Laboratories

Analyte	First Event Percent of Failures		Second Event Percent of Failures		Third Event Percent of Failures	
	Other	POLs	Other	POLs	Other	POLs
Hemoglobin	1	4	1	3	1	3
Culture identification	9	15	7	14	2	6
Cholesterol	4	10	3	10	4	10
Glucose	4	10	2	8	2	7

From Department of Health and Human Services, Health Care Financing Administration: Proficiency Testing. CLIA-Approved Proficiency Testing Programs. 1994 Comparison of Results by Physician Office Laboratories (POLs) Versus Other Laboratories. Baltimore, February 1995

some level of ongoing surveillance on every laboratory's current level of effectiveness.

Great effort has been made to make a relatively easy transition into CLIA '88. For example, because of the language of the law, almost all physicians qualify automatically as a laboratory director by virtue of their experience in running their own laboratory or their training in residency.

Also, all POLs, including those performing highly complex tests, can continue using their current testing personnel as long as the personnel have at least a high school diploma and training for the laboratory work that they are performing and are adequately supervised. By 1997, those personnel would be expected to have attained a minimum of an associate degree in medical laboratory technology.

Clinicians, however, have raised a tremendous furor over the need for their being under the jurisdiction of CLIA '88. In 1994, HCFA compared POLs versus other

laboratories on the basis of proficiency testing performance. Table 22–2 illustrates the major findings of that study. The total number of participants included 89,230 POLs (58.5%), 8,834 hospital laboratories (5.8%), and 5,767 independent laboratories (3.8%) among a total of 152,423.[29] The CDC also reported that, in 1996, "POLs and other newly regulated testing sites had higher rates of unsatisfactory PT performance than previously regulated hospital and independent laboratories."[30]

From a slightly different perspective, Table 22–3 provides a 1994 comparison of the total number of CLIA inspection deficiencies versus the number of "condition-level" deficiencies.[31] These deficiencies are of such importance as to warrant the most severe of CLIA sanctions—the rescinding of certification. Table 22–4 illustrates a HCFA summary of the improvement of CLIA-regulated laboratories in terms of 1994 zero and condition-level deficiencies.[24]

HCFA also has published some of the leading 1994

Table 22-3
Health Care Financing Administration Summary of Physician Office Laboratories (POL) Improvement Following 1994 CLIA '88 Inspections

	First Inspection	Second Inspection	Percent Improvement
Total POL deficiencies	1,886	1,449	23
Average deficiencies per POL	5.5	2.7	51
Total POL condition-level deficiencies	175	129	26
Average condition-level deficiencies per POL	.12	.09	25

Department of Health and Human Services, Health Care Financing Administration: Improvement in Physician Office Laboratories Between First and Second CLIA Inspections. Baltimore, CLIA Data Bank, 1995

Table 22-4

Health Care Financing Administration Summary of Condition-Level Deficiencies Following 1994 CLIA '88 Inspections

	After 1st Cycle	After 2nd Cycle
Laboratories without deficiencies	684 (6%)	3236 (30%)
Laboratories with condition-level deficiencies	1042 (10%)	734 (7%)

Department of Health and Human Services, Office of the Inspector General: CLIA's Impact on the Availability of Laboratory Services. Washington, DC, June 1995

CLIA inspection testing deficiencies. Summarized in Table 22–5, those data include POL deficiency incidence rates compared with rates of other laboratories.[29] A separate state of Washington inspection program has confirmed HCFA findings regarding improvement of previously unregulated laboratories (ie, POLs).[32]

In assessing these HCFA surveys, there have consistently been indications of higher patient risk from test results produced by POLs. For whatever reason, POLS have not adhered as closely to the standards of practice as do other types of laboratories. There is active study underway of the unique quality control and quality assurance needs of the POL environment.[33]

The data indicate that CLIA '88 has produced a positive effect on *all* types of laboratories. There is always some room for improvement when inspecting or surveying any laboratory. However, CLIA's impact on POL improvement has been particularly significant.

Since the tightening of federal regulatory control, physicians in support of POLs have attempted to regain exemption from governmental regulatory control. Advocacy support has been provided by various groups, including the Practicing Physicians Advisory Council, the American Medical Association (AMA), and most of the clinical specialty and subspecialty associations. Among several arguments, these practitioners have stated that the regulation of POLs has limited clinical physician access to office laboratory testing. In June 1995, the Office of the Inspector General of the DHHS published the results of its study of this issue. Its final conclusion was that "the number of physicians with access to office laboratories has remained unchanged since 1988."[24]

Thus, a political tug-of-war is likely to continue between various health-care factions over certain aspects of laboratory regulation. Diametrically opposite opinions will continue to prevail, particularly between laboratorians and the private physicians who run POLs. Basically, it is a matter of laboratorian concern about operational effectiveness and reliable patient care versus private physician concern about operational efficiency and economics. There is no question that a philosophy of professional and economic independence courses deeply through the fabric of American health-care politics.

Both clinical laboratory and clinical physician fac-

Table 22-5

Health Care Financing Administration Summary of Major 1994 CLIA '88 on-Site Inspection Deficiencies Comparing Physician Office Laboratories (POLs) and Other Laboratories

Problem	Failure Rate		
	POL	Hospital	Independent
No assessment of test accuracy	34%	13%	23%
Manufacturer's instructions not followed	28%	12%	21%
Appropriate personnel training, written procedures, or testing oversight not provided	19%	12%	14%
Did not verify reactivity of reagents used in microbiology	9%	2%	5%
No system to ensure reliable identification of patient specimens	12%	6%	9%

From Department of Health and Human Services, Health Care Financing Administration: Proficiency Testing. CLIA-Approved Proficiency Testing Programs. 1994 Comparison of Results by Physician Office Laboratories (POLs) Versus Other Laboratories. Baltimore, February 1995

tions have significant political influence on Capitol Hill. To a large extent, these issues even divide along major political party lines, and whichever party is in power in Congress determines which faction has the advantage.[24,34]

To reach some compromise, HCFA and most peer review organizations are incorporating interim self-inspections into the certification/accreditation system. Referred to as the CLIA Alternate Quality Assessment Survey (AQAS), this approach is predicated largely on the credence paid to proficiency testing performance.[35,36]

The CAP pioneered the use of interim self-inspection as an important component of its inspection and accreditation program in the 1960s. This approach is finally becoming a feasible possibility due to the extent of "over-the-shoulder" scrutiny that is becoming available through modern telephonic computer system linkage. If implemented, the AQAS could reduce the frequency and expense of on-site visits, especially if followed suit by all other subsidiary certifying/accrediting organizations with deeming authority.

FOOD AND DRUG ADMINISTRATION

As illustrated previously (see Fig. 22–1, page 378), the three administrative components of the DHHS—FDA, CDC, and HCFA—impact significantly on health-care in the United States. Of the three, the FDA regulates the market entry of clinical laboratory instruments, reagents, and systems that are manufactured by the medical device industry.

Stemming originally from the Food and Drug Act of 1906, the FDA was officially created in 1931 and is a major component of the DHHS. The FDA derives its present authority from the Food, Drug, and Cosmetic Act of 1938 (FDCA '38). Closely related laws include the Public Health Service Act of 1944 and the Medical Devices Amendments of 1976 and 1990.[37]

The FDCA '38 is cited in 21 CFR. Chapter I of the law is divided into the following parts:

Parts 1 to 99: General regulations
Parts 100 to 169: Food regulations
Parts 170 to 199: Food additives regulations
Parts 200 to 299: General regulations for drugs
Parts 300 to 499: Drugs for human use regulations
Parts 500 to 599: Drugs for animals regulations
Parts 600 to 799: Biologics and cosmetics regulations
Parts 800 to 1299: Medical devices, mammography and radiological health regulations

It is important to understand the structure of this law, especially when the discussion turns to blood banking regulations. The main thrust of all of these reg-

ulations is that the FDA is entrusted to protect the public by regulating clinical laboratory devices and blood manufacturing facilities and ensuring the practice of current good manufacturing practice (CGMP), the resultant device or blood product being safe and effective.

Safe is the state in which there is "reasonable assurance that . . . the probable benefits to health outweigh any probable risks" (21 CFR Part 860.7[d][1]).

Effective is the state in which there is "reasonable assurance that in a significant proportion of the target population, the use of the product will provide clinically significant results" (21 CFR part 860.7[e][1]).

CGMP is defined by 21 CFR 211 and 21 CFR 606. Part 211.12 describes a "quality control unit," Parts 600.10 and 606.20 describe the "responsible head," and Part 820.20 describes the "quality assurance supervisory." These are essential elements of quality management in understanding CGMP rules and regulations.

Regulation of In Vitro Diagnostic Devices

The FDA regulates clinical laboratory devices and blood and blood products. A device is defined by section 201(h) of the FDCA as "an instrument, apparatus, implement, machine, contrivance, implant, in vitro reagent, or other similar or related articles, including any component, part or accessory which:[38]

- Is recognized in the official National Formulary, or the United States Pharmacopeia, or any supplement to them,
- Is intended for use in the diagnosis of disease or other conditions, or in the cure, mitigation, treatment, or prevention of disease, in man or other animals, or
- Is intended to affect the structure or the function of the body of man or other animals
- Does not achieve any of its principal intended purposes through chemical action within or on the body of man or other animals and which is not dependent upon being metabolized for the achievement of its principal intended purposes.

Enhancing the FDAC of 1938, the Medical Devices Amendments of 1976 initiated regulations to guide the medical device manufacturing industry. These amendments expanded the definition of device to include:[38]

- Devices intended for the use in the diagnosis of conditions other than disease, such as pregnancy
- In vitro, diagnostic products, including those previously regulated as drugs.

The Safe Medical Devices Act of 1990 expanded the responsibility of the FDA to regulate medical devices, providing more specific oversight stipulations.

FDCA '38 requires the FDA to classify all manufactured devices sold for the intention of human use into three classes—I, II, and III. This registration and classification process has been under the direct scrutiny of the FDA's Division of Clinical Laboratory Devices (DCLD) since 1995.

Class I includes devices that have been found "substantially equivalent" to a legally marketed device. They are subject to only the most general of controls that would still adequately ensure safety and effectiveness. This class comprises about 46% of all in vitro diagnostic (IVD) devices. The industrial controls required for these devices would include appropriate registration; protection against illegal copies (adulterated or misbranded); labeling; notification procedures for risks, repairs, or refunds; restrictions of sale, distribution, or use; and oversight of good manufacturing practices, records, reports, and inspections.

Examples of Class I devices include a routine dipstick urinalysis procedure or immunohistochemicals (IHCs) that are well established through long-time usage and provide only adjunctive diagnostic information that may be included in a pathologist's report but not as independent findings (eg, markers that differentiate between squamous and adenomatous cell lines, such as antikeratin).[41,42]

Class II includes devices that are also substantially equivalent but are more complex, requiring specific controls or "performance standards" deemed necessary to provide adequate assurance of safety and effectiveness. This class comprises about 47% of all IVDs. Such performance standards are established specifically for each device in this class. Thus, in addition to the general controls listed previously, Class II devices involve a more recent, complex technology that requires special standardization devices or procedures. Class II devices are being triaged in three "tiers" to facilitate their processing.

Examples of Class II devices include a blood chemical testing system using routine photometric analysis (eg, calcium) or IHCs that provide pathologists with adjunctive diagnostic information that is ordinarily reported as independent diagnostic information to the ordering clinician (eg, for immunologic detection and semiquantitative measurement of specific ligand markers of cellular proliferation, such as the $Ksub[K_i]$ form of antikeratin).

Class III includes all new, innovative devices for which insufficient information exists to ensure that general controls and performance standards would provide reasonable assurance of safety and effectiveness. Thus, these devices are subject to the most stringent PMA review process to provide adequate assurance of safety and effectiveness.

This class comprises about 10% of all IVDs. This potentially lengthy control process is necessary for devices that are used to sustain life, are implanted in the body, or pose any other unreasonable risk of iatrogenic illness or injury. Such devices ordinarily have insufficient data immediately available to ensure that general controls or performance standards would provide reasonable assurance of safety and effectiveness.

Often, Class III devices are investigational, requiring extensive field studies, scientific review by FDA personnel, specially appointed peer review advisory committee members and consultants, ancillary government personnel (eg, [CDC], the National Committee on Clinical Laboratory Standards [NCCLS], and the Health Industry Manufacturers' Association). Thus, in addition to the general controls and performance standards determined for the first two classes of devices, Class III devices require much more extensive investigation and control procedures. Some applicants might be awarded an investigational device exemption if the device is not used to produce results used for clinical care.

Examples of Class III devices include a new *Herpes simplex* virus antigen testing system, an IHC marker for estrogen, and a progesterone receptor marker; a device to detect clinically significant mutations that appear normal by conventional microscopy; or an antigen capture assay for detecting *Plasmodium falciparum* infection.

Every establishment involved in the manufacture, preparation, propagation, compounding, assembly, or processing of a device intended for human use must register annually with the FDA. Registered manufacturers must submit an up-to-date listing on every device marketed by the firm.

An aspiring manufacturer of any new device must notify the FDA of its intent to market the device by one of two pathways. Premarket notification (PMN) is required to introduce a new product on the market that is a version of a device already in the marketplace (referred to as a "me too" device). Such devices are cleared by the PMN process as being in the Class I or II category.[39,40]

The second pathway is that of premarket approval (PMA) for any entirely new, innovative device. The PMN process addresses the approval of all Class III devices.

The DCLD reviews over 1700 device applications per year. The length of time required for PMN clearance or PMA approval depends on the complexity of the test device in question. For example, the classification of a class I device might take 180 days, whereas a class III device might take up to 3 years. The FDA publishes final approval notices in the Federal Register and follows up with marketing and postmarket performance surveillance.

Future issues to be addressed by the FDA and its DCLD include how to classify the "home-brew," point-of-care, and for-home-use testing systems that are beginning to enter the market. Additionally, new technologies are clearly visible on the developmental horizon, such as miniaturized computerization, programmable robotics, micromachines, activity-based ion-selective electrodes, polymerase chain reaction, nonradioactive labeling of nucleic acid probes, DNA amplification using microfabricated reaction chambers, nucleic acid hybridization, immunosensor technology, optimal immunoassay, and immunodiffraction grating techniques.

How the FDA copes with these new testing systems will impact on the conventional clinical laboratory's ability to vie for its share of the economic market while striving continually to provide the most efficacious clinical laboratory service to the clinical patient.[43]

As we poise on the brink of a new century, the regulation of clinical laboratory technology is being aimed at controlling technical quality and productivity.[44,45] In due course, the industry should come full circle in considering defect rates and process stability, reminiscent of Shewhart's teachings in the early 1930s.[46]

Regulation of Blood and Blood Components

Since Landsteiner's initial studies of ABO blood antigen groupings at the beginning of the 20th century, blood banking in this country has undergone immense regulatory changes. Most of the new rules have been intended to control the transmission of infectious diseases through blood transfusion.

The threat of spirochaetal and bacterial contamination of preserved blood and its components has been recognized for many decades, presaging the modern threat of transfusion-associated hepatitis and retroviral disease. In 1941, donor blood became required to undergo serologic testing for syphilis. Accreditation standards also required safeguards against bacterial contamination.

In the 1960s and 1970s, blood banking began to be a focus of the civil court system subsequent to the rising threat of transfusion-transmitted hepatitis. This legal activity was paralleled by the equally rapid response by the industry to develop the technology required to test human blood adequately for hepatitis infectivity.

In 1971, the viral era began with the testing of donor blood for hepatitis B surface antigen. In 1985, human immunodeficiency virus-1 (HIV-1) antibody testing began. In 1988, there was the onset of testing for the human T-lymphocyte virus I and II antibody.

1990 marked the testing for anti-hepatitis C virus antibody. In 1994, protozoan agents became an issue with the risk of donor malarial transmission being raised. Testing for HIV-1 antigen began in 1996.[47]

Since the 1980s and the advent of HIV-1 transfusion-transmitted disease, there have been many legal battles with some important judicial findings, and millions of dollars have been won by lawsuit. To protect public safety, the federal government has rigorously stepped up the regulation of the manufacture and use of human blood and its components, and many blood banking licenses have been lost due to failure to comply.

In 1970, the PHS Act was amended to stipulate that biologics also included blood and blood components or derivatives. It also added "responsible head," biennial inspections, label control, and additional registration requirements.

In 1973, a National Blood Policy was formulated. In the same year, the FDA began to intensify further its public scrutiny of the manufacturing and use of human blood by requiring all blood banks to register as drug manufacturers. Up to that time, only 199 licensed blood banks had been under surveillance; then, more than 7,000 facilities were compelled to register and expected to meet specific CGMP regulations. Thus, the FDA began to regard not only blood and blood components as biologics, but also blood banks and transfusion services as pharmaceutical manufacturing and distribution facilities.[17,47,48]

As a biologic, blood had already been regulated under the statutes and regulations of 21 CFR Parts 600 to 680 of the Food, Drug, and Cosmetic Act. The law defines biologic products as "any virus, therapeutic serum, toxin, antitoxin, or analogous product applicable to the prevention, treatment, or cure of diseases or injuries of man." Thus, whole blood or plasma, or any organic constituents derived from whole blood, plasma, or serum are considered to be biologic products.

According to 21 CFR, Part 606, federal licensing also requires that there be CGMP for blood and blood components as outlined for biologics. Pursuant to Section 351 of the Public Health Service Act (42 USC Part 262), control of these regulations falls under the purview of the Center for Biologics Evaluation and Research of the FDA.

As a drug, blood and its components are considered to be "intended for use in the diagnosis, cure, mitigation, treatment, or prevention of diseases in humans" as defined in Section 201(g) of the Food, Drug, and Cosmetic Act. As a drug, blood and its components should be considered adulterated if "the methods used in or the facilities or controls used for its manufacture, processing, packing, and holding do not conform to or are not operated or administered in conformity with current good manufacturing practice to assure that each drug meets the requirements of the Act."

Thus, the regulations in Parts 210 to 226 and 600 to 680 of the Food, Drug, and Cosmetics Act are considered to supplement each other. In addition, in the course of its activities, FDA recognizes the five major areas of compliance of CLIA '88.

Adherence to CGMP is essential to ensuring the continued safety of the nation's blood supply. CGMP implies that a comprehensive quality management system is in place that provides effective control over all manufacturing systems, programs, and processes, as monitored through operative-level quality control and administrative-level quality assurance. Such a management system should include the surveillance of key critical control points (Box 22–14). In 1980, the FDA and HCFA signed a memorandum of understanding that the FDA would not inspect hospital transfusion services performing only compatibility testing.[49]

OCCUPATIONAL SAFETY AND HEALTH ADMINISTRATION

During World War II and the subsequent aftermath of labor union advocacy, significant concern has arisen over employee safety and welfare, including all health-care workers at any level of responsibility. In the 1940s, one of the first issues was air purity, which led to the development of high-efficiency particulate air filters for use in the manufacturing environment.

In the clinical laboratory, automatic pipetting began to be used in 1958, precluding the practice of mouth pipetting of toxic or infectious materials. In the mid-1960s, biological safety cabinets were required. In 1968, the Radiation Control for Health and Safety Act was enacted, requiring controls for x-ray and laser-emitting medical devices.

In 1970, the Occupational Safety and Health Act (29 CFR) was passed. The law created the Occupational Safety and Health Administration (OSHA) under the Department of Labor. A steady stream of regulation has followed, covering a wide spectrum of employee safety and health-related issues (Box 22–15). In many cases, these safeguards have required the joint involvement of OSHA, the CDC, or the FDA.[50]

Almost all of the enacted regulatory controls have improved the working environment. In a few cases, the regulations have been overzealous in an attempt to make a political statement. For example, as this chapter goes to press, there is considerable controversy about proposed tuberculosis controls. First proposed by OSHA in 1995, these regulations now are too much too late. The rising incidence of pathogenic *Mycobacterium* species noted during the 1980s and early 1990s has abated due to controls already recommended by the CDC. However, OSHA persists in trying to enact stricter, more costly controls even though the public health problem has largely been addressed. This is a matter of proposed legislation looking for a problem to solve. If enacted, OSHA's new rules will most likely be over-

---

Box 22•14

Key Control Points for Current Good Manufacturing Practice

- Quality control and assurance system
- Donor suitability system
- Blood collection system
- Component manufacturing system
- Product testing and compatibility system
- Lot release system
- Storage and distribution system
- Report evaluation system
- Computer system

Box 22•15

Occupational Safety and Health Administration Requirements

- Eating and smoking in the laboratory (1970)
- Acid bottle carriers (1972)
- Centrifuge safety protecting against aerosol contamination (1973)
- Safety shields protecting against splashing, aerosolized, and flying blood and body fluids (1975)
- Classification of patient examination gloves as Class I medical devices (1980)
- Hepatitis B vaccine (1981)
- Sharps disposal (1983)
- Universal precautions to prevent transmission of blood-borne pathogens (1983)
- Formaldehyde handling (1987)
- Hazardous waste disposal and spill response (1989)
- Hazardous chemical exposure (1990)
- Blood-borne pathogens standard (1991)
- Needlestick prevention (1993)
- Respirators (1994)
- Personal protective equipment (1994)

Box 22•16

Government Agencies Involved in Regulation of Clinical Laboratory Operations (Beside the Occupational Safety and Health Administration)

- Environmental Protection Agency for hazardous waste disposal; for example, in 1990, 500,000 tons of regulated infectious medical waste produced in the United States yearly by about 380,000 regulated generators. This was equivalent to 0.3% of the 158 metric tons of waste generated overall.[51]
- Department of Transportation (DOT) for safe packaging, labeling, and transportation of biological products. For example, in 1991, the DOT issued its Final Rule on Performance-Oriented Packaging Requirements for Medical Waste.
- Department of Justice and the Federal Trade Commission for antitrust oversight

---

kill—adding to the burden of already established regulatory controls that have been effective in solving the problem at hand.

Aside from OSHA, other government agencies are involved in regulation of clinical laboratory operations (Box 22–16).

INTERNATIONAL ORGANIZATION OF STANDARDIZATION

In addition to continually burgeoning federally mandated requirements, voluntary international standards are emerging through the efforts of the International Organization for Standardization (IOS), based in Geneva, Switzerland. The IOS is a worldwide federation of national standards bodies that includes the American National Standards Institute (ANSI). The IOS's Technical Committee 212 (TC 212) addresses standards for clinical laboratory testing. Other IOS committees are addressing quality management, medical devices, and reference systems.[52]

The ANSI has delegated its medically related duties concerning the IOS for clinical laboratory standardization to the NCCLS. NCCLS administrates the United States Technical Advisory Group (TAG). This TAG provides United States representation to the IOS's TC212, appoints members of working groups, and develops American positions on laboratory-related issues.

During recent years, the IOS has developed a growing series of manufacturing and performance standards. American laboratories engaged in international commerce are already familiar with the ISO 9000 standards, and the volume of in vitro diagnostic test system commerce is expected to expand significantly. In that process, interchangeability of test results will become a problem to be resolved, along with many other control and assurance issues set on the stage of the global market.

Technical committees of the IOS are at work formulating clinical laboratory standards that include quality management, reference systems, and in vitro diagnostic products. For example, one committee is designing standards on clinical laboratory testing and in vitro diagnostic test systems. Another committee has been addressing quality management of medical devices. In response to these international activities, the federal government is beginning to meld the language of United States law with that of international standards through appropriate legislation. It should be expected that various components of the FDA will remain prominent in international regulatory control and other clinical laboratory reform issues of the future.

STATE AND LOCAL REGULATION OF CLINICAL LABORATORIES

Both Medicare/Medicaid and CLIA '88 regulations mandate that all participating laboratory facilities must be in compliance with the state and local laws of the locality in which they operate. Such laws may include personnel licensure, facility licensure, fire safety requirements, and other related health and safety requirements. As discussed previously, most states have licensure or other types of requirements for clinical laboratories or their personnel. Some states have proficiency testing programs. Local regulations vary widely from state to state and even in major cities within a state, thus adding further complexity to an already confusing laboratory regulatory climate.

PEER-LEVEL ASSURANCE INSPECTION AND ACCREDITATION OF CLINICAL LABORATORIES

Abraham Flexner's report on *Medical Education in the United States* in 1910 was a landmark peer study. It was the initial springboard for significant reformation and standardization of American and Canadian health-care education and practice for the 20th century. Spurred on by the Flexner Report, the 1912 Third Clinical Congress of North America called for the development of a standardized program of medical education.[52–54]

Also based on the impact of Flexner's report, the American College of Surgeons (ACS) was founded in 1913, funded by a gift from the Carnegie Foundation, to enhance the quality of institutional patient care nationwide. The ACS's early emphasis was on the adoption of a uniform medical record format that would facilitate accurate recording of the patient's clinical course to measure surgical outcomes or clinical course. The ACS recognized that such a program also involved setting standards for hospital services.

In 1917, the ACS established its Hospital Standardization Program for voluntary hospital survey. In 1918, it published its first "Standard on Efficiency." In 1919, field trials revealed a pass rate for that standard of only 89 out of 692 hospitals of 100 beds or larger. In 1924, the ACS adopted its five-part "Minimum Standard." Even then, one of the five standards was concerned with the availability and function of clinical laboratory and pathology services in the hospital. By 1951, the ACS had approved more than 3,000 American hospitals—this amounted to over 50% participation.[55]

Unlike the voluntary inspection and accreditation programs which originally evolved from the desire of the laboratory professionals to improve medical care, peer-level review has become more mandatory. This has come about by the pervasiveness of CLIA '88 and the fact that the JCAHO (and other peer organizations) have sought and received deeming status to perform CLIA inspections of their organizational members or clients. The members would rather receive a CLIA inspection by their peers than by state- or federal-level regulatory agency inspection teams.

Survey, inspection, and accreditation programs for clinical laboratories have become well established. A number of voluntary programs have been a major factor in the attainment of the high standards of quality that characterize laboratory medicine in the United States today.

Joint Commission on Accreditation of Healthcare Organizations

The JCAHO is an outgrowth of the ACS hospital standardization program that was launched in 1917. In 1950, the size, scope, and expense of the ACS inspection program had grown beyond the resources that one organization could sustain. Thus, the Joint Commission on Accreditation of Hospitals (JCAH) was created.

The founding members were the ACS, the American College of Physicians, the AMA, the Canadian Medical Association (CMA), and the American Hospital Association. In 1980, the CMA withdrew, and the American Dental Association was added to the organization in 1980. In 1987, the JCAH reorganized as the JCAHO.

As the JCAH, the organization began to offer accreditation to hospitals in January 1953. Currently, the JCAHO surveys more than 5,000 health-care organizations a year and has its own full-time field staff to carry out this mission.

In 1979, recognizing the complexity and growth of laboratory medicine, the JCAHO agreed to work with CAP in updating and refining the standards that the JCAHO had adopted for hospital laboratories. As a result this coordination, the laboratory requirements became more uniform, and there was an agreement that the JCAHO would waive its inspection of the hospital laboratory during the course of the general survey of the hospital departments if the laboratory had been previously accredited by the CAP. A major exception to this waiver has been in the areas of quality assurance and safety, which the JCAHO team has maintained as part of its overall survey of the hospital.

Such joint arrangements between the JCAHO and CAP have continued with the advent of CLIA '88. CLIA has become the universal gold standard for minimal operational personnel, quality control, and quality assurance requirements. Both the JCAHO and CAP have become deeming authorities and continue to work together to avoid unnecessary overlap of accreditation requirements.

The JCAHO survey process is based on an accreditation manual that the JCAHO reviews, updates, and revises yearly. The JCAHO *Accreditation Manual for Hospitals* (AMH) began as a department-focused collection of standards. However, based on JCAHO's 1987 *Agenda for Change*, they have extensively reorganized the AMH into a performance-oriented collection of standards that are universally applicable to any hospital department and any other type of health-care organization.

Of key importance has been the evolution of the JCAHO's philosophy on quality management. Unfailingly, the JCAHO has placed strong emphasis on the importance of the general concepts of total quality management and continuous quality improvement. In the course of developing its overall approach, the JCAHO has moved from the concepts of quality assurance, to quality assessment and QI, to improving organizational performance. This is a never-ending process, and we can only expect new developments as the JCAHO continues on its journey.

Just as it responded to passage of the Medicare law, PL 89-97, in 1965, and to a limited extent, CLIA '67, the JCAHO has responded to meeting regulatory changes of CLIA '88. As a deeming authority, the JCAHO may inspect and accredit member hospitals or other laboratory organizations.

College of American Pathologists

The Laboratory Accreditation Program of the CAP came into being in November 1961 when an *ad hoc* committee on laboratory accreditation and the Board of Governors of the CAP implemented a program for the voluntary inspection and accreditation of clinical laboratories, which primarily focused on hospital laboratories. Over the past four decades, the CAP has developed the largest single voluntary laboratory improvement program in the world.

The CAP program owes its genesis to the hospital accreditation program of the ACS, which had included clinical laboratory services in its standards. However, over the years, clinical laboratories grew in size, organizational sophistication, and technical complexity. Thus, it became increasingly clear that even the general JCAHO inspection was inadequate to ensure the highest technical laboratory standards and that a specialized accreditation program was needed. The CAP responded to this need with its laboratory accreditation program. As mentioned previously, the CAP program has received deeming status from DHHS and HCFA and sub-deeming status from the JCAHO.

The CAP standards of performance and the inspection process are developed, initiated, and updated through continuous performance review and education. There has been a constant need to keep in step with CLIA '88 requirements, JCAHO standard changes, and other federal- and peer-level developments. Key areas of recent interest have been:

1. Amplifying the laboratory director's responsibilities
2. Improving quality assurance
3. Providing uniform standards for all laboratories
4. Dealing with ancillary and point-of-care testing programs
5. Adopting a standard format for all technical procedure manuals

6. Developing alternative quality control approaches (eg, electronic)

The CAP accreditation program continues to be a voluntary program with heavy emphasis on improvement through peer review and education. The heart of the program is the corps of trained volunteer inspectors who are practicing pathologists and medical technologists.

The standards are supplemented by an extensive checklist that is used by each inspector and the subject laboratory to review laboratory performance in great detail. These checklists are developed and approved by various CAP committees, which cover each laboratory discipline and represent the state of the art in each subspecialty of laboratory medicine. The checklists are frequently revised in response to the burgeoning scope of laboratory testing and regulatory demands.

American Association of Blood Banks

A third voluntary inspection and accreditation program is the AABB, which has been actively evaluating and accrediting blood banks and hospital transfusion services since 1947. The AABB bases its inspection process on its *Standards for Blood Banks and Transfusion Services*. During the 50 years of its existence, the AABB standards manual has become recognized as the single most authoritative source for evaluating the practice of blood banking and transfusion medicine.

The AABB standards address every conceivable aspect of blood banking and transfusion service at every level of technical complexity. Their standards and publications have continuously remained on the cutting edge, extremely timely, and up-to-date.

Volunteer inspectors conduct on-site surveys of member blood banks and transfusion services using an extremely complete and up-to-date checklist. The AABB is recognized as having deeming authority, and the organization recognizes CLIA and FDA regulatory requirements as minimal standards.

It is possible that a hospital clinical laboratory blood bank and transfusion service might be inspected by the FDA, JCAHO, CAP, and AABB during the normal course of licensing and accreditation of the overall laboratory. The potential for confusion and misunderstanding among these parties is addressed through the appointment of liaison members from the FDA, JCAHO, CAP, the American Red Cross, and the Department of Defense to the AABB Committee on Standards.

Of some import is the AABB's method of dealing with the FDA's CGMP requirements and 1995 quality assurance guideline. The result has been the development of the AABB quality program (QP). The QP is a quality management matrix used to identify key quality indicators of the operational path of work flow (ie, preanalytical, analytical, and postanalytical) matched against the key policies, plans, procedures, manuals, forms, and reports that document the pre-established expectations and ongoing quality of those key indicators.[56-59]

This brings this chapter on regulatory control of clinical laboratories to a close. Suffice it to say that most regulatory control is brought on us by the need to protect public health while protecting a health-care economic market in a free, democratic society. By virtue of our dealing with human endeavor, the outcome is not always as desired. Thus, some control is needed.

However, there will always remain the constant quandary as to just how much regulation is really necessary before it becomes an inappropriate burden.[60]

REFERENCES

1. Senhauser DA: Laboratory accreditation, licensure, and regulation. In Snyder J, Senhausen DA (eds): Laboratory Administration and Management. Philadelphia, J.B. Lippincott, 1983
2. O'Leary DS: The Joint Commission looks to the future. JAMA 58:951–952, 1987
3. Morgan AE: Microscope on Washington. The movement toward managed care. Lab Med 26:498–499, 1995
4. Clark G: Systematic Quality Management. Chicago, ASCP Press, 1995
5. Continuous Quality Improvement: Essential Management Approaches and Their Use in Proficiency Testing. Proposed Guideline GP22-P. Wayne, PA, National Committee on Clinical Laboratory Standards, 1996
6. Kessler G: Personal communication. Flemington, NJ, Health Care Direct, Inc, 1997
7. Buxton FL: Healthcare reform hits the laboratory. What (almost) happened in California. Lab Med 26:113–117, 1995
8. Feichter M: Microscope on Washington. Keys to understanding state licensure. Lab Med 26:238–239, 1995
9. 1995 Public Policy Sourcebook for Laboratory Medicine. Washington, DC, American Society of Clinical Pathologists, 1995
10. A Guide to State Licensure and Certification of Medical Technologists and Other Laboratory Personnel. Washington, DC, American Society of Clinical Pathologists, April 1996
11. Snyder J: The pros and cons of licensure: Accountability and the medical laboratory. Lab Med 25:355–356, 1994
12. Shimberg B, Roederer D: Questions a legislator should ask. Lexington, KY, The Council on Licensure, Enforcement, and Regulation, 1994
13. Castleberry B: Personal communication. Chicago, IL, American Society of Clinical Pathologists Board of Registry, 1995
14. 1997 Procedures for Examination and Certification. Chicago, American Society of Clinical Pathologists Board of Registry, 1997
15. Hargis DM: The health provider: Liability implications. In Howanitz PJ (ed): Conference Proceedings on Quality Assurance in Physician Office, Bedside, and Home Testing. Atlanta, GA; Skokie, IL, College of American Pathologists, April 2–4, 1986
16. Miller RD: Problems in Hospital Law. Rockville, MD, Aspen Systems, 1983
17. Solomon JM: The evolution of the current blood banking regulatory climate. Transfusion 34:272–277, 1994
18. CLIA '88 Regulatory Handbook. Abbott Park, IL, Abbott Quality Institute, 1994
19. Public Law 100-578, October 31, 1988; 102 STAT 2903-2915, Congressional Record 134:1988
20. Final rules for CLIA '88. Fed Reg February 28:7137–7243, 1992
21. ASCP Statement before the Practicing Physicians' Advisory Council, July 22, 1996
22. CLIA Q and A. Melvern, PA; Washington, DC, Clinical Laboratory Management Association and American Association of Clinical Chemists 1993
23. CLIA '88 Statistics. Baltimore, Department of Health and Human Services, Health Care Financing Administration, Center for Laboratories, April 1996
24. CLIA's Impact on the Availability of Laboratory Services. Washington, DC, Department of Health and Human Services, Office of the Inspector General, June 1995
25. Larison J: Laboratory practice: Personnel competency assessment. Clin Lab Science 6:13–14, 1993
26. CLIA Watch: Which labs fare best; worst on PT? National Intelligence Report, 1996;10:80
27. A Summary of Major Provisions of the Final Rules Implementing the Clinical Laboratory Improvement Amendments of 1988. Washington, DC, American Society of Clinical Pathologists and College of American Pathologists, 1992
28. Colorado CLIA Certified Laboratories. Denver, CLIA Unit, Division of Laboratories, Colorado Department of Public health and Environment, July 1995
29. Department of Health and Human Services, Health Care Financing Administration: Proficiency Testing. CLIA-Approved Proficiency Testing Programs. 1994 Comparison of Results by Physician Office Laboratories (POLs) Versus Other Laboratories. Baltimore, February 1995
30. Clinical laboratory performance on PT samples. MMWR, March 1996
31. Department of Health and Human Services, Health Care Financing Administration: Improvement in Physician Office Laboratories Between First and Second CLIA inspections. Baltimore, CLIA Data Bank, August 16, 1995
32. LaBeau KM: Laboratory testing in previously unregulated laboratories. Washington State's experience. Lab Med 26:64–69, 1995
33. Baer DM, Belsey RE: Limitations of quality control in physicians' offices and other decentralized testing situations: The challenge to develop new methods of test validation. Clin Chem 39:9–12, 1993
34. Mahkorn S: Cutting Red Tape on Clinical Labs: Why Congress Should Deregulate Doctors. In The Heritage Foundation Backgrounds. Washington, DC, The Heritage Foundation, October 10, 1995
35. Supporting Statement for the Clinical Laboratory Improvement Amendments (CLIA) Revised Flexible Survey Protocol Form (HCFA-667) Now Titled the Alternate Quality Assessment Survey (AQAS). Baltimore, Department of Health and Human Services, Health Care Financing Administration, July 1995
36. Form HCFA-667. Clinical Laboratory Improvement Amendments (CLIA) Alternate Quality Assessment Survey. Baltimore, Department of Health and Human Services, Health Care Financing Administration, February, 1996
37. Department of Health, Education, and Welfare; Food and Drug Administration: 21 CFR parts 16, 20, 860; Fed Reg 1977;42:46028-46039.
38. Everything You Always Wanted to Know About the Medical Device Amendments . . . and Weren't Afraid to Ask. Rockville, MD, Public Health Service, Food and Drug Administration, Center for Devices and Radiobiological Health, March 1984

39. Thomas J: Microscope on Washington. The path to FDA device approval. Lab Med 25:424–425, 1994

40. Thomas J: Microscope on Washington. FDA regulation of monoclonal antibodies. Lab Med 25:616–617, 1994

41. Department of Health and Human Services, Food and Drug Administration: 21 CFR Part 864. Medical devices; classification/reclassification of immunohistochemistry reagents and kits. Fed Reg 61:30197–30200, 1996

42. FDA issues IHC proposal. ASCP Washington Report 14:1, 1996

43. Aziz KJ: CLIA and future applications of technology. Clin Lab Man Rev September/October:515–523, 1994

44. Thomas J: Microscope on Washington. Changes underway in medical device approval process. Lab Med 26: 562–563, 1995

45. Aziz KJ, Gutman SI, Sliva CA, Uettwiller-Geiger D: New approaches to the evaluation of in vitro diagnostic devices by the Food and Drug Administration. J Clin Ligand Assay 18:255–258, 1995

46. Shewhart WA: Economic Control of Quality of Manufactured Product. New York, Van Nostrand, 1931

47. Sazama K: Bacteria in blood for transfusion: A review. Arch Pathol Lab Med 118:350–365, 1994

48. Sazama K: Impact of legal and regulatory changes during the past decade. In Nance ST (ed): Blood Supply: Risks, Perceptions, and Proposals for the Future. Bethesda, American Association of Blood Banks, 1994

49. Proposed Guideline for Quality Assurance in Blood Establishments. Rockville, MD, Department of Health and Human Services, Food and Drug Administration, Center for Biologics Evaluation and Research, July 11, 1995

50. Yablonsky T: How safe is laboratory practice? Lab Med 27: 92–98, 1996

51. Agency for Toxic Substance and Disease Registry: The Public Health Implications of Medical Waste: A Report to Congress. Washington, DC, U.S. Department of health and Human Services, September 1990

52. Flexner A: Medical Education in the United States and Canada. New York, Carnegie Foundation for the Advancement of Teaching, 1910

53. Pena JJ, Haffney AN, Rosen B, Light DW: Hospital Quality Assurance. Rockville, MD, Aspen Press, 1988

54. Raffel MW: The U.S. Health System Origins and Functions. New York, John Wiley and Sons, 1980

55. Roberts JS, Cook JG, Redman RR: A history of the Joint Commission on Accreditation of Hospitals. JAMA 258: 936–940, 1987

56. Berte LM, Nevalainen DE: Managers' roundtable. Quality management for the laboratory. Lab Med 27:232–235, 1996

57. Berte LM, Nevalainen DE: Managers' roundtable. Documentation pyramid for a quality system. Lab Med 27: 375–377, 1996

58. Berte LM, Nevalainen DE: Managers' roundtable. Writing standard operating procedures. Lab Med 27:514–516, 1996

59. Berte LM, Nevalainen DE: Managers' roundtable. Self-assessment in a quality system. Lab Med 27:655–658, 1996

60. Pelehach L: The quandary over quality. Lab Med 28: 182–189, 1997

23

Quality Management in the Laboratory

Lucia M. Berte

The definition of quality in the laboratory depends on who is defining it. Laboratory pathologists or technologists are likely to place words such as accuracy, reliability, and clinical applicability high on their lists. Nurses, unit clerks, and patient care technicians may define laboratory quality as test result timeliness, ease of ordering, courtesy of laboratory personnel, and ability to answer questions. Physicians are likely to define laboratory quality as test result timeliness, clinical utility, and availability of pathologist consultation; in their minds, accuracy is understood. Hospital administrators may think of laboratory quality as cost effectiveness, physician satisfaction, and exemplary inspection performance.

These definitions of laboratory quality remind one of the group of blind people asked to describe an elephant by touching it. Each "sees" a different part of the whole elephant. For the laboratory, no single description is completely correct, yet taken together, they provide a comprehensive overview of laboratory quality.

The quality aspects most important to laboratory customers are not the first on the laboratory's list. This means that the laboratory expends significant quality effort on activities such as accuracy and precision that the customers take for granted. The importance of the laboratory's quality program becomes aligning the laboratory's quality efforts with the customer's expectations for timeliness, courtesy, and consultation.

A BRIEF HISTORY OF LABORATORY QUALITY EFFORTS

Quality Control

Surveys conducted in Pennsylvania in the 1940s showed that laboratories had serious proficiency problems and demonstrated the need for laboratory accuracy comparisons on a large scale.[1] In 1950, Levey and Jennings modified the manufacturing industry's basic statistical quality control (QC) practices for laboratory chemical tests.[2] Before this time, the laboratory staff depended solely on its analytical skill and feedback from the medical staff. The introduction of a daily laboratory QC program by medical technologists Freier and Rausch in 1958 furthered laboratory quality efforts.[3] Modern instrumental tolerance levels and multirules proposed by Westgard and colleagues reflect today's changing resources and technology.[4]

Educational programming sponsored by the American Society of Clinical Pathologists promulgated QC techniques and concepts throughout clinical laboratories. In 1972, the College of American Pathologists (CAP) began its interlaboratory comparison (proficiency testing) program, which is now a fundamental part of the regulated laboratory's QC program.

Defined as the periodic systematic surveillance of people, tools, methods, and reagents, QC guarantees the laboratory's stated limits of precision with some reassurance of accuracy. QC does not, however, inquire into the appropriateness of tests ordered and performed and does not inquire into the efficiency with which the laboratory has been used.[5]

Quality Assurance: The Joint Commission on Accreditation of Healthcare Organizations Enters the Picture

Quality assurance (QA) by the peer review process received the greatest impetus from Medicare legislation of the late 1960s and early 1970s. The subsequent adoption of the prospective payment system by means of diagnosis-related groups provided further stimulus for QA efforts. In this environment, critics have alleged that cost-containment incentives based on prospective payment systems and capitated reimbursement methods could compromise patient care because necessary care and services may not be provided.[6]

The Joint Commission on Accreditation of Healthcare Organizations' (JCAHO) response to these allegations was to modify its hospital survey program to encompass the broader scope of health-care organizations. It shifted its focus away from "Can the facility provide quality services?" to "Does it provide quality services?" and required objective evidence of improved quality in health-care services. Because of the potential for nonaccreditation and loss of Medicare funding, hospitals complied with requirements for more stringent review of care and services. This requirement was extended to include the laboratory through the inclusion of a new laboratory standard in 1988: "As part of the hospital's quality assurance program, the quality and appropriateness of pathology and laboratory medicine services are monitored and evaluated and identified problems are resolved."[7]

In response to this laboratory standard, laboratory programs were to have three components: monitoring of important aspects of care and outcomes, problem solving to ensure actions were taken to improve care and outcomes, and documentation and reporting of activities.

The JCAHO subsequently added the "10-step process" as a model format designed to facilitate uniform monitoring, evaluation, and problem solving. The model became the framework for planning, implementing, and documenting most laboratories' QA programs. Step 3 of the 10-step process asked laboratories to identify the important aspects of care from the high-volume, high-risk, problematic activities in which the laboratory was involved. Those aspects of care formed the basis from which indicators were derived. Indicators are well-defined objective variables used to monitor the quality and appropriateness of an important aspect of patient care.[8] Indicators of the quality of laboratory patient care support reflected one of Donabedian's classical elements of quality—structure, process, or outcome.[9]

The indicators were to be defined, identified, and outlined as the laboratory's QA plan. The laboratory monitored its performance on the selected indicators, implemented improvement efforts when necessary, and reported its progress to hospital QA committees as required.

The College of American Pathologists Joins in

In 1987, the CAP introduced laboratory standard III aimed specifically at laboratory QA. That standard remains unchanged a decade later.[10] To assist laboratories in identifying indicators that have high relevance to patient outcome, the CAP introduced Q-Probes, a subscription service for QA monitors, in 1989. Q-Probes investigate the structure, process, and outcome of laboratory services. This subscription service provides a set of studies in clinical and anatomic pathology to systematize benchmarking practices. Laboratories perform the Q-Probes study over a given time, submit their results, and receive a critique, a peer comparison, and recommendations for quality improvement (QI). Q-Probes are meant to assist laboratories in their QA programs, not to be the sole source of QA activities. The CAP's other voluntary programs for interlaboratory peer oversight include proficiency testing surveys, the laboratory management index program, and on-site laboratory accreditation.

Written laboratory QA plans, required by the CAP standards, are as variable as the pathologist involvement in laboratories that developed them. Numbers of indicators range widely. Distribution of the indicators into structure, process, and outcome aspects of patient care varies. Monitoring schedules are different, and documentation of improvement actions is not standardized. This diversity of QA programming allows a wide latitude for laboratories to design what has been easiest for them to assimilate. In addition, the random selection of laboratory QA indicators has created a piecemeal approach to QI efforts. Without a "big picture" view of total laboratory QI, one must wonder how random improvements can really contribute to patient care quality.

The Health Care Financing Administration

The 1988 amendments to the Clinical Laboratory Improvement Act of 1967 (CLIA '67) cover all entities testing human specimens for the purposes of clinical decision making, regardless of where the testing is performed. CLIA '88 contains quality standards for QC, proficiency testing, patient test management, personnel standards, and QA. The regulations constitute a series of baseline standards that are intended to ensure the accuracy, reliability, and timeliness of clinical laboratory testing. Overall, these regulations have focused visibility on laboratory quality at a level not previously seen.[11]

MOVING BEYOND QUALITY CONTROL AND QUALITY ASSURANCE

Current laboratory QA programs and accreditation activities with their related checklists are organized within and along laboratory clinical specialties, for example, anatomic pathology, chemistry, hematology, microbiology, and blood banking. However, reengineering, downsizing, merging, joint ventures, point-of-care testing, and other health-care reform activities are changing the ways laboratories are organized within and outside of the hospital and how laboratory work is accomplished. The traditional walls separating clinical specialties—and in some cases, the actual walls—are being removed. Concepts such as core, stat, and immediate response laboratories; point-of-care testing; and cross-training have blurred the traditional lines of distinction. Because laboratories themselves are organizationally changing, there is a need for quality efforts to do so and to assure continuing contribution to high-quality patient care and outcomes.

The JCAHO has taken the first step by applying performance-based, functionally organized standards to the laboratory accreditation process. Seven dimensions of performance are framed against eight important laboratory functions. This framework is applied to the laboratory as a whole, and the JCAHO standards are no longer separated into clinical specialties.[12]

The JCAHO laboratory standards prescribe what the laboratory's quality program should include but does not describe how those activities should be carried out. This permissiveness allows laboratories to design their own quality programs, resulting in considerable diversity. Some laboratories will have comprehensive quality plans, while others will be at a loss as to how to proceed. Many laboratories will continue to do what they have always done until forced to change.

Clark has developed a comprehensive laboratory quality measurement system from a foundation of JCAHO QA principles.[13] This approach brings more structure to laboratory quality management and provides a comprehensiveness not seen in individual laboratory programs. The system consists of three programs: team building (quality actualization), strategic planning (quality anticipation), and quality assessment and QI. A key tool for facilitating the implementation of the system is quality profiling. This spreadsheet-like matrix matches the laboratory path of work flow against an improvement process. The activities described comprise a portion of the JCAHO's 10-step process of monitoring, evaluation, action, and assessment. Figure 23-1 depicts the expansion of laboratory quality efforts in the last 5 decades.

The Food and Drug Administration and the American Association of Blood Banks Adopt Quality Systems

The era of acquired immunodeficiency syndrome heralded a new intensity on the scrutiny of the safety of the blood supply in the United States. Manufacturers hastened to prepare tests to detect antibody to the human immunodeficiency virus (HIV) in donated blood as a screening measure to remove tainted donations and improve transfusion safety. Between 1985 and 1990, the blood banking community added tests for antibody to

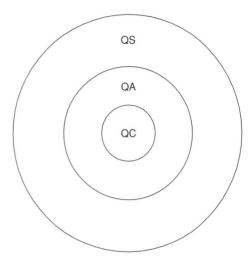

LABORATORY QUALITY
Doing Things Right

QS

QA

QC

FIGURE 23-1. In the last 5 decades, quality in the labotatory has expanded from quality control to quality assurance and now to quality systems. (Used with permission from the Abbott Quality Institute)

HIV, alanine aminotransferase (a liver enzyme), antibody to hepatitis B core antigen, antibody to human T-cell lymphotropic virus I and II, and antibody to hepatitis C virus to the traditional blood donation testing for hepatitis B surface antigen and syphilis.

The additional testing increased record keeping and computer software burdens on facilities that tested blood donations. In its periodic unannounced inspections of blood donation establishments, the Food and Drug Administration (FDA) began to find serious record-keeping errors, some of which could have had potential effects on transfusion safety. The FDA then started to apply good manufacturing practice (GMP) regulations for the pharmaceutical industry to blood establishment inspections. What they found was a need for QA in blood establishments that was more far reaching than current blood banking accreditation programs required. Adapting models from business and industry, the FDA released its *Guideline for Quality Assurance in Blood Establishments* in 1995.[14]

Concurrent with the FDA QA guideline finalization, the American Association of Blood Banks (AABB) convened a special committee to expand the concepts of that guideline into a practical working model for blood centers, hospital blood banks, and transfusion services. The resulting quality program is offered to institutional members as a model from which they can design their own QA programs.[15] Both the FDA and the AABB require facilities that draw and transfuse blood to have written quality programs.[14,16]

A MODEL LABORATORY QUALITY SYSTEM

A modification to the AABB quality program model has been made that provides direction and structure to the design of a laboratory quality system.[17] Thus, laboratories now have the benefit of the health-care organization-wide approach supported by the JCAHO and the structure with "how to" guidance specific from a laboratory's perspective. Figure 23-2 depicts a framework for a laboratory quality system. The left side of the table has been slightly modified from the AABB version but includes 11 important quality principles generic to laboratory processes. Across the top of the table is the laboratory's path of work flow, defined as the sequence of activities for specimen analysis or laboratory testing. The general path of work flow—preanalytical, analytical, postanalytical—has been further subdivided into 10 laboratory processes (operating systems) that are generic within any laboratory clinical discipline. Therefore, the quality system model can be used to coordinate quality activities within and across the entire laboratory or just within one section. The quality system described in the following pages includes all CLIA '88 (Health Care Financing Administration), GMP (FDA), JCAHO, CAP, and Commission on Laboratory Accreditation laboratory regulations and standards.[18]

To transition the laboratory quality system framework from a table on paper into an actual working reality, some specific activities are necessary. The activities correspond to those taken in business and industry to implement the ISO 9000 series quality standards.[19] They include the formation of the quality system manual, the reorganization of laboratory technical operating procedures, the redesign of the internal assessment (currently QA) program, and the application of continuous QI techniques to problem solving.

The Quality System Documentation Pyramid

A simple diagram of a laboratory quality documentation system is shown in Figure 23-3. Note that the documentation levels correspond to their respective sections of the quality system table in Figure 23-2. Level I documents are written policy statements that describe the laboratory's mission, goals, and objectives with regard to the 11 quality activities represented on the left side of the table (the quality system). Level II documents expand the quality policy statements into quality system

procedures that describe how the quality policies are accomplished laboratory wide. Level III documents are the standard operating procedures (SOPs) that laboratory employees follow to perform the tasks within the path of work flow operating systems. Level IV documents are the forms, records, labels, tags, and other items generated to document the results of performing operating procedures.[20]

The Quality System Manual

The guidance for the laboratory's quality program is embodied in the laboratory's quality system manual, which includes statements of the laboratory's policy with regard to the quality system activities. Each activity is conducted uniformly across the path of work flow. Therefore, a quality policy for personnel training would apply to all laboratory employees whether they collect specimens, work with the information system, or perform laboratory testing in any clinical laboratory discipline. The policy describes "*what* will be done"—that training is provided, competent trainers are used, training is documented, personnel must successfully complete training before performing tasks in the laboratory environment, and competence to perform job tasks will be assessed. The level II quality procedures describe in detail "*how* it will be done"—how training is conducted and documented, how competence is assessed, and how continuing education requirements are met and documented. Another example of a quality policy directs that the laboratory employees will report deviations from expected process results so that analysis of the deviations can provide information on where the laboratory may need to improve its processes. The accompanying quality procedure would describe how the employees use the laboratory-wide occurrence reporting mechanism to capture the relevant information that is further analyzed to identify opportunities for improvement. Figure 23-4 shows the relationship of the quality policies and procedures to the operations systems.

Compilation of the quality manual constitutes the development of a written laboratory QA plan/program as required by CLIA '88, JCAHO, CAP, AABB, and the FDA. The quality manual format clearly and concisely demonstrates to regulators and accreditation inspectors what the laboratory's quality system is, how it applies to the entire laboratory, and how it is implemented. Reports of the results of the self-assessment of QA monitors indicate the effectiveness of the quality program. Table 23-1 shows a listing of the quality policies and procedures that should be included in the quality manual.

A brief description of the quality policies and procedures in each of the 11 sections of the quality manual follows.

A QUALITY SYSTEM FOR THE LABORATORY

QUALITY PLAN	PRE-ANALYTICAL				ANALYTIC		POST-ANALYTIC		DATA SYSTEMS	
	Test Results	Specimen Collection/ Labeling	Specimen Transport	Specimen Receipt/ Processing	Testing/ Review	Interpre-tation	Results Reporting	Post-Test Specimen Management	Lab Information System	Information Management
LEVEL I										
1. Quality Program Organization										
LEVEL II										
2. Personnel										
3. Process Validation										
4. Calibration and Preventive Maint.										
5. Proficiency Testing										
6. Customer and Vendor Issues										
7. Process Control										
8. Documents and Records										
9. Incidents, Errors, and Accidents										
10. Internal Assessment										
11. Process Improvement										
LEVEL III										
Work Instructions (SOPs)										
System CCPs, KEs and SCs										
LEVEL IV										
Forms, Documents & Records										

FIGURE 23-2. The model laboratory system frames universal quality elements against the path of work flow common to all laboratory disciplines. (Used with permission from the Abbott Quality Institute)

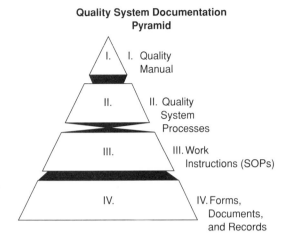

Quality System Documentation Pyramid

I. Quality Manual

II. Quality System Processes

III. Work Instructions (SOPs)

IV. Forms, Documents, and Records

FIGURE 23-3. The laboratory quality system can be documented in a hierarchy of quality policies, quality processes, standards operating processes, and related forms. (Adapted from: ISO 9000 Compendium, 6th ed. Geneva, Switzerland; International Organization for Standardization, 1996)

Quality Program Organization

The policy for this section includes a written statement about how the laboratory has organized its quality program. The policy should state the laboratory's quality goals and objectives, the identification of a designated function or person to coordinate laboratory QA efforts, how the quality program is documented, and how assessment findings and follow-up actions are communicated to the organization's QA function. A copy of the laboratory organization chart with a description of reporting relationships should be included. The quality procedure for this section describes the process for periodic review and revision of the quality program.

Personnel Selection, Training, and Education

The policy for this section includes a written statement that the laboratory provides job descriptions, orientation, training, competence assessment, and continuing education to all laboratory employees. Quality procedures describe how the orientation, training, competence assessment, and continuing education activities are conducted and documented.

Processes Validation

The policy for this section includes a written statement that new equipment, test methodologies, and computer system upgrades will undergo a validation process prior

to performance of patient testing. Validation provides evidence and assurance that the process will perform to its predetermined specifications before patient testing is conducted. The quality procedure describes how a validation process is conducted and documented.

Calibration and Preventive Maintenance

The quality policy for this section states that the laboratory will have a written program for the calibration and preventive maintenance activities required by laboratory regulations or accreditation standards. Quality procedures describe how equipment is identified and how procedures for calibration and preventive maintenance activities are written, results are documented, and the results periodically reviewed.

Proficiency Testing

The quality policy for this section states that the laboratory will participate in proficiency testing when required for all regulated analytes and describes its participation. The quality procedure describes how proficiency testing samples are received, distributed to testing personnel, and tested. The same or another quality procedure describes how results will be reviewed, investigated if found to be variant, and such reviews documented.

Customer and Vendor Issues

The policy for this section states that the laboratory will assess proposed suppliers of critical materials and services based on objective criteria. The laboratory will maintain a listing of approved suppliers, review contracts for critical supplies and services, and has a system to receive, evaluate, and inventory incoming critical materials. Quality procedures describe how each of these activities is carried out.

Process Control

The quality policy states that all laboratory processes are recorded on a flowchart to determine where prevention steps can be built in to reduce error and minimize variations. The policy also states that the laboratory has a written, active QC program for instruments, test methodologies, and reagents. Quality procedures describe how statistical process control measures are used to monitor and document processes in laboratory operating systems and how the QC program is implemented.

Documents, Records, and Reviews

The quality policy states that the laboratory will have a mechanism to control how procedures are developed, managed, revised, and archived and will also have a

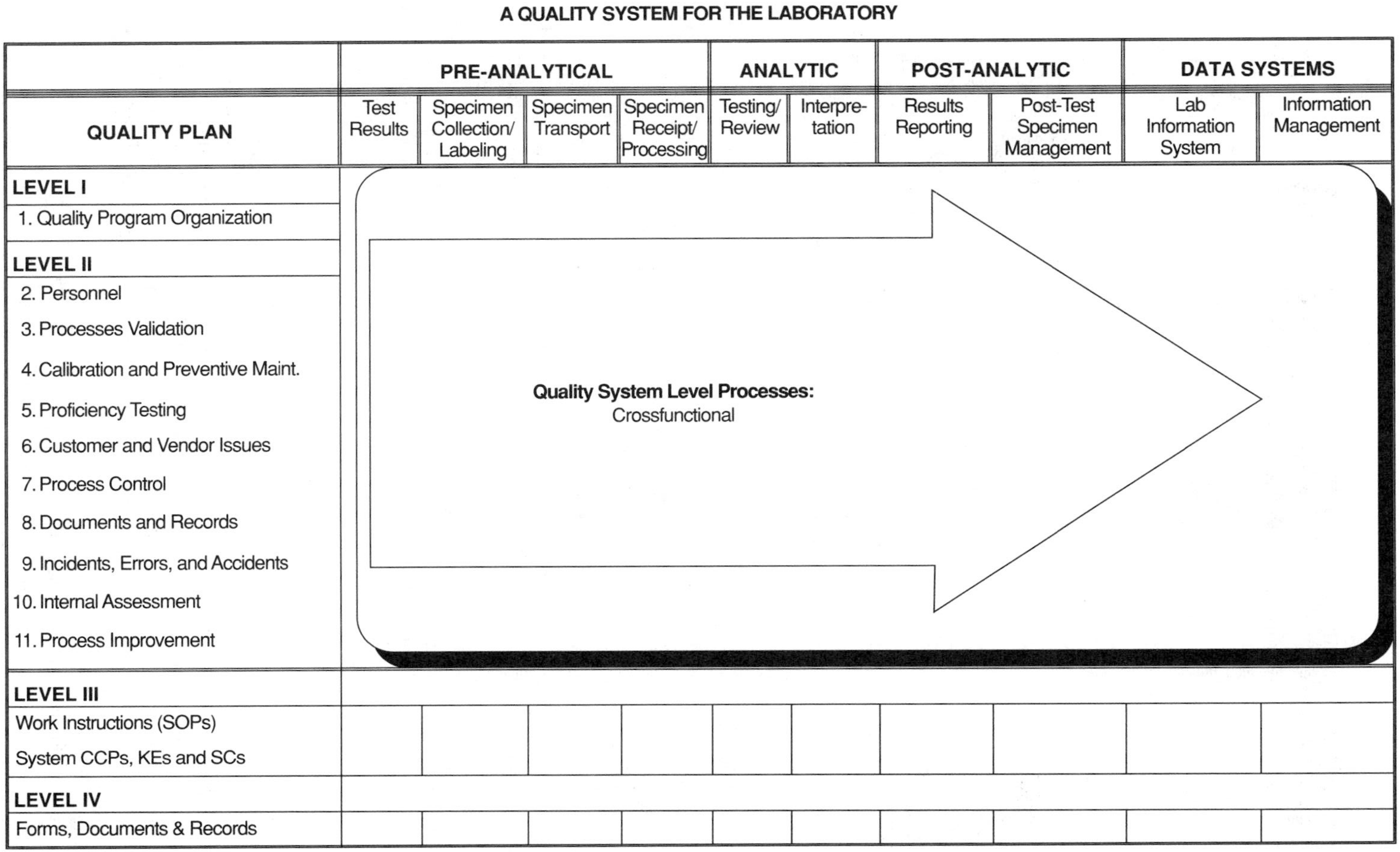

A QUALITY SYSTEM FOR THE LABORATORY

QUALITY PLAN	Test Results	PRE-ANALYTICAL			ANALYTIC		POST-ANALYTIC		DATA SYSTEMS	
		Specimen Collection/ Labeling	Specimen Transport	Specimen Receipt/ Processing	Testing/ Review	Interpre-tation	Results Reporting	Post-Test Specimen Management	Lab Information System	Information Management
LEVEL I										
1. Quality Program Organization										
LEVEL II										
2. Personnel										
3. Processes Validation										
4. Calibration and Preventive Maint.										
5. Proficiency Testing										
6. Customer and Vendor Issues										
7. Process Control										
8. Documents and Records										
9. Incidents, Errors, and Accidents										
10. Internal Assessment										
11. Process Improvement										
LEVEL III										
Work Instructions (SOPs)										
System CCPs, KEs and SCs										
LEVEL IV										
Forms, Documents & Records										

Quality System Level Processes: Crossfunctional

FIGURE 23–4. Laboratory quality procedures are applied to all personnel and processes in the path of work flow. (Used with permission from the Abbott Quality Institute)

Table 23-1
Policies and Procedures in the Quality Manual

Quality Policies	Quality Procedures
1. Quality program organization	Annual review of quality program
2. Personnel selection, training, education	Laboratory orientation Training Competence assessment Continuing education
3. Process validation	Validation protocol for new/revised methods/procedures
4. Calibration, preventive maintenance	Calibration program for laboratory equipment Maintenance program for laboratory equipment
5. Proficiency testing	Proficiency testing program
6. Customer and vendor issues	Qualifying laboratory suppliers Reviewing laboratory contracts Receipt and inspection of incoming materials
7. Process control	Building process controls into laboratory procedures Quality control of laboratory instruments, equipment, and reagents
8. Documents and records	Writing standard operating procedures Writing training guides Document change control program Record control program
9. Incidents, errors, accidents	Occurrence reporting
10. Internal assessment	Monitoring laboratory quality improvement indicators Preparing laboratory quality improvement reports
11. Process improvement	Corrective action Using quality improvement tools and techniques

mechanism for generating, reviewing, and storing records. Quality procedures describe how laboratory procedures are written and approved, reviewed and revised, managed and archived. Other quality procedures include instructions for how record reviews are conducted and documented and how records are stored and retrieved.

Occurrence Review

An occurrence is defined as anything that happens that was not the expected outcome. Occurrences are later classified as incidents, errors, or accidents. The quality policy states that the laboratory will have an active occurrence management process in place to detect, report, and categorize incidents, errors, and accidents and will coordinate its efforts with the organization's risk management function. The policy also states that the laboratory will use the findings from occurrence analysis and trending to identify opportunities for improvement. The quality procedures describe how occurrences are documented, reviewed, classified, and followed up.

Internal Assessment

The quality policy states that the laboratory has identified quality indicators for key functions and systematically monitors, documents, and reports its performance as scheduled and required by the organization. The quality procedures describe how data are captured, documented, reviewed, and followed up.

Process Improvement

The quality policy states that the laboratory will use the results of internal (self-conducted) and external (inspection and survey) assessments, the results of occurrence analysis, and customer feedback to improve its performance and will work within the organization's total quality management/continuous improvement process to plan and implement needed improvements. The quality procedure describes how the reports are written and how QI teams (if used) conduct and document their activities.

Reorganizing Technical Operating Procedures

Quality system level III documents are step-by-step work instructions for specific laboratory tasks, known commonly as SOPs. These operating system procedures are required to be in substantial compliance with a specified format; the National Committee for Clinical Laboratory Standards (NCCLS) guideline is recommended.[21] The latest version of the NCCLS guideline for writing laboratory procedures (GP2-A3) allows laboratories to design its policies and procedures within a quality system.[22]

The SOPs are to be available to personnel at the work stations to provide direction and reduce performance variations that can cause errors. Each operating system in the laboratory path of work flow has its own set of level III procedures as shown in Figure 23-5.

To ensure uniformity in writing procedures, training, test performance, and occurrence investigation, all laboratory technical procedures should be written in a specified format following the instructions given in a laboratory quality procedure for SOP development. This "SOP for SOPs" is used laboratory wide and allows personnel at any job level in any operating system to produce uniform documents. Other quality procedures provide instructions for review, revision, removal, and archiving of SOPs. There should be an approved document identification system that allows the laboratory to track the status and location of any level II or III procedure. This document control system ensures that the laboratory can track the development, use, revision, removal, and retrieval of any laboratory procedure and its related forms and is a valuable component of the laboratory's risk management activities.

An added benefit of uniform procedures is the ability to develop a uniform training system and its supporting documentation. The written procedure is used as a template to design a training document that combines learning objectives with required training activities and procedure performance. NCCLS Guideline GP21-A describes a training verification system for laboratory personnel.[23] The AABB has published a model for SOPs, training guides, and competence assessment tools that can be adapted for use in other parts of the laboratory.[24]

The Internal Assessment Program

This segment of the laboratory quality system involves identifying QI indicators for all key laboratory processes and procedures, monitoring to assess performance, reporting the findings to the laboratory's top management and the organization as required, and developing corrective action plans for areas needing improvement. This portion of the laboratory quality system is most similar to current laboratory QA programs. One significant difference is that quality system indicators are organized by path of work flow activity rather than within clinical discipline. This reorganization standardizes the indicators across clinical disciplines, thus allowing a "big picture" view of how laboratory processes are functioning.

Quality indicators have been derived by mapping the accreditation standards of the JCAHO and CAP and the regulatory requirements of CLIA '88 to the quality system table.[18] Table 23-2 is an example of the major system activities and QI indicators for one laboratory path of work flow system.

Presently, laboratories choose which QI indicators they will monitor and the monitoring frequency. Ideally, all QI indicators should be monitored all of the time. Realistically, however, laboratories need to choose indicators that represent the biggest impact on the quality of laboratory service in patient care. The organization's quality priorities, previously identified problem areas, and current quality initiatives may dictate what indicators laboratories monitor and when. However, a subset of QA indicators derived from the laboratory quality system should form the core of every laboratory's internal assessment program. Clark discusses this subject in detail and suggests that laboratories determine early in planning the quality assessment program how many quality indicators the laboratory can realistically monitor on an ongoing schedule and arrange the schedule depending on priority and characteristics of the given indicators. He suggests that laboratories can also begin modestly and build more comprehensively after time and practice.[13] Table 23-3 is a listing of minimum core quality indicators organized by operating system. Each clinical discipline can collect data appropriate for its activities that can be combined into the laboratory's periodic quality report.

Process Improvement

Laboratories receive input about the quality of their processes and any problem areas from three different means: internal assessment (QA monitoring), the occurrence reporting process (incidents, errors, accidents, customer feedback), and external assessment (labora-

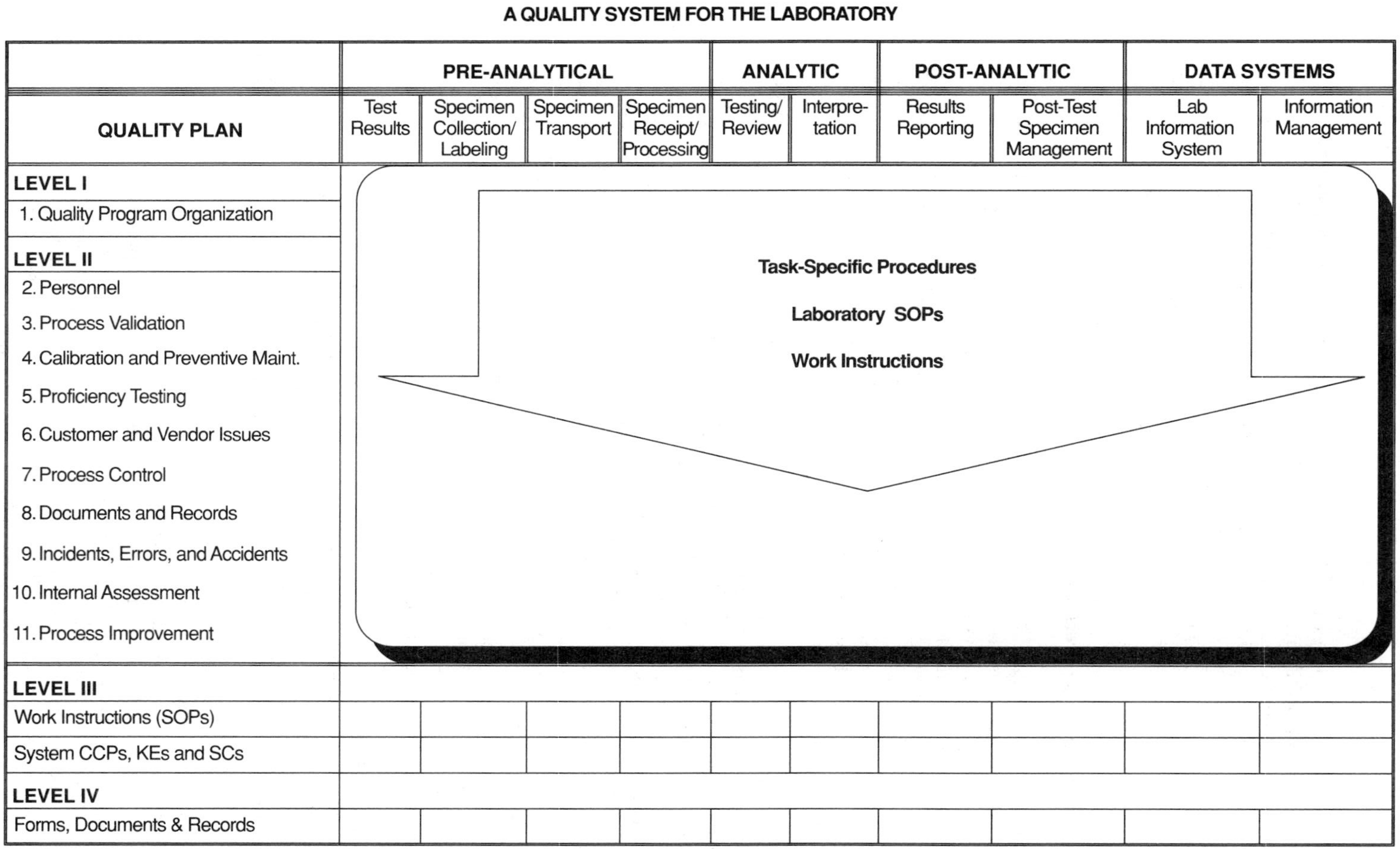

A QUALITY SYSTEM FOR THE LABORATORY

QUALITY PLAN	Test Results	PRE-ANALYTICAL			ANALYTIC		POST-ANALYTIC		DATA SYSTEMS	
		Specimen Collection/ Labeling	Specimen Transport	Specimen Receipt/ Processing	Testing/ Review	Interpre- tation	Results Reporting	Post-Test Specimen Management	Lab Information System	Information Management
LEVEL I										
1. Quality Program Organization										
LEVEL II										
2. Personnel										
3. Process Validation										
4. Calibration and Preventive Maint.										
5. Proficiency Testing										
6. Customer and Vendor Issues										
7. Process Control										
8. Documents and Records										
9. Incidents, Errors, and Accidents										
10. Internal Assessment										
11. Process Improvement										
LEVEL III										
Work Instructions (SOPs)										
System CCPs, KEs and SCs										
LEVEL IV										
Forms, Documents & Records										

Task-Specific Procedures

Laboratory SOPs

Work Instructions

FIGURE 23–5. Laboratory standard operating procedures are written for each laboratory operating system in the path of work flow. (Used with permission from the Abbott Quality Institute)

Table 23-2
System Quality Improvement Activities and Respective Indicators for Specimen Receipt

Laboratory Operating System: Specimen Receipt/Processing		
Critical Control Points	Key Elements	Systems Checks (Quality Improvement Indicators)
CCP-1 specimen receipt	1. Requirement for all specimens to be accompanied by an acceptable requisition 2. Mechanism to ensure inclusion of specimen date and time, when appropriate 3. System to document specimen receipt, time of receipt by laboratory and specimen condition	1. Number of specimens arriving without properly prepared requisitions 2. Number of specimens arriving without specimen date and time 3. Periodic audits that system captures laboratory receipt time and specimen condition
CCP-2 specimen acceptance/rejection	1. Criteria for the rejection of unacceptable specimens 2. Criteria for the handling of suboptimal material 3. Mechanism to document disposition of unacceptable specimens	1. Annual review of specimen rejection criteria 2. Annual review of suboptimal specimen handling criteria 3. Number and source of unacceptable specimens
CCP-3 specimen accessioning	1. System to accession appropriately all specimens received 2. System to ensure continued specimen identity, integrity, and security	1. Number of inappropriately accessioned specimens noted by testing laboratories 2. Periodic tracking of specimen through accession process

tory inspections). The findings from these activities are likely to reveal areas of less-than-acceptable laboratory performance and must be acted on to effect real process improvements. Laboratories have a number of methods and tools available to undertake improvement efforts.

Team Methods

Juran's Journey

Juran's journey is a generic approach. The diagnostic journey involves three steps of *understanding* the symptoms of the problem, *theorizing* the causes, and *testing* the theory. The remedial journey steps include *formulating* the remedy, *testing* the remedy, and *establishing* checks and controls to sustain the gain.[25]

Joiner Process

The Joiner process consists of five steps: (1) *Understand* the process in question; (2) *eliminate* errors in the process; (3) *simplify* the process by removing unnecessary steps; (4) *reduce* variation in the process by establishing statistical control; and (5) *plan* for continuous improvement through the use of the Shewhart cycle.[26]

FADE

Organizational Dynamics, Inc. has published their four-step FADE process: (1) *Focus* by prioritizing a number of opportunities for improvement to a single choice; (2) *analyze* by collecting data and determining the means for improvement; (3) *develop* by planning a remedy for improvement; and (4) *execute* by aligning organizational commitment, activating the plan, and monitoring the outcome.[27]

FOCUS-PDCA

The Hospital Corporation of America developed its FOCUS-PDCA process by adding to the original Shewhart cycle. The FOCUS phases include (1) *finding* a process to improve; (2) *organizing* a team that understands the subject process; (3) *clarifying* what is known about the process; (4) *understanding* the causes of process variation; and (5) *selecting* a plan for improvement. The Shewhart cycle, originally published for industry in 1932, is the basis for practically every modern assessment and improvement process, including the Levy–Jennings laboratory QC program described previously. The PDCA cycle includes (1) setting improved expectations (plan); (2) implementing improved process (do); (3) measuring performance (check); and (4) evaluating and learning (act).[28]

Table 23-3
Selected Quality Indicators for Laboratory Operating Systems

Laboratory Operating System	Sample Quality Indicator
Test requests	Number and source of inadequately prepared test requests
Specimen collection and labeling	Number and source of patients without proper identification at the time of specimen collection
Specimen transport	Number and source of specimens that exceeded maximum transportation times
Specimen receipt	Number and source of any unacceptable specimens
Testing and review	Number of test results and reasons for exceeding maximum allowable turnaround times
Interpretation	Number of disparities between frozen section and final diagnosis
	Number of disparities between histologic and cytologic findings
Results reporting	Number of times critical values were not communicated or documented
	Number of and reasons for reports exceeding established turnaround times
	Number and severity of reporting errors
Post-test specimen management	Number of times a retained specimen cannot be located on retrieval attempts
Laboratory information system	Number of times and reasons for unscheduled downtime
Information management	Performance in external database comparisons

Note: This list is not meant to be all-inclusive.

Analytical and Graphic Tools

Table 23-4 describes eight commonly used tools for problem identification, analysis, and evaluation.[29] These tools are helpful in statistical process control monitoring, problem solving, and follow-up evaluations to see that the corrective action implemented has indeed reduced or eliminated the problem.

BEYOND LABORATORY WALLS

The laboratory quality system described thus far is only part of a comprehensive approach to quality, measuring only how efficiently and effectively the laboratory performs the functions within the path of work flow. As personnel, facility, and equipment resources dwindle in a managed care environment, an organization's performance will also be measured on how it chooses only efficacious procedures and interventions, selects the appropriate procedures or interventions for a specific patient, and makes the procedure or intervention available

to the patient.[30] Appropriate use of laboratory testing by the medical staff is as important to laboratory testing as having an effective quality system. Working with the medical staff to order the right tests for the right reasons takes place outside the path of work flow and is primarily the responsibility of the pathologist laboratory director.

Laboratory Quality: The Right Information at the Right Place at the Right Time

How can the internal laboratory quality system and the external utilization issue be integrated to contribute positively to patient outcomes? The key is to pursue actively two important quality objectives: Do the right things, and do those things right.

Doing the Right Things

One of the most important problems faced in today's laboratories is the need to do the same or more work—of which a fair amount is unnecessary, redun-

Table 23-4
Eight Commonly Used Tools for Problem Solving

Tool	Description and Use of the Tool
Flowchart	A pictorial representation showing all steps of a process to document a program and examine how various steps are related
Cause and effect diagram	Represents the relationship between some effect and all the possible causes influencing it, sorted by people, materials, methods, and machinery; commonly called a "fishbone" diagram
Run chart	Points plotted on a graph in the order in which they become available to see whether or not the long range average of a process is changing
Control chart	A run chart with statistically determined upper and lower lines drawn on either side of a process average used to discover how much variability in a process is due to either random variation or unique events
Check sheet	A form on which to record the answer to the question, "How often is [this event] happening?"; used to gather data based on sample observations
Histogram	A vertical bar graph that shows the frequency with which certain events occur; used to discover and display the distribution of data
Pareto chart	A special form of vertical bar graph that displays the relative importance of all the problems to help determine which problems to solve in what order
Scatter diagram	A graph plotting the measurement values of one variable on the horizontal axis against the measurement values of the second variable on the vertical axis that displays the existence and strength of a relationship between the two variables

dant, and inappropriate[31]—with fewer resources. The key is to do mostly or only what is necessary for optimal patient care and positive patient outcome. The pathologists, as medical leadership in the laboratory, should support the building and maintenance of the quality system, but more importantly, they need to participate actively in medical staff development of practice guidelines and clinical pathways so that the "right things" are ordered from the laboratory. These measures are becoming more popular as a means to select prudently the correct laboratory testing protocol for a given patient condition.

PRACTICE GUIDELINES

Practice guidelines specify for physicians the proper indications for performing medical procedures and treatments and the proper management of specific clinical problems. They are a means of reducing inappropriate care, controlling geographic variations in practice patterns, and creating effective use of health-care resources.[32,33] Despite concerns about restrictive application of guidelines by third-party payers, malpractice courts, regulators, health administrators, utilization re-

viewers, and others, the current growth of interest in practice guidelines suggests that they will play an increasingly prominent role in the day-to-day practice of medicine. Practice guidelines are in the novice stage of development as physicians and heath-care practitioners debate the issues and practicalities of implementation. The laboratory is an important link in the development and execution of practice guidelines because testing is frequently performed to assess a patient's condition before choosing the next practice step. Many practice guidelines developed by interspecialty physician committees have been published. The future role of laboratory involvement in practice guidelines is likely to include ways to implement practice guidelines, particularly by maximizing their potential in laboratory computerization.[34]

CLINICAL PATHWAYS

The terms "practice guidelines" and "clinical pathways" are sometimes incorrectly used interchangeably. Clinical pathways, also called critical paths, are clinical management tools that organize, sequence, and time interdisciplinary processes to achieve patient outcomes

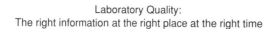

Laboratory Quality:
The right information at the right place at the right time

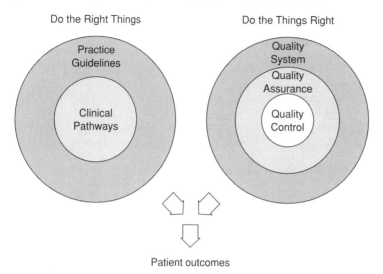

Patient outcomes

FIGURE 23-6. The right information at the right place at the right time is necessary for the laboratory to make a positive contribution to patients' outcomes. (Used with permission from the Abbot Quality Institute)

while appropriately managing cost.[35] A clinical pathway defines a set of expected interventions that is used to move a patient progressively through a defined clinical experience, for example, the course of inpatient care for a surgical procedure. When developing a clinical pathway, an interdisciplinary team of health-care personnel and medical staff members craft a schedule of the current interventions, such as tests, procedures, treatments, diet orders, and medications a patient experiences for a given diagnosis, treatment, or procedure. Patients are placed on the pathway, and the actual interventions, timing, and frequency are documented and compared with those expected. Patient outcomes are combined with information from the previous step to understand how the interventions relate to the outcomes. Opportunities usually exist for modifying the current pathway to improve the process of patient care and potentially reduce cost. The objective is to decrease the numbers and types of interventions and treatments that do not positively affect patient outcome and to increase the effectiveness of those remaining.

Laboratory participation is vital to answer questions regarding the appropriateness, frequency, and timing of laboratory tests and to assist in developing a cost-effective laboratory test ordering protocol for the clinical pathway's particular diagnosis, treatment, or procedure.

Doing Things Right

The laboratory quality system provides the means to ensure that the laboratory does things right. Policies and procedures are in place, people are trained and competent, processes are assessed for weaknesses, and corrective action is taken when problems are identified. Process controls and process improvement measures help the laboratory attain the higher quality goal of doing it right the first time as the laboratory further strives to make its outputs error free. Administrative laboratory leadership therefore needs to provide the operational resources to build and maintain the quality system and take timely, appropriate action on problem areas revealed in the assessment process, particularly when problems are interdepartmental.

Figure 23-6 demonstrates the relationship of doing the right things right. When laboratory testing is ordered from accepted guidelines and pathways and there is a structure to provide efficient and effective internal operations, laboratory pathologists and staff can build error-proof processes to deliver high-quality, reliable results expediently; improve the portion of patient care under their direct control; and make a positive contribution to the patient's outcome.

Dennis O'Leary, long time president of the JCAHO, wrote into the foreword of the 1993 JCAHO laboratory standards, "For the patient, doing the right things and doing them well begins with selecting the appropriate tests and concludes with accurate and helpful results that can be used to guide sound diagnostic and therapeutic determinations by the responsible practitioner."[36]

REFERENCES

1. Belk WP, Sunderman FW: A survey of the accuracy of chemical analysis in clinical laboratories. Am J Clin Pathol 17: 853–861, 1947
2. Levey S, Jennings ER: The use of control charts in the clinical laboratory. Am J Clin Pathol 20:1059–1066, 1950
3. Freier EF, Rausch VL: Quality control in clinical chemistry. Am J Med Technol 24:195–207, 1958
4. Westgard JO, Barry LB, Hunt MR, Groth T: A multi-rule Shewhart chart for quality control in clinical chemistry. Clin Chem 27:493–501, 1981
5. Diamond I: Quality assurance and/or quality control. Arch Pathol Lab Med 110:875–876, 1986
6. Maxwell KR, Stevenson TD: Quality assurance and peer review in the clinical laboratory. In Snyder JR, Senhauser DA (eds): Administration and Supervision in Laboratory Medicine, pp 369–372. Philadelphia, J.B. Lippincott 1989
7. Accreditation Manual for Hospitals, pp 125–129. Oakbrook Terrace, IL, The Joint Commission on Accreditation of Healthcare Organizations, 1988
8. Fromberg R (ed): Monitoring and Evaluation: Pathology and Medical Laboratory Services. Chicago, IL, Joint Commission on Accreditation of Healthcare Organizations, 1987
9. Donabedian A: Characteristics of clinical indicators. Qual Rev Bull November:330, 1989
10. Standards for Laboratory Accreditation. Skokie, IL, College of American Pathologists, 1988
11. Yost JA: Quality—a regulatory view. Clin Lab Man Rev 8: 43–48, 1994
12. Comprehensive Accreditation Manual for Pathology and Clinical Laboratory Services. Oakbrook Terrace, IL, Joint Commission on Accreditation of Healthcare Organizations, 1996
13. Clark GB: Systematic Quality Management. Chicago, IL, American Society of Clinical Pathologists, 1996
14. US Food and Drug Administration: Guideline on Quality Assurance in Blood Establishments. July 11, 1995
15. The Quality Program. Bethesda, MD, American Association of Blood Banks, 1994
16. Klein H: Standards for blood banks and transfusion services, 17th ed. Bethesda, MD, American Association of Blood Banks, 1996
17. Berte LM, Nevalainen DE: Quality management in the laboratory. Laboratory Medicine 27:232–235, 1996
18. Nevalainen DE, Berte LM: Pounding the drum for quality: A new beat. CAP Today 11(3):10–20, 1997
19. ISO 9000 Quality Management Compendium, 6th ed. Geneva, Switzerland, International Organization for Standardization, 1996
20. Berte LM, Nevalainen DE: Documentation pyramid for a quality system. Laboratory Medicine 27:375–377, 1996
21. Commission on Laboratory Accreditation. Inspection Checklists. Northfield, IL, College of American Pathologists, 1996
22. Clinical Laboratory Technical Procedure Manuals, 3rd ed. Approved Guideline Document NCCLS GP2-A3. Wayne, PA, National Committee for Clinical Laboratory Standards, 1996
23. Training Verification for Laboratory Personnel; Approved Guideline Document NCCLS GP21-A. Wayne, PA, National Committee for Clinical Laboratory Standards, 1995
24. Transfusion Service Manual of Standard Operating Procedures, Training Guides and Competence Assessment Tools. Bethesda, MD, American Association of Blood Banks, 1996
25. Juran JM: Juran on Leadership for Quality. New York, The Free Press, 1989
26. Scholtes PR: The Team Handbook: How to Use Teams to Improve Quality. Madison, WI, Joiner Associates, 1989
27. Quality Action Teams. Burlington, MA, Organizational Dynamics, 1991
28. Shewhart WA: Economic Quality Control of Manufactured Product. New York, Van Nostrand, 1931
29. Brassard M: The Memory Jogger Plus + : Featuring the Seven Management and Planning Tools. Methuen, MA, GOAL/QPC, 1989
30. Clark GB, Schyve PM, Lepoff RB, Reuss DT: Will management paradigms of the 1990s survive into the next century? Clin Lab Man Rev 8:426–433, 1994
31. Peterson SE, Rodin AE: Prudent laboratory usage, cost containment, and high quality medical care: Are they compatible? Hum Pathol 18:105–108, 1987
32. Woolf SH: Practice guidelines: A new reality in medicine. Arch Intern Med 150:1811–1817, 1990
33. Lohr KN: Guidelines for clinical practice: What they are and why they count. Journal of Law, Medicine & Ethics 23: 49–56, 1995
34. Friedberg RC, Moser SA, Jamieson PW, Margulies DM, Smith JA, McDonald JM: Automating clinical practice guidelines: A corporate-academic partnership. Clin Lab Man Rev 10:120–123, 1996
35. Clark KM, Steinbinder A, Anderson R: Implementing clinical pathways in a managed care environment. Nursing Economics 12:230–234, 1994
36. Accreditation Manual for Pathology and Clinical Laboratory Services. Oakbrook Terrace, IL, Joint Commission on Accreditation of Healthcare Organizations, 1993

24

Medicolegal Concerns in Laboratory Medicine

Daniel I. Labowitz

Laws govern the relationship among individuals and between an individual and society itself. The proper management of a clinical laboratory requires that the supervisor and the technologist be aware of the laws affecting that laboratory and its operation. This chapter is concerned with the controls on the operation of the laboratory and discusses the responsibilities and liabilities of the laboratory technologist within society. Specific coverage is given to possible areas of negligence liability, how to recognize problems before they give rise to a lawsuit, and how best to handle a problem that may have already occurred. As society becomes more involved with lawsuits for various reasons, the technologist may be called on as a witness in court. This chapter discusses how to respond to a subpoena; how to prepare for the court appearance, either as a fact witness or as an expert; and how best to present testimony. One of the most important areas of laboratory management, from a medical and from a legal viewpoint, is the keeping of proper and accurate records. The legal problems of record keeping will be developed to allow proper planning by the supervisor. The material presented in this chapter is intended as a guide and cannot be considered to be legal advice because of the constantly changing laws on this subject and the diversity among the many jurisdictions in the United States. If the administrator or supervisor has a specific problem, legal counsel should always be sought to ensure proper action.

LEGAL LIABILITY

A proper understanding of why a laboratory may become liable for the actions of its personnel requires a basic knowledge of the law involved. This area is known as tort law and involves three types of wrongful conduct: intentional acts, strict liability, and negligence. Intentional acts are those that a person intends to commit and intends to result in harm to someone else. Intentional acts, such as the willful falsification of laboratory records, would leave an individual, but not the laboratory, liable and are not covered here.

Also, areas covered by the doctrine of strict liability are not applicable to the clinical laboratory, because the doctrine applies to product liability and not to the performance of a service. This doctrine does become involved with the blood bank and is discussed in that section. A *tort* can be defined as a civil wrong or injury, not arising from a contract, and *negligent acts* are defined as the failure to do something that a reasonable man, guided by the considerations that ordinarily regulate human affairs, would do, or the doing of something that a reasonable and prudent man would not do. The standard against which all action must be measured is this mythical "reasonable man," or in the case of the laboratory, the "reasonable, trained technologist." Bad results sometimes occur when the proper procedures have been followed and the mythical standard person would have acted in the same manner. Not all bad results make the technologist or the laboratory liable.

To prove that a negligent act has been committed and to prove liability, the injured party, known as the plaintiff, must prove to the court each of the following elements:

The laboratory had a specific duty to which to conform. The injured party must prove that a duty of care existed and that the laboratory was obligated under that duty to the plaintiff to perform under a set standard of care. In the case of *Lauro v. Travelers Insurance Company*, 261 So. 2d 261 (1972), a pathologist, on examining a

411

frozen section cut on a freezing microtome, diagnosed the tissue sample as scirrhous carcinoma, and the surgeon performed a radical mastectomy. When a paraffin section was examined the following day, the diagnosis was changed to granular cell blastoma, not a malignancy. In reviewing a jury verdict for the pathologist, the court said a pathologist was not to be held to the highest degree of skill but to the ordinary level of skill used by other pathologists in good standing. The trial evidence supported the procedure followed by the defendant and found that he did not vary from the duty to conform to a specific standard of care. In addition, the court held that a freezing microtome, although not as advanced as a cryostat, was scientifically acceptable and that the standard of care did not require the use of a cryostat. If the laboratory procedure followed is acceptable to the scientific community, an element of negligence cannot be proven and no liability will result against the technologist or laboratory.

The accepted standard of care must be followed. Once the plaintiff establishes a standard of care, the fact that the laboratory fails to conform to that standard is the next element of proof. It must be shown that the laboratory did not follow the established, accepted scientific practice or performed it in an erroneous manner. As an example, in the *Lauro* case cited above, if the testimony had been such that a freezing microtome was an acceptable procedure but an ordinarily skilled pathologist would not have made the same diagnosis as the defendant, an element of proof of negligence would exist. In some instances, a plaintiff would be able to prove this element by establishing the standard of care and claiming that the result obtained by the laboratory was not possible if the procedure had been performed properly. The legal doctrine applicable here is called *res ipsa loquitur*, which means "the thing speaks for itself." Under this doctrine, the plaintiff alleges that because the procedures were under the total control of the laboratory and because the results obtained were in error, the procedures could not have been followed, and, therefore, the laboratory was negligent. This doctrine has been barred in many states from being raised in medical negligence cases. If this doctrine is unavailable, the plaintiff must prove by the use of evidence and expert testimony exactly what was done and why that failed to conform to the scientifically acceptable standard of care. This may be accomplished by

testimony of the technologist as to what was done and by an expert witness that the procedure was not acceptable in a similar scientific community. If the technologist performed according to accepted standards, there is no liability. Perhaps technology should be mentioned at this point, because an often-raised issue is that the laboratory failed to use the most up-to-date or state-of-the-art equipment to perform the procedures. In the legal setting, the idea that "newest is best" does not apply. Concern in a court of law is that a procedure is acceptable, accurate, and reliable, not necessarily the newest or fastest means of obtaining the same results. If either procedure is acceptable, reliable, and accurate, then either will be a valid standard of care for the court to apply in the case before it. The technologist has cause for concern if the procedure used is not accurate or reliable, because the question of liability will arise.

The failure to conform to the standard of care must be the direct cause of the injury. The legal concept called *proximate cause* means that a causal chain must exist from the breach of duty by the laboratory to the injury suffered by the plaintiff. Even if the technologist failed to follow an accepted procedure, no liability may exist if that error does not have a direct link to an injury to another person. This chain from laboratory to plaintiff may be broken by another party or by an intervening act of negligence. Courts have generally held that a treating physician who should have realized the laboratory results were in error, owing to his own standard of care, becomes such an intervening factor to break the causal chain. However, in determining proximate cause, the court is not limited as to time or number of intervening factors. In the case of *Renslow v. Mennonite Hospital*, 367 N.E. 2d 1250 (1978), the Supreme Court of Illinois allowed a child born in 1974 to sue a hospital for a negligent blood transfer in 1965. The negligence consisted of failing to notify the mother that she had been sensitized with Rh-positive blood, which caused a hemolytic disease process in the child. As remote as this may seem and with 9 years intervening between the negligent act and the injury, the court found proximate cause to exist. A federal court in Florida in *Givens v. Lederle*, 556 F 2d 1341 (1977), allowed a mother to recover from the manufacturer of an oral polio vaccine given to her child because the child contracted the disease and the mother had not been warned of that possibility. The opposite situation, where no proximate cause was held to exist, may be exemplified by the Georgia case of *Lankford v. Trust Co. Bank*, 234 S.E. 2d 179 (1977), which is not medically based but illustrates the point. The plaintiff had lost his charge card and notified the bank of the loss, yet the bank paid a hotel bill charged by a person who had obtained the card and then billed the plaintiff. Plaintiff's wife saw the hotel bill, and despite her husband's explanations, a divorce resulted in which she was awarded alimony and child support. The plaintiff sued the bank for the loss resulting from his divorce, but the court held the divorce was not in the relationship of having been proximately caused by the bank's negligent billing. This is a bit farfetched, perhaps, but it is an actual case that exemplifies how far some people will go to attempt to recover on a lawsuit. When the question of laboratory liability exists, proximate cause is always involved because of the frequency with which the laboratory deals indirectly with the patient and because the results of its procedures are interpreted by a physician.

The plaintiff must have damages. The term *damages* does not refer to the specific injuries suffered by a person, but rather to a probable amount of money to pay for the value of those physical injuries. Because no possibility exists to return the plaintiff to a physical or mental condition that existed prior to the wrong done, some measure of reparation must be found. Damages have two categories: special and general. The easier to determine are the special damages, which include such items as medical and hospital bills and related expenses. Little question exists as to these amounts because they have been billed to the plaintiff and are a known amount. General damages raise a different question, because they encompass the pain and suffering of the plaintiff, future loss of income, and future expenses necessitated by the physical or mental loss. Any injury to the plaintiff must be converted into a sum of money either for amounts due in the past or that may be due in the future. Any future amounts must be based on current injuries and not on possible future injuries that are speculated on the plaintiff. If no monetary damages can be proven—and this possibility has occurred—then even if the three other elements are proven, the laboratory will not be held liable.

When considering the possible liability of the clinical laboratory, the technologist must consider the elements of proof required to establish that liability before a court of law. An error by the technologist may not give rise to automatic liability, because of the many variables to be considered and proven by an injured party. The most important factor is that the procedures followed were accurate, reliable, and acceptable to the scientific community and that all ancillary functions were performed as a reasonable and prudent technologist would perform them. One additional factor in the question of laboratory liability is the legal doctrine of *respondeat superior*, which is concerned with the liability of the employer for acts of the employee. The employer, whether the laboratory director or the hospital (usually both), is generally held liable for negligent acts of the employee that are performed while the employee is performing the duties for which he was hired or is reasonably expected to perform. The technologist is not relieved of personal responsibility; rather, the supervisory chain to the employer will be made responsible in addition because a supervisor is responsible for the work of those under him. The Texas Court of Civil Appeal in *Wilson N. Jones Memorial Hospital v. Davis*, 553 S.W. 2d 180 (1977), held a hospital liable for the negligent acts of an employee on the basis that the employee had lied on his employment application as to his qualifications, and the hospital had failed to check out the history. The hospital could not claim the employee was performing outside of his training when they failed to confirm the extent of that training and assigned the tasks to be done by him. The manager, therefore, should be certain of the background and training of people employed in the laboratory, because he will be responsible for their actions. This doctrine provides sufficient basis for managers to consider the possible liabilities of their laboratory operations and act to prevent them.

Problem Areas

Direct exposure to the patient raises the possibility of a liability suit. Laboratory personnel involved in obtaining the specimen from the patient must be aware of the problems involved in patient contact and liability. An incident that in itself is not negligence, yet causes panic among most technologists is the breaking of a syringe needle during the collection of the specimen. Needles do break for various reasons, many of which do not result in the liability of the technologist; however, liability may result if the technologist fails to react properly. Preventing the broken part from traveling in the vein is the first concern. The second is obtaining assistance. Remaining calm and professional is the best method of avoiding liability. Another common problem in venipuncture is not being able to find a vein from which to draw the specimen. It is more difficult to do this with some people than with others, so failure is not negligence. What may cause the patient to bring a lawsuit is the "patient pincushion syndrome," in which the technologist, on failing to obtain a vein, continues to probe until one is obtained. The patient is outraged and injured because of apparent ineptitude. Again, reasoned thinking and seeking assistance would possibly avoid a lawsuit, whether negligence existed or not. In *Leiman v. Long Island Jewish Hillside Medical Center-South Shore Division*, 401 N.Y.S. 2d 562 (1978), the New York Court held that expert testimony was required to prove negligence when a patient claimed damage to a median nerve from numerous venipuncture attempts during which the patient suffered extreme pain. The Louisiana Court of Appeals in *Sugulas v. St. Paul Insurance Company*, 347 So. 2d 855 (1977), held that a large hematoma and false aneurysm caused by a punctured artery during an intravenous pyelogram was not due to the negligence of the physician. The court, relying on expert testimony, said that even the most skillful practitioner may have results such as this and that it is a risk of the procedure.

Although not thought of as relating to venipuncture, the problems associated with the fainting patient are easily prevented yet if not anticipated, may expose the laboratory to liability. The technologist should assume that all people are subject to fainting when the specimen is being drawn and should take precautions, including using a patient chair with arms or having the side rails up on a patient-transfer cart. The negligence is not in the fainting; it is in allowing the patient to fall and become injured when basic precautions have not been taken. The same can be said of any other patient reactions, which, by asking the patient or reviewing the chart, can be avoided. This brings us to the question of consent. Normally, this is not a problem for the laboratory, but it may become so with patient contact. The treating physician should have informed the patient that a specimen would be drawn and obtained consent prior to the request of the laboratory. The simple precautionary measure of reminding the patient of the physician's request and explaining what is going to occur should solve this problem. If, however, the patient objects to the sample being drawn, it is advisable to proceed no further before clarifying the issue with the treating physician. An annoyed patient is more likely to bring a lawsuit than one who is treated with kindness and concern.

The questions of blood samples drawn at the request of police officers should be considered. Under implied-consent laws enacted in each state, a person is deemed to have given consent to a blood-alcohol test by operating a motor vehicle on the highways of that state. A police officer, after arresting a person for driving while intoxicated or under the influence, may request a blood test to determine a blood-alcohol level. Some states allow a conscious person to refuse the test and suffer the loss of driving privileges. However, if the person consents or is unconscious, then the specimen may be drawn for analysis. The United States Supreme Court in the landmark case of *Schmerber v. California*, 384 U.S. 757 (1966), allowed a blood sample to be taken from a person who was conscious and protesting on the grounds that the sample was evidence that could cease to exist if not taken then and that therefore a search warrant was not necessary. The court did hold that removal of a blood sample was a search and seizure subject to the protection of the Fourth Amendment to the United States Constitution and would be valid if certain provisions were met. These provisions are that the blood must be drawn by medical personnel, standard medical procedures must be followed, and no physical force may be used if the person gives physical resistance.

Laboratory personnel, when requested to obtain a blood sample by a police officer, should be concerned with the last provision, because the first two are only good medical practice. If the person gives physical resistance, do not get involved. Let the police handle the matter, and then the laboratory will not face a possible liability suit. Local laws vary, and the laboratory should have a policy developed after consultation with an attorney.

Related to the topic of specimen collection are three other problem areas of which the laboratory manager should be aware. Specimens have been lost and will continue to be lost, often owing to no act of negligence on the part of the laboratory. The problem arises when the technologist attempts to cover up the loss and hopes that the specimen will be forgotten. In most situations, a new specimen can be obtained for analysis, and if done quickly, no harm will occur. If the specimen cannot be obtained again, as with a biopsy, then the submitting physician must be notified immediately on the discovery of the loss to plan a different approach to a diagnosis. A specimen that is wrongly identified is as good as lost until the error is corrected. When obtaining the specimen, personnel should ensure that it is correctly labeled and that it has been obtained from the correct patient. Use of good labeling procedures and labels that will remain on the container should avoid problems of erroneous identification and specimen loss. If the laboratory is using reusable glassware, proper sterilization techniques and documentation must be used to prevent contamination and subsequent error in test results. A well-thought-out application of common laboratory sense should avoid exposure to liability for problems in obtaining the specimen.

After the specimen has been brought to the laboratory, the next area of concern is the one where most supervisory attention is directed: the analysis performance, the main function of the clinical laboratory. Already mentioned but still of prime consideration is the problem of contamination of glassware, instruments, and the laboratory itself. Establishing and using procedures to ensure that all equipment and work areas remain free from contaminants are the best ways to avoid a liability claim. A poorly run laboratory or a sloppy work area will lead to legal problems for all personnel. All decontamination procedures and preventive measures must be documented in the laboratory as *standard operating procedure* and fully recorded on a regular basis. The use of knowns and blanks must be documented to establish that such precautions were taken and that the erroneous result claimed by the plaintiff was not caused by the laboratory. An area that may cause a laboratory to be made the defendant in a lawsuit is an erroneous analysis caused by failure of instrumentation used. The failure itself is usually not negligence unless caused by improper operation by the technologist, but failure to realize an error has occurred and failing to take corrective measures may be negligence.

If the failure was caused by a design error or if the manufacturer failed to notify the laboratory of a problem with a procedure, then the manufacturer, rather than the laboratory, is the negligent party. This principle may be exemplified by the case of *Kind v. Hycel, Inc.*, 372 N.E. 2d 385 (1977), in which the Illinois Court of Appeals upheld a verdict against the manufacturer of a blood-sugar test. The patient had suffered several fractured ribs and subsequently showed signs of fat embolism, for which he was treated with dextran. Another physician ordered a blood-sugar test about the time the dextran was discontinued, and the test results were 2,000 mg glucose. (A normal readying would be between 65 and 110 mg.) To counter this reading, the patient was given insulin, which brought the reading to 24 mg. The part that dextran played in the reading was realized too late to save the patient, who became comatose and eventually died. A lawsuit was brought against the physicians, the laboratory, the hospital, and the manufacturer. The jury held the manufacturer liable but not the others on the evidence that no instructions were made available as to the interference problem caused by recent doses of dextran with the blood-glucose test. The results were in error, but the error was not due to any negligence of the laboratory, which was absolved of any liability.

On discovery of an instrument failure, the technologist should document what occurred, determine whether any analysis results were released that were possibly in error, and determine why the instrument failed. If results have been given to a physician, he must be notified immediately of the error and given possible corrective measures, if any. If it is determined after examination of the malfunctioning instrument that the error was due to a manufacturing fault or a component failure, this should be documented by an independent source, not laboratory maintenance or the manufacturer. The independent evaluation should assist the laboratory in avoiding liability and possibly shifting it to where it may belong: with the reagent or equipment manufacturer. The instrument should *not* be used until a complete check has been made and it is again certified as performing properly.

With the increased use of electronic calculators and computers in the laboratory, and for personal use, mathematical errors have decreased. The ever-present decimal point will continue to float to places it does not belong, and each person's handwriting may be given to interpretation; therefore, the technologist must remain aware of the imperfection of numbers and the possibility of transposition. Double-checking figures, taking extra care in writing them down, and maintaining automatic printers to provide for a clear, readable numeral printout are the best means of avoiding liability for simple computation errors. The technologist should remember the requirement for test reliability discussed previously as it is re-emphasized now. If the technologist is scientifically satisfied that the method of analysis is reliable and accurate, then this method should be used. Reliability must be documented should it need to be proven to a court of law. When performing any test, document the method of analysis used and the accuracy of the equipment. This is best done by daily or weekly logs showing when blanks and knowns were run and the result obtained. If done on a regular basis, these logs are admissible as evidence of the reliability and accuracy of test procedures and equipment.

One legal doctrine that must be followed if any specimens are retained at the laboratory that are known to be evidence is called the *chain of custody*. This means that the evidence must be accounted for from the time it is obtained by the laboratory until it is delivered to the court or its agent. If these specimens are kept frequently, then a locked refrigerator and a limited-access policy should satisfy the requirements of the chain of custody. If the situation is unique, a locked container in the normal specimen refrigerator should suffice. The purpose of being able to account for the sample is to assure the court that the correct specimen was analyzed and to allow its identity to remain out of question. Whether dealing with an evidence sample or a normal specimen for analysis, the laboratory manager should establish standard procedures for the handling of all biologic materials brought into the laboratory to assure anyone as to exactly what chain of events occurs from acceptance of the sample, through analysis, to disposal or storage. A well-established procedure will aid in avoiding liability and providing for an efficiently run laboratory.

After the analysis has been performed, the next step is reporting the results, which also has problem areas to be aware of in the attempt to avoid liability. The case of *Jones v. French Drug Company*, decided by the Massachusetts Court of Appeals in 1977, exemplifies what can occur when documents are illegible or unclear in their meaning. The plaintiff was given a prescription for the circulatory drug Ethatab, and the pharmacist filled it with Estratab, a female hormone. The injuries suffered by the 51-year-old male plaintiff included memory lapse, enlarged and tender breasts, loss of hair and sex drive, and various personality changes. The court awarded the plaintiff $135,000 in damages.

Legibility and transposition of figures are the leading causes of laboratory liability in the reporting of results to the contributor. Caution should be taken to ensure that the proper patient's records receive the analysis results. The laboratory's responsibility here is not to maintain patient records, but to be certain that the correct patient name and number are on the reports that are sent out of the laboratory. This will avoid any question of laboratory negligence if the physician is notified, the patient's records are annotated, and the patient is injured as a result of the misrouting error. If an error is noted in a laboratory report, all copies must be corrected immediately and anyone who has been informed of the results told of the correction. It is for this reason that telephone notifications of initial results may cause problems: It is not known to whom results may have been reported. It is suggested that if telephone reports are made, a single person in the laboratory be authorized to do so and that this person should keep a log book listing who was notified and what information was given. This will allow corrections to be given rapidly to the proper person and control access to medical records, a topic that is covered later in this chapter. If written reports have left the laboratory and must be corrected, the proper method to do this is to cross out the erroneous data and write in the correct data and date the new entry. The use of erasures or correction fluid raises questions as to alteration of medical records, which in most cases reflect badly on the laboratory.

The final area of laboratory operation is the one in which the largest number of lawsuits have been brought, although it is not necessarily the area that is most open for liability: blood banking. As mentioned previously, the doctrine of strict liability is involved in blood-bank liability. This doctrine comes into play in some states that consider the provision of human blood for transfusions the sale of a product. When blood is considered a product, the "seller" or blood bank is held to be strictly liable on its applicability and fitness for the purpose for which it was "sold." If the blood causes an injury to the person who receives it under this doctrine, the liability of the blood bank is assumed, and the only remaining question is that of the amount of damages. The contraction of hepatitis is the major injury suffered, and because of the relative difficulty of screening blood completely to avoid this problem, the doctrine of strict liability can cause definite problems for the blood bank. Fortunately, many state legislatures have passed laws that hold the provision of blood for transfusions as a service, which is not subject to the doctrine of strict liability, because no warrants of merchantability go with a service as they do with a sale. This is supported by the case of *Warvel v. Michigan Community Blood Center*, 253 N.W. 2d (1977), in which evidence was presented that laboratory tests for hepatitis in blood were only 45% to 60% effective. State law was such that if no valid test existed to test the fitness of whole blood, the furnishing of blood became a service and not the sale of a product. It must be noted that without statutory protection, most courts would hold that the furnishing of blood was a sale and subject to strict liability. This was laid down by the Florida Court of Appeals in *Lewis v. Associated Medical Institutions, Inc.*, 345 So. 2d 852 (1977), where the transfusions were made before the status of transfusions as a service became effective, and hepatitis was discovered afterward. The court held that the discovery of the disease was made after the law changed and that therefore it would not allow the lawsuit based on strict liability. This situation does not absolve a laboratory from bad results in the furnishing of blood for a transfusion, because a plaintiff can still allege negligence in the testing of the blood, obtaining data as to the donor's health, or storage procedures in the blood bank. Following proper scientific and laboratory procedures should avoid a holding of liability in this area. The procedure of requesting an emergency supply of blood that has not been cross-matched to a patient may open up the blood bank for liability. If the request is truly for an emergency and plasma will not suffice until a cross-match has been done, then as a general rule no court will hold a laboratory liable in providing whole blood. There have been occasions, however, when the request was not an emergency, but the result of the surgeon or nurse having neglected to request a cross-match in sufficient time or having requested an insufficient supply be set aside. The best procedure to cut down on the number of "emergency" requests for other than true emergencies is to require the requester to sign a form that states that the need is truly an emergency and that the laboratory is absolved of all responsibility in providing blood that has not been cross-matched to the patient. While this may not remove the laboratory's responsibility to the patient, it should reduce the number of "emergency" requests and also would be looked on favorably by a court of law should a question arise.

THE SUBPOENA

If a laboratory becomes a defendant in a negligence case or a technologist has become so knowledgeable in the field that his testimony is needed at another trial, the first knowledge of involvement may be the delivery of a legal document known as a *subpoena*. This document may be in any one of numerous forms and says that the person subpoenaed must appear at a specified place and time to provide testimony on a case of which he has knowledge. A subpoena may be one or both of two types: One calls for personal appearance for giving testimony, and the other asks for records to be delivered to the proper party. Most frequently both are called for when the clinical laboratory is involved. A request for records is called a *subpoena duces tecum*.

On receipt of any subpoena, the first thing you should do is notify the laboratory director and the attorney for the laboratory. Time is normally short on the response to a subpoena, and your attorney will need all the time he can get to prepare for the court proceedings or to make arrangements if you cannot be available at the time and place requested. A subpoena is a *command* by a court, which must not be taken lightly. Failure to obey the command of the court (or of a grand jury, which also has subpoena power) could put a person in contempt of that court. In contempt-of-court proceedings, a judge may order the person he holds in contempt to go to jail or to pay a fine. Although this rarely occurs in civil cases, there is no excuse for not answering a subpoena or making arrangements with all parties to appear at a different time or date, if necessary. On rare occasions, a subpoena may arrive with little or no time left before the court appearance date. At such times, contact with your attorney is essential in avoiding the anger of the court and being allowed to present your case fully. When the laboratory is a party to a lawsuit, you should be told in advance what is happening and when you will be required to testify. You should still check with your attorney on receipt of the subpoena to confirm what it is for and what you are to do. If the subpoena is for a criminal action—for example, a case in which a blood sample has been analyzed for blood-alcohol content—you should contact the person who sent the subpoena and your attorney. In criminal cases, your attorney will have little to do with the prosecutor who will be presenting the case. Above all, when you receive a subpoena, do not file it away to be looked into tomorrow or in the future, but look into it immediately. Receipt of a subpoena is not cause for panic, but it does require actions not within most technologists'

normal operational habits and should be a cause for concern. Remember to call your attorney, check to see whether you have the materials requested, refer to your notes or log books on the case, and approach the subject of testimony with scientific caution, and no problems need arise.

THE TECHNOLOGIST AS WITNESS

If a person makes an observation of an occurrence that later becomes important in a civil or criminal court proceeding, that person is subject to being called as a witness to testify in court. Any person who has knowledge of an event that was gained by that person's own observations is called an *ordinary* or *fact witness*. Such a witness is limited in the testimony given to the facts so obtained and may not venture an opinion except in limited circumstances. An ordinary witness may give an opinion only if formed on his own experience. A common example is observation of intoxication, if the witness has a basis on which to make that conclusion. A technologist would be a factual witness if he were to testify regarding facts obtained from observations made in the laboratory. These could include the procedure for a specific analysis in question or the operating procedure for handling reports in the laboratory. There is no limit to what such a witness may testify to as long as the information sought is relevant to the issue at the trial; however, such a witness may not give an opinion as to whether the analysis was done within acceptable scientific guidelines or whether the procedure was proper. This opinion calls for the testimony of an *expert witness*. A technologist may be very well qualified as an expert in the laboratory, but until that person qualifies as an expert before the court, an opinion on the science or procedure involved may not be given. Why do courts require expert testimony? When the knowledge involved is outside the common understanding of the finder of fact, whether the jury or the judge, an expert witness is necessary to establish the fact or knowledge. The field of medicine and laboratory science is outside such a common understanding and requires that an expert form an opinion and testify as to that opinion, which may not be based on personal knowledge gained by the witness. An expert witness is allowed to form an opinion based on "reasonable scientific certainty" from facts or information provided from another source. The case of *Todd v. Eitel Hospital*, 237 N.W. 2d 357 (1977), illustrates the need for expert testimony in medical cases. The court stated "where the conduct of the physician involves complexities of pathological diagnosis, we are not persuaded that nonmedically trained jurors are competent to pass judgment." Expert witnesses were held to be necessary to establish the standard of care; the jury could not establish one without such assistance. Expert testimony is the only time such testimony is admissible as evidence in a court of law. This opinion is just that, an opinion, but it must not act as a determination of guilt or liability, because that is the sole prerogative of the finder of fact. An expert opinion may be based on a hypothetical question formulated for the jury that requires an opinion on facts alleged in that sometimes lengthy question. Facts in evidence must be used in such a question, and the opinion must be based on those facts to be allowed. A question such as this is most often used by the opposition attorney in an attempt to get the expert to change the opinion based on a slight change of fact in his client's favor. That is an acceptable form of examination of an expert in most jurisdictions and should be expected by an expert witness.

An expert witness is distinguished from a fact witness in that the expert is arranged for beforehand by the attorney and is paid for his expertise and time, rather than receiving a set witness fee for the court appearance. The amount the expert charges will vary among communities and among experts of various levels of experience and knowledge. Determination of a fee based on an hourly rate should include research time, preparation time, and time in court and should be discussed with the attorney at the time the expert is hired. The expert is being paid for his time and experience, and the testimony is not being bought. Another point that was made by the United States Court of Appeals for New York in 1977 should be kept in mind. That court approved a local rule barring the payment of contingent fees to expert witnesses. A contingent fee is one of which the expert would receive a percentage of the award if the party on behalf of whom he testified won the lawsuit. If that party (usually the plaintiff) did not win, the expert would receive nothing. Such arrangements are common in negligence suits where the plaintiff shares his proceeds with the attorney, because this allows a person to obtain a lawyer without having to produce a fee and allows less wealthy people to bring a lawsuit. However, when the expert witness has an economic interest in the outcome of the lawsuit, he loses all scientific objectivity, becomes an advocate for that party, and ceases to be a proper scientific expert. Whether barred by a jurisdiction or not, do not become an expert on a contingency-fee basis.

Trial Preparation

Whether a technologist is testifying as a fact or as an expert witness, he should always prepare for that testimony even if he has testified numerous times before. The first step is to meet with the attorney who will be presenting the testimony, not just to establish fees for the expert but to discuss the entire case and learn the part the witness plays in the attorney's presentation. Determine from the attorney who is to obtain records and other necessary materials on which an expert opinion will be formed. Also determine whether the attorney is aware of whatever laboratory records you have that are pertinent to the case. If unaware of what the attorney is attempting to prove with expert testimony, do not be afraid to ask and to provide advice to help him understand the science and laboratory procedures involved. Treat the relationship as a partnership in the effort to present the complete case to the jury, and you will have the proper attitude. On obtaining all of the records and reports, review them thoroughly, even if you are already familiar with them. Your testimony will be based on the record, and you must be as knowledgeable of it as possible to do your best as a witness. If further records are needed, obtain them so that you will have a complete understanding of the case and all of the possible issues involved.

In your review of the case materials, it is not advisable to discuss them with other technologists unless they have been involved in the case also. The testimony you will give must be your own, and if others have been consulted, explain why and what assistance they provided. This may appear to the jury as a means of reassuring yourself as to your testimony or even worse, an attempt to develop a better story for the witness stand. These problems may easily be avoided by limiting your consultations with nonwitnesses and other experts who have not been retained to testify. While reviewing the case material, also review the literature on whatever science or procedure is involved to become as current as possible on the subject. The opposing attorney and his experts will do this, and your preparedness will enable you both to advise the attorney with whom you are working and to respond to questions on cross-examination. This review is especially helpful if some new technique has been reported, and you are able to discuss it and its effect, if any, on the case at hand. Frequently, these issues are raised in an attempt to have the jury believe that the procedures followed were not the latest or best. This is usually a smokescreen, and your preparation with the latest literature will avoid problems at trial.

After your initial review of all of the records and all the literature with the attorney, another review is necessary. The first review is to assist you; the second is to allow you to educate the attorney about what he must know to question you properly and to rebut any claims by the opposition's attorney. Your assistance is invaluable in the attorney's preparation of a cross-examination if any experts testify for the opposition. It is at this stage that you can best provide that assistance.

Because you must qualify as an expert at the trial to be allowed to give an opinion on a scientific matter, frequently your training and experience will be an issue as a fact witness if the question of proper procedure and analysis is raised. For this reason, you should thoroughly review your *curriculum vitae* and be prepared to explain what your duties were at various places of employment or your course of study at school or continuing education courses. The opposition attorney may waive your qualifications, and your attorney may still put them in to show the jury that you are an expert and impress them with your education and experience. Thorough familiarity with your *curriculum vitae* and what went into it is an important asset for your attorney in either establishing your expertise or as a good basis for your knowledge of how a specific analysis is performed. The important factor is not to allow the opposing attorney to raise any doubt about your qualifications or your knowledge. If your attorney approves, and never without his approval, bring all the records to the trial. This will speed the procedure if you have to refer to them and will allow for a more professional presentation. However, in some jurisdictions, the records may not be available to the opposition, and they should not be brought to court without the attorney's approval.

As an expert witness, the technologist has agreed to review the records, advise the attorney, and present testimony in court if the need should arise. Not all lawsuits result in a court trial. Rather, the minority do; therefore, many attorneys will rely on an expert's advice on the validity of the allegations about the scientific aspects of the case. As an expert, if you believe that the case as portrayed by the attorney is not coordinated with the science and is therefore difficult to prove, let him know. If the science is either nonprovable or not supportable from a legal viewpoint, then the attorney should attempt to obtain an out-of-court settlement of the case, rather than expending time, effort, and the hopes of his clients on a weak or nonexistent case. The sooner he knows this, the easier it is for him to work out an amicable settlement.

The only other obligation of the expert witness is to fulfill the agreement and appear to give testimony when called. The New Jersey Superior Court in the 1976 case of *Lapham v. Dingawall* allowed a plaintiff to recover a monetary award from an expert witness who failed to come to the trial and thereby caused the plaintiff to receive a lower award at trial. If you fulfill your agreements, there is no cause for worry. After a thorough preparation and evaluation of the records, the next step is to present the testimony if the case goes to trial.

Presentation of Testimony

As a general rule, witnesses are not allowed in the courtroom while other witnesses are testifying, so you will not be able to observe the trial at which you are to testify before your turn arrives. If you are unfamiliar with the courtroom, ask you attorney if you can see it when a case is not being presented so you can sit in the witness chair and become acquainted with your surroundings. If possible, observe another trial in which your attorney is involved to see how questioning is done. This pretestimonial familiarization will help to alleviate any fear or nervousness you may have as a new witness. A witness who is comfortable in the courtroom will present a more relaxed and professional appearance and will be able to concentrate on the questions and answers. The technologist should strive to present a professional appearance, both in clothing and demeanor. Do not try to act out a preconceived notion of what a professional looks like. Rather, be yourself, and seek your attorney's advice if you have any problems. Casual clothes are usually not the proper attire for testifying, but neither is a three-piece suit if you are not accustomed to it. Self-assuredness will allow you to keep mentally alert, the most important item to remember when testifying.

After you are called and take the witness chair, listen carefully to each question before you respond. Do not anticipate questions and thereby shut your mind down while you give a prepared answer. Wait until the question has been completed before answering. Especially on cross-examination, attorneys may hesitate in their questioning, hoping to get a response to an incomplete question, and thereby throw the witness off the issue concerned and cause him to worry about what was done or said. If you wait and listen until the question is complete, you should have no problem. Always speak clearly, distinctly, and with understandable language. Avoid the use of technical slang or abbreviations, which confuse a jury composed of people with no knowledge of the laboratory. Explain terms you must use in your testimony. If the witness were to think of himself as a teacher and the jury as students, the relationship would be easier to comprehend. Do not talk down to the jury, and do not present an attitude of preacher expressing dogma, but explain the science in clear, understandable language, and they will appreciate it. Do not go far afield in responding to a question, and do not volunteer information not requested. Confine your response to the question asked, unless you do not believe that you will be able to do so. If you must explain further, tell the judge that this is the case, and seek permission before you begin your response. In addition, if you do not understand a question, say so, and ask for clarification. Do not appear argumentative or uncooperative but professional and unwilling to respond incorrectly to a question you believe cannot be answered properly. If you cannot answer a question because you do not know the answer, do not be afraid to say "I don't know," which is a valid and acceptable response. This does not weaken your expertise or knowledge in the eyes of the jury; it makes you appear human and more believable. You should keep in mind why the testimony is being given, keep alert mentally and physically, and remain professional in all ways to be an effective witness in a court of law.

RECORDS

One area of the clinical laboratory that causes many questions to be asked is that of records keeping and the quality of those records. The legal aspects of medical records are briefly discussed here to enable the technologist to understand better the responsibilities and liability involved.

The prime consideration is the ethical, and in many jurisdictions legal, requirement of confidentiality of medical records. Either by agreement between the patient and the laboratory or by stature, confidentiality requires that these records not be released to anyone outside the laboratory, except the treating physicians, without the patient's consent. There are a few exceptions, such as in response to a valid subpoena, to the next of kin of a deceased patient, or to an attorney of the patient. The exceptions vary between jurisdictions and should be listed in any statutory "privacy act." A laboratory would be liable if it released information to a person without authority. This liability could be just to the patient, if injury could be proven, or in the form of a fine to the state if the statute so provides. Therefore, access to laboratory medical records should be limited and controlled to avoid the unauthorized release of analysis results and other patient information. As stated previously in this chapter, a telephone request is the easiest way for information to be released to a person without authority to be obtaining it. A single authorized person responsible for telephone requests who also maintains a log book for such requests will eliminate much of the problem. In addition, a system of callbacks, whereby the laboratory will call back the requester at a valid number, rather than giving the data at the requester's call, will cut down appreciably on the frequency of giving data to unauthorized people. Do not let so-called freedom of information statutes confuse you as to which takes precedence, privacy or freedom of information. In the federal act (US Code Svc. Tit.§552), as in many state acts, medical records held by a governmental agency are exempt from disclosure and protected by the privacy act (US Code Svc. Tit.§552a). When in doubt as to whether or not records should be released, consult your laboratory administrator and legal counsel before releasing them.

A phrase heard frequently regarding records is that they are privileged and therefore not releasable. This term relates solely to the use of medical and laboratory information at a trial and is a legal principle that would ban its admissibility as evidence if the information fell within this classification. To be so classified, records must have the following four elements:

A patient–physician relationship must exist. This relationship includes the entire health-care team, not just the treating physician. The laboratory qualifies here whether the analysis has been run at the request of the treating physician or another outside medical source. A test requested by a police officer does not qualify for the privilege because no physician–patient relationship exists.

The information was obtained during treatment.

The information was necessary for diagnosis and treatment. Even if a patient–physician relationship existed, if the information given by the patient was irrelevant to the treatment, no privilege exists. The laboratory would rarely come under this exception, because by the very nature of its function, any information it receives and any reports generated are necessary for diagnosis and treatment of a patient. The only exception would be if the laboratory accepted specimens from nonmedical sources for analysis for reasons not needed or outside a physician–patient relationship.

The interest of society in keeping information privileged outweighs any instant interest to release it. The privilege has been established by statute passed by the legislature, speaking for society, saying that the need to have a free flow of information from patient to physician for treatment is superior to anyone else's interest in knowing what was said. All privileges (except for attorney–client) are established by statute and may be eliminated by statute. It should be noted that no physician–patient privilege is recognized in the federal courts. The privilege belongs to the patient, and the patient must waive the privilege and allow the other party to release the information at trial. The patient cannot use the privilege to the disadvantage of others, such as by claiming certain medical status and barring the release of his medical information. In such cases where the laboratory is the subject of a lawsuit brought by the patient, the privilege is waived by the patient's actions and the information may be testified to in court. Therefore, if you are called to testify regarding patient information and the patient or his representative is not bringing the lawsuit, check to determine whether a waiver has been made; if not, you are barred from testifying about that information. This is another reason you should consult an attorney on receipt of a subpoena for laboratory records.

Finally, who owns medical records? This question has given some cause for concern when patients want to transfer records to another physician, or a laboratory consolidates with another and the question of patient files is considered. The general legal proposition is that a practitioner owns the files he has maintained regarding his patients. He may do as he would with them, keeping within any restraints set up by statute and ethical considerations. The major consideration is that on request of a patient, he must transfer these records to another physician with the promise that the patient is not in debt to that physician. Also, hospital records are the property of the hospital when an agreement between a physician and the hospital modifies that general rule. Laboratory records, therefore, generally are the property of the laboratory or of the hospital if the laboratory is owned by the hospital. Frequently, clinical laboratories are operated on a contractual basis for one or more hospitals; the contract should cover who has control over laboratory records. It must be noted that the ownership of the records is to be contrasted with the ever-expanding right of the patient to have access to the information in his records.

The legal aspects of laboratory administration and practice are not intended to confuse the practitioner nor difficult to understand if common sense is applied to a problem and an objective viewpoint is taken. The practices and procedures of the laboratory, whether scientific or record keeping, are subject to the ultimate review of a panel of jurors who are not scientists and must be instructed by experts about the correct procedure. This perspective should help any laboratory ad-

ministrator or supervisor avoid liability, both personally and on behalf of the laboratory.

ANNOTATED BIBLIOGRAPHY

The Citation. Chicago, American Medical Association (semi-monthly)

This text is a compilation with synopses of court decisions affecting medical practice with an interpretation of the meaning of the decisions. It is an excellent means for updating the legal aspects of laboratory medicine with actual court decisions.

Feegel J: Legal Aspects of Laboratory Medicine. Boston, Little, Brown, 1973

Of interest to the pathologist; in particular, coverage of the areas of records keeping, consent, blood banking, and testimony in court would be of general interest to the laboratory supervisor. A general guidebook for the pathologist in those areas of practice concerned with legal matters.

Hoyt E: Medicolegal Aspects of Hospital Records. Berwyn, H: Physician's Record, 1977

This book is intended for people who deal in the maintenance and release of hospital records. It is an excellent text for laboratory supervisors who are more and more becoming concerned with record-keeping problems. Specific coverage of the legal system, evidence, trial practice, and the right to privacy should be helpful to the laboratory technologist.

Laboratory Regulation Manual. Germantown, Aspen Publications

Updated on a regular basis, this is an extensive resource for the laboratory director or supervisor. Although its prime interest is in government regulatory rules, three chapters of its three volumes deal with business conduct, laboratory employees, and malpractice.

Warren DG: Problems in Hospital Law, 3rd ed. Germantown, Aspen Publications, 1978

This book is a general treatise on the legal problems applicable to all aspects of hospital operation. Although it is not concerned with laboratory operation, Chapter 7, "Principles of Liability," and Chapter 9, "Collection and Disclosure of Patient Information," should be of interest to the laboratory supervisor.

25

Managing Point-of-Care Testing

Susan E. Perkins

Clinical laboratories have witnessed and initiated many changes in clinical testing as a result of technologic advances. One important change witnessed in recent years has been the evolution of point-of-care testing (POCT)—from satellite laboratories, to hybrid laboratories, to bedside testing. Point-of-care technology is changing the future of laboratory operations, providing an opportunity to restructure responsibilities and improve the way in which clinical customers are served. During this change, the clinical laboratory was often left out of the process of developing the protocols for testing performed on nursing units and clinics within their own institutions. A laboratory managed POCT program can remedy this situation.

POINT-OF-CARE TESTING DEFINED

Clinical Laboratory Improvement Amendments of 1988 (CLIA '88) defined laboratory testing as analytical testing on specimens withdrawn from patients, such as blood, urine, stool, ascites, fluid, sputum, vaginal secretions, and biopsy samples. The law also classified tests by their complexity level. POCT is any laboratory testing, at any complexity level, performed and documented within the hospital at sites that are located outside the central laboratory. POCT is also called new patient testing, ancillary testing, decentralized testing, and bedside testing. The central criterion is that it does require permanent, dedicated space.

Initiating a POCT program requires some careful interdepartmental planning to ensure that laboratory standards of excellence relative to quality, regulatory compliance, billing, medical record documentation, and safety are achieved. To initiate a management program that provides consulting or resource services from the laboratory not only requires cooperation, but also administrative support. CLIA regulations have created a window of opportunity for the laboratory administration to offer the same services to their own institution

that many laboratorians have offered through the creation of consulting services for physician office laboratories (POLs).

Issues in Point-of-Care Testing

Regulations

To meet federally mandated standards, accrediting agencies with Health Care Financing Administration deemed status, must follow CLIA '88 requirements when evaluating POCT. The three principal organizations currently inspecting and accrediting POCT programs include the Joint Commission on Accreditation of Healthcare Organizations, the College of American Pathologists, and the Commission on Office Laboratory Accreditation.[1]

For these deemed status agencies, a POCT program must address direction and supervision of the program, procedures performed, proficiency testing, quality assurance, quality control, procedure manuals, specimen handling, results reporting, reagents, calibration and standards, instrument selection and maintenance, personnel requirements training and competence, and safety (Box 25-1).[1]

Driving Incentives

Rapid turnaround time (TAT) between test ordering and receipt of results is perhaps the strongest driving force behind POCT. While rapid TAT is beneficial for emergency situations, critical care areas, and surgical areas, the POCT trend is also fueled by changes in laboratory technology, laboratory use, and a changing health-care environment sensitive to costs associated with length of stay. In addition, quicker results have been linked to customer satisfaction.[13] Reports in the literature generally note that costs increase for testing done by POCT technology when compared with costs for centralized testing.[3,13] However, few studies balance costs associ-

423

Box 25·1

Waived Testing Accreditation Agency Regulations

CLIA '88

Adhere to good laboratory practice and follow manufacturer's recommendations

JCAHO

Responsible individuals are identified
Documentation of training and periodic verification of competency
Written procedures manuals
QC performed according to manufacturer's recommendations (two levels of control each day of use for glucose meters)
Correlation of QC records, instrument problems, and individual patient results

CAP (SELECTED ITEMS)

Testing performed under the supervision of the laboratory
Responsible individuals are identified
Documented training and periodic verification of competency
Written procedures (NCCLS format)
QC performed, documented, and evaluated each day of patient testing (two levels of control each day of testing)
Documentation of glucose meter performance
Linearity checked initially and semiannually
CAP PT Surveys
Policies for positive identification of patient specimen and results report
Policies for safe handling and disposal of patient specimens and infectious waste

JCAHO, Joint Commission on the Accreditation of Healthcare Organizations; QC, quality control; CAP, College of American Pathologists; PT, proficiency testing.

ated with a POCT program and outcomes in terms of overall care improvement.[11,13] A reduction is length of stay with no increase in cost has been shown in some reports when POCT was implemented,[3,13] but decreased therapeutic TAT through decentralization and improved specimen transit were observed in another report.[9]

Analytes for Point-of-Care Testing

Box 25-2 lists a variety of analytes reported in the literature for POCT.[2–6,8,13] This list is generally based on tests for which a 5-minute or less TAT is necessary for effi-

cient care. Obviously, the technology to accomplish such a TAT using a microspecimen is key to analytes on the list.[3]

Technology for Point-of-Care Testing

Advances in technology that have enabled POCT include whole blood biosensors, ion-selective electrodes, substrate-specific electrodes, and amperometric and impedance electrodes.[4,6] Miniaturization, accompanied by microchemistry, microelectronics, and microprocessing, has enhanced the mobility of testing technology in the form of transportable and hand-held units.[4] Selection of technology to support POCT is a critical consideration.[6,8,12] Box 25-3 lists criteria for "ideal" POCT analyzers.

Data Management in Point-of-Care Testing

A particular challenge to realizing the full benefit of POCT is data management. Laessig and Ehrmeyer note that, "once data are acquired through POCT devices, they must be assimilated into a logical framework, communicated to practitioners, routed to patient charts, and filed in patient records to be available for a variety of purposes."[7] Different settings (eg, critical care unit versus a general hospital unit) require different data management strategies.[4,7]

Box 25·2

Analytes for Point-of-Care Testing

Cooximetry
Occult blood
Glucose
Hematocrit or hemoglobin
Ionized calcium
Ionized magnesium
Partial thromboplastin time
pCO_2
pH
pO_2
Potassium
Pregnancy test
Prothrombin time
Sodium
Urine chemistry
Urine-specific gravity (refractometer)

Adapted from Jacobs E: Total quality management and point-of-care testing. MLO Suppl 25(95):4, 1993

Criteria for the "Ideal" Point-of-Care Testing Analyzer

- Requires minimal or no routine of preventive maintenance
- Is a self-contained system
- Interfaces with laboratory information system
- Has a flexible test menu
- Requires minimal training and troubleshooting
- Uses whole blood
- Is precise and accurate
- Has bar code capability for test packs, controls, and specimens
- Has controlling software that allows:
    Automatic one- and two-point calibration
    System lockouts for:
        Quality control not run or failed
        Patient identification not entered
        Validated user identification not entered

Source: Jacobs E: Total quality management and point-of-care testing. MLO Suppl 25(95):6, 1993

Critical Path Analysis

No doubt some of the rationale behind rapid TAT is based on care plans for specific medical conditions. Enhancement of POCT can be accomplished by mapping performance and quality paths for patient-focused care.[4,5]

Point-of-Care Testing Personnel

Often POCT is performed by nonlaboratory personnel who may be cross-trained for this function.[2,8,13] Consequently, the laboratory staff must be prepared to provide training, technical assistance, and supervisory oversight of this ancillary testing.[6] Key to training is assurance with documentation of operator proficiency.[12,13]

Box 25-4 summarizes these and other issues in the form of guidelines for POCT.[5] The goals of the patient care area need to be considered by a multidisciplinary group of stakeholders. Strategies to operate and manage the POCT operation need to be identified. Insight into quality POCT from a laboratory medicine perspective also needs to be addressed.[5]

IMPLEMENTING POINT-OF-CARE TESTING

The development of an effective and efficient POCT program can be fraught with many hurdles.[2,3,10,12] The evolution can be facilitated by understanding a model of POCT and steps to make the transition. The remainder of this chapter provides just that. First, however, it is appropriate to recognize that the managing laboratorian assigned as the point-of-care coordinator is actually an "in-house" technical consultant:

- We *are* accountable by regulatory agencies.
- *We* have the expertise.
- *We enhance our position* within the institution providing this as customer service.
- We should *embrace and manage* the POCT concept.

Quality Testing Outside the Laboratory

The Point-of-Care Testing Policy Committee

This committee can be formed in many ways. To have authority and regard from the rest of the institution, it needs full support from senior administration. The chair should be held by a laboratory pathologist. This position and membership can be held for a specific term or be permanent. The members of the committee should be representatives from the areas affected by POCT. Some suggestions are as follows:

Laboratory administration
Pathology
Point-of-care coordinator
Medical nursing
Surgical nursing
Ambulatory nursing
Purchasing or distribution
Hospital information services
Risk management
Medical staff
Diabetes education and training

Other personnel could be involved on an ad hoc basis as subjects are brought up concerning their area of care (ie, specific testing in a neonatal intensive care unit). Smaller task force groups may be formed to deal with specific issues, such as the variety of urinalysis strips and tablets used throughout the institution. The goals of the committee are listed in Box 25-5.

With the authority and support of the laboratory and POCT policy committee, the person can be chosen from the laboratory staff to be the coordinator of the

Box 25•4

Guidelines for Designing Hybrid Laboratories for Patient-Focused Care

MATCHING THE GOALS OF THE PATIENT-FOCUSED CARE CENTER

1. Customize for specific patient-focused care centers that may have different objectives requiring different levels of testing and speeds of response.
2. Involve physicians and care teams early and continuously.
3. Integrate planning carefully with the care paths (care plans) used by the physician specialists to decrease the time spent on the bottleneck route.
4. Decentralize testing, and select test clusters to meet the clinical needs of the specialty and to improve the performance of quality paths.
5. Provide direct patient care according to the needs of the patients as determined by a consensus of the care team.
6. Create ways to reduce non–value-added activities (e.g., scheduling, traveling, waiting, delaying, documenting, repeating) in testing cycles, work flow, and laboratory functions.

ADDRESSING MANAGEMENT AND OPERATIONS STRATEGY

1. Obtain a strong leadership commitment and use consensus to reach agreement on the use of laboratory resources for the entire hospital.
2. Set up task-oriented groups strong in process and maintenance abilities to formulate a decision process for space, testing levels, and work flow.
3. Integrate services within the patient-focused care center, between care centers, and among all hospital laboratories.

4. Evaluate the relative performance of quality paths periodically to improve continuously the quality of patient care.
5. Use multiskilled clinical and technical partners to help perform laboratory work and cross-cover patient care functions.
6. Distribute computer resources to each care suite (room), integrate fully with all laboratories, and incorporate new informatics (eg, pen-based notepads) and bedside technologies (eg, hand-held instruments).

IMPLEMENTING LABORATORY MEDICINE PRINCIPLES

1. Ensure proximity to patients, accessibility to caregivers (eg, adequate hours of operation), and efficient communication (eg, results broadcast and message pagers).
2. Use hand-held, portable, transportable instruments and mobile instrument workstations because these significantly improve performance levels and patient outcomes.
3. Fulfill accreditation requirements viewed from the institution as a whole.
4. Meet federal regulations, state laws, and licensing requirements, but seek waivers or exceptions when these are inappropriate or outdated.
5. Include transport systems located appropriately for use with nonroutine tests and when tests cannot be performed at the point of care.
6. Develop contingency plans defining two levels of testing for routine tests, additional backup levels for critical tests, and redundant pathways for disasters.

Source: Kost GJ, Lathrop JP: Designing diagnostic testing for patient-focused care. MLO Suppl 25(95):21, 1993

Box 25•5

Goals of a Point-of-Care Testing Committee

1. To ensure compliance with the requirements of the regulatory agencies (eg, Clinical Laboratory Improvement Act [CLIA] of 1988, FDA) and the accreditation agencies (eg, JCAHO, CAP) in regard to point-of-care testing
2. To serve as an advisory resource on point-of-care testing issues, such as test and instrument choices, documentation, cost versus benefit analysis, affect on length of stay, test implementation and QC and QA issues; all of these issues need to be considered whether the laboratory testing is performed under the CLIA license held by the main laboratory or under a separate license.
3. To assist in the evaluation of new technology, instrumentation, and supplies and make recommendation as appropriate
4. To determine the policies governing point-of-care testing within the institution

The point-of-care testing policy committee can assume the responsibility for ensuring the review and approval of all new requests to add instruments or testing outside the main clinical laboratories. The committee can also provide advice, assist in development of correspondence to ensure regulatory compliance, and develop protocols to meet accrediting agency regulations. The committee can advise senior management, as appropriate, of changes in regulations that affect hospital point-of-care testing.

---

program. It is also useful to have a nursing liaison for fostering a cooperative environment.

The Discovery Tour

To begin a quality management program of the testing performed at bedside, one first must determine what is being performed within the institution. Contact should be made with each nursing unit and clinic to assess the testing being performed. A survey form could be used for a large institution, but nothing can supplant the personal contact with the area supervisor and visual observation of the circumstances of the testing in each area. The implementation of new testing, such as glucose meters or other point-of-care analyzers, creates the perfect opportunity to bring other testing up to the same compliance required for new testing.

Because some of this testing has been used on nursing units for many years, the addition of a quality assurance plan can be met with some skepticism or resistance if not handled with tact and support from the laboratory. One example of this testing is macroscopic urinalysis with various dipsticks. A review of the products in use through the stockroom can give an idea of what check. Checking products in use for outdates is suggested. An ad hoc committee formed with the authority of the POCT policy committee should propose the policy for determining areas in which this testing is appropriate and should be continued and those in which use of dipsticks or tablets should be limited.

Many patient care areas use hydrometers or refractometers, which could be replaced with a dipstick that includes a specific gravity. The point-of-care coordinator then assumes review and management of the testing. Another test done on most nursing units is for occult blood. The use of the performance monitors with each test and proper documentation of the test result and the performance monitors in the nursing record should be encouraged. Proper storage of test cards is an issue to which users need to pay attention. Clinics that send test cards home with patients must use postal service–approved envelopes for mailing the cards back to the hospital. Occult blood in gastric samples needs a separate testing card product. Education and support to ensure this testing is performed with site-neutral quality are responsibilities of the point-of-care coordinator.

Creating a list of testing sites and the testing being performed is necessary before any management can be initiated (Table 25-1). From this point, any additional testing will be initiated with the full support and the same quality of the central laboratory.

Building Bridges

Just as a POL consultant would establish a good working relationship with the personnel in the physician's office and keep the physician apprised of areas needing improvement and areas doing a good job, it is good practice to build good working relationships with the appropriate nursing personnel and keep the quality assurance (QA) committees and POCT policy committee

Table 25-1
Point-of-Care (POC) Testing Location Overview

Hospital Location	Tests Performed	Technical Consultant
Renal—chronic	ACT, whole blood glucose	POC coordinator
Renal—acute	ACT, whole blood glucose	POC coordinator
East 1	Whole blood glucose Hemoccult, gastroccult	POC coordinator
East 2	Whole blood glucose Hemoccult, gastroccult	POC coordinator
Neighborhood health clinic	Whole blood glucose Occult blood, Hct Pregnancy test, rapid *Streptococcus* KOH wet preps Urinalysis dipstick	POC coordinator
Endoscopy	Whole blood glucose Hemoccult, gastroccult Clo test	POC coordinator
East 3	Whole blood glucose Hemoccult, gastroccult	POC coordinator
Chapin 3	Whole blood glucose Hemoccult, gastroccult	POC coordinator
East-4 ADOL	Whole blood glucose Hemoccult, gastroccult	POC coordinator
Medical daystay	Whole blood glucose	POC coordinator
East 5	Whole blood glucose Hemoccult, gastroccult	POC coordinator
East 6—PACU	Whole blood glucose	POC coordinator
Daystay main 5	i-STAT	POC coordinator
Cardiac catherization laboratory	ACT	POC coordinator

ACT, activated clotting time; Hct, hematocrit; KOH, potassium hydroxide.

apprised of compliance with QA guidelines. The mechanism for withdrawing testing privileges from any areas comes from the authority of the POCT policy committee and the point-of-care coordinator. Building quality into the program can be achieved only with a team effort by all personnel involved. A description of the point-of-care coordinator role is provided in Box 25-6.

The point-of-care coordinator must act as the resource person and technical consultant to ensure that each area supervisor understands the responsibilities involved in the decision to perform any laboratory testing in his area (Box 25-7).

Vendor Policy

Vendors who market laboratory test kits, reagents, and instruments should be required to present any new products to the laboratory for review, evaluation, and recommendation before purchase or acquisition of each item. If vendors make their initial contact with medical, nursing, or ancillary staff (eg, respiratory therapy, pharmacy), the vendor should be referred to the laboratory as well.

Equipment

Equipment used for POCT should be limited to that approved by the point-of-care policy committee.

Cessation of Testing/New Testing

Cessation of testing should occur when QA guidelines are not properly followed. Standard policies for implementing new tests should be followed when the point-

Box 25•6

Point-of-Care (POC) Coordinator Responsibilities

1. Determine quality assurance (QA)/quality control protocols for each test that will effectively monitor all aspects of the testing that is also based on accrediting agency requirements.

2. Prepare procedures in NCCLS format for all tests done in each area. A manual clearly labeled *Point-of-Care Testing* (POCT) should be placed in each area performing laboratory testing. These procedures should contain information on patient identification, patient preparation, specimen collection and handling, and test policy and procedures for each test. This manual is also a good place to maintain the list of certified or trained personnel for any testing. QA reports from the point-of-care coordinator, communication, any memos or newsletters pertaining to POCT, quality control, and maintenance documentation should also be available in this manual. Perform and document an annual review of all procedures, and ensure distribution and knowledge of any revisions.

3. Documentation that all personnel who are performing any laboratory testing have received adequate training is a primary requirement for quality performance of any laboratory procedure. The routes taken to ensure this are varied and may need to be adapted to fit the circumstances unique to each institution. Vendors are often willing to provide training. This is a good cost-saving measure as long as the laboratory POC coordinator is able to determine the content, consistency of sessions, and post-training quizzes or observation for competency. In other situations, the POC coordinator can conduct the training sessions by training all the testing personnel or by training the trainers using nursing educators.

4. Determination of appropriate proficiency testing programs may be based on the complexity of the testing. Some programs may be tested with in-house specimens, and others may be appropriate for commercial programs. The programs available for physician office laboratories may be just what is needed for a clinic that performs primarily waived testing and some tests classified as moderately complex.

5. Ensure that specimen collection techniques for both capillary and venous collection are adequate to provide a quality specimen.

6. Familiarity with accrediting agency regulations to ensure appropriate compliance in each area.

   Any testing of a moderate complexity requires a more diligent training program and more diligent oversight by the laboratory to ensure the quality of the program. Usually, testing on this level is for electrolytes or blood gases. With new technology, the manufacturer takes a greater responsibility for building in quality control functions into the instrumentation usage by nonlaboratorians. These are tests for which turnaround time has always has been an issue with the main laboratory. In the current environment in which length of stay is a vital concern to the efficiency of the institution, if this testing can be performed with a quality program managed by the laboratory, everyone can benefit.

7. Arrange for all employees who could be performing testing to be tested for color discrimination at their new employee physical.

8. Billing for laboratory testing should also be site neutral. Therefore, the laboratory should also put in place mechanisms to ensure that all tests are appropriately billed. Summations of this billing by each area should be available for the POC coordinator to review and prepare a periodic report. The laboratory should be familiar with proper billing codes.

Box 25•7

Area Supervisor Responsibilities

1. Maintain documentation of all personnel certified to perform point-of-care testing (POCT), with operator identification codes when appropriate; a copy should be sent to the point-of-care coordinator.
2. Ensure participation and documentation of quality control, remedial action for out-of-range controls, maintenance and proficiency testing programs by all certified personnel.
3. Ensure proper documentation of patient test results.
4. Review and retain area performance reports, and prepare corrective action plans when there is a failure to meet quality assurance guidelines.
5. Ensure all testing done is accompanied by documentation of the person who performed the test.

---

of-care policy committee approves requests for new tests. The protocol is the same as it would be to implement any new testing or instrument in the main laboratory. Determination of accuracy and precision, comparisons with primary laboratory instrumentation, and establishment of test ranges and linearity are examples of the appropriate laboratory section to ensure this is done. The hospital area that will be performing the testing should be informed of the results of these studies. Box 25-8 is an example of a request and resolution.

Continuous quality improvement projects enhance POCT programs. The cooperative efforts of these programs lend themselves to assessment for the ways and means to improve the procedures on an ongoing basis.

SUMMARY

Managing POCT is a complex and fairly new area for many laboratory managers. This chapter begins by citing some of the key issues in this new arena. Box 25-9 summarizes the operations management issues in POCT. The latter portion of the chapter provides some

---

Box 25•8

Point-of-Care Testing: Case Example

The labor and delivery floor of our institution wanted to perform a scalp pH. This testing had been problematical for some time. Specimens were collected and sent to a stat laboratory on another floor for testing. Specimens were often inadequate, either quantity not sufficient or already clotted. One of the physicians had seen an instrument in use in another institution that only required 15 µL of whole blood and was easy to operate. The physician submitted a proposal to the point-of-care testing policy committee, and the request was considered. The pathologist on the committee discussed the request with the manager of the chemistry service in the laboratory for input and suggestions. With the submission of that report, the vote to obtain analyzers for trial passed. All studies were conducted by the laboratory. The test results were adequate, and although the cost per test was higher than that done by the main laboratory, all felt that the quality of the service for the patient would be improved. The analyzer was purchased by the labor and delivery department. House staff and residents were required to attend training sessions on performing patient tests and quality control tests. The surgical technicians from the labor and delivery surgical area were trained to perform quality control procedures. The point-of-care coordinator prepared a written procedure in standard laboratory format and quality control log sheets. Copies of the procedure were distributed during the training sessions. During the first month of use, the electronic quality control cartridge that cost $300 was accidentally thrown away, and testing was stopped until a new one was purchased and available for use. The area nursing supervisor informed the point-of-care coordinator when the cartridge was lost. A special container well labeled with instructions to be sure to replace quality control cartridge has prevented any further problems. The point-of-care coordinator reviews the quality control log sheets weekly.

insight using examples of one institution's experience developing a POCT program.

REFERENCES

1. Carlson DA: Point of care testing: Regulation and accreditation. Clin Lab Sci 9:298–302, 1996
2. Harris CH, Letz C, Gibson C: A path-free inauguration of point-of-care testing. MLO 27(6):41–43, 1995
3. Jacobs E: Total quality management and point-of-care testing. MLO Suppl 25(95):2–6, 1993
4. Kost GJ: The hybrid laboratory: Shifting the focus to the point of care. MLO Suppl 24(95):17–28, 1992
5. Kost GJ, Lathrop JP: Designing diagnostic testing for patient-focused care. MLO Suppl 25(95):16–26, 1993
6. Kerec AS: Implementing point-of-care testing. Clin Lab Sci 6:225–227, 1993
7. Laessing RH, Ehrmeyer SS: Data management of POCT: The vision. MLO Suppl 27(95):2–6, 1995
8. Lyneh SP: Point-of-care testing in pediatric hospitals. MLO 27(11):36–41, 1995
9. Mohammad AA, Summers H, Burchfield JE, et al: STAT turnaround time: satellite and point-of-care testing. Lab Med 27:684–688, 1996
10. Pelchach L: Focus on the patient: The rewarding, challenging and sometimes frustrating world of patients focused care. Lab Med 26:512–518, 1995
11. Rabbitts DG: Point-of-care testing: Needs and cost-benefit analysis. Clin Lab Sci 6:228–230, 1993
12. Roby PV, Kenny MA, Garen D: The laboratory outside the laboratory: Our role in point-of-care testing. Clin Lab Sci 6:222–224, 1993
13. Yablonsky T: Point-of-care testing: The evolving role of the medical technologist. Lab Med 25:777–780, 1994

Box 25•9

Essential Factors to Address in Point-of-Care Operations Management

Instrumentation
- Mobility, maintenance, and backup
- Point-of-care operator protocols
- "Fast QC" pattern recognition

Education
- Resources and documentation
- Clinician certification courses
- Annual renewal plan

Patient results
- Verification and reporting
- Communication and computerization
- Notification of critical results

Critical path analysis
- Transport systems
- Response times
- Emergency preparedness

Source: Kost GJ: The hybrid laboratory: Shifting the focus to the point of care. MLO Suppl 24(95):26, 1992

26

Marketing Clinical Laboratory Services

Carolyn C. Hart • Sharon S. Gutterman

Until the 1980s, the word "marketing" was not used to describe business-building activities in health care. Many hospitals had a public relations department whose job was to disseminate information about special events and procedures in the hospital, but marketing as a strategic planning tool was virtually unknown. In fact, to many health-care professionals, the word *marketing* was synonymous with *advertising* and, therefore, considered unethical. Codes of ethical conduct, established by professional associations, prevented professionals from engaging in any active solicitation of new patients. To hospital boards, the thought of marketing smacked of crass commercialism. Attitudes changed as decision makers began to understand the meaning of marketing, the changes in health-care economics, and the potential benefits to the hospital.

In recent years, competition in delivering health-care services has increased sharply. Providers of medical services now see themselves as serious business people and recognize the need to use the same tools that other businesses use. Hospitals are looking for profit centers, and laboratory services present a revenue-producing opportunity. Administrators understand that marketing activities are necessary to provide people with satisfying goods and services.

It is clear that managed care and capitation are affecting the volume of laboratory tests ordered. For some hospital laboratories, declining volume and declining reimbursement have led to excess personnel and equipment capacity.[6] While one solution may be to downsize the work force, a baseline of testing and staffing is required to keep the laboratory functioning to meet patient and physician services. An alternate solution is to increase the number of outpatient tests performed by developing an outreach program or negotiating laboratory services for managed care contracts.[6] Doing either of these requires marketing.

The basic constructs that define marketing are quite compatible with the goal of offering excellent service to consumers. In fact, chances are that you already perform marketing activities but never think about them as such. Posting signs to help outpatients find the laboratory, extending hours of service to accommodate patients and physicians, and telephoning results are outcomes of marketing planning.

DEFINING THE MARKETING CONCEPT

"Professional services marketing consists of organized activities and programs designed to retain present clients and to attract new clients by sensing, serving, and satisfying needs through delivery of appropriate services, on a paid basis, in a manner consistent with credible professional goals and norms."[5] The marketing concept can be summarized in three patient-oriented words: *sensing, serving,* and *satisfying*. Marketing plans begin with sensing what needs in the marketplace are not currently being met.

Sensing market needs can be achieved by using sophisticated market research methods or more informally by listening to people's questions and requests. The business that is attuned to what its audience needs and wants has a greater chance of succeeding in a competitive environment. Data are gathered, processed, and interpreted to improve managerial decision making.

Serving refers to developing and implementing the marketing program. Decisions concerning personnel tasks and which laboratory service to promote must be addressed.

Satisfying involves ensuring that purchasers of the laboratory service have their expectations met. A satisfied customer is the goal.

Marketing, then, focuses the health-care provider's attention to the needs and desires of the potential buyer as the starting point for planning. The range of activities that brings the buyer and seller together for their mutual benefit is the marketing function.

433

An organization must try to identify and satisfy the needs of customers, clients, or patients by coordinating a set of activities that concurrently allows the organization to achieve its own goals. When the business learns what will satisfy customers and creates products and services accordingly, then the business must continually monitor the environment to adapt its services to changing desires and preferences.

It should be clear by now that marketing refers to much more than the words *selling* or *advertising*. There is a strong research component necessary to identify customer needs, competitors' offerings, and environmental trends. In general, more research and program development have been done on how to market *goods*. As the dollars spent by Americans continue to increase—for health care, entertainment, repair services, airlines, and so forth—there is an accompanying need to learn whether the approach to marketing *services* parallels the approach to marketing *products*. In other words, is services marketing different?

According to Leonard L. Berry,[2]

> A good is an object, a device, a thing; a service is a deed, a performance, an effort. When a good is purchased, something tangible is acquired, something than can be seen, touched, perhaps smelled or worn or placed on a mantel. When a service is purchased, there is generally nothing tangible to show for it. . . Services are consumed but not possessed.

Berry continues by discussing how service delivery is perceived as an intrinsic part of the "product." For example, clinical laboratories have an ongoing internal process to control the quality of the results; the patient, however, may evaluate the quality of the laboratory on the basis of the pleasantness and skill of the phlebotomist. Physicians may evaluate the laboratory on the basis of the turnaround time. Clearly, the performance is part of the laboratory "product."

The communication component of marketing is composed of the techniques a business uses to tell potential buyers what it has for them. Human beings constantly scan their environment looking for reliable ways to satisfy needs. Promotional communication methods attempt to inform and persuade customers to choose their company's products and services. Market research methods can reveal buyers' television show preferences, magazines they read, radio programs they listen to, and newspapers they buy.

MARKET RESEARCH

Market research methods provide vital information to assist in making marketing decisions. Research and information storage systems provide feedback to the organization. Strategic planning is influenced by the opinions expressed by members of the target market. Consider the hospital laboratory, for example, that wants to market routine chemistry tests and blood counts to physician offices. The market research indicates that the physicians are very satisfied with the commercial service. The hospital laboratory cannot compete with the price the physicians are getting from the commercial laboratory. To compete on strictly business terms, the hospital laboratory would have to provide the physicians equivalent service at a lower price or additional needed services for the same price. The decision not to enter the market when the chance for success is borderline can result from market research.

Although marketing managers rely on gathering systematic, objective data, intuition also plays a role. Marketing managers may make decisions because "it feels right." Experience and personal judgment are valuable inputs. Scientific research and intuition meld in reaching a decision.

A number of research techniques and resources are available: conducting surveys, documenting direct questions and observations, reviewing records, and using sources of stored data. Survey methods include questioning people by mail, in person, and by telephone. The market researcher carefully designs a research problem based on what he or she wants to determine, designates the population to be reached, and recommends the methods to be used. In a mail survey, questionnaires are sent to representatives of the target market, who are encouraged to complete and return the survey instrument. For telephone surveys, respondents answer questions posed by the telephone interviewer, and their answers are recorded. Personal surveys conducted face-to-face are highly favored but may be difficult to obtain because people's schedules and lifestyles are so varied. A variation of the personal survey is the focus group interview, which consists of approximately 10 people who share characteristics of the market one wants to reach. The group is given an incentive to meet with a trained moderator and answer questions and express opinions about the product or service undergoing scrutiny.

Observation methods include quietly observing what is occurring in the setting by recording information from an unobtrusive spot. If the presence of an observer might bias behavior, then devices such as cameras, recorders, counting machines, and other mechanical equipment may be used.

Sources of stored data include reviewing records in the hospital, studying census tract information, and identifying other public records resources in the community. In addition, companies sell data about people and their buying habits. Many insights can be gleaned from going to these sources, and the cost of "secondary data" is far less than if one had to generate information by developing one's own study.

Selecting the appropriate market research instrument and developing, administering, and evaluating it require skills that are usually not part of the medical technology curriculum. Laboratories in larger hospitals may get help from the professional marketing staff employed by the hospital. When that support is not available, contracting for consulting services with an independent marketing firm can be worthwhile.

MARKET SEGMENTATION

Marketing experts recognize that the general population is composed of groups of people, or "segments," who share certain similar characteristics. These segments become target markets for business planning. Groups of people can be segmented according to any variable that has relevance for the business.

Health-care services are segmented into specialty areas. People sharing certain medical needs go to physicians who specialize in a particular area. A laboratory may segment the market in the same way, for example, by developing a set of services to meet the special needs of a group of patients, such as oncology patients.

A laboratory may also segment the market on the basis of the requirement for specialized skills or equipment. Virology and toxicology are examples of this kind of segmentation.

Two major ways of segmenting a market are by grouping people according to demographic variables and by psychographic variables.

Demographic Variables

Consumer buying habits correlate with characteristics such as age, sex, address, income, occupation, and education. Women over the age of 40 having regular mammograms are an example of market segmentation using demographic data.

Psychographic Variables

Behavioral and psychological attributes can be used to segment the population. Psychographic variables include identifying lifestyle activities, interests, values, attitudes, and opinions. Although it would be difficult for a hospital laboratory to segment the market using psychographic variables, laboratory participation would be important for some hospital programs that segment the market this way. Sports medicine, weight reduction, and wellness programs would fit this category. A hospital's affiliation with a religious group would also tend to segment the population by psychographic variables.

THE MARKETING ENVIRONMENT

Although a need for services may have been identified, forces in the environment also influence business decisions. External environmental forces are called "uncontrollables" because the individual business cannot immediately change what is occurring. Uncontrollables are trends, and to change these trends in one's favor requires time and support from many groups of people. The decision to market laboratory services is complex and must take into account pressure from environmental forces beyond the control of the individual hospital.

Economic Forces

The economic condition of the marketplace affects the size and strength of demand for goods and services. The state of the nation's economy has bearing on the buyer's ability and willingness to make purchases. During times of prosperity, buying power is increased. During recessionary periods, buyers are cautious about their limited buying power.

Technologic Forces

New technology has a direct impact on consumer buying behavior. Technologic developments affect our standard of living as thousands of new products and services are introduced each year. The speed at which new laboratory procedures are introduced can make previous methods appear slow and even obsolete. Consider, for example, that the time-consuming isolation and identification of some microorganisms are no longer performed because new immunologic techniques take only a few minutes. In addition, some laboratory services that were only performed in hospitals are now being performed routinely in outpatient service centers or even by the patient at home.

Legal Forces

Marketing decisions must be sensitive to laws that restrain and control certain business activities. Laws are enacted to preserve a competitive marketplace or to protect consumers.

Regulatory Political Forces

Regulatory units at the local, state, and federal levels affect marketing decisions. Trade commissions and special-interest associations exert pressure on businesses to inhibit undesirable behaviors.

Societal Forces

Shifts in population, dual-career families, and lifestyle and life-cycle preferences are some of the forces to which marketing must be attuned. Increased spending for services continues in the United States economy. In their book, *The Service Society,* Gersuny and Rosengren[4] comment on social change and the growth of services.

American society is marked by the emergence of secularized services rendered outside the family. A service revolution has, in fact, followed on the heels of the industrial revolution. This service revolution brings with it not only great new markets for the distribution of intangibles, but a new and highly significant dimension in the division of labor—the active participation of the consumer in the production of many services.

THE MARKETING MIX: THE CONTROLLABLES

What variables are available to the marketing planner? Over which factors does he or she have more direct control? The marketing mix consists of five major components, which, although affected by the general marketing environment at large, can be modified to fit business goals. The marketing-mix variables include product, distribution, place, promotion, price, and people. It quickly becomes obvious that there are limits to how controllable these variables really are. For example, a laboratory is not free to adjust prices whimsically on a daily basis because of economic conditions or government regulations. In addition, promotional campaigns must adhere to certain guidelines and cannot be changed overnight. Although the hospital can control the hiring and firing of staff, the marketing manager cannot always control workers' behavior or productivity. A major goal is to adjust marketing-mix variables to create and maintain satisfying goods and services.

Product refers to goods, services, and ideas an organization provides. Naturally, the decision about which laboratory services to market is tempered by what the competition is doing and other broader environmental forces; however, the final decision is ultimately one's own. New products are introduced in the marketplace all the time. It is the marketing department's responsibility to monitor its success and to de-

cide when it is necessary to eliminate them. Market researchers attempt to discover wants and needs so that they can modify goods and services to meet the desired characteristics. For example, a laboratory may alter the format of the requisition form or the written reports to make them more convenient for the physician to use.

Place refers to the site of the physical facilities. This may be the hospital, a satellite laboratory, or perhaps a remote blood-drawing station.

Distribution involves the logistic arrangements required physically to get the goods from the manufacturer to the point at which they are sold. Laboratory equipment and supplies pass through many distribution points before ultimately reaching a hospital laboratory. Selecting wholesalers, developing and maintaining inventory, and managing transportation and storage systems are within the realm of the marketing manager. The logistics of marketing laboratory services, picking up specimens, and delivering reports in an efficient and timely manner may be the most difficult part of the service process.

Promotion is the variable that usually comes to mind when one thinks about marketing. The goals of promotion are to inform, persuade, and remind buyers about a business and its services. The word *promote* is derived from the Latin word meaning "to move forward."

Personal selling, advertising, sales promotion, publicity, and packaging design comprise the "promotional mix." A major decision for service businesses is determining which vehicle in the promotion mix should be emphasized. Someone within the hospital or an outside agency assumes overall responsibility for coordinating the promotional mix. Too frequently, promotional activities involve different goals and vague personal accountability. A promotion program must be integrated into the organization. For example, assume the laboratory develops a direct-mail campaign. The people working in the laboratory and any sales staff must be aware of the advertising message so that they can reinforce the message when they come in contact with potential clients.

Advertising is a paid form of communication, and the sponsor of the message is clearly identified. Advertising messages are presented to large numbers of people by television, radio, direct mail, billboards, newspapers, and magazines.

Personal selling is a closer interpersonal interaction. It may be accomplished face to face or by telephone (telemarketing).

Public relations activities attempt to create awareness and a positive image for the company with its constituent groups. Although a public relations agency may be hired to represent the business to the media, the publicity message itself is free. Newspaper stories about newsworthy events, tours of facilities, and even thank-you letters are included in the realm of "good" public relations.

Sales promotion techniques include incentives to influence consumer action directly. Contests, trading stamps, premiums, and trial-size displays are examples.

People are an important variable in the marketing mix. They must be trained to communicate the image of the hospital. They need to understand the rules and regulations and have a general knowledge of the tests and services the hospital wants to sell.

THE MARKETING PLAN

The successful marketing of clinical laboratory services requires the same careful, thorough planning as the development of any kind of business, especially in light of today's competitive health-care environment. There is a series of logical steps in developing a marketing plan: developing a mission statement, formulating goals and objectives, conducting a study of internal strengths and weaknesses, analyzing the competition, and finally preparing a plan. A football game analogy is helpful in defining these terms. The mission statement describes the general task, to win the game. Goals are steps necessary to accomplish the task, getting the ball over the goal line as frequently as possible. Objectives are even smaller steps, stated in measurable terms, that are designed to help meet the goal. In football, an objective would be keeping possession of the ball by moving it at least 10 yards in four tries. In football, as in business, studying the competition is important. The final plan is the amalgamation of all of the information that describes who is going to do each task and when it is going to be done—in other words, the game plan.

The first step is the development of a mission statement. It encompasses the criteria against which one will measure the appropriateness of proposed activities and should be worded so that it gives guidance without being too limiting. The mission statement does not need to be a lengthy, complicated treatise but should clearly spell out the nature of the business and the reason for that business. One way to start developing this is to examine the mission statement or philosophy of the parent organization. The chances of success will be greater if the statement developed is congruent with the written mission of the institution and if it is also consistent with the mission of the institution as perceived by those associated with it, such as physicians, other health professionals, patients, the community, and the administrative or governing boards. Without the support of any one of these groups, it may be difficult to grow.

The goals and objectives of the enterprise should

Box 26•1

Mission Statement and Goals of a Marketing Plan

The mission of this venture is to create the most efficient, profitable, and progressive clinical laboratory possible.

Goal 1: Acquire two major instruments per year.
Objective: To increase test volume by 10% to justify the acquisition of new equipment
Goal 2: Increase market share to 40%.
Objective: To achieve competitive prices by selecting instruments that increase productivity and take advantage of the economics of batch testing

---

also be part of the mission statement. These describe what one is going to do to accomplish the mission. They may be stated in terms of revenue or may reflect where that revenue will be beneficial. Box 26–1 is an example of a mission statement and goals. The mission of Box 26–1 is general, but the goals and objectives are more specific and can be measured.

The next step in the marketing process is the research component. The major questions that need to be answered can be divided into several general areas: the internal strengths and weaknesses, the market's wants and needs, the competition's ability to satisfy the market, and other factors in the market environment that may affect business activity. These areas are addressed in a stepwise manner, but the information for all areas can be collected simultaneously.

Internal Strengths and Weaknesses

Conducting an objective study of one's own institution can be satisfying and painful. Traditionally, laboratories have evaluated themselves on the speed and accuracy of their work within a well-defined internal system of receiving a specimen, producing the requested result, communicating that result to the appropriate person, and doing whatever is necessary to be financially compensated for the service. The same steps are necessary in the commercial environment, but there are more potential complications, because the laboratory does not have the same degree of control over the external part of the process. The evaluation of the internal operation of the laboratory should answer questions about services that one has to offer. The following questions address broad major areas. Each institution will have a unique set of questions.

What Does it Cost to Perform the Tests That Are Currently Being Done in the Laboratory?

Other chapters of this text deal with laboratory finance and how to determine these costs. Remember that one will have some costs in addition to the cost of performing the test. These costs cannot be calculated until the extent of services to be provided is actually determined. For example, printing special forms and providing a courier service would be additional expenses. This information is crucial in pricing services.

Are the Testing Methods Currently Being Used Cost-Effective and Efficient?

The instrumentation in some laboratories was selected to serve a hospital population whose needs may be different than the needs of the external market. The hospitalized patient may need rapid results, whereas the outpatient may be more concerned about low-priced testing. For example, the instrument that provides rapid turnaround time for an individual test may not be able to provide the efficiency of an instrument designed for high-volume batch testing. Obviously, if one is using inefficient testing methods, it will be difficult to compete in the marketplace on the basis of price.

Does the Laboratory Have Excess Capacity in Terms of Personnel and Instrumentation? Is There Adequate Backup Capability? Can You Get Additional People, Equipment, or Space When Needed?

These are critical questions for any laboratory considering marketing its services. A service cannot be produced and stored in a warehouse like goods can, but it is produced when the customer needs it. This presents a major difficulty in planning.[1] Excess capacity and backup capability enable one to provide consistent service. If one has gone to considerable effort to market services and then cannot consistently provide those services, the customer may look for another provider. Not only is it difficult to get customers back once they have become dissatisfied, but they may tell potential customers about the problem.

What is the Attitude of the Laboratory Staff Toward Marketing Laboratory Services?

Laboratories may have to change staffing patterns to satisfy customers' needs, for example, increasing the evening shift to process a larger volume of work arriving late in the afternoon. Demands made on the staff will increase, and a laboratory is truly fortunate if the staff sees this venture as an opportunity to expand services, increase job security, or benefit in other ways. An internal program to communicate the plans for the venture and the importance of the staff's involvement may increase the morale and job satisfaction in those who will be affected by this effort.[1]

What Is the Reputation of Your Laboratory Within the Target Area?

Are there areas of the laboratory that are recognized by the users in the community for their excellence? Conversely, are there areas that need to be improved? These questions help to determine one's market position or what attributes the marketplace ascribes to one's organization.[7] The answers to these questions will be more objective if they are compiled from information from a variety of sources. It is important to separate perception from actuality. If the perception is inaccurate, it may be necessary to develop a strategy to change that belief.

Does the Marketing Effort of the Laboratory Have the Full Support of the Administration of the Hospital?

Ideally, the marketing process is a part of the overall strategic planning and budgeting process of the organization. Even though written plans and budgets for the implementation of the new venture may be in place, the people who have control of the finances must understand the potential changes that may occur if one's efforts are successful. They may have to make special arrangements to increase orders for supplies and reagents. Additional people may need to be hired, or equipment may need to be replaced sooner than planned. The revenues from the marketing effort should justify increases, but institutions generally budget once a year, and it could be difficult to make requests heard in the middle of a budget cycle. The ability to respond quickly to customer needs will be important in maintaining customer satisfaction.

Is the Internal System for Handling the Clerical Work Adequate to Handle an Increased Workload?

The paper flow is extremely important because it is the interface with the customer. Delays and confusion in this area can be a major cause of customer dissatisfaction. It is crucial to ensure that clerical work affecting the workload of other departments be well planned. Patient billing frequently falls into this category.

The Market

Market needs are determined by using a multifaceted study designed to answer a variety of questions about potential customers themselves, their current needs, and possible future needs. Unclear or incomplete information about the needs and wants of prospective customers is the reason many plans fail during implementation.[9]

Who Is the Customer?

This question may seem to have an obvious answer, but in reality, there are many choices: the patient, the physician, another laboratory, industry, or third-party payers, such as insurance companies and government agencies. It is equally important to identify the decision makers, the decision influencers, and the criteria used to make the decision. For example, a physician may select a laboratory on the basis of the convenience to his staff. The staff would be decision influencers, and it would be important for one to talk with them to determine their needs.

What Range of Service Is Required for the Laboratory to Compete?

The services required will, of course, vary with the size and nature of the customer. Some services may not be feasible now but could be areas for future development. Consider a large nursing home that now has phlebotomy service, courier service, stat service, and printer on site. These services are costly and would require a large testing volume to justify them. Most businesses cannot be all things to all customers; rather, they try to find their niche. O'Donnell defines *niche* as the set of needs that the hospital chooses to fill.[7] Finding an unsatisfied need or detecting a new trend can help discover a unique place in the market.

What Is the Market Potential?

Several other questions need to be answered before determining the probability of a profitable venture. What is the volume of testing in the target market? What percentage or share of the market would have to be captured for a profit to be made? Is it realistic to expect to get that share of the market? In general, laboratory services provided by one organization increase at the expense of another similar organization because the market is shrinking.

The Competition

Who Is the Competition?

The list of those trying to capture the dollars spent on laboratory testing includes not only commercial laboratories and hospitals, but also physicians. Even patients are trying to avoid the cost of laboratory services by doing some tests at home. The competition is also a potential market if they have testing needs that are currently unmet.

What Are They Charging for Their Services?

In general, businesses charge whatever the market will pay. Most laboratories have a published list price and discount from that for larger accounts according to their volume. The price of any given test, therefore, may vary considerably. A more key question is how much they can lower the price and remain profitable. Cutting prices is a strategy used in some industries to discourage new competitors. That is one reason for considering factors in addition to price in the marketing mix when planning the strategy for a new venture.

Does the Competition Have any Problems Providing Service to the Target Area?

Laboratories may produce accurate test results and may still not be able to serve customers adequately. For example, if the location is remote, they may not be able to provide stat service, or the area may not fit into the courier schedule at a time that is desirable for the customer. The market survey should help to uncover information that will help the company or laboratory be more competitive in variables other than price.

Other Important Factors

How Will Current Medicare and Other Regulations Affect the Marketing Effort?

In his article "Independent Laboratory or Hospital Laboratory: What Difference Does it Make?" Barry[2] discusses the Medicare treatment of both kinds of laboratories. He states, "there is wide disparity in the way carriers and intermediaries apply Medicare rules. Before deciding on a particular course of action it is advisable to consult with knowledgeable carrier and intermediary personnel." State laws, tax laws, and antitrust statutes should be reviewed before implementing any marketing activity. The more creative your efforts, the more carefully antitrust statutes should be examined. According to Polk,[8] such practices as joining with competitors to divide markets or to allocate customers, controlling

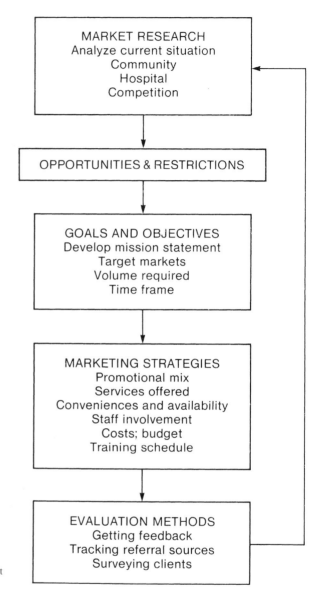

FIGURE 26–1. Marketing process overview. (Copyright Gutterman Associates, 1987)

market prices, boycotting third parties, "tying" the sale of one product to the separate purchase of another, and forming group purchasing agreements that unreasonably restrain trade have generated controversy.

The information gathered in the above process is used to answer the primary question: Can the institution profitably satisfy the needs of the target market? The marketing process is summarized in Figure 26–1. This overview emphasizes that marketing is a process that is constantly being reviewed and evaluated to detect changes in the marketplace. Change implies not only challenge, but opportunity. It is through the marketing process that laboratories prepare to meet the challenges and take advantage of the opportunities.

REFERENCES

1. Albers J, Vice JL: Strategic planning. American Journal of Medical Technology 49(6):411–414, 1983

2. Barry DM: Independent laboratory or hospital laboratory: What difference does it make? Pathologist February:31–36, 1985
3. Berry LL: Services marketing is different. Business Magazine May–June, 1980
4. Gersuny C, Rosengren WR: The Service Society. Cambridge, Schenkman Publishing Company, 1974
5. Kotler P, Conner P: Marketing professional services. Journal of Marketing January, 1977
6. Nigon DL: Economics of outreach testing in the hospital laboratory: Part I. Clinical Laboratory Management Review 7: 283–291, 1993
7. O'Donnell M: Finding you niche in the marketplace. Optimal Health September/October:20–24, 1985
8. Polk LT: Avoid conflict: Know the legal complications. Pathologist August:546–548, 1983
9. Portugal B: Strategic planning for outreach laboratory services. Pathologist August:537–540, 1983

ANNOTATED BIBLIOGRAPHY

Hillestad SG, Berkowitz EN: Health Care Marketing Plans: From Strategy to Action. Homewood, Dow Jones–Irwin, 1984
This book identifies and applies marketing techniques for improving the effectiveness and profitability of health-care organizations. The focus is on integrating planning with marketing, and a step-by-step approach to setting and achieving objectives is presented.

27

Consulting to Physician Office Laboratories

Diana Mass

During the 1980s, economic and regulatory incentives and technologic innovation in instrumentation and test methodology significantly changed the delivery of laboratory services. The diagnosis-related group payment plan for Medicare patients altered the financial posture of hospital-based clinical laboratories from an income center to a cost center. Capital for new laboratory instrumentation became a rare commodity, and the laboratory manufacturing industry was forced to look elsewhere for financial gain. At the same time, congress passed direct billing laws that eliminated the customary practice of physicians' markup of laboratory charges for Medicare patients. If physicians were to profit from Medicare patient laboratory testing, the testing would have to be performed within the physician's practice site.[1,2] Thus, new incentives were created for the laboratory manufacturing industry to develop instrumentation and simpler testing methodology for a new market—the physician office laboratory (POL).

In the ensuing years, these two regulatory changes would forever alter the history and practice of laboratory services and would play a major role in the development and transformation of the Clinical Laboratory Improvement Amendments of 1988 (CLIA '88) regulations. All these forces have shaped and created a new role for the clinical laboratory scientist—that of a consultant.

CONSULTATION PROCESS AND ROLES

Consultants are individuals with recognized expertise who are asked by a client to apply their knowledge and skills to a given situation. The consultation process generally involves the functions listed in Box 27–1.

Consultants are hired to perform a specific function agreed on in advance. The expectations of both consultant and client are outlined in an initial letter of agreement or contract. After the consultant delivers a final report that includes recommendations, the relationship usually terminates.[3]

Consulting is aimed at helping a person or a group to deal with problem confrontations and change efforts. Change is the operative word, because consultants deal primarily with the effect of change on an organization and its personnel. Effective consultation requires that change occur. In this capacity, consultants act as change agents and must consciously create an environment in which change choices occur.[4]

A consultant is a facilitator, an observer, and a specialist in how to diagnose needs and how to identify resources. During the consultation process, consultants are confronted with a series of decisions and possible alternatives. The primary value of a consultant lies in the expertise to identify, analyze, and resolve accurately the real problems and needs of the client. It is not unusual for the problem identified by the client to be overshadowed by a more significant and complex one. Thus, the consultant must explore and identify all facets of the problem thoroughly before attempting to suggest a solution.[3,5,6] Box 27–2 lists typical consultative roles, which are correlated to problem-solving activities. A consultant's proper diagnosis of the client's needs and problems determines the appropriate role for a given situation.[7]

THE NEED FOR LABORATORY TESTING AND CONSULTANTS IN THE PHYSICIAN OFFICE LABORATORY

Just as physicians have guarded their role, so has the clinical laboratory community with respect to ownership of laboratory testing. There has always been con-

Box 27·1

Functions of the Consultation Process

- Evaluate
- Research
- Advise
- Plan
- Supervise
- Train

cern about laboratory testing in the physician's office practice. However, there is a good case for testing in this environment—the need for timely, effective, and efficient patient care. The medical evaluation of a patient is expedited when test results are available on-site, thus allowing for the prompt establishment of treatment plans. Physicians can order further diagnostic studies, if needed, while the specimen is still available. In addition, office testing is convenient for patients. When patients present acute symptoms, they can be evaluated in the office rather than being referred to a hospital emergency room, which generally results in higher costs and delays in alleviating pain. Also, many patients are anxious as they await the results of laboratory work, and having test results while the patient is in the office, or shortly thereafter, significantly reduces their anxiety. In this light, the consultative role of the laboratory scientist can make a major and positive impact not only on the patient, but for the total health-care delivery system.[8,9] With the growth of POL testing and implementa-

tion of CLIA '88, consultants will be needed to advise physicians on quality assurance measures to meet the standards for laboratory accreditation. CLIA '88 requires the POL to maintain quality control and quality assurance programs, to keep appropriate records, to employ personnel who meet Department of Health and Human Services (DHHS) qualifications, and to participate in DHHS-approved proficiency programs.[10]

CONSULTATION SERVICES

Consultants for POLs can advise physicians in several ways. First, they can help the physician develop specific policies and procedures to ensure accurate results. A consultant's technical expertise can prove invaluable in developing procedure and safety manuals and designing appropriate documentation for patient results, quality control, instrument maintenance, and problem solving. In addition, evaluations of instruments and test kits may be more cost effective and better focused under the direction of consultants familiar with the physician's test menu needs and volume and with the education and skills of the personnel who will perform the testing. Consultants can also play a major role in selecting, evaluating, and training these personnel. Moreover, with continuous changes in clinical laboratory technology, qualified consultants can assist physicians with new methodologies, reimbursement practices, and regulatory changes. The federal government has emphasized the importance of proficiency testing to ensure quality, and consultants can provide any needed support to perform follow-up assessments, corrective procedures, and training.[8,9] Clinical laboratory scientists can provide a variety of services for a physician. These are outlined in Box 27–3.[8] Individuals with knowledge and experience in these areas can perform an invaluable service.

Another important role and contribution that laboratory consultants can provide is improving test use and thus promoting better integration of laboratory services into the patient care process. To implement this new role, we must understand the "traditional" laboratory, which is changing, and the "new" laboratory, which is emerging.[11]

The traditional laboratory model (Fig. 27–1) is a flow process of one activity preceding the next activity. The only concern in this series of events is in the quality of the test performance and in the internal organization and production features of the laboratory. Our focus as clinical laboratory professionals in this model is on the science and technology and skill of test performance. In the traditional laboratory, communication is almost nonexistent prior to the test order being received or after the result is released. In this model, the emphasis is on the quality of the test performance. Neither clinical

Box 27·2

Typical Consultation Roles

1. The fact finder gathers data and stimulates thinking.
2. The informational expert provides policy and practice decisions.
3. The advocate proposes guidelines, persuades, or directs the problem-solving process.
4. The objective observer raises questions for reflection.
5. The process counselor observes the problem-solving process and raises issues.
6. The joint problem solver offers alternatives and participates in decisions.
7. The trainer/educator trains the client.

Box 27·3

Services Typically Provided by Physician Office Laboratory Consultants

- Laboratory development
  Evaluate laboratory facility:
    Space and design
    Staff needs
  Evaluate product availability:
    Instruments
    Reagents/controls/calibrators
    Test/kit systems
    Information systems
  Perform cost analyses.
  Implement cost-effective purchasing/leasing.
  Perform work flow analysis.
- Test selection and performance
  Advise on in-house test menu.
  Analyze test results.
  Correlate results with clinical data.
  Evaluate discrepancies.
  Advise on test use and interpretation.

- Personnel management
  Write job descriptions.
  Evaluate/supervise personnel.
  Design/deliver in-service training.
  Monitor safety policies.
- Quality assurance
  Develop/implement procedure manual.
  Develop/implement quality control procedures.
  Design/implement laboratory record system.
  Monitor calibration, maintainance, problem solving, and repair of instruments.
  Evaluate proficiency testing.
  Advise on procedure/system changes.
- Regulation and reimbursement:
  Advise on state/federal regulatory requirements.
  Monitor and report on reimbursement policies.
  Coordinate inspection/regulatory compliance.

Modified from Crowley JR, Oliver JS: The physician office laboratory. In Davis BG, Bishop, ML, Mass D (eds): Clinical Laboratory Science: Strategies for Practice, p 981. Philadelphia, J.B. Lippincott, 1989

---

appropriateness nor interpretation of test results is considered a major concern of the clinical laboratory.

The new laboratory model is an interactive process. In this model, the scope of laboratory practice is broader. Here the focus is not only on the quality of test data generated (process), but also on the clinical appropriateness of test requests (input) and the proper interpretation of the laboratory information (output). Our involvement in the total sequence of events will improve the clinical relevance of the laboratory's service (process).

The three phases of laboratory use as it occurs in the new laboratory is described by Barr's[11] model (Fig.

27–2). Briefly, in the "input" phase, one must question if the test is appropriate for the clinical condition and if the specimen at its time of collection is correct. During the "process" phase, one must determine if, within clinically relevant guidelines, the test result is accurate and precise and the process is responsive to the turnaround time needs of physicians. Finally, in the "output" phase, one must evaluate if the results are properly interpreted and integrated into patient care or if data overload is confusing or misleading physicians.[11] CLIA '88 regulations identify these three phases as preanalytical, analytical, and postanalytical.[10]

The model of laboratory use identifies the factors

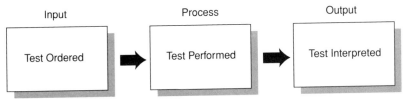

FIGURE 27–1.   Traditional laboratory model. (Davis GD, Bishop ML, Mass D: Clinical Laboratory Science: Strategies for Practice. Philadelphia, J. B. Lippincott, 1989)

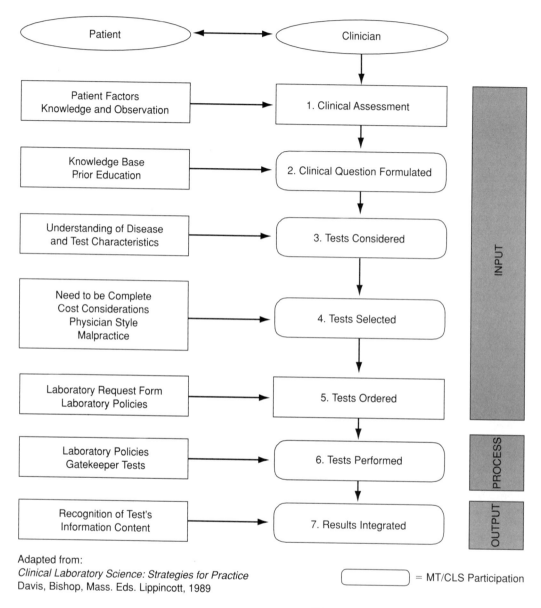

Patient ←→ Clinician

Patient Factors Knowledge and Observation	→	1. Clinical Assessment
Knowledge Base Prior Education	→	2. Clinical Question Formulated
Understanding of Disease and Test Characteristics	→	3. Tests Considered
Need to be Complete Cost Considerations Physician Style Malpractice	→	4. Tests Selected
Laboratory Request Form Laboratory Policies	→	5. Tests Ordered
Laboratory Policies Gatekeeper Tests	→	6. Tests Performed
Recognition of Test's Information Content	→	7. Results Integrated

INPUT

PROCESS

OUTPUT

Adapted from:
Clinical Laboratory Science: Strategies for Practice
Davis, Bishop, Mass. Eds. Lippincott, 1989

⬭ = MT/CLS Participation

FIGURE 27–2. Model of laboratory utilization.

that affect the clinician's decisions or actions at each step of the laboratory use process. It also demonstrates the appropriate role, if any, for the medical technologist at each step of this process. Starting with the clinician's assessment of the patient's condition, the laboratory use process proceeds in seven steps, which results in the application and integration of the test result into patient care. In step 1, the clinician assesses the patient's status and formulates the clinical questions that must be answered in step 2 to guide further management of the patient. Many tests are considered in step 3 that might be used to answer the questions. Step 4 involves the mental selection of a specific test(s). In step 5, the cognitive selection is converted into the placement of an order for the selected test(s). In step 6, a specimen is collected, and the laboratory conducts the analysis. Step 7 involves the integration of the results with the patient's condition. Steps 1 through 5 are part of the input phase; step 6 is the process; and step 7 is the output phase.[11]

All three phases are critical. If a test is not clinically indicated, the laboratory's precision is beyond that needed for clinical judgments, or the result was misinterpreted, then an accurate and precise laboratory result is of no value. It must be acknowledged that such tests are of no value because they unnecessarily consume the limited health-care resources and may potentially lead to patient harm.

This new consultative role will challenge medical technologists to accept new responsibilities that are beyond the process of producing a test result. Now an additional set of skills is also valued in the new laboratory: skills to determine whether a test should be done at all and that assist physicians to use the laboratory appropriately. In the new laboratory, only tests that actually contribute to effective and efficient diagnosis will be performed. Those that contribute nothing to the diagnosis or that confuse the issue because they address the wrong clinical question are not performed. In the new laboratory, the medical technologist's role will be to focus on the patient and to take an integrated view of the laboratory data as a means to an end rather than an end in itself.[12]

Unfortunately, laboratory professionals have abrogated this critical role in the past. Accelerating this new role and service is the Health Care Financing Administration (HCFA) and other third-party payers who want to reimburse only for tests that are medically necessary. In April 1994, HCFA, along with the American Clinical Laboratory Association and the American Medical Association, sponsored a consensus conference to discuss the appropriate use of laboratory testing. These discussions may ultimately result in medical necessity guidelines that laboratory professionals must be prepared to evaluate regarding their efficacy.[13]

CLIA '88 TECHNICAL CONSULTANT

The creation of the position of technical consultant in moderate-complexity laboratories by CLIA '88 has legitimized the role of clinical laboratory professionals as consultants. The technical consultant is responsible for the technical and scientific oversight of the laboratory. This individual does not have to be on site at all times while testing is performed; however, the consultant must be available either on site, by telephone, or by electronic consultation. Box 27–4 is a list of the technical consultant responsibilities and qualifications as identified by the CLIA regulations.[10] Although the labo-

---

Box 27•4

CLIA '88 Technical Consultant Responsibilities and Qualifications for Moderate Complexity Laboratory

RESPONSIBILITIES

- Selecting test methodology
- Verifying test procedures (precision and accuracy)
- Enrolling and participating in an HHS approved proficiency testing
- Establishing a quality control program
- Resolving technical problems and ensuring that remedial actions are taken
- Ensuring that patient test results are not reported until all corrective actions have been taken
- Identifying training needs and ensuring that each individual performing tests receive training appropriate for the services performed
- Evaluating the competency of all testing personnel and ensuring that the staff maintain their competency
- Evaluating and documenting the performance of individuals responsible for moderate-complexity testing

QUALIFICATIONS

- MD, DO, or DPM and certified in anatomic or clinical pathology by ABP, AOBP, or equivalent qualifications
- MD, DO, or DPM and 1 year laboratory training/experience in the designated specialty/subspecialty of responsibility
- Doctorate in chemical, physical, biologic, or clinical laboratory science or medical technology and 1 year laboratory training/experience in the designated specialty/subspecialty of responsibility
- Master's degree in clinical laboratory science, medical technology, or chemical physical, or biologic science and 1 year training/experience in the designated specialty/subspecialty of responsibility
- Bachelor's degree in medical technology or chemical, physical, or biologic science and 2 years laboratory training/experience in the designated specialty/subspecialty of responsibility

ratory's medical director can qualify for this role, it is unlikely that this physician has been trained to fulfill the role. If POLs are to comply successfully with the CLIA standards, they will require assistance from clinical laboratory professionals.

In 1992, in response to a growing need to recognize qualified technical consultants, the American Soci-

---

Box 27•5

Consultant Competencies

KNOWLEDGE AREAS

- Foundation in administrative philosophies, policies, and practices
- Knowledge of educational and training methods
- An understanding of the stages in the growth of individuals, groups, organizations
- Knowledge of how to design and help a change process
- Knowledge and understanding of human personality, attitude formation, and change

SKILL AREAS

- Communication skills: listening, observing, identifying, and reporting
- Teaching and persuasive skills: ability to impart new ideas and insights effectively
- Counseling skills to help others reach meaningful decisions on their own power
- Skill in designing surveys, interviewing, and other data-collecting methods
- Skill in using problem-solving techniques and assisting others in problem solving
- Ability to work with groups and teams in planning and implementing change
- Ability to be flexible in dealing with all types of situations
- Ability to form relationships based on trust

ATTITUDE AREAS

- Attitude of a professional: competence, integrity, feeling of responsibility
- Maturity: self-confidence, willingness to take necessary risks, ability to cope with rejection, hostility, and suspicion
- Open-mindedness, honesty, intelligence
- Possession of a humanistic value system

Source: Adapted from Mass D, Clinical laboratory scientists as consultants to physician office laboratories. Clinical Laboratory Sciences 5(5):284–287, 1992

---

ety for Clinical Laboratory Science (formerly known as the American Society for Medical Technology) and the American Society of Clinical Pathologists-Associate Member Section jointly developed qualifications and competencies for this CLIA personnel position (Box 27–5).[14]

CONSULTANT CHARACTERISTICS COMPETENCE

Consulting involves dealing with people as opposed to dealing with machines or mathematical solutions. Thus, there is a great need to acknowledge the personality characteristics and job requirements of the professional and successful consultant. Successful consultants commonly are innovative, creative, and flexible; can deal with conflict, confrontation, and ambiguity; can plan, communicate, and make decisions; can adapt to unfamiliar circumstances; have a high frustration level; are willing to take risks; and are future oriented.[12,13,15,16] In the search for consultative competency, Lippitt and Lippitt surveyed successful consultants to identify the factors that distinguish competence and clustered their responses according to knowledge, skills, and attitudes. Box 27–6 identifies these competencies.[7,17] A list of success factors for the medical technologist/clinical laboratory scientist would be very different. This is to be expected, because the traditional role and environment of the medical technologist/clinical laboratory scientist are remarkably different from that of the consultant. Consulting is based on the behavioral sciences, an area that is not stressed in the highly technical education of the medical technologist/clinical laboratory scientist.[14,15,17,18]

BASIC CONSULTATION SKILLS

A combination of interactive skills makes a successful consultant. One area where one must excel is technical knowledge and skill. In addition to this area of expertise, a successful consultant must be on the leading edge of the client's technology. The consultant should be pursuing state-of-the-art concepts and techniques. Successful consultants translate expert knowledge into useful application. However, if they have the best information and approach or the most effective solution to a problem but not the ability to work with their client and client's personnel, then the result is negative, and failure is inevitable. Therefore, the second area in which the consultant must excel is the entire realm of interpersonal skills. This area includes skills in communication, leadership, being a team player, understanding value structures, and conflict resolution.

Another important area is the requirement for good conceptual skills. A consultant must be able to see be

Box 27·6

Competency Statements for Personnel Financial, Operations, and Quality Management of the Laboratory

1. Prepare job descriptions.
2. Recruit, interview, and select new employees.
3. Develop a wage and salary administration program.
4. Develop a system to evaluate and document competency of testing personnel, and ensure that the staff maintain their competency to perform test procedures and report test results promptly, accurately, and proficiently.
5. Develop and present a program to identify training needs and ensure that each individual performing tests receives appropriate training for the type and complexity of the laboratory services performed.
6. Evaluate and counsel employees.
7. Develop a test request and reporting system that ensures that patient test results are not reported until all corrective actions have been taken and the test system is functioning properly.
8. Develop procedures for patient identification, specimen collection, handling, and processing.
9. Prepare work schedules.
10. Prepare and update procedure manuals.
11. Develop procedures for calibration, operation, and preventive maintenance of laboratory instruments.
12. Design and maintain an inventory control system for laboratory.
13. Develop system for labeling, handling, and storing reagents and materials.
14. Evaluate and recommend reference laboratory services.
15. Design a billing and procedure coding system to obtain appropriate reimbursement.
16. Evaluate and recommend appropriate test methods, including reagents, supplies, and equipment, that are cost effective and appropriate for the clinical use of the test results.
17. Establish reference ranges for tests.
18. Resolve technical problems and ensure that remedial actions are taken whenever test systems deviate from the laboratory's established performance specifications.
19. Verify the test procedures performed and establish laboratory test performance characteristics, including the precision and accuracy of each test and test system.
20. Evaluate and recommend an HHS-approved proficiency testing program that is commensurate with the services offered.
21. Establish a comprehensive laboratory safety program to comply with federal, state, and local regulations.
22. Develop, implement, and monitor a quality control program that is appropriate for the testing performed and establishes the parameters for acceptable levels of analytical performance and ensures that these levels are maintained throughout the entire testing process, from the initial receipt of the specimen through sample analysis and reporting of test results.
23. Monitor and evaluate compliance with federal, state, and local regulations.
24. Establish procedures to evaluate the validity of the test results in terms of reference intervals (normal ranges), reportable ranges, quality control data, analytical system performance, correlations and interpretations with other test data, and clinical significance relative to patient status.
25. Develop a test priority list that ensures that workload is arranged to optimize patient care.
26. Evaluate and organize work flow to ensure maximum efficiency.
27. Design a system to monitor process improvement constantly using continuous quality improvement, total quality improvement, or total quality management techniques.

yond the immediate problem, relate all of the pieces, and then integrate them into a conceptual working whole. Immediate problems are usually symptoms of a real problem. All changes in an organization have a ripple effect. If a recommendation is implemented that solves only an immediate problem, then negative consequences may result that far exceed any potential gain to the client's organization.[5,7,15,16]

REFERENCES

1. Title VI, Section 1886(d), Prospective Payment or Inpatient Hospital Services, Social Security Amendments of 1983 (P.L. 98-369), enacted April 20, 1983
2. Title III, Division B, Deficit Reduction Act of 1984, The Medicare and Medicaid Budget Reconciliation Amendments of 1984 (P.L. 98-369), enacted July 18, 1984
3. Siebert ML, Price G: Consulting as a professional role for the clinical laboratory scientist. In Davis BG, Bishop ML, Mass D (eds): Clinical Laboratory Science: Strategies for Practice, pp 3–12. Philadelphia, J.B. Lippincott, 1989
4. Ellis J, Helbig S: The Health Care Consultant as a Change Agent, pp 1–134. Chicago, American Medical Record Association, 1986
5. Gallessich J: The Profession and Practice of Consultation, pp 1–85. San Francisco, Jossey-Bass, 1982
6. Turner A: Consulting is more than giving advice. Harvard Business Review Sept/Oct:120–129, 1982
7. Lippitt G, Lippitt R: The Consulting Process in Action, pp 1–108. La Jolla, CA, University Associates, 1978
8. Crowley JR, Oliver JS: The physician office laboratory. In Davis BG, Bishop ML, Mass D (eds): Clinical Laboratory Science: Strategies for Practice, pp 975–984. Philadelphia, J.B. Lippincott, 1989
9. Mass D: Laboratorians As Consultants to Physicians and POLs, Test Trends. Roche Diagnostic 4(2), 1990
10. Final regulations, Clinical Laboratory improvement Amendments of 1988. Fed Regist 1992 (Feb 28).
11. Barr JT: Clinical laboratory utilization: The role of the clinical laboratory scientist. In Davis BG, Bishop ML, Mass D (eds): Clinical Laboratory Science: Strategies for Practice, pp 31–46. Philadelphia, J.B. Lippincott, 1989
12. Mass D: Medical technologists of the future: New practice, new service, new functions. Laboratory Medicine 24(7): 402–406, 1993
13. Bongiorno P: National affairs: Lab payment consensus conference. Management Briefs 16(11): 1, 6, 1994
14. Headley D: POL forum: CLIA '88 regulations provide a new opportunity for technologists. Laboratory Medicine 24(1): 46–48, 1993
15. Kelley RE: Consulting, pp 1–40. New York, Charles Scribner & Sons, 1986
16. Meredith GG, Nelson RE, Neck PA: The Practice of Entrepreneurship, pp 1–36. Geneva, Switzerland, International Labour Organization, 1982
17. Mass D: Clinical laboratory scientists as consultant to physician office laboratories. Clinical Laboratory Sciences 5(5): 284–287, 1992
18. Mass D: The clinical laboratory scientist's transition to consulting. In Crowley JR (ed): A Manual for the Clinical Laboratory Scientist Consultant, pp 1–16. Washington, D.C., The American Society for Medical Technology, 1988

28

Assessing Laboratory Operating Performance: The Laboratory Management Index Program

Thomas M. Sodeman

Management concepts for the laboratory are changing. There is a demand that laboratory management systems relate to organizational systems in the hospital and be easily verifiable. With today's increased emphasis on staff reduction, cost containment, and use control, modern management requires evaluation of every aspect of operations that influences the laboratory's and the hospital's fiscal viability. Data analysis should take into consideration the effect of management decisions. An efficiently managed laboratory, with a focus on cost-effective quality patient care, can be a hospital's most valuable asset. In the past, management programs evaluated the productivity of bench technologists and instrument systems in the laboratory. How the management decision process affected that productivity, the financial performance, and the impact of physician use on productivity and cost were not considered.

BACKGROUND AND INTRODUCTION

In the early 1970s, the College of American Pathologists' (CAP) Workload Recording Method (WLRM) was used to measure productivity and assess laboratory staffing needs. However, in the past few years, the program became increasingly difficult to maintain. The process of assessing work unit values was cumbersome and difficult to validate, and rapid technological advances and introduction of new equipment forced laboratory personnel to assign arbitrary and often unreliable values for testing activities. The arbitrary nature of counting allowed laboratory managers to game the system. Hospital administration was unable to verify the data provided by the laboratory. It was obvious that a more modern tool was required, capable of assessing not only productivity, but also cost-effectiveness and use of laboratory services. It was essential that the tool measured the performance of management and how the decision process affected the productivity and cost effectiveness of the laboratory.

In October 1990, CAP introduced the Laboratory Management Index Program (LMIP), which is a structured approach to laboratory management using a series of ratios derived from daily operational data. The program was to step past the traditional workload unit and look to a broader approach for evaluating management performance. The program was to integrate use and cost-effectiveness programs, be simple to collect, and generate only essential data with clear target monitors that permit continuous quality improvement (CQI) of management decisions. Because the data were developed around the "billed test," hospital administration could relate laboratory operational performance to hospital data systems. Initially, LMIP limited its analysis to the global performance of the laboratory. As an example, it evaluated the balance of technical to nontechnical personnel in the laboratory but did not provide staffing guidelines for individual laboratory sections.

With the discontinuance of the WLRM in 1993, LMIP was expanded to include evaluation of individual laboratory sections. Analysis of the productivity data in LMIP demonstrated that to replace WLRM, it would be essential that the measures of overall productivity related to the specific laboratory sections individually: chemistry, microbiology, transfusion medicine, hematology, urinalysis, immunology, anatomic pathology, and specimen procurement.

THE LABORATORY MANAGEMENT INDEX PROGRAM

The Laboratory Management Index Program is a peer comparison program of productivity, use, and financial operation. The program has 1,000 participants, including small hospital laboratories that produce approximately 300 tests per day and large laboratories that produce 3,000 tests per day. The program groups laboratories together based on the number of billable tests produced in a quarter. Four peer groups have been developed on this basis. Laboratories submit 20 data elements that are converted to a series of 20 ratios. Information is reported back to the individual participants giving their ratios and a peer ranking. The 25th, 50th, and 75th percentiles are reported in a graphic representation.

With a current database of more than 1,000 participating laboratories, the LMIP provides interlaboratory comparison of participant data that can assist managers in decision making by allowing laboratories to compare their operating performance with other laboratories of similar function and structure. This is accomplished through LMIP's unique methods of peer grouping.

Hospital peer groups are established based on the volume of billable tests performed (billable groups 1–4) and laboratory complexity (complexity groups I–V). Billable groups are defined by quartiles with respect to ranges that reflect the number of billable tests performed per quarter (Box 28-1).

An analysis of laboratory services, specialty functions, employee skill mix, intricacy of testing, and laboratory organizational structure is used to produce a *complexity index;* laboratories are then assigned to one of five complexity groups. If a laboratory is found to be performing outside the range of its billable group (based on test volume), it could examine the extent and complexity of services performed to see whether greater complexity accounts for the level of perfor-

---

> **Box 28•1**
>
> ### Billable Groups 1 Through 4
>
> Billable group 1: 0 to 44,948
> Billable group 2: 44,949 to 86,728
> Billable group 3: 86,729 to 152,410
> Billable group 4: > 152,410

---

mance. Because the two sets of groups (billable and complexity) have different statistical bases, a particular laboratory might be classified in complexity group III but billable group 4 (a laboratory with high volume in terms of billable tests but low complexity in terms of test mix and institutional need). However, while differences in the makeup of these groups may occur, several expected and logical observations are noted for both: labor, billable test volume, and consumable expenses increase in general with increases in billable and complexity group number, as does use of laboratory services. In general, larger laboratories are more complex than smaller laboratories.

Interlaboratory comparison and regular monitoring of individual performance with respect to these peer groups can assist in establishing benchmarks or targets, identifying areas of variance, and analyzing reasons for this variance. In all cases, participating laboratories are supplied a percentile ranking of their performance in relation to their peers by size and complexity. The program suggests that participants use the data to identify areas for potential improvement, that is, to identify ratios that are most at variance with peer laboratories, to find explanations for the variance, and to develop processes most likely to lead to continuous improvement.

The LMIP also conducts periodic focus studies to investigate specific areas of laboratory operations indepth or to review a particular aspect of laboratory management not addressed in the routine data collection activities. Focus studies allow review of laboratory operations that are of interest to laboratory management and for which trend data are not important. Results of some of these studies are discussed later. To assist laboratories in understanding and applying the management approaches in LMIP, each participant receives an LMIP Users Guide that describes the operations and uses of the program and its components in more detail.

Laboratory Management Index Program Design

Basic LMIP consists of three modules that deal with laboratory operation. These modules contain management ratios that are used as performance indicators. The ratios are built on groups of output and input units. The calculation of ratios is a simple task performed in many laboratories. When done internally, it provides a tracking system of performance. Performance ratios similar to those designed for LMIP should be tracked regularly by laboratories. The establishment of targets based on ratio analysis can provide an indication of improvement and a positive performance tool for employee morale. *LMIP provides the added feature of peer grouping of data to permit judgment of performance in relation to a similar laboratory.* As such, LMIP is a basic quality improvement tool for management.

The LMIP is divided into three sections, productivity, cost effectiveness, and laboratory use. While the output units vary depending on the variables for analysis and the laboratory subsection, the basic output units for productivity are the billable and total test. The input units are labor, full time equivalent (FTE), and financial costs (salary, consumable, and equipment). Productivity is examined in the broadest context, using both financial and labor elements. Basic LMIP centers around the total laboratory and requires each participant to submit 25 pieces of information.

Individual productivity modules are available for a series of standard sections. These sections are listed in Box 28-2.

Participants provide raw data specific to their section. The data are converted to productivity comparison ratios. Peer group analysis is structured in two groups, billable groups and complexity groups, and takes into account the variability between sections in laboratories.

A central core of input data and production ratios exists for each section of specific modules (Box 28-3).

As a group, these ratios provide a study of the productivity of personnel, instrumentation, laboratory policies and procedures, salary dollar use, physician use,and organizational benefits. They are indicators of management decisions and as such, provide a CQI tool.

Basic LMIP gives information on general staffing,

Box 28•2

Standard Sections

1. Chemistry
2. Microbiology
3. Hematology
4. Blood bank
5. Immunology
6. Anatomic pathology
7. Urine
8. Specimen procurement

Box 28•3

Input Data and Production Ratios

DATA INPUT ITEMS

Section on-site billable tests, by inpatient,
   Outpatient and nonpatient
   Section technical FTEs
   Section total FTEs
   Section paid hours
   Section worked hours
   Section technical FTE paid hours
   Section salary expense
   Section consumable expense
   Section equipment depreciation expense
   Hospital discharges
   Hospital outpatient visits

These input data will provide a central core of information to calculate productivity, use and cost-effectiveness ratios. In addition, each section has specific ratios related to its subspecialty testing.

PRODUCTIVITY RATIOS

Section on-site total billable tests/section
   technical FTE
Section on-site total billable tests/section total
   FTE
Section technical FTE/section total FTE
Section worked hours/section paid hours
Section on-site total billable tests/section paid
   hours

USE

Section in patient on-site billable tests/discharge
Section outpatient on-site billable tests/outpatient
   visit

COST EFFECTIVENESS

Section Nonpatient on-site billable/Tests/section
   on-site total billable tests
Section total expense/section on-site total billable
   tests
Section total labor expense/section on-site total
   billable tests
Section total expense/discharge
Section total expense/outpatient visit

that is, the number of technologists required for the billable tests generated in the total laboratory. The specific sectional modules are required to determine staffing needs for the sections. There is marked variation in the number of billable tests that can be produced by a technologist in each section as seen in Box 28-3. The efficiency of the procedures varies from section to section, for example, 0.79 billable tests per total test in chemistry versus 0.39 in microbiology. Peer grouping at the section level is essential. One does not have to use a detailed, labor-intensive workload system to determine staffing needs. The other elements in the core ratios provide data on the effectiveness of management decisions on the productivity of labor, dollars spent, and physician use. Because peer grouping does include acuity measures, the complexity or lack of complexity is not an excuse for variation within a peer group.

Measuring Productivity

For years, laboratory labor output units were measured in terms of CAP workload units. This unit, a measure of defined activity, required engineering time studies for measurement and varied by instrument and procedure. A standardized protocol was developed by CAP to establish the time for each step in an analysis. The variations in application of methods by different laboratories are reflected in the CAP unit as an average, not an absolute value. This average inflates or deflates productivity, depending on the specific procedure in use in a laboratory.

The number of studies performed to calculate the CAP unit was frequently limited and in many cases extrapolated from like instruments or methods without performing a formal time study. The program was falling behind in measuring new technology, restudy of prior work, and conversion of extrapolated units to hard data. An example of the need for restudy of even the most basic CAP workload unit is evident from the results of one of the last restudies, the manual differential unit. This resulted in the CAP unit changing from 11.0 to 6.0 units per slide. Given the number of manual differential studies performed in this country, a change of this magnitude suggests that staffing, when based on CAP workload units, is significantly inflated in hematology. In actuality, while the number of CAP units may fall with the new CAP unit, the actual work will not decrease. For example, a hospital performing 39,000 manual differentials a year should adjust staff down 1.57 FTEs to account for the drop in workload units. A similar adjustment of workload units in the 1980s for microbiology caused an immediate negative reaction for the program. While these adjustments brought the system closer to truth, the management implications hurt the system's

credibility. Management of productivity requires a stable output unit to ensure year-to-year comparisons.

The workload system was a method of product evaluation rather than a measure of technologists' performance. It reflected differences in performance characteristics of methods and instrument systems. Subtle variations in measurement gave a tremendous marketing advantage to a product.

The accumulated problems with the CAP units resulted in laboratories adding fudge factors or altering units to achieve staffing necessary for output. The complexity of application of the system required laboratory information systems (LIS) for accurate capture of units and often manual procedures to supplement the LIS. The raw data are massive, leading to analysis generally of only summarized data. The relationship of CAP units with other productivity factors has shown a divergence. Studies in the Veterans system[1] have particularly amplified this problem. A common variance is the relationship between the number of workload units to billable tests when trended over time. The CAP workload system required laboratories to update programs yearly, and the failure to do so increased the lack of continuity in the system.

The LMIP model uses a basic *production output unit* rather than minutes of activity to determine the productivity of personnel. It relies on the *average* output, as workload relied on the *average* number of minutes to produce a test. It does not require expensive and lengthy time studies to determine the unit as with workload units. It is not subject to the difficulties of converting raw counts to total workload units or of having to measure and collect individual parts of a test system. In the workload system, one major problem was how to account for time not measured by CAP units. LMIP looks at the global environment and measures how many FTEs are required to produce a billable test. This incorporates both workload measured time and nonworkload time.

Unlike CAP workload units, in which the benchmark for comparative analysis is a minute of effort for a specific method, ratios use a peer group. The productivity of management decisions on instrument selection, laboratory policies, and procedures is evident within a billable peer group. Individual laboratories can determine how their management decisions in a section affect staff production (billable test/FTE) in relation to a peer group producing similar numbers of billable tests. The goal is to manage the total process, of which the number of FTEs is only one component. A laboratory that is unhappy with its position in relation to its peer group should examine the full testing process before deciding that staffing alone is excessive or insufficient. The number of billable tests per FTE is influenced by many management decisions, including test load, personnel efficiency, available time for test production, and instrument performance.

The LMIP productivity module uses the billable and total test count as its basic output unit. Both are carefully defined for the participants in a list of definitions of terms. Billable tests are equated to ordered tests for laboratories that do not bill. It reflects an almost universal unit in hospital and independent laboratories. It is a unit that is easily understood, requires no special methods to determine (unlike the workload unit), and is tracked by the financial systems of most institutions. It is a unit understood and accepted by nonlaboratory management. It is verifiable through the financial systems of institutions and is not subject to internal manipulation by laboratory management or section personnel. The billable test is considered equal to the CPT code count. The CPT code system, developed and managed by the American Medical Association, consists of a test list that has been assigned a specific code and is in general use as a billing code. In CPT code procedure laboratory profiles are assigned a single number. In LMIP, production output units are related to a variety of input units to determine productivity, use, and cost effectiveness. The major difficulty with the billable test for interlaboratory comparison lies in the method by which profiles are counted. Some laboratories break profiles into individual reportable units. This results in an inflated number, in relation to those laboratories that count the profile as one billable unit. Consequently, the LMIP advisory committee elected to count the profile as a single billable unit, not its components. This decision was based on the concept of counting the specimen load. Usually one sample is required for a single profile. Labor and costs of modern instrumentation requires little additional effort to perform multiple tests in profiles, as shown by earlier workload studies. Most profiles are grouped around instrumentation. Some packaging of multiple profiles does take place in the market, and a laboratory should consider breaking multiple profile packages into the their unit profiles before counting billable units. This decision to use the billable test is compatible with the CPT coding system in which profiles are provided single codes and not counted by their components. It provides a uniform counting system. Blood and blood components are not counted as a billable test.

Managing Productivity

A relationship must be established between workload (output) and the laboratory work force (input) to measure laboratory productivity. In LMIP, productivity is measured using on-site billable and total tests as the output units and labor expense and personnel time (ex-

cluding pathologists) as the input units. Personnel time is defined in terms of FTEs and worked and paid hours. An FTE is equivalent to one person working 40 hours per week for 52 weeks per year, or 2,080 paid hours per year. FTEs in LMIP are defined as technical or nontechnical. A technical individual is one who actually performs test procedures (eg, medical technologists or technicians, histologists). Nontechnical individuals do not perform tests but are involved in administrative, clerical, or support activities (eg, supervisors, secretaries, couriers, morgue attendants).

As noted previously, LMIP provides productivity comparison ratios for evaluating laboratory productivity (Box 28-4).

On-site billable tests per total FTEs is a gross measure of laboratory staff productivity. However, because not all employees are directly involved in performing tests, the ratio on-site billable tests per technical FTE is more meaningful in representing the output produced by the bench labor force. It is not diluted by the variation in types of nontechnical staff present in a laboratory, and it eliminates differences among the laboratories using support personnel, such as couriers or phlebotomists.

The ratio of technical to total FTEs decreases as laboratory size increases. As laboratory size and workload increase, the requirement for administrative functions also increases. Larger laboratories are also more likely to have other nontechnical employees, such as couriers and phlebotomists. Similarly, independent laboratories usually require nontechnical staff to do business functions, such as billing, collections, and marketing, functions seldom found in hospital laboratories.

The LMIP also examines productivity in terms of worked hours and paid hours. The number of billable tests performed in a paid hour is an indication of the productivity of a single hour of time in the laboratory. However, it is diluted by vacation time, personnel leave, and other non–test-productive activities (employee benefits). In contrast, the *on-site billable tests per*

Box 28•4

Productivity Comparison Ratios

On-site billable tests per total FTEs
On-site billable tests per technical FTEs
Percent technical FTEs per total FTEs
On-site billable tests per worked hour
On-site billable tests per paid hour
Worked to paid hours ratio
Percent on-site billable tests/total billable tests

worked hour ratio represents the productivity of employees in terms of actual working hours.

The on-site billable tests per worked hour ratio when examined with the *on-site billable tests per technical FTE* ratio can provide an idea of the productivity (volume produced) per hour for the technical employees actually involved in the testing process.

The *worked to paid hour* ratio provides laboratories with an estimate of the benefit package offered by the laboratory and hospital facility compared to other hospitals. A laboratory with a relatively stable, long-term staff; low personnel turnover; and generous benefit package of vacation and holiday leave will have a lower worked-to-paid hour ratio than a new laboratory, one with high personnel turnover, or one with a more restrictive leave policy.

While the *on-site billable tests per technical and/ or total FTE* ratios demonstrate the productivity of the laboratory staff, the *percent of on-site billable tests per total billable tests* ratio reflects the proportion of testing that is performed at the hospital rather than sent to off-site or reference laboratories.

Data such as these can assist laboratory administration in forecasting necessary staffing adjustments needed to accommodate changes in the workload. By monitoring individual laboratory sections, management can also observe the influence or contribution of each on total laboratory operations.

Managing Cost Effectiveness

Funding in laboratories has undergone a tremendous change since the introduction of prospective reimbursement. Hospitals are no longer simply able to pass through costs to third-party payers. Managed care and other forms of contract medicine further strain the resources of hospitals and commercial laboratories. Laboratories are in a global fight for dollars with other healthcare services.

Evaluation of a laboratory's costs in relation to its peer group can assist in identifying areas where potential cost savings may be achieved. In combination with management insights, such evaluations may provide reasons for variance from peers. As noted previously, the LMIP collects data for the cost-effectiveness ratios listed in Box 28-5.

These ratios allow management to paint a picture of the laboratory's costs in relation to its peer group, which is essential for fiscal viability in today's healthcare environment.

Total laboratory expense per discharge and per patient day increases as billable group size and complexity group increase. In both cases, the increase observed with increase in group number is consistent with other data that show that patients who are more acutely ill

---

Box 28•5

Cost-effectiveness Ratios

Consumable expense per on-site billable test
Depreciation expense per on-site billable test direct
Expense per on-site billable test
Total labor expense per on-site billable test
Technical labor expense per on-site billable test
Total laboratory expense per discharge
Total laboratory expense per patient day
Referred billable test expense per referred billable test
Total laboratory expense per total billable test
Cost of blood as a percent of total laboratory expense

(higher case-mix indices) require more services, resulting in more costs to the hospital.

The largest portion of laboratory expense is labor. Total labor expense includes the total cost of wages and benefits paid to technical and nontechnical staff. LMIP data reveal that the expense for the technical labor pool is much higher than that for the total employee pool and that both increase across the billable groups. These increasing expenses may reflect requirements for more highly skilled technologists or more extensive benefit packages in larger and more complex institutions. The seniority of the staff and regional salary differences are other variables that must be considered when evaluating these ratios.

The LMIP data also show that *labor and direct expenses per on-site billable test* decrease as the number of billable tests increases, reflecting an increasing level of automation, batching of tests, and generally improved efficiency. Total labor expense accounts for 66% of the direct expense (the sum of total labor expense, consumable expense, equipment maintenance and rental expense, and equipment depreciation expense) per billable test. LMIP data can be used to indicate how a laboratory's labor expense differs from peer laboratories with respect to total and individual laboratory sections.

Total labor expense per on-site billable test decreases as the number of tests increases. More efficient use of personnel and changes in the blend of clerical and technical personnel may be factors in the decrease in this ratio for the larger laboratories.

A study on the percent of supervisory time spent on the bench has revealed that supervisors in laboratories that perform more procedures spend less time performing tests. This is probably due to increases in complexity of operations and in the number of people supervised.

Consumable expense, which is second only to labor as a percentage of direct costs, includes reagents, controls, disposables, and computer and other laboratory supplies. On the average, consumables account for 29% of the direct expense of a billable test in LMIP. Consumable expense is directly related to laboratory volume. LMIP data support the concept that bulk purchasing reduces costs—the *consumable expense and direct expense per on-site billable test* ratios drop as the volume increases. Federal laboratories apparently have greater success in negotiating discounts for reagents and supplies than the private sector.

Managing Use

The experience of LMIP in its first 2 years emphasizes that the greatest cost and productivity benefit lies in control of use. As an example, the study of one moderate-sized hospital in the LMIP program demonstrated that physician use patterns of laboratory tests was of greatest value to control costs. In this hospital, the physicians order 15 fewer tests per discharge than the mean for its peer group. The hospital discharges 5,810 patients each quarter. From the LMIP data, a billable test in that laboratory costs $8.49. This hospital experiences a $793,903 saving per quarter in relation to the peer group mean. The average salary per FTE in that laboratory is $8,563 per quarter. To achieve a similar saving by labor reduction would require eliminating more than 25 FTEs. A reduction of one test per discharge in this hospital equates to a potential saving of $49,325 in laboratory costs.

As competition in health care becomes more intense, the cost of laboratory testing per episode of care will be a primary focus in health system reform. Effective laboratory use involves maximizing the value to patients of the episode of care by ordering only tests that contribute most to diagnosis and necessary treatment at the least total cost. Use data reflect laboratory production in relation to hospital census days and discharges, and reflect physician ordering patterns and patient acuity. Teaching hospitals with acute or complex patients tend to have higher use, placing them at a potential cost disadvantage to other hospitals.

Increasingly, physicians' ordering patterns will be evaluated in relation to patient outcomes, adherence to practice guidelines, ordering standards, and cost. Physician laboratory use patterns clearly influence the overall cost of patient care. Inappropriate or unnecessary use patterns can be altered by educational efforts and by payment incentives. In a risk-based situation (eg, Medicare diagnosis-related grouping or capitation), this difference translates to a potential savings of more than $700,000 per quarter to the hospital, assuming patients

of similar acuity being treated. Average reductions of as little as one test per discharge have significant cost-reduction consequences.

Laboratory administration can indirectly influence the use of its services by documenting the impact of certain hospital practices on its operating budget. This can be accomplished by using the LMIP to monitor the following use comparison ratios.

Inpatient billable tests per patient day
Inpatient billable tests per discharge
Percent billable stat tests per on-site billable test

Inpatient billable tests per patient day and *inpatient billable tests per discharge* reflect the medical staff's use patterns, intensity of service, and patient acuity. It is, therefore, expected that figures for these ratios would increase across the billable groups with increasing size and complexity of operations. *Percent billable stat tests per on-site billable tests* defines one aspect of intensity of use and complexity. Higher levels of stat testing increase unit cost. The need to respond with rapid turnaround impacts instrument purchasing and buying decisions as well.

Physician use of laboratory services can be examined with respect to the amount of work that is performed on-site in the laboratory department as a whole and more specifically, within laboratory sections. Based on data collected in LMIP pilot studies of discipline-specific modules for on-site billable tests, inpatient activity in transfusion medicine constitutes between 73% and 84% of all transfusion medicine on-site billable tests. Microbiology inpatient activity comprises between 47% and 66%, and hematology inpatient activity accounts for 46% to 60%.

When compared to *total* laboratory tests reported for participants submitting data for each of the respective disciplines, transfusion medicine accounts for 2% to 9% of total on-site billable tests, microbiology accounts for 7% to 10%, and hematology contributes between 22% and 30%. As expected, transfusion medicine and microbiology make up a lower volume of outpatient and physician referral testing than hematology. Clearly, hematology accounts for a greater percentage of the work performed on-site than either transfusion medicine or microbiology.

Peer Grouping

Benchmarking as a method to improve specific elements of an operation represents a new trend. Benchmarking, however, does not mean necessarily the operation with the lowest costs, as some management programs propose. Rather, it refers to maintaining quality, productivity, and cost through analysis of successful operational management. The determination of a benchmark for laboratory management is difficult unless quality parameters are also included in the evaluation.

The LMIP used the billable test initially to peer group laboratories. The demographics of hospital beds no longer can be used as a comparative tool to determine either personnel or financial productivity. Many hospitals run a census considerably below bed rates. The move to outpatient units in hospitals has resulted in a dramatic growth in laboratory work that has little relationship to hospital bed rate. In LMIP, outpatient testing is running approximately 20% of laboratory work for medium to large hospitals. Outreach programs for nonpatients is similarly growing for hospitals. The experience of LMIP for interlaboratory comparison of productivity is unmatched.

CONCLUSION

Efficient and effective management of the clinical laboratory in today's health-care climate requires knowl-edge of where and how resources are used, evaluation of laboratory performance against standards and benchmarks, and planning, implementing, and monitoring change. It involves management decisions based on review of every aspect of laboratory operations, including the forces that drive the costs, and those that generate income for support of laboratory and hospital services.

In the current environment of health system reform, emphasis has been placed on cutting costs. Cutting costs does not necessarily result in efficient operations. Effective use of all laboratory resources balances laboratory costs and quality of patient services. The LMIP will not remove the challenges facing laboratories today, but it can serve as a quality improvement tool that provides continuous assessment of performance and facilitates effective management of the total laboratory process.

REFERENCE

1. Travers E: CAP Today, p 84. Northfield, IL, College of American Pathologists, 1993

Principles of Laboratory Finance

29

Introduction to Laboratory Financial Management

David J. Fine • Barbara Caldwell Salmon
• Rohn J. Butterfield • Justin E. Doheny

FINANCING HEALTH CARE

Medicare, Medicaid, prospective payment, diagnosis-related groups (DRGs), preferred provider organizations (PPOs), health maintenance organizations (HMOs), managed care systems, payback, fiscal intermediary, return on investment, not for profit—the financial side of the health-care industry possesses a vocabulary that is, for the most part, unknown to the medical technologist. The financing of hospitals and laboratories is as strange to the laboratorian as a type and cross-match is to the hospital financial officer. However, to succeed as a laboratory manager, one must be able to understand both sides of the many complex issues. One must be as concerned about positive cash flow and controlling the laboratory's costs as one is about quality assurance and procedure controls.

The objective of this chapter is to provide the reader with a general understanding of hospital finance, an appreciation of how the laboratory fits into the overall picture, and an introduction to the tools of the financial manager. Readers are not expected to master each of these subjects, but it is hoped that they will become knowledgeable enough to use certain of the techniques and gain sufficient insight into the world of financial management to serve as an interface between the laboratory and the financial stewards of the hospital.

Industry Overview

The health-care industry is among the largest in the country, and it is second only to defense in its share of the gross national product (GNP). In 1994, health-care expenditures accounted for 16% of the GNP,[4] an increase from 10.8% in 1984.[3]

Historically, hospitals have been a growing segment of the health-care sector and have been a major driving force in the expansion of overall health-care costs. In 1965, 33.3% of national health expenditures were for hospital services; by 1994, this had grown to 48.6%. Expressed on a per capita basis, $1,580 was

459

spent on health care in 1984, of which, $645 was for hospital services,[3] as compared to a per capita expenditure in 1994 of $3,068 for health care and $1,492 for hospital services.[4]

These figures demonstrate that hospitals are big business. There are, however, several unusual characteristics of hospitals that affect their performance and behavior. First, while many people consume health-care services, few pay the bills directly. The number of uninsured people is increasing because of lack of comprehensive insurance plans available at a cost affordable to the working poor, but most people in the United States are beneficiaries of health or hospital insurance of some sort. It is the insurers, including the federal government, who pay most of the health bill. In 1994, 20.3% of the country's population was covered under a managed care program in which patients may have restricted access to physicians and diagnostic services.

Most hospitals in this country are tax exempt, so called *not for profit*, meaning that no profits or earnings are distributed to owners of the hospital. Thus, hospitals have not historically been as profit conscious as other corporations, and their success or failure has been judged not so much on profitability as on a number of other considerations. In recent years, there has been an increase nationwide in the number of tax exempt hospitals being purchased by *investor-owned* health-care corporations. This group of hospitals is particularly cost conscious while maintaining a competitive level of service and quality.

In the past, these factors significantly modified the traditional free-market competition concept governing most United States industries. While profitability may not have been a prime concern for hospitals in the past, the unique characteristics of the hospital industry cited previously have been modified or eliminated by massive changes in the financial incentives created for hospitals, physicians, and their patients by the public and private health insurance industry. These changes are described in some detail below and represent the most dramatic alteration of the nation's health delivery system since the Medicare and Medicaid legislation of 1966. With some assurance, one may point to these changes as the major causal factors for the retardation of the rate of health-care expenditure growth noted since 1984 as opposed to the inexorable rise in costs experienced before 1984.

Medicare and Medicaid

Prior to 1983, the single event having the greatest impact on the health-care marketplace was the enactment and implementation of Medicare and Medicaid in July 1966.

This legislation, also known as Title XVIII and Title XIX of the Social Security Act, was perhaps the most significant piece of social legislation since the original Social Security Act of the 1930s, because it established a mechanism for financing the health care of the elderly and poor.[2]

Medicare eligibility is limited to those 65 years and older or to those who meet other criteria related to disability or chronic renal disease. Medicaid eligibility is based on a number of criteria established by the individual states within a framework established by the federal government. It is the intent of the Medicaid program to pay the health-care costs of the poor or medically indigent.

The Medicare program is split into two parts: Part A provides payment for inpatient services in a hospital or skilled nursing facility or to a home health agency after discharge from a hospital or skilled nursing facility. Part A will pay for laboratory tests, along with a long list of other covered services. Part B helps to pay the bills from physicians, hospital outpatient visits, and certain other medical services and supplies not included in Part A coverage.

Figure 29–1 indicates the dramatic increase in federal financing of health care, owing largely to the advent of Medicare and Medicaid. One can also see a reciprocal drop in direct payments made by individuals. There has also been a significant increase in private health insurance payments.

Before 1983, all Part A payments to hospitals by Medicare were based on the hospital's actual and imputed costs. Under such a reimbursement system, there were strong economic incentives for hospitals to sacrifice cost-containment efforts to provide the highest quality patient care and technology possible. This incentive, along with absolute growth in the amount of services provided to the newly enfranchised elderly population, were the primary factors driving the tremendous growth in federal expenditures for health care. Also during this era, Part B payments to physicians were made on the basis of reasonable charges. Among other services, Part B paid professional fees charged by a pathologist for laboratory and pathology procedures.

In October 1983, based on a growing national concern over health-care costs in general and hospital expenditures in particular, Medicare began implementation of a completely new method of payment to hospitals called the prospective payment system (PPS) for covered inpatient Part A services. Essentially, the thrust of the PPS was to ensure that hospitals assumed financial risk for their costs in exchange for Medicare payments.[7]

Medicare established 468 DRGs; that is, patient diagnoses were grouped according to the diseases affecting specific organ systems of the body. The basis of

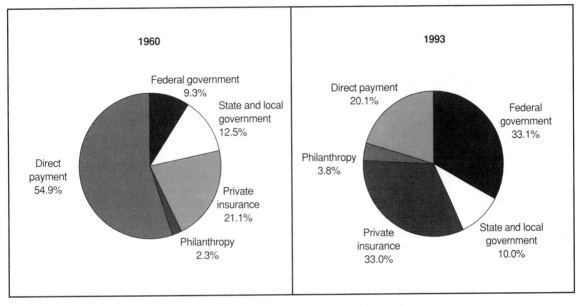

1960

Federal government
9.3%

State and local
government
12.5%

Direct
payment
54.9%

Private
insurance
21.1%

Philanthropy
2.3%

1993

Direct payment
20.1%

Federal
government
33.1%

Philanthropy
3.8%

Private
insurance
33.0%

State and local
government
10.0%

FIGURE 29–1. A comparison between personal health-care expenditures in the United States in 1960 and 1993 (excludes prepayment and administration expenses and government public health activities). (From Health United States 1994: Hyattsville, Department of Health and Human Services, 1994)

payment was the discharge, which was classified into one of the DRGs. Payments per discharge in a specific DRG were set prospectively based on average historical Medicare costs for discharges in that DRG. The change-over from the cost-based system to the DRG-based PPS was to be completely phased in by 1988.[7]

The effects of the change from a *retrospective cost-based reimbursement* system to a *prospective price-based payment* system were immediate. The federal government had, for the first time since Medicare was enacted, introduced competitive principles into the health-care marketplace. For example, prior to the PPS, if a hospital's cost for a particular Medicare discharge was $5,000, this cost would have been reimbursed in full by Medicare. Under the PPS, by contrast, Medicare may have set the DRG price for that discharge at $4,000, regardless of the hospital's actual cost. In this example, the hospital would lose $1,000 for every discharge in that DRG unless the cost of delivering care to patients in that DRG could be reduced. For the first time, hospitals were forced to look at reducing costs to remain within the DRG reimbursement payments. Conversely, if the hospital's cost was $3,000, the hospital would realize a $1,000 surplus. In short, the risk for health-care costs under the PPS shifted from Medicare to the hospital and established Medicare as a "prudent buyer"

of health-care services, as opposed to the government's formerly passive funding role.[6]

Under the PPS, then, hospitals are attempting to define and control the cost of delivering services to an extent unknown just a few years ago. As a result, the laboratory, for Medicare purposes at least, becomes a true cost center and just one of the variables whose cost must be controlled for realization of a net surplus from the patient's stay in the hospital.

Part B changes affecting pathologists' professional fees were also enacted in the early 1980s before PPS. Medicare contended that certain payments to hospital-based physicians (including pathologists) under Part B should more properly be paid to hospitals under Part A (for activities such as supervision of laboratory personnel and hospital administrative duties) and that Part B payments should be related only to physician services requiring clinical judgment for which the physician had been uniquely trained. Therefore, reasonable charges paid under Part B were limited to clinical activities deemed appropriate by Medicare (eg, written laboratory and pathology consultations), and the balance of Part B payments were to be factored into Part A DRG discharge payments on full implementation of the PPS.

Although this change had little impact on other hospital-based physicians, pathologists were greatly affected, because professional fee charges rendered to Medicare for most clinical laboratory tests would no longer be paid under Part B but would be paid to the hospitals under Part A. The amount of Part B dollars to be incorporated into Part A DRG payments has been reduced by restricting the procedures for which Medicare will pay clinical pathologists for professional interpretive fees.

It is difficult to make generalizations about payments under the Medicaid program because the specific eligibility requirements and services covered are defined by the various states. In most cases, charges by pathologists and hospitals related to laboratory tests are included.

It should be noted, however, that many states have taken Medicare's lead and have adopted competitive models of Medicaid payment, including contracts for discounted charges, DRG-based payments, and capitated managed care.

In the 1990s, Medicare began to look at outpatient laboratory testing and has suggested a parallel plan to inpatient DRGs. These ambulatory patient groups would motivate improved cost control in the outpatient setting, which is steadily increasing in volume as more illness episodes are managed outside of the hospital.

Private Health Insurance

Although local, state, and federal governments account for nearly 43% of all health-care expenditures, private insurance policies and plans account for the balance of insured health care and comprise more than 33% of all health-care costs. Included among the list of nongovernmental health insurers are Blue Cross and Blue Shield. These insurance plans have grown significantly since the establishment of the first Blue Cross plan in 1929. Today there are approximately 80 separate Blue Cross corporations providing hospitalization insurance benefits to their subscribers. Blue Cross was established to pay hospital bills, and Blue Shield was established to pay physician fees. Commonly thought of together, they are generally separate corporations, although in certain areas, they are one legal entity. Until recently, Blue Cross usually paid hospitals on a negotiated cost basis, whereas Blue Shield paid physicians on some basis related to charges.

Although slow to respond to the competitive forces initiated by Medicare, both Blue Cross and Blue Shield have established a number of alternative payment and delivery systems in recent years. These include negotiated discounted price contracts with hospitals and physicians alike; the creation of PPOs, which contract on a discounted basis with low-cost providers and include

certain restrictions; and managed care plans, which are really insurance organizations that pay a set price to providers on a per member (capitation) basis. Managed Care plans use primary care physicians to monitor and control the patient's use of more expensive providers of care, such as hospitals and physician specialists. In addition to these newer systems, most insurance beneficiaries have witnessed an increase in deductions and coinsurance percentages in traditional indemnity policies and increased coverage for outpatient medical and surgical care, both of which are intended to guide and control consumer choice regarding cost and use patterns.

In contrast to Blue Cross and Blue Shield, which are generally not-for-profit organizations, the private, for-profit insurers have diversified rapidly. In addition to the alternative delivery systems and other changes noted previously, these firms have merged or joint-ventured with investor-owned hospital chains and voluntary hospital groups in an attempt to create integrated health-care systems on a national or regional basis to include insurance plans, wide-ranging availability of services, and centralized management of resources. Consolidation of health-care providers and insurers will continue as competitors scramble to maintain and improve on their traditional share of the market through enhancement of economic clout.

The Future

What is the effect of the changes in health-care financing for hospitals and their laboratories? With the passing of the "quality at any cost" philosophy that dominated previous decades, the challenge for hospitals in the 1990s and beyond is to provide lower prices and easy access to services while reducing per capita cost and maintaining high standards of quality. Central to this strategy is the redefinition of the hospital's business and diversification away from high-cost, inpatient care.

As more of the decisions regarding the cost and volume of health services to be delivered move from the physician and hospital to the purchasers of care and the growth of managed care systems accelerates, hospitals have focused increasing energy on accounting for and managing inpatient costs and diversifying into outpatient care as a lower cost method for ensuring market share. In either case, the economic mission of the hospital laboratory has shifted from revenue generation *per se* to both the revenue and cost sides of the equation. Mirroring the larger health-care industry, hospital laboratories have increasingly replaced labor with technology; creatively dealt with productivity issues;

merged, consolidated, regionalized, and joint-ventured to achieve economies of scale and market share improvements; and generally become more complete participants in the marketplace.

These trends, of course, make the laboratory's responsibilities considerably more challenging than in the past. The financial techniques, strategies, and approaches discussed in this chapter and the next are now more important than ever, because the laboratory, along with all other hospital departments, is required to be considerably more discerning in its consumption of ever-scarcer resources. Price competition is a reality, and the laboratory must become more productive by producing more with the same or fewer materials and human resources. Familiarity with the types and interrelationships of production costs will be essential to the achievement of higher productivity through cost-containment.

COST, VOLUME, AND REVENUE RELATIONSHIPS

Fixed and Variable Costs

Operating expenditures in a laboratory may be divided into the broad categories of fixed and variable costs. This classification reflects the sensitivity of costs to in-creases or decreases in clinical volume. If a cost changes in more or less direct proportion to volume, it is *variable*. If a cost remains unchanged in total for a set time despite fluctuations in volume, it is *fixed*. Examples of fixed costs include supervisory and custodial wages and benefits required regardless of volume and depreciation of plant and equipment. Variable costs include technologist wages and benefits, reagents, controls, proficiency testing, disposable supplies, and forms. Figures 29–2 and 29–3 graphically display the behavior of variable and fixed costs.

These costs are often difficult to classify definitively. Clerical staff can be reduced given a decrease in clinical activity, but a certain number of such people is required regardless of volume. These are called *mixed costs* and compose a third, more subtle, classification of cost. In addition, fixed costs hold constant only over a *relevant range* of activity. If volume increases or decreases dramatically, all fixed costs become variable to some extent. For instance, even supervisors may be laid off in the event a hospital is compelled to close a substantial number of its beds because of a downturn in business fortunes, consolidation, or mergers.

For the purposes of this discussion, all costs are assumed to be either fixed or variable, and variable costs are assumed to vary in a direct linear relationship with volume. Given these assumptions, Figure 29–4 dis-

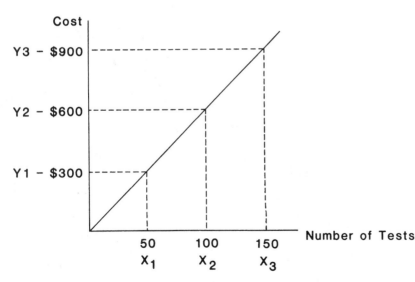

FIGURE 29–2.   Behavior of variable costs. In this figure, a simplifying assumption is made that total variable cost varies directly with the number of tests. For example, as volume increases from X_1 to X_2 total variable cost also increases by the same percentage amount. Thus, $\frac{X_2}{X_1} = \frac{Y_2}{Y_1}$.

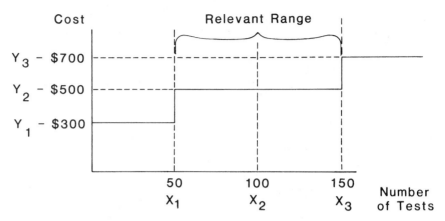

FIGURE 29–3. Behavior of fixed costs. Total fixed cost remains constant at \$500 (Y_2) over all three levels of volume (50, 100, 150 tests) within the relevant range (see Table 29–1). However, should volume drop below X_1 or increase above X_3, associated total fixed cost may decline to Y_1 or rise to Y_3, respectively. The step phenomenon reflects the fact that certain costs remain fixed over large ranges of volume but ultimately become variable to some extent.

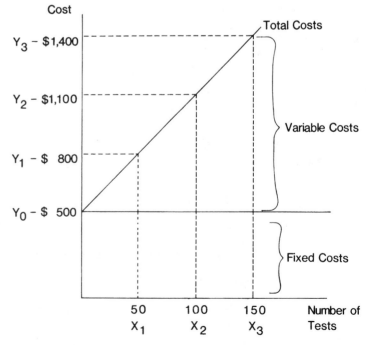

FIGURE 29–4. Total cost curve. In constructing a total cost surve, total fixed cost is assumed to remain at Y_0 (\$500) over all levels of volume, forming the base to which the total variable cost curve is added. For example, if volume increases from X_1 to X_2, total cost will increase from Y_1 to Y_2, and $\frac{X_2}{X_1} = \frac{Y_2 - Y_0}{Y_1 - Y_0}$. Notice that the same variable cost and volume relationship exists in the total cost curve as in Fig. 29–2, except that the constant, Y_0, is subtracted from each cost level. This can be verified by referring to the data in Table 29–1.

plays how fixed and variable components compose total cost. Many factors may affect their behavior, and if the cost of labor, supplies, and other variable operating expenses rises, then total cost will rise, regardless of volume changes. If the diagnostic composition of the patient population changes, costs may rise or fall accordingly. Seasonality may affect volume levels, because there are certain periods when the census is higher or lower than the average.

Direct and Indirect Costs

Direct and indirect costs are another discrete categorization of total costs. All costs that can be specifically linked to a test are *direct costs*. Those costs not directly traceable to the test but included in total laboratory expense are termed *indirect costs*, or *overhead*. Examples of direct costs include technicians, supervisory and clerical personnel, overtime, on-call payments, and reagents and supplies related to the test. Examples of indirect costs include depreciation, building and equipment maintenance, insurance, utilities, housekeeping, purchasing, and billing services.

Unit Costs

For many of the laboratory manager's financial decisions, *unit costs* are crucial. Their analysis helps to identify fluctuations in the cost to produce a given unit of service, thereby permitting measurement of productivity. The first step in calculation is to identify the unit of measurement, usually an individual laboratory test. Many laboratories also use relative value units, discussed in the next two chapters, as the unit of measure.

Next, unit costs are classified into fixed and variable components. Variable costs per unit generally remain the same regardless of volume. Fixed costs per unit, on the other hand, are reduced as the total fixed cost is spread over more tests (Fig. 29–5). Graphically, these illustrations are different from those describing fixed, variable, and total costs. This is because there is a conceptual difference between total costs and total cost per unit. Table 29–1 demonstrates how costs behave as total costs and total costs per unit.[1] As volume increases, variable cost increases by the same percentage, yet on a per-unit basis, variable cost remains unchanged. Likewise, fixed costs remain the same regardless of volume increases, whereas on a per-unit basis, they decline. As can be inferred from Table 29–1, the higher the volume of tests, the lower the total unit cost.

This illustrates the economies of scale available in the active laboratory.

Interaction and Control of Types of Costs

As demonstrated, total variable and fixed costs may be recast to form unit costs. In addition, direct and indirect costs interact with fixed and variable costs. For instance, supervisory personnel are considered a fixed and direct cost of operation. Thus, there are fixed and variable direct costs and fixed and variable indirect costs. Generally, however, direct costs are coincident with variable costs, and indirect costs are consonant with fixed costs. The reader is cautioned not to apply this rule of thumb blithely.

Costs are subject to varying degrees of management control. In general, variable and direct costs are controllable by the manager, and fixed and indirect costs are uncontrollable. However, as noted previously, in unusual circumstances, fixed costs may become variable. The laboratory manager must be continually sensitive to opportunities to control any and all costs, regardless of formal classification.

Accumulation of Direct and Indirect Costs

There are two basic methods for accumulating direct and indirect costs in the laboratory.[5] The first method, *direct costing*, assigns all direct costs to the laboratory. Generally, a *chart of accounts* is used to delineate the appropriate categories within which costs are to be assigned. These natural classifications may be detailed or very broad. For instance, the major direct expense categories are labor and supplies. However, many subdivisions of these broad categories are possible and desirable for analytical purposes. These categories are discussed in greater detail in the next chapter.

The second method, *full costing*, attempts to allocate indirect costs to the hospital laboratory to achieve accumulation of total operating costs. In industry, indirect expenses are transferred to the affected department or allocated on some reasonable basis when the service performed cannot be directly linked to a specific department. Once full costing is completed, *standard costs* are developed that reflect what an efficient department should cost in total, and this costing system is compared with actual costs through *variance analysis*. As such, the cost-accumulation system also serves as a measure of cost effectiveness. In hospitals, the industry norm has been traditionally eschewed for various cost-finding methods. The literature, however, has emphasized the benefits of standard costing and variance analysis for

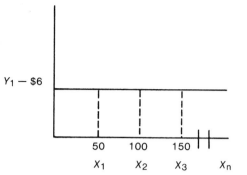

A

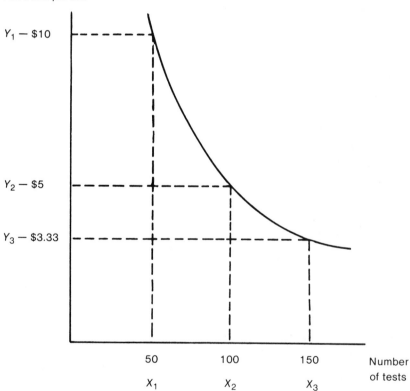

B

FIGURE 29–5.   Graphic representation of units costs. (*A*) Variable cost per unit, Y_1, holds for all levels of activity (Table 29–1). Thus, for X_1, X_2, X_3, . . . , X_n, Y_1 is the variable cost per unit. As volume increases from X_1 to X_3 (*B*), fixed cost per unit decreases from Y_1 to Y_3 (Table 29–1). This is the component of total unit cost that yields economies of scale at higher levels of production.

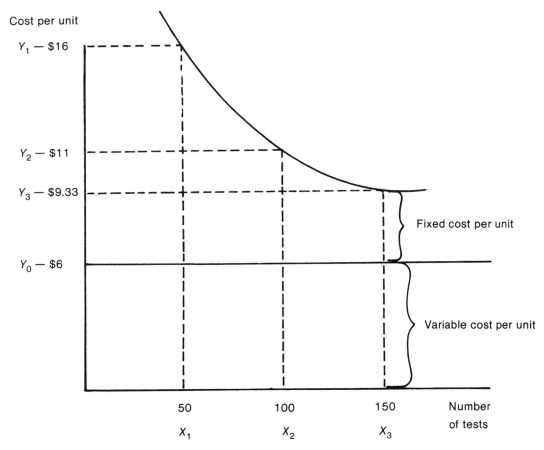

FIGURE 29–5. *continued* Because variable unit cost remains constant at Y_0 (C) over all levels of activity, this cost forms the base on which fixed costs are added. The result of this addition is the total cost per unit curve. Note that as volume increases, total cost per unit declines (Table 29–1).

controlling costs.[5] The reader is encouraged to become familiar with this approach, even though it may not be feasible currently. Although complicated to implement, this system will become more popular as cost-containment pressures increase.

Indeed, several cost-accounting systems used in private industry have been adapted for hospitals and are being incorporated into hospital automated accounting systems. Once implemented, such improvements should help to mitigate a major weakness of current hospital ledger systems: the inability to identify specific unit costs and the concomitant inability to price units of service on a precise costing basis.

Assuming the hospital has not yet attained improved identification of costs through more sophisti-

cated accounting systems, there are generally four methods of cost finding: *direct apportionment, the step-down method, double step-down,* and *algebraic apportionment.* Application of these methods is a task for the hospital finance officer. Should the reader want to explore cost finding in more detail, refer to Berman and Weeks.[2]

Although the laboratory manager may not be involved in the apportionment of indirect costs to cost centers, to the extent that the manager is responsible for setting prices for services provided in the laboratory, a working knowledge of cost-accounting techniques is helpful, because fixed and variable costs of direct and indirect expenses are often identified in the more sophisticated systems.

Table 29-1
Behavior of Total Costs and Unit Costs

	Number of Tests		
	50	100	150
Total Cost			
Variable cost	$300	$600	$900
Fixed cost	500	500	500
Total cost	$800	$1,100	$1,400
Unit Cost			
Variable cost per unit	$6	$6	$6
Fixed cost per unit	$10	5	3.33
Total cost per unit	$16	$11	$9.33

The Break-Even Point

The *break-even* point is the point of laboratory test volume where total revenues equal total costs, and there is neither a profit nor a loss. This point is the baseline for evaluation of changes in revenue, costs, or volume.

In an accounting sense, *net income* equals total revenue less bad debts and allowances minus all variable and fixed costs. Because of the peculiarities of the hospital field, gross charges rarely yield a 100% return in revenue. Reimbursement based on cost, reductions in payments based on discounted charges, and charity care result in deductions from gross charges and are often termed *allowances*. The resulting revenue actually received is gross charges less allowances and bad debts. Any rate setting based on required revenue must take these circumstances into account to ensure that prices are realistic. The subject of price setting is discussed in some detail in the next chapter. The following equation formally defines net income:

Net income = Revenue (gross charges less allowances and bad debts) − Variable costs − Fixed costs

Revenue, then, may be stated as follows:

Revenue = Variable costs + Fixed costs + Net income

If net income is set at zero (ie, no profit or loss), equality between revenue and costs is attained, and the break-even point can be calculated:

Let x = The break-even point in number of tests

   r = Revenue per unit

   v = Variable cost per unit

   f = Total fixed cost

   c = Net income contribution

Then the general formula for the break-even point is as follows:

$$rx = vx + f + c$$
$$rx - vx = f + c$$
$$x(r - v) = f + c$$
$$x = \frac{f + c}{r - v}$$

With the example presented in Table 29–1, v = $6 and f = $500. If we set the unit revenue (r) at $10 and c at zero, then

$$x = \frac{500 + 0}{10 - 6} = \frac{500}{4} = 125 \text{ tests}$$

Thus, 125 tests must be performed to break even. Graphically, the break-even point just calculated is illustrated in Figure 29–6. Note that the break-even point is the intersection of the total cost line and the total revenue line where total cost equals total revenue. The shaded area below the break-even point is the area of net loss; the area above the break-even point is the area of net income.

As stated previously, total revenue is not a 100% reflection of total charges. For instance, if a hospital receives as revenue 80% of total charges, then the hospital must charge 25% more per test, or a total of $12.50, to ensure recovery of the $1,250 required to cover the total fixed and variable costs of producing 125 tests.

Sensitivity Analysis

Assume for the moment that a hypothetical laboratory is currently operating at the break-even point determined in Figure 29–6. What happens if volume, cost, or revenue increases or decreases next year? The method most often used for exploration of future outcome questions is *sensitivity analysis*. This is a "what if" technique that uses data provided from the break-even point analysis and informs the manager about the effects of changes in costs, revenues, volumes, or net income. Several specific examples cited in Box 29–1 illustrate the usefulness of this technique for the laboratory manager.

As can be seen, almost any future situation may be analyzed with the use of current data. Although, at one time, laboratories could produce a net contribution to help cover losses experienced in other revenue-producing departments and to provide for future economic growth of the institution, this is less often the case today.

Although sensitivity analysis is appealing because of its simplicity, caution must be exercised for the same

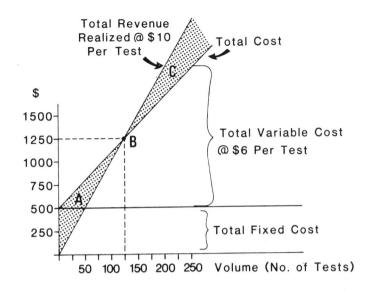

FIGURE 29-6. The break-even point. Break-even occurs at point B where 125 tests are performed. In zone A the test is losing money, and in zone C it is showing a profit.

reason. Remember that before the analysis, all costs were categorized as either variable or fixed (ie, no mixed costs), variable costs were defined as *directly* proportioned to volume, and a relevant range was assumed to exist for all levels of activity. These simplifications make the analysis possible, but they should also temper the manager's interpretation of analytical results. A realistic attitude toward the analysis of costs, especially as they pertain to the unknowns of the future, will serve the prudent manager well. Of course, sensitivity analysis is also useful for evaluating negative trends in operations, including increased costs and volume reductions.

Generally, the easiest variable to affect positively is the containment of costs. Many laboratories now experience strong price competition, and hospital use review can produce a downward trend in the number of tests ordered. Internal laboratory use is an issue that must be addressed: repeats, confirmations, instruments that require more quality control and more calibration than others, and duplicate testing. These are a few of the items the laboratory manager must control.

THE CLINICAL LABORATORY IN HOSPITAL CONTEXT

Role of the Laboratory Manager

The role and responsibility of the laboratory manager will vary depending on the placement of the laboratory and the laboratory manager within the hospital organization structure. Normally the clinical laboratories will be considered one department of the hospital. The per-

son responsible for the management of the laboratory will then report to a member of the hospital administrative staff. Although often a pathologist, the manager can be an administrative technologist or a trained business administrator.

The laboratory manager often will be caught between the competing goals of quality and cost: He or she will be held responsible by the hospital to operate within the budget and professionally obligated to achieve the highest possible level of quality. In the real world, a compromise of cost and quality must be achieved, and this is the province of the laboratory manager.

Laboratory managers must understand what responsibilities they hold for the financial performance of the laboratory and the many other aspects of laboratory management. Who proposes and approves price changes? Who approves adding or deleting a procedure, and what criteria are used to make this decision? Is the revenue budget as much the responsibility of the laboratory manager as is the expense budget? Is the laboratory manager to determine the staffing pattern of the clinical laboratories? These questions and others must be answered before one can comprehend the role of the laboratory manager in a particular setting and fully understand the manager's financial responsibility.

Planned Service Capacity

It is often said that there are distinctions and similarities between the hospital-based clinical laboratory and its free-standing counterpart. However, no single distinc-

Box 29·1

Examples of Sensitivity Analysis

1. Assume that a 20% increase in volume is predicted.

    Because variable costs are assumed to vary directly with volume, variable costs will also increase by 20%. Fixed costs may realistically increase by a small percentage, but in this example they can be assumed to remain constant. Because total revenue also varies directly with volume, total revenue will increase by 20%.

Component	Current	+20% Volume
Volume	125	150
Total revenue @ $10/test	$1,250	$1,500
Variable cost @ $6/test	$750	$900
Fixed cost	$500	$500
Net income	$-0-	$100

    Thus, the volume increase contributes $100 to the hospital's operating surplus. If management does not require these funds, assuming no bad debts or allowances, the test price may be reduced from $10 to 9.33. In a price-competitive market, this reduction could result in a significant market advantage and help to ensure the predicted volume increase. As a practical matter, some midpoint price would probably be selected. In a capitated market, the hospital profit margin would increase, all other factors held constant.

2. Assume a price increase that produces a 20% increase in revenue, again assuming no bad debts or allowances. In this case, volume and all costs are assumed to remain at the current level.

Component	Current	+20% Revenue
Volume	125	125
Total revenue	$1,250	$1,500
	(@ $10/test)	(@ $12/test)
Total Cost	$1,250	$1,250
Net income	$-0-	$250

    The net income contribution can either be added to hospital surplus or it can be a reserve against misestimated volume levels or an unexpected increase in costs. Such a scenario is merely hypothetical in the health-care marketplace of the 1990s.

3. Assume that it is possible to produce the same number of tests with 20% less variable labor, unit revenue remaining the same.

Component	Current	−20% Labor
Volume	125	125
Total revenue @ $10/test	$1,250	$1,250
Variable cost	$750	$600
	(@ $6/test)	(@ $4.80/test)
Fixed cost	$500	$500
Net income	$-0-	$150

    Hence, by virtue of productivity improvement, the laboratory realizes net income in the amount of $150.

4. Finally, assume that management requires a $400 net income, that total costs can be increased a maximum of 18%, and that volume will increase 8%. What price must be charged per test if the laboratory recovers 80% of charges in actual revenue?

Component	Current	Future
Volume	125	135
		(+8%)
Total revenue	$1,250	?
Total cost	$1,250	$1,475
		(+18%)
Net income	$-0-	$400

Total revenue required = Total cost + Net income

$$= \$1,475 + \$400$$

$$= \$1,875$$

$$\text{Unit revenue required} = \frac{\text{Total revenue}}{\text{Volume}}$$

$$= \frac{\$1,875}{135}$$

$$= \$13.89$$

Price per test that must be charged at 80% recovery

$$= \frac{\$13.89}{0.8}$$

$$= 17.36$$

tion so affects the operating cost of the laboratory as its planned service capacity. *Planned service capacity* can be defined as the anticipated volume, time distribution, and array of procedures the laboratory will perform. It is the level to which the laboratory is designed and staffed.

Planned service capacity is often outside the control and influence of the hospital laboratory manager but is determined by such parameters as the parent hospital's goals and objectives, the spectrum of medical and surgical specialties the hospital provides to its community, or its operation as a teaching institution. The clinical laboratory is asked to be all things to all people and to provide each medical discipline with the laboratory diagnostic capabilities it requires and to do so at a moment's notice.

The free-standing laboratory can generally reject such demands on economic grounds alone, but the hospital-based laboratory must come up with a different answer, one that requires all the analytical and political skills the laboratory manager can muster.

Physician demands for service further exacerbate these issues in the laboratory given the advent of DRGs, because any costs assignable to the laboratory, beyond the minimum necessary to care for a patient adequately, expose the hospital to potential operating losses. While the portfolio of tests to be offered to physicians is the one factor most controllable by the laboratory, active education of the hospital's medical staff regarding diagnostic and therapeutic laboratory testing requirements may also be helpful in controlling use. In addition, levels of service beyond the test itself may also be negotiable. For instance, is 24-hour phlebotomy necessary? What tests can and should be batched that were formerly produced on a stat basis? While change in these areas is far more problematic in the hospital environment, the laboratory manager should be alert to all opportunities to reduce costs while still providing effective service at an acceptable quality level.

It is by establishing new in-house procedures only when there is a sufficient cost/benefit justification that the laboratory can maximize its use of resources. New services must be added in a way that maximizes the diagnostic ability of the attending physician and minimizes additions to planned service capacity. Any procedure that cannot achieve its break-even point is a new cost burden to be carried by other procedures. The laboratory manager must always evaluate whether a test can be done more economically. Should a contract with a reference laboratory be undertaken? Is there another

laboratory that has or can develop this expertise and with which a reciprocal relationship can be developed?

These and other questions should be asked and answered as the proposal for establishing a new test is prepared. It is in this process of judicious addition of new or deletion of old procedures that staffing can best be controlled, capital equipment can best be used, and operating expenses can best be contained. It is through this financial and clinical decision-making process that laboratory managers can make their contribution to the health of the clinical laboratory.

REFERENCES

1. Anthony RN, Reece JS: Accounting Text and Cases, 7th ed. Homewood, Richard D. Irwin, 1983
2. Berman HJ, Weeks LE: The Financial Management of Hospitals, 8th ed. Ann Arbor, Health Administration Press, 1994
3. Health United States, 1985. Hyattsville, U.S. Department of Health and Human Services, 1985
4. Health United States, 1994. Hyattsville, U.S. Department of Health and Human Services, 1994
5. Managerial Cost Accounting for Hospitals. Chicago, American Hospital Association, 1980
6. Managing Under Medicare Prospective Pricing. Chicago, American Hospital Association, 1983
7. The Medicare Prospective Payment System (E & W No. J58475). Chicago, Ernst and Whinney, 1983

ANNOTATED BIBLIOGRAPHY

Berman HJ, Weeks LE: The Financial Management of Hospitals, 8th ed. Ann Arbor, Health Administration Press, 1994
    This source presents a complete overview of the major topics confronting health-care financial managers. The discussion includes sources of revenue, budgeting, financial planning, and the management of working capital. See Chapter 6 on Medicare and Medicaid and Chapter 7, Appendix 7.A on cost analysis.
Cleverley WO: Essentials of Health Care Finance. Rockville, Aspen Publishers, 1992
    This is a "how-to" book for those who want to have a better understanding of hospital finance.
Health United States, 1997. Hyattsville, U.S. Department of Health and Human Services, 1997
    This report, prepared annually, presents a wealth of statistical information regarding the status of health care in the United States.
Managerial Cost Accounting for Hospitals. Chicago, American Hospital Association, 1980
    This publication introduces modern cost accounting principles for the management of today's more complex institutions. Major topics include cost classification and behavior, cost analysis, standard costs, variance analysis, and flexible financial reporting.

30

Budgeting Laboratory Resources

David J. Fine • Barbara Caldwell Salmon •
Rohn J. Butterfield • Justin E. Doheny

THE OPERATING EXPENSE BUDGET

Why Have a Budget?

Thirty years ago it was not uncommon for hospitals to operate through an informal process of matching revenues and expenditures without a specific budget. This simple approach to management would seem amazingly primitive for today's health-care executive. Budgeting in businesses of all kinds has matured rapidly in sophistication in recent decades and is now one of the most fundamental building blocks of the well-managed organization. Many factors contribute to the prominence of the budget. Principal among them is the planning and control capability that the carefully formulated budget represents. As an instrument through which the manager projects the near term or longer term revenues and expenses of the entire business entity, or any of its departments, the budget is a guidepost against which actual performance can be measured. A budget agreed to by department manager, administration, and, as appropriate, the governing board, is considered to be the principal tool through which the various levels of an organization achieve financial accountability to one another.[8]

In recent years, as health-care organizations have been called on to be increasingly cost-effective, the expense associated with services rendered has come to receive as high a profile in public policy debates as their quality. Because of this, the budget, which is a systematic expression of the institution's operational plan, is used by external regulatory and reimbursement agencies and by internal management.

It was the Medicare-enabling legislation that first required participating institutions to have a budget. Section 234 of Public Law 92-603 required the following:

An annual operating budget, including income and expenses

A 3-year capital expenditure plan
Annual review and revision
Governing board, medical staff, and administrative participation in the budgeting process

In this context, our discussion focuses on the planning, organizational, and control characteristics of the laboratory budget.

The Budget Forecast and Narrative

The development of a sound budget is highly dependent on clearly stated institutional goals and objectives within which the laboratory has a known role and on which it can base its own specific objectives.

The budget is also dependent on historical data and projections of future activity. For the laboratory, a desirable database would include a weighted procedure volume report for the most recent 5 years or more (Fig. 30–1). Such a weighting sets forth the relative value of each procedure through a process more fully discussed in Chapter 29. Set forth in graphic format (Box 30–1), the data permit trend analysis by the manager.

In addition, the laboratory manager should expect to receive budget guidelines from the institution's financial officer that would include expected inpatient and outpatient census for the budget year, demographics of the patient population, and a concise statement of any anticipated changes in the total service program of the organization. Illustrative of this point might be the creation of a new cancer center, which would result in a significantly expanded load of oncology patients who would require frequent laboratory monitoring. A doubling of capitated managed care resulting in stricter utilization review would be another good example.

The laboratory manager should expect to provide the financial officer with a brief statement of program

473

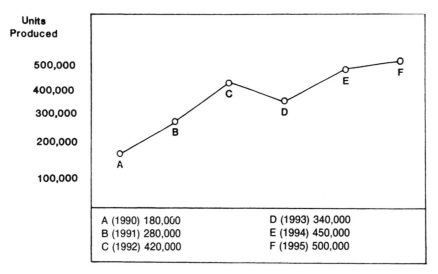

FIGURE 30–1. Procedure volume trend analysis. Here the manager can visualize the growth in relative value units produced from 180,000 in 1990 to 500,000 in 1995. Although steady growth has been experienced, the rate of increase has declined markedly. The conditions contributing to a drop in volume in 1993 should be reviewed to assist in the accurate projection of 1996 volume.

changes that should be planned for as a result of changes in laboratory science or to explain any unusual volume effects resulting from new programs or service needs. Examples of such changes would include procedures that will be diminishing in volume because of obsolescence or physician education, volume estimates for newly implemented procedures, and a technology forecast underlining any predictable changes in laboratory practice for the coming year.

Once these matters have been established, the laboratory manager is in a good position to state the expected volume of activity in terms of procedures per patient day in the least complicated budget approaches, or with more meaning to the laboratory, a specific enumeration of the expected number of procedures by type in each laboratory section in the more advanced methodologies. Although physical counts of procedures may be the practical limit for some organizations, those who are making use of relative value units can avail themselves of a far more useful tool.

The budget presentation is often the only time of year the laboratory manager enjoys a thorough review of operations by the senior management team; therefore, preparation of a budget narrative outlining in a candid way the operational successes and failures of the concluding budget year and a statement of the principal goals and objectives of the coming year are often in order.

Once this basic information has been compiled, the more advanced budget program will often incorporate volume projections specifically by month and day of the week. This ultimately permits far greater sophistication in laboratory staffing and cost analysis. When evaluating staffing, always be aware that key staff members must always be present regardless of volumes. Examples might include a blood bank technician on a second or third shift.

TYPES OF BUDGET

Broadly speaking, institutions select their budgeting approach from among three general systems: the appropriation budget, the fixed forecast budget, or the variable or flexible budget.

Appropriation Budget

This budget is most common to government institutions depending on periodic appropriations from central authorities. Typically, this form of budget will assign a fixed sum to each department. Often expressed in terms of expenditure authority, the appropriation-oriented budget is characterized by inflexibility as a function of

Box 30•1

Natural Classification of Expense—Typical Budget

SALARIES AND WAGES

Regular pay
Overtime pay
Shift differential
Supplemental pay/on call
Personnel/sick leave
Temporaries

EMPLOYEE BENEFITS

FICA
Retirement plan
Health insurance
Dental insurance
Life insurance
Worker's compensation

OPERATING EXPENSES

Departmental supplies
Postage
Data processing
Publishing, printing, photography
Cost of blood
Reference laboratory
Subscriptions
Conference registration
Employee relocation
Job-applicant expense
Equipment rental
Data processing
Repair and maintenance
Travel expense
Medical and clinical contracts
Memberships/dues
Office supplies
Papers/fax/printers
Dietary
Minor equipment
Cylinder gas
Laboratory information system supplies
Microfilm
Reagent rentals
Other expenses
Utilities

clinical volume and poor incentive or reward for the manager.

In the event that expenses run below appropriated levels, the laboratory may have little incentive to return funds to the central authority, because this can often lead to lower appropriations in subsequent years. In the unhappy circumstance of expenses that are higher than budget, any number of authoritarian controls may be imposed.

Fixed Forecast Budget

This budget is probably the most common form in use today and differs in concept from the appropriation budget only in the ease of making programmatic adjustments without resorting to approval from external authorities. In this approach, typically an annual negotiation of expenditure levels is subject to recasting in the event operating assumptions change.

Variable or Flexible Budget

This budget is a more creative tool than either of the traditional approaches mentioned heretofore. Such a budget is developed with the assumption that certain operating expenses are relatively fixed for a given range of clinical activity, whereas others vary directly with the level of activity. Identification of cost elements associated with each component of the budget is often difficult and therefore requires greater data management sophistication.

Once established and given the fine tuning of experience, this approach is an excellent way to set realistic expenditure expectations for the laboratory that obviate the need for frequent renegotiation as the fiscal year progresses. Once the variable and fixed components of cost are negotiated by the laboratory manager, the variable elements will be expressed in terms of expense per unit of output, and the fixed elements will be budgeted in the traditional fashion.[7]

In recent years the *limited-term budget*, generally cast for a single fiscal year, has been replaced by the *continuous budget* in a relatively small number of organizations. In this approach, the manager is continuously updating the budget, replacing the concluding month with a new one so that there is always a 12-month expense forecast. Although the broad applicability of this approach has not yet been established, it is possible to predict that its combination with the variable budget will become increasingly popular with the wider dissemination of computerized financial reporting systems.

The budget is typically segmented into categories of expense called *natural classifications*. Although considerable latitude exists in most instances, some states with significant health-care regulatory activity have mandated classification systems. The objective of the natural classification is to group like expenditures together, with the result that the departmental budget is neither too detailed nor too summarized. Box 30–1 provides a sample natural classification system often used by laboratories. Some institutions will use even more detailed breakdowns, and others may simply divide expenses into the two broad zones of salaries/wages and supplies/materials.

In addition, the total hospital budget is divided into cost centers to permit the accounting process to follow responsibility lines within the organization. For hospitals with more than 250 beds, the laboratory budget usually results in separate cost centers for chemistry, hematology, the blood bank, microbiology, immunology, anatomic pathology, and perhaps others.

Budgeting for Personnel Expenses

Having established the staffing levels required for efficient laboratory operation (see Chap. 13), the budget preparation cycle requires the translation of full-time equivalents (FTEs) into dollars and cents. A necessary first step will be to compare expected laboratory workload for the coming fiscal year as developed in the budget forecast with current staffing levels, making upward or downward adjustments as necessary.[5] This process yields a staffing plan. Although the marginal capacity of laboratories to absorb increased volume without staffing changes in heavily automated areas is high, in manually oriented sections, this is often not the case. Because the effects of understaffing and overstaffing are equally bad for the employee and for the organization, great care must be taken in casting the personnel requirements.

In a typical hospital, personnel expenses constitute almost 60% of total expenditures (Fig. 30–2), and therefore control of this area is fundamental to the efficiency and resulting cost effectiveness of the organization. In addition, assembly of the proper mix of appropriately certified personnel is essential to the assurance of a quality product.

Development of the staffing plan for budgeting purposes is a process entirely separate from scheduling. As a result, it is not appropriate to base the new fiscal year budget on current work schedules. Rather, the reverse is true, and the schedule would be derived from the staffing plan.

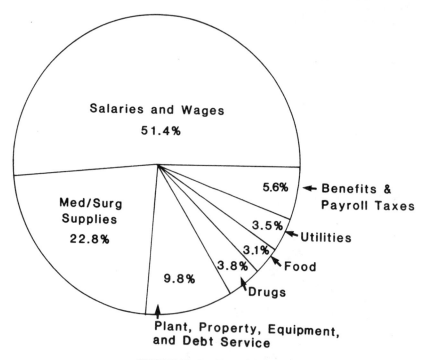

FIGURE 30–2. Typical distribution of hospital expenditures.

Having determined the numbers and types of personnel required, the next step in budgeting is to identify the wage level that will be required to attract qualified individuals in the marketplace. In most instances, the laboratory manager can depend on the personnel department to conduct timely compensation surveys for this purpose. However, the laboratorian may more readily sense shifts in the labor market as a result of wage increases at competing institutions and should communicate this to those charged with administering these matters.

As illustrated in Box 30–1, the personnel budget is divided into several categories. Projection of salaries and wages is an arithmetic process derived from the number of workers in a given category and their hourly, weekly, or monthly wages.

Employee benefits in most organizations are derived by formulas linked to a percentage of wages. As a result, social security insurance, health and life insurance, pension funds, worker's compensation, and other fringes will often be calculated by the financial officer on the basis of departmental wage and salary budgets. The treatment of vacation, holiday, and sick leave for budget purposes will vary from organization to organization as a function of the policies governing their accrual and payment. When employees have no limitations on accrual and are eligible to be paid for unused time off, it is often necessary to budget these benefits specifically. Box 30–1 does not take this approach.

Because of their particular characteristics, most departments are asked to budget overtime and shift differentials separately from regular pay. Shift differentials are reasonably straightforward and are usually a function of the institution's personnel policies. Overtime, however, is often a sensitive matter, and highlighting it in the budget typically results in lengthy management debate.

The obligation to pay overtime wages is defined in the Fair Labor Practices Act and is administered by the Federal Department of Labor. Although the cost premium involved in this payroll category is desirable to avoid, it is in actuality unlikely that the laboratory can function efficiently without some scheduled overtime. In many instances, modest amounts of scheduled overtime are a less costly alternative to adding another employee with attendant training, supervision, and benefit costs. Unscheduled overtime is also a reality in the laboratory, because peak workload levels must be staffed and illnesses covered, and compensatory time off is not an alternative for the nonexempt employee. These issues notwithstanding, the effective manager schedules in a fashion to minimize the number of these high-cost hours.

Administrative costs for part-time employees are slightly higher because of supervision, training, and miscellaneous paperwork. However, their judicious use is one of the manager's creative opportunities to staff for average levels of workload and still meet anticipated peaks on high hospital admission and surgery days, cover vacations, and provide for on-call technologists to cover for sick employees. The advantages of this approach are the avoidance of premium overtime pay for the full-time staff and, in general, limited benefit payments.

Budgeting for Supplies, Materials, and Other Operating Expenses

Box 30–1 suggests the array of expenditure classifications that may be found in a typical laboratory in which detailed budgeting is being emphasized. While all laboratories will not have budget entries in every category, many of them will be used.

Successful budgeting for operating expenses is dependent on the laboratory manager's detailed knowledge of the material ingredient costs of each procedure (see Chap. 35), his accurate estimates of repair and maintenance costs (see Chap. 20), and his determination of employee development standards, including attendance at outside seminars, travel, and other factors.

Probably most significant in the difficult projections required to predict operating expenses is the estimate of price changes that will occur during the fiscal year. When budgeting, it is always important to check with vendors on increases expected during the fiscal year. Projects for new testing or programs must also be budgeted by forecasting expected volumes and the costs associated with these. The prudent manager must plan to provide sufficient funds for such eventualities. Although the materials manager or purchasing agent may be called in for support, the laboratory manager's role in negotiating with vendors cannot be overstated. This is particularly true when product evaluation may permit the substitution of lower cost items or when decisions concerning reusables versus disposables must be made.

Several techniques are used to estimate price escalation of supplies; most common among them is the consumer price index (CPI) to laboratory operating expense ratio.[5] As illustrated in Figure 30–3, operating expenses in the laboratory for supplies and materials are plotted against the CPI. Once derived, the ratio can be applied to the CPI forecast issued quarterly by the federal government.

Perhaps the best means of taking the uncertainty out of supply prices is the fixed price contract through which the laboratory manager can set prices of high-use items for a given length of time, usually 1 year, with succeeding extension years. Although many hospitals still undertake contracting on their own, more are enter-

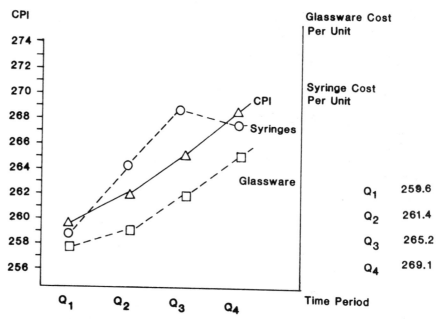

FIGURE 30–3. Ratio of consumer price index (CPI) to laboratory operating expenses. The CPI can be plotted by calendar quarter ($Q_1 \ldots Q_4$) and then compared with the unit cost trend line of a given supply item over the same period. For example, by simultaneously plotting the unit cost of glassware, a manager can establish the historical relationship of the CPI and laboratory glassware. If the two are synchronous, federal government projection of the CPI can be used to project future glassware expenditures at constant levels of volume. Certain supply items, including petroleum derivatives, such as syringes, often do not lend themselves to such a predictive formulation.

ing into consortia for group purchasing, which permits even greater buying leverage and often results in fractional-cent savings on every item used. Mergers and acquisitions by hospital systems have also encouraged large new national purchasing relationships.

The budgeting approach for operating expenses usually begins by projecting the actual expenses of the current year to a full 12 months. From this baseline, the next fiscal year is budgeted by adjusting for anticipated volume and estimated price changes.

Assessing Performance Relative to Budget

As previously mentioned, the budget is a planning document and a control document. To maximize its use as a tool through which control is exercised, it is important to have a financial reporting system that will track actual expenditures against budgeted figures. The financial officer of the organization should be expected to produce a variety of timely reports at the close of each operating

period, usually a calendar month.[2,10] The most common reports are discussed below.

The *departmental trend summary* (Table 30–1) displays the month's expenditures relative to budget and year-to-date totals. In advanced budgeting systems, departments can divide their annual expenses in ways other than $\frac{1}{12}$ for each month to reflect more accurately anticipated clinical activity differences from month to month or an uneven pattern of expense disbursement (eg, maintenance agreements paid semiannually or annually). Also included in this report are workload measures. Sometimes called a general ledger, this report is often presented with monthly columns totaled for the year to date with calculation of percent variation from budget.

The *work force analysis* shows the number of FTEs employed in the cost center, along with an analysis of productive time and overtime. The data in Table 30–2 illustrate a laboratory's chemistry section now at full staffing following 1 year of below-budget salary expenses. The productivity coefficient, 0.82, for the full

Table 30-1
An Abbreviated Departmental Trend Summary for a Clinical Laboratory

Natural Classification	September Budget	September Actual	August Actual	July Actual	YTD Actual	YTD Budget	Variance ($)	Variance (%)
Salaries and Wages								
Technical personnel								
Regular pay	29,500.00	26,686.42	25,923.41	25,761.38	78,371.21	88,500.00	(10,128.79)*	(11.4)†
Overtime pay	1,700.00	2,602.38	2,200.67	1,906.41	6,709.46	5,100.00	1,609.46	31.5
Total	31,200.00	29,288.80	28,124.08	27,667.79	85,080.67	93,600.00	(8,519.33)	(9.1)
Employee Benefits								
Retirement	2,360.00	2,134.91	2,073.87	2,060.91	6,269.69	7,080.00	(810.31)	(11.4)
Health insurance	875.00	807.32	723.22	706.41	2,236.95	2,625.00	(388.05)	(14.8)
Total	3,235.00	2,942.23	2,797.09	2,767.32	8,506.64	9,705.00	(1,198.36)	(12.3)
Operating Expenses								
Repair and maintenance	2,100.00	2,383.46	1,680.44	2,707.39	6,771.29	6,300.00	471.29	7.5
Medical contracts	800.00	627.91	627.91	627.91	1,883.73	2,400.00	(516.27)	(21.5)
Cylinder gas	200.00	198.37	177.62	163.69	539.68	600.00	(60.32)	(10.0)
Other supplies	14,900.00	16,575.64	15,982.21	15,631.13	48,188.98	44,700.00	3,488.98	7.8
Total	18,000.00	19,785.38	18,468.18	19,130.12	57,383.68	54,000.00	3,383.68	6.3‡
Total	52,435.00	52,016.41	49,389.35	49,565.23	150,970.99	157,305.00	(6,334.01)	(4.0)
Workload units	41,650	43,621	40,790	41,000	125,411	124,950	(461)	(0.4)

* Parentheses denote favorable variance.
† This department is 11.4% below budget in technical personnel. The strong clinical volume supports the 31.5% higher than budgeted overtime and suggests the manager may be facing some technician recruitment difficulty.
‡ Operating expenses are running 6.3% above budget, owing primarily to supplies. This figure is not consistent with workload and suggests either unusually high purchasing levels in the current period, price increases that have not been properly planned for in a budgeting sense, or extraordinary utilization. Management intervention is indicated to establish the cause and to take appropriate corrective action.
YTD, year to date.

year is a manager's index to the percentage of paid time consumed by training, illness, vacation, and other non–production-oriented functions. For obvious reasons, it would be unusual to see a figure above 0.90.

Perhaps the most important report for the cost-conscious manager is the *profit and loss statement* (P&L). As more fully set forth later in this chapter, revenue is budgeted and actual collections can be plotted against actual expense to yield the profit-or-loss position of the laboratory. As in any business, a certain profit margin is necessary to provide for capital improvements and program development, and the P&L is the acid test of the manager's performance in this regard. Income and expenses that are out of synchrony are the inevitable alarm signal for the department head. An example of a P&L for a pathology department is shown in Table 30–3.

Table 30-2
Work Force Analysis—Chemistry Section

Period	Full Time Equivalent		$		Overtime			Productivity
	Budget	Actual	Budget	Actual	Hours	$ Budget	$ Actual	
June	14.9	14.9	20,179	19,920	0	800	0	0.85
YTD	14.9	12.4	242,148	205,826	973.8	9600	11,245	0.82

YTD, year to date.

Table 30-3
Profit and Loss Statement—Pathology—For the Nine Months Ending March 31

	This Month			*Year to Date*		
	Budget	Actual	Variance	Budget	Actual	Variance
Gross revenue	395,000	407,058	+12,058*	3,400,000	3,630,044	+230,044
Allowances	15,000	28,494	−13,494†	136,000	181,502	−45,502
Net revenue	380,000	378,564	−1436	3,264,000	3,448,542	+184,542
Salaries and benefits	159,316	148,000	+11,316	1,433,844	1,375,422	+58,422
Operating expenses	76,596	85,000	−8404	703,872	758,733	−54,861
Total direct expenses	235,912	233,000	+2912	2,137,716	2,134,155	+3561
Overhead (0.32)	74,761	74,560	+201	684,069	682,930	+1139
Surplus (deficit)	69,327	71,004	+1677	442,215	631,457	+189,242

* The + denotes favorable variance.
† The − denotes unfavorable variance.

Although administrative practices vary a good deal from organization to organization, today's laboratory manager should seek accountability for what is known as bottom-line performance, another term for profitability or net income. In too many organizations, the laboratory manager is held accountable only for adequate control of expense. It is the authors' opinion that this traditional approach fails to offer the department head sufficient understanding of the laboratory's contribution to the hospital as a whole.

Many other financial reports are produced regularly, including balance sheets, fund-balance statements, and cost reports. Because these have less direct applicability to the laboratory manager, they are not discussed here. For further information, consult the sources listed in the chapter bibliography.

CAPITAL DECISION MAKING

Preliminary Considerations

In addition to the need for careful operational budgeting, some method must be developed to allocate resources for major investments in buildings and equipment. This process is called capital budgeting. There is a dependent relationship between the operating and capital budgets, because efficiency of operations may largely depend on the wisdom of capital-acquisition decisions.

The capital-budgeting decision is important for another, more obvious reason. As Berman and Weeks have noted, "If an error in judgment is made, the costs of the decision error can be expected to be incurred over a considerable length of time."[3] For instance, if the purchased equipment does not operate efficiently or is underused, a high cost may be incurred over time in lost revenue and increased expenses.

In accounting terms, a capital item is generally called a fixed asset expected to provide service for more than 1 year.[1] This general definition of a capital item can lead to confusion about what should properly be classified as capital, and some additional guidelines may be helpful:

Repair and maintenance costs should be differentiated from improvements. Maintenance and repair work keeps the equipment in good condition and is treated as an expense in the operating budget. Improvements or upgrades that make equipment better than when it was purchased are treated as a capital expenditure.

Generally, the replacement of an entire fixed asset is a capital expenditure; the replacement of a component part is an operating expense. Some institutions place a maximum dollar limit on component parts under which replacement is an operating expense and over which, a capital expense.

There are subtleties in types of leasing arrangements that define an expense as either a capital or an operating item.

Relatively low-cost items that meet the 1-year criterion are often classified as capital expenditures initially but are treated as operating expenses when replaced (eg, furniture and items under $500 or some other set dollar figure).

Given the critical nature of capital decisions for laboratories and for any business enterprise using high-cost equipment, it is incumbent on the laboratory manager to be fully cognizant of the methodologies used in analyzing capital-investment alternatives.

Before applying precise decision techniques, the hospital clinical laboratory should first determine a budgeting period. In the case of capital equipment, there are usually two periods: a short-term, or 1-year, horizon and a long-term, or 3- to 5-year, horizon.

As in operational budgeting, it is also necessary to identify clearly the goals and objectives of the laboratory. Goals should be specific and based on planned new programs and projections of future workload. Objectives of the laboratory should be consonant with hospital goals and objectives, with consideration given to information regarding new hospital services that impact the laboratory's capabilities. Laboratory capital decisions are then examined in light of the needs specified in the department's goals and objectives. A word of caution must be interjected here. The viability of a long-range set of goals is largely dependent on the accuracy of prediction. The longer the time horizon, the more likely it is that predictions will fall prey to the risks inherent in the basic uncertainty of the future. Therefore, a flexible attitude toward the capital plan must be assumed, and at least annual review of the plan must take place.

Another major intervening factor in the capital-budgeting process is the inevitable political reality of prioritization of competing demands. A prioritized departmental capital-acquisition list, which has already weathered departmental and sectional politics, must then be cast in with other departmental lists for prioritization at the institutional level. While the ideal situation would be a simple matching of institutional goals with departmental requests and available funds, projects of influential departments, particularly at medical centers, may often appear as non sequiturs on the capital plan of the hospital. This does not necessarily imply that projects have been considered capriciously; there are usually solid reasons for the ultimate decision. The point is made primarily to emphasize the enormous complexity involved in making such important determinations.

Finally, development of a detailed hospital long-range plan involves significant expense and may include extensive marketing studies. Because not all organizations are able to afford such research, hospital long-range plans are quite variable in their relative sophistication. These cautionary notes should not dissuade laboratory managers from attempting to develop a worthwhile long-range plan for the laboratory. On the contrary, reduction of risk associated with capital decisions is, to a great extent, a function of the rigor with which the capital budget is developed.

Capital Budget Categories

The capital budget is generally divided into two categories. The first is composed of relatively low-cost items, perhaps under $5,000, for which the level of analysis is normally minimal. All that is typically required is a simple outline of the costs involved; classification of the request as a replacement, new item, renovation, or improvement; and a brief narrative justification. Items in this category may be given simple numeric priority rankings or classified into groups[3] (Box 30-2).

In this manner, decisions may be made either sequentially through priority rankings or categorically. Some consideration might be given to both methods to ensure greater flexibility.

The other major category of the capital budget is for all items over $5,000. This category usually is split into yearly purchase requests over a 3- to 5-year period. It is at this point that the level of analysis must increase significantly. While the basic classification format for high-cost items remains the same as for low-cost items, support documentation becomes more detailed and specific[3] (Box 30-3).

The last two elements are often difficult to estimate. Data on expected cash inflows and outflows, however, are crucial to the analytical techniques to be used in the evaluation of capital alternatives, and a few guidelines should aid in their identification.[11]

Consider only incremental amounts. What *additional* cash outflows and inflows will occur as the direct result of this project above and beyond those that would occur anyway?

Only *cash* inflows and outflows should be counted. Accounting statements of revenue and expense are generally unreliable as estimates of actual cash generated or spent, unless accounting is on a cash

---

Box 30•2

Categories of Capital Budget Items

1. Capital expenditures necessary for continuance of present service or new equipment required for volume growth
2. Capital items that represent a cost savings or profit with the present service volume and mix
3. Capital items that represent an improvement in the quality or effectiveness of present services
4. Capital items related to new programs or improvement of existing programs

basis. The ideal to be sought here is the actual change in cash that occurs because of the project, not what the accountant will report as expenses and revenues.

Data Analysis Techniques

After the major capital list has been prioritized on the basis of perceived need, supporting data must be gathered for further refinement of priorities. Because capital items are so important in providing for the financial strength of the hospital laboratory and in helping to ensure the viability of future growth, an attempt must be made to ensure a reasonable return on the investment. Generally, the hospital's financial officer will provide the laboratory with a return percentage, called a *required rate of return*. In the following discussion, a 15% rate is used.

The actual required rate of return on a project may be based on a number of single factors or be a combination of all factors. Elements generally considered are listed in Box 30–4.

Depreciation is another datum required for the analysis of capital alternatives. Depreciation recognizes the fact that fixed assets have a limited useful life. Therefore, depreciation is an accounting method whereby "a fraction of the cost of a fixed asset is properly (charged) as an expense in each of the accounting periods in which the asset is used."[1] Because useful lives of assets

are difficult to establish accurately, the fraction expensed each year is generally an estimate.

Standard accounting practices sanction several methods for determining the size of the fraction expensed. *Straight-line depreciation* is the most commonly recognized means of expensing fixed assets. In this method, the estimated useful life in years is divided into the total acquisition cost of the item, expensing the result in each period:

$$\frac{\text{Item's acquisition price} = \$10,000}{\text{Estimated useful life} = 10 \text{ years}}$$

$$= \$1,000 \text{ per year expensed as depreciation}$$

A case example demonstrating the evaluation of a capital purchase is shown in Box 30–5. As noted previously, cash inflows must be incremental. In the case of the hypothetical automated differential counter, year 1 cash inflows and outflows are estimated to be \$75,000 and \$25,000, respectively. The inflow figure reflects cash that would not be realized if the counter were not purchased. Likewise, the outflow figure represents cash that would not be spent if the counter were not purchased. Outflows are then subtracted from inflows to yield a net cash-flow figure to be used for future decision analysis. This same calculation is performed for all remaining years of the equipment's useful life, yielding a complete net cash-flow schedule.

Finally, in the case of the differential counter, cash outflows increase over time, and cash inflows decrease over time. While this need not be the case for all projects considered, it is a fairly typical pattern for capital investments. For instance, as the differential counter gets older, repair and maintenance costs can be expected to

Box 30·5

Case Example—Purchase of an Automated Differential Counter

An automated differential counter is purchased for $125,000. The equipment's useful life is estimated to be 5 years. Yearly depreciation is established at $25,000 with the straight-line method. Estimated yearly cash inflow generated by the machine is hypothetically as follows:

Year 1 = $75,000
Year 2 = $75,000
Year 3 = $67,000
Year 4 = $60,000
Year 5 = $50,000
Total = $327,000

Estimated yearly cash outflows related to the machine are estimated to be as follows:

Year 1 = $25,000
Year 2 = $25,000
Year 3 = $30,000
Year 4 = $35,000
Year 5 = $40,000
Total = $155,000

Calculated net cash flow for each year is then as follows:

Year 1 = $50,000 ($75,000 − 25,000)
Year 2 = $50,000 ($75,000 − 25,000)
Year 3 = $37,000 ($67,000 − 30,000)
Year 4 = $25,000 ($80,000 − 35,000)
Year 5 = $10,000 ($50,000 − 40,000)
Total = $172,000

Purchase Price
$125,000
Cash Flows
Year 1 = $50,000
Year 2 =   50,000
Year 3 =   37,000
              $137,000
Payback
$50,000 + $50,000 + $25,000
Year 1 + Year 2 + 0.58 years = 2.68 years

rise. Resulting downtime from this activity will generally yield some loss in revenue. In addition, equipment purchased in future years may replace or negatively affect procedure volume performed on the differential counter or use patterns may change, rendering it underused or obsolete.

Payback Analysis

The *payback method* is examined first because it is the simplest approach and has retained some value over time. This method calculates the point in the useful life of the differential counter when the original investment is recovered from cash flows. Alternative capital projects can be ranked, and the shortest payback is the most desirable financially.

This method has received much criticism because it does not recognize the time value of money (discussed in succeeding paragraphs) and ignores cash flows beyond the payback period. While these are certainly valid points, there are significant benefits to this approach as well.[9] The method is useful for comparing projects having roughly the same benefits and economic life and is valuable as a crude measure of risk, because it favors projects with a short time horizon for payback. Specifically, this reduces the impact of uncertainty inherent in longer time horizons.

Average Rate of Return

A second method has been termed *average rate of return* (ARR).[11] In this approach, an attempt is made to average the initial investment over the useful life of the project and compare this with the average investment return over the same period. Average annual investment return divided by average annual investment yields the ARR (Box 30–6).

The concept of average annual investment may be somewhat confusing, because it does not represent an actual cash flow in each year, as does the average annual investment return. For purposes of analysis, average annual investment means the average amount of the original investment still tied up in the differential counter each year. Conservative calculations of ARR use the initial investment as the denominator. Thus,

$$ARR = \frac{\text{Average annual investment return}}{\text{Initial investment}}$$

$$\frac{\$ \ 34,400}{\$125,000} = 27.5\%$$

Box 30·6

Calculation of Average Annual Investment Return

Sum of cash flows = $172,000
Useful life = 5 years
Average annual investment return =

$$\frac{\text{Sum of cash flows}}{\text{Useful life}} = \frac{\$172,000}{5 \text{ years}} = \$34,000$$

CALCULATION OF AVERAGE ANNUAL INVESTMENT

Initial investment = $125,000
Annual depreciation (straight line) = $25,000
Investment in counter over six years =
Year 1 = $125,000
Year 2 = $100,000
Year 3 = $75,000
Year 4 = $50,000
Year 5 = $25,000
Year 6 = $-0-
Sum of years 1 through 6 = $375,000
Average annual investment =

$$\frac{\text{Sum of years 1 through 6}}{6} = \frac{\$375,000}{6} = \$62,500$$

CALCULATION OF AVERAGE RATE OF RETURN

$$\text{ARR} = \frac{\text{Average annual investment return}}{\text{Average annual investment}} = \frac{\$34,400}{\$62,500}$$

$$= 5.5\%$$

If cash flows in this example had actually been equal for each year of the useful life (ie, $34,400 for years 1 through 5), payback would have been 3.63 years. ARR would then simply have been the reciprocal of payback, or 1 ÷ 3.63 27.5%.

Regardless of the ARR approach used, alternative projects considered are ranked, the highest ARR being most desirable. Although this method does make an attempt to account for all cash flows, its major weakness is a lack of recognition for the impact of time. Thus, taking an extreme example, two proposals may be calculated to have the same ARR, but one project may return all of its investment in the first year and the other in the last year. In such a case, the former project would be more desirable because funds would be freed sooner for other investments. Averaging blurs this important decision criterion.

The Concept of Present Value

The time factor has been demonstrated to be of importance when considering investment proposals. The time value of money is sometimes difficult to understand intuitively and is worthy of some exploration prior to discussing analytical techniques using the concept.[1]

When growing up, many people were taught to save money in their piggy banks. They were congratulated when the bank was opened and the coins counted. At that time, they learned implicitly that it was better to have money in the future than in the present, that the value of money in the present is less than its value in the future.[1]

In business, however, the values are different. The expectation in this arena is that money invested today should *increase* in value in the future, that a return on today's investment must be realized. Thus, money that is available for investment today is more valuable than an equal amount of money that will not be available until some point in the future. As a result, the manager values an amount of money in the present more than the same amount in the future.

The concept of present value is so important to capital investment analysis that it deserves precise definition. Anthony and Reese[1] provide the following: "The present value of an amount that is expected to be received at a specified time in the future is the amount which, if invested today at a designated rate of return, would cumulate to the specified amount." The formula for calculating the present value of $1.00 to be received *n* years in the future at a required rate of return *i* is

$$\frac{\$1.00}{(1 + i)^n}$$

The numerator is generally referred to as the *future value*, because it is the amount to be received in the future, in this example, $1.00.

Because in the example of the counter, cash flows will be received at the end of a number of periods, the additive effect of multiple periods must be calculated. For equal yearly cash flows, the general formula for present value is

$$PV = CF \left[\frac{1 - (1 + I)^{-n}}{I} \right]$$

where PV present value of all cash flows and CF yearly cash flow. For unequal yearly cash flows, as in the counter, the general formula is

$$PV = \frac{CF_1}{(1 + i)^1} + \frac{CF_2}{(1 + i)^2} + \frac{CF_3}{(1 + i)^3} + \dots \frac{CF_n}{(1 + i)^n}$$

where $CF_1 \dots n$ = cash flows in year 1 to n.

It is not necessary to undertake this calculation manually because present value tables exist for this purpose, and modern financial calculators are preprogrammed for this use.

Net Present Value

The first method using the time value of money is the technique of *net present value* (NPV). NPV is the present value of all cash flows minus the initial investment. If the NPV is positive or zero, then the project is generally considered financially acceptable. This is because all future cash flows have been converted into current dollars, with the use of a pre-established required rate of return and then have been compared with the initial investment. However, small negative NPVs should also be examined for possible inclusion in the list of acceptable projects, because other factors may influence acceptability, including risk inherent in the project, size of initial investment, and benefits to patients. Returning to the case of the automated differential counter, Box 30–7 demonstrates how NPV is calculated.

Given the decision rule, the project could be rejected. In practice, given the small negative result and the large investment cost, the project might usefully be accepted as financially viable given a 15% required rate of return. Aside from this subtlety, the manager must also evaluate investment size with respect to competing alternatives. A large investment ranking the same as a small investment in terms of NPV may not be as wise as the smaller project, because it involves the commitment of considerably more absolute dollars for the same return. This may be rectified by constructing *profitability indices*1 and ranking projects accordingly. This is done by dividing present value by initial investment, the highest index being most desirable.

Also, given varying useful lives of alternative projects, some method must be found for equating useful lives to ensure proper comparison. There are several sophisticated methods for approximating equal useful lives, but a crude technique[1] is to take the shortest useful life, say 5 years, and use only the first 5 years of longer lived projects for comparative purposes. Cash flows beyond year 5 would be treated as part of the cash flow in year 5.

Time-Adjusted Return Method

Another method using the time value of money may be termed the *time-adjusted return* method. This technique does not require the selection of a required rate of return. Instead, it "computes the rate of return which equates the present value of the cash flows with the amount of the investment; that is, that rate which makes the net present value equal zero."[1] The resulting rate is termed the *internal rate of return* (IRR). Alternative project proposals are then ranked from highest to lowest IRR, highest being most desirable. Those projects not meeting management's preset required rate of return, in this case 15%, may be discarded after review.

Calculation of the IRR for a project is relatively simple for even yearly cash flows, because present value tables may be used. For uneven cash flows, however, the rate must be determined through a time-consuming iterative mathematic process. Many current financial calculators quickly compute IRR, and this has simplified the process enormously.

With the use of a calculator, the IRR for the differential counter under consideration can be determined as 14.949%. The accuracy of this figure can be verified by referring to the discussion of NPV, where NPV nearly equaled zero at the 15% required rate of return.

The major potential weakness of this method is that an implicit assumption is made that all cash flows are reinvested for the rest of the project's useful life at the same IRR.[9] This is not a problem if the laboratory realizes a 14.949% return on all of its other investments. However, if the average return is only 10%, the reinvestment assumption of 14.949% is unrealistic. Because the NPV method uses a common required rate of return, it is not subject to the same criticism and is therefore generally the method of choice.

Table 30–4 presents a comparison of each of the analytical techniques discussed and may help to put the four methods into perspective.

Box 30•7

Calculation of Net Present Value

Initial investment = $125,000. Required rate of return, I = 15% n = 5 years

Year 1 = $50,000
Year 2 = $50,000
Year 3 = $37,000
Year 4 = $25,000
Year 5 = $10,000
PV − Initial investment = PV − $125,000

Where PV = $124,879
NPV = $124,879 − $125,000 = −$121

Table 30-4
Data Analysis Techniques—Alternative Project Evaluations

Method	Calculation	Ranking System	Decision Rule	Benefits	Deficiencies
Payback	Years until original investment recovered from cash flows	Shortest to longest payback in years	Shortest payback best	Useful for comparing projects with similar useful lives A crude measure of risk	No recognition of time value of money Ignores cash flows beyond payback
Average rate of return (ARR)	Average yearly return as percentage of average yearly investment	Highest positive to lowest positive ARR	Highest ARR best	Accounts for all cash flows	No recognition of time value of money Blurs differences in timing of cash flows
Net present value (NPV)	PV minus initial investment	Highest positive to lowest positive NPV	Highest NPV best	Accounts for time value of money Evaluates projects at same required rate of return	Ignores differences in investment size Comparison of projects with different useful lives difficult
Time-adjusted return (TAR)	Rate of return at which NPV equals zero; result is internal rate of return (IRR)	Highest to lowest IRR; rejected it below required rate of return	Highest IRR best	Accounts for time value of money	Usefulness questionable if IRR is substantially different from actual expected return on reinvestment

Capital Budgeting—The Decision Process

While all of these techniques are useful in the financial evaluation of proposed projects, final prioritization of projects for the capital budget must address other factors as well. Each of the classifications in the section on capital budget categories may be examined. Projects in the first category may not require detailed financial analysis, because they are required to maintain the existing level of service. On the other hand, projects in the second category, those that increase profit or produce a cash savings given present service levels and patient mix, are particularly well suited to financial evaluation. Those projects improving the quality or effectiveness of present services and those relating to new programs should generally be subject to financial and benefit

analysis. Benefit analysis, not considered here, is often highly problematic and subjective, but efforts have been made to quantify the evaluation and link it with the financial analysis to achieve an overall ranking of such projects. The reader is referred to Berman and Weeks[3] for a good discussion of this technique.

Once all four categories have been adequately ranked, the stage is set for final determination of items to be included in the capital budget. Generally, projects in the first category should be funded first, followed by second, third, and fourth category projects. However, the laboratory manager or the capital planning committee of the hospital may want to pick some projects from each category, depending on the overall needs of the laboratory or hospital and the available funding resources.

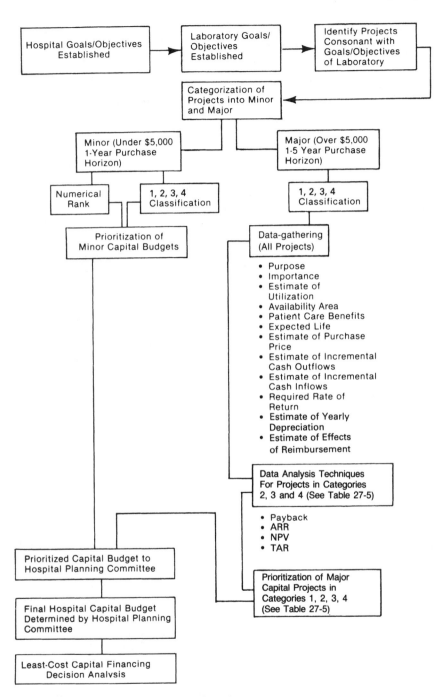

FIGURE 30–4. Capital decision-making flow chart.

While it must be re-emphasized that the decision phase of capital budgeting is subject to considerable adjustment of priorities, the decision makers will have the best available objective data if one of the above formulations is used. A schematic representation of the capital budgeting process is shown in Figure 30–4.

Alternative Choice Financing Decisions

Once the decision to acquire capital items has been made, financial analysis techniques may be used again to evaluate the least costly financing alternative.[4] A common decision of this type for the laboratory manager is the lease-or-buy decision, which is an example of present value analysis. Basically, there are two kinds of leases: cancelable and noncancelable. If the laboratory can cancel the lease and stop making payments at any time, the lease is treated as an operating expense according to generally accepted accounting principles. This is termed an operating lease. If a lease is noncancelable for the period of the lease and there is an option to purchase, it is viewed as a form of borrowing for a purchase and is treated as an asset, or capital acquisition, for accounting purposes. Such leases are termed capital leases and are included in the capital budget.

While this distinction has important implications for operating and capital budgets, it does not affect the basic lease-or-buy decision. Generally, the three choices open to the laboratory manager are to purchase from internal funds, to borrow funds, and to obtain a lease. With the present value technique, costs associated with each alternative need to be analyzed. A general example follows:

Purchase From Hospital Funds

Present value = Initial investment

Five-Year Lease

Present value = Annual lease payments discounted at the
                 hospital's required rate of return for period
                 of the lease

Borrow Funds

Present value = Annual loan payments and associated inter-
                 est, discounted at the hospital's required rate
                 of return for period of the loan

With this general example in mind, the automated differential counter is examined in Box 30–8. Given the results, the 5-year lease is the best method of financing the counter's acquisition because it is the lowest cost financing alternative.

At this level of analysis, the alternative with the *lowest* present value is the best method of financing the acquisition.[4]

Box 30•8

Case Example—Financing of Automated Differential Counter Acquisition

PURCHASE WITH HOSPITAL FUNDS

Cash outflow = <u>$125,000</u>

FIVE-YEAR LEASE

Required rate of return = 15%
Annual lease payment = $30,000
Present value of 5-year lease discounted at 15%
   = <u>$100,565</u>

FIVE-YEAR LOAN AT 12%

Required rate of return = 15%
Annual loan payment at 12% interest = $30,961
Present value of loan payments discounted at 15%
   = <u>$103,786</u>

Assuming the hospital has decided on a noncancelable lease and does not have access to a salvage market at the end of the lease, the analysis ends at the level described in the example. If the hospital does have a salvage market, there is a simple method by which one can further analyze the viability of the lease or purchase.

First, the manager subtracts the present value of the lease from the present value of the purchase. Given that the lease was chosen, the resulting number will be positive and represents the present value of the amount that must be provided from future resale. Then the required future resale price is calculated and compared with the manager's best estimate of future market conditions. If the manager believes the item can be sold for more than the required future resale price, then purchase is the correct decision; if the item cannot be sold at the required future resale price, leasing is the best alternative. The same procedure may be used in lease-or-loan decisions. An example of this analysis in the case of the differential counter is shown in Box 30–9.

REVENUE BUDGET AND RATE SETTING

Revenue Budget

As will be recalled from the discussion of the breakeven point and sensitivity analysis in Chapter 29, there is a crucial relationship among volume, cost, and revenue. While the expense budget outlined in this chapter incorporates the volume and cost factors to yield an oper-

Box 30•9

Case Example—Financing of Automated Differential Counter Acquisition with Availability of a Salvage Market

LEASE OR PURCHASE

Present value of purchase = \$125,000
Present value of lease = \$100,565
Present value of resale = Present value of purchase −
Present value of lease = \$125,000 − 100,565 = \$24,435
Required future value of resale to provide for present value of resale = PV $(1 + 1)^1$
where PV = Present value of resale = \$24,435
   i = Required rate of return = 15%
   n = 5
Required future
value of resale   = \$24,435 $(1 + 0.15)^3$
            = \$24,435 $(1.15)^5$
            = \$24,435 (2.01)
            = $\underline{\$49,148}$
The required resale price at the end of period 5

LEASE OR LOAN

Present value of loan = \$103,786
Present value of lease = \$100,565
Present value of resale = \$103,786 − 100,565 = \$3,221
Required future   = \$3,221 $(1 + 0.15)^5$
value of resale   = \$3,221 (2.01)
          = $\underline{\$6,479}$
The required resale price at end of period 5

FINANCING DECISIONS BASED ON RESIDUAL MARKET ANALYSIS

Resale Price Assumption	Appropriate Decision
\$0–\$5,478	Lease
\$6,479	Indifferent to lease or loan
\$6,480–\$49,147	Loan
\$49,148	Indifferent to lease or purchase
\$49,149+	Purchase

ating plan, some mechanism must be developed for forecasting the revenue required to ensure institutional viability.

The *revenue budget* is a forecast of expected gross charges, deductions from gross charges, and resulting revenue. The forecast revenue requirements may take many forms given the goals and objectives of the institution.

In many institutions, the expense budget is completed prior to the revenue budget. However, it is often more logical to project revenue first. Most hospitals find there are always more requests than can be reasonably supported from available revenue. Given a preliminary revenue projection, expenses can be budgeted hospital wide to meet that projection. This permits the overall budgeting process to be iterative, giving a target for the expense budget. Many prospective reimbursement plans are just that; hospitals negotiate a fixed level of revenue from a given third-party payer and then must perform their service within that previously negotiated limit. This, of course, is also true of Medicare's prospective payment system (PPS), except that the established price is not negotiable.

Regardless of whether the expense or revenue budget is prepared first, they both must be matched to produce a positive net income. If the expense budget is so large that it cannot be supported by expected revenue and revenue cannot be further increased, then reductions must be made in the expense budget. This may necessitate two or more cycles in preparation of the expense and revenue budgets. In many institutions, the successive budgeting cycles will be completed by senior management without the involvement of the laboratory manager; however, a number of hospitals now include their managers in the later stages of budgeting to ensure a sense of ownership for the budget by the departmental executive and because they often have the best knowledge of service needs.

Rate Setting

Rate setting in the health-care field is the subject of much study and recent progress. Certain basic principles are generally accepted, and there are a limited number of approaches to determining rates in the laboratory. The basic philosophy underlying rate setting is that there should be equity among all patients. This means that the charge for a given service should reasonably reflect the cost of providing the service.[6]

The second principle is that aggregate rates must cover all costs. Expressed in another way, rates must be structured to meet the full financial requirements of the institution. In Chapter 29, the various components of cost were defined. These components include direct costs, such as personnel, supplies, and reagents, and indirect costs, such as heat, light, administration, and others. In addition to these costs, a variety of other expenses must be covered by revenue, including bad debts, charity care, and the cost of capital acquisition. The laboratory will usually be allocated a specific dollar amount of these expense items to support from its revenue. In the for-profit sector of the health-care field, return to the investors must also be taken into account.

The third principle is that profit centers, departments that generate income over and above their level of direct and indirect expense, must support departments that do not cover the full costs of delivering their services. It was once commonplace for hospital administrators to require that the laboratory and other service areas, such as pharmacy, radiology, central supply, and the operating rooms, operate at a profit to offset losses in other areas, such as labor and delivery and the emergency room. This required contribution would vary, depending on the financial requirements of the individual hospital. However, it can be expected that the surcharge would fall in the range of 10% to 90% of direct and indirect cost, although a higher percentage may be required. With the onset of managed care, the laboratory can no longer, in many cases, provide this contribution. As a result, hospitals are looking at methods of reducing costs, which may include consolidations, flattening of organizations, and seeking outside revenues.

Although these principles hold true in the main, there is a corollary to the third principle: When payment to the hospital for laboratory services is not based on a test as the unit of service, test prices set by the hospital are diminished in importance. For instance, under the PPS, Medicare payments are based on the discharge as the unit of service, and all hospital services become cost centers in relation to the single discharge profit center. In some cases, health maintenance organizations pay hospital expenses on a *per diem* or per stay basis, again focusing attention on the cost of producing a day's care or a patient stay in relation to the overall negotiated price. In such cases, all the rate-setting principles are still applicable to the specified unit of service; however, laboratory tests are but one of the costs of producing that unit, and the tests are not priced units per se.

Managed care systems in some parts of the country represent the majority of admissions at hospitals and are growing rapidly in importance. Regardless of the method of payment for laboratory tests, however, the incentives to identify and control costs effectively to ensure market competitiveness are pervasive.

Rate-Setting Techniques

Three rate-setting mechanisms are recommended by the American Hospital Association for use in ancillary service areas. They are hourly rates, surcharge, and the weighted-value basis.[6] The weighted-value method is most frequently used in laboratories, but the other approaches are worthy of comment and brief description.

The hourly rate method is useful in departments where the service provided to the patient can be reasonably correlated to the time required for the procedure. This method is commonly used in the operating room and may be used in labor and delivery and apheresis sections of some laboratories. This method requires the calculation of the total cost of the department, including direct and indirect costs. A projection of the hours the facility is used is then made, and the charges are billed on the basis of cost per hour.

The cost-plus, or surcharge, approach is useful in departments such as pharmacy and central supply, where the supply cost is high compared with the labor cost involved in providing a service. This method requires the identification of the cost of supplies to be sold to patients, other costs in the department, and determination of a ratio between the two (ie, other costs to billable supplies). The cost of an item is then increased by the calculated percentage. This method can be further modified by introducing a variable surcharge based on variability in costs associated with handling different classes of supplies.

It is not uncommon to find these two methods used together in single departments. A prime example is the operating room. While the department may use an hourly rate to charge for time in the room, use of manpower, and routine supplies, it may also use a surcharge method for unusual supplies, such as pacemakers or artificial joints. This helps to allocate the burden of these costly devices equitably to the people who benefit from them, rather than distributing their costs to all patients.

Weighted-Value Basis

Of most interest to the laboratory manager is the weighted-value, or relative-value, basis of rate setting. This method is also useful in other areas where different types of procedures are done, including radiology, cardiography, and encephalography. In this approach, each procedure is assigned a relative weight based on the direct costs of performing the procedure. This value is multiplied by the number of times the procedure is performed, and one arrives at a total number of weighted units produced in an accounting period. Weighted units for all procedures are added together, and the total is then divided into the total financial requirements of the laboratory for a cost per weighted unit. The cost per weighted unit is then reapplied to the specific procedures based on the relative weight assigned in the first step of the method to yield a price. A brief example is shown in Box 30–10. A more detailed explanation of this subject is provided in Chapter 31.

In the past, laboratories used the College of American Pathologists' (CAP) relative values as published in their *Laboratory Workload Recording Method* as the basis for establishing the relative weight. However, this

Box 30·10

Weighted-Value Basis of Rate Setting

Test	Number Performed	Relative Weight	Weighted Units
Irregular antibody screen	300	1.2	380
Complete blood count	750	0.6	600
.	.	.	.
.	.	.	.
.	.	.	.
Chemistry, profile	1,000	2.3	2,300
Luteinizing hormone and follicle-stimulating hormone	325	4.5	1,462.5
Total number of weighted units produced			47,220.0

FINANCIAL REQUIREMENTS

Direct costs =	$435,000
Indirect costs (28%) =	121,800
Required contribution (10%) =	55,680
	$612,480

COST PER WEIGHTED UNIT

($612,48 ÷ 47,220)   12.97

Test	Relative Weight	Cost/ Weighted Unit	Price
Irregular antibody screen	1.2	$12.97	$15.56
Complete blood count	0.8	12.97	10.36
.	.	.	.
.	.	.	.
Chemistry, profile	2.3	12.97	29.83
Luteinizing hormone and follicle-stimulating hormone	4.5	12.97	58.37

method was not intended to be used for establishing rates and provides relative values based only on the productive time required to perform a given procedure. Since 1994, the CAP workload program has been replaced by a variety of other comparison groups. One need only consider the vast difference in supply expense between a complete blood count and a flow cytometry panel for CD 34 cells to understand the problems with assuming supply expense is equally distributed among procedures.

The weighted-value basis of rate setting is recommended for the laboratory because it provides a mechanism of apportioning the financial requirements of the laboratory equitably across the consumers of its services. Additionally, this method provides the basis for beginning to measure the productivity of the laboratory to determine how effectively the laboratory manager is using the resources at his disposal. Although the method is relatively difficult to implement because of the great variety of procedures completed in today's clinical laboratory, it is preferred because of the logical, cost-oriented foundation it establishes for rate setting.

The Realities of Rate Setting

This section has addressed the rationale and theory of rate setting in the ideal world. Unfortunately, the practice of rate setting requires that theoretically ideal rates be adjusted to fit reality.

Now that health-care costs are no longer simply passed on to businesses, individuals, and the government without scrutiny by these constituencies, virtually all purchasers of care have become prudent buyers searching for the best price for equivalent services. As a result, laboratory prices have become increasingly more sensitive to competition for market share among numerous suppliers. Nowhere is this competition more highlighted than in the market for outpatient testing, where consumer choice is more readily exercised than in the inpatient setting, and out-of-pocket costs to the consumer are still significant as compared with hospital care. To illustrate, if a routine urinalysis costs $12.50 in the hospital outpatient department, why should local physicians refer their patients to the hospital instead of a local private laboratory, which perhaps charges only $8.00? For procedures sensitive to the marketplace, it may well be a good strategy to set a price below the ideal and make up the revenue difference by charging more for a less price-sensitive procedure. A basic rule of thumb, however, should be to set the price no lower than the direct cost level, because on a per-test basis, the institution will lose money for every unit priced below direct costs. When this is not possible, cost shifting, cost reduction, or deletion of the test from the price list is generally the alternatives of choice, all other factors being equal.

Alternatively, the laboratory manager may consider establishing a separate outpatient laboratory to compete with the private laboratory. Under this scenario, the outpatient laboratory would offer a limited array of procedures priced to compete successfully, while the inpatient laboratory would establish prices at a level sufficient to recover its full financial requirements. Such a device permits the laboratory to compete on a price basis in the outpatient setting and set its inpatient rates recognizing that they are not as price sensitive nor as subject to direct competition. Another contemporary alternative is the consolidation of several laboratories into one outpatient setting. This often permits economies of scale and a subsequent cost reduction on a per-test basis. Consolidated laboratories can often negotiate a better contract with an outside reference laboratory for tests subsequently sent out because of increased contract volumes. In a similar vein, third-party payers who base their payments on area-wide norms may stimulate upward or downward price adjustments by hospitals who attempt to maximize their reimbursement from these sources.

As can be seen from the foregoing, rate setting is a complex process requiring certain inputs from the financial officer and certain inputs from the laboratory manager. Although it is always desirable to relate properly relative value and the rate schedule, marketplace realities will often require strategic readjustments. The laboratory manager should be an active participant in this process and should expect to be the hospital's expert in the pricing practices and cost structures of the competition.

REFERENCES

1. Anthony RN, Reese JS: Accounting Text and Cases, 7th ed. Homewood, Richard D. Irwin, 1983
2. Beck DF: Basic Hospital Finance Management. Germantown, Aspen Systems Corporation, 1980
3. Berman HJ, Weeks LE: The Financial Management of Hospitals, 8th ed. Ann Arbor, Health Administration Press, 1994
4. Boer GB: Analysis of equipment leases. In Bennington JL, Boer GB, Louvau GE, Westlake GE (eds): Management and Cost Control Techniques for the Clinical Laboratory, pp 199–208. Baltimore, University Park Press, 1977
5. Budgeting Manual. Sacramento, California Hospital Association, 1974
6. Cost Finding and Rate Setting for Hospitals. Chicago, American Hospital Association, 1968
7. Deason JM (ed): Flexible budgeting. Topics in Health Care Financing 5(4), 1979
8. Griffith JR, Hancock WM, Munson FC (eds): Cost Control in Hospitals. Ann Arbor, Health Administration Press, 1976
9. Hunt P, Williams CM, Donaldson G: Basic Business Finance, 4th ed. Homewood, Richard D. Irwin, 1971
10. Lusk EJ, Lusk JG: Financial and Managerial Control: A Health Care Perspective. Germantown, Aspen Systems Corporation, 1979
11. Silvers JB, Prahalad CK: Financial Management of Health Institutions. Flushing, Spectrum Publications, 1974

31

Laboratory Cost Accounting

David W. Glenn

PURPOSE, USE, AND HISTORY

A laboratory manager has many tools available to help in making decisions affecting the future existence and growth of the laboratory. A staff medical technologist has quality control statistics to help assess the acceptability of patient results. Similarly, a laboratory manager can use cost accounting information to evaluate the financial performance of the laboratory.

The financial impact on the laboratory caused by government programs like the disease-related groups and Clinical Laboratory Improvement Amendments of 1988 (CLIA '88) has been significant. However, the recent development of managed care programs is having an even larger impact on laboratories that are bidding for provision of laboratory services. If an institution is bidding to provide laboratory services on a capitation basis (set fee for laboratory services per member per month), it is imperative that the laboratory management and institution administration know the true costs of providing these services. Some laboratories have given low-ball bids ($0.50 or less per member per month) and won contracts that lost the laboratory so much money that they had to drop the contract after 1 year.[1] The administration of a hospital may be looking only at the extra cost of reagents when bidding on such contracts. It is up to laboratory management to be aware of what projects the institution's administration may be considering, which could impact the laboratory, and the laboratory manager must be aware of all costs in the laboratory and assist administration so appropriate bids are made.

The purpose of cost accounting is to identify the costs involved in a specific set of activities. Accurate cost accounting data are needed to track, monitor, and control the costs of laboratory operations. Cost accounting is also vital for making informed decisions about personnel staffing, capital equipment acquisition, instrument/method comparison, fee setting, competitive bidding, and which tests to perform in house or send to a reference laboratory.

Cost accounting data are not precise to the nearest penny of all costs involved in operating a laboratory. However, an accurate estimate of costs can be achieved to meet the needs of laboratory management. In a physician office laboratory serving only two or three physicians, the cost accounting system may be rather simple. A large hospital or reference laboratory may use a complex computerized system. The manager of a large hospital laboratory may receive information from the administration regarding payroll, purchasing, financial statements, and budget analysis.

The size or complexity of the cost accounting system is not as critical as is how appropriately that information meets the needs of management in making financial decisions. In fact, the larger, more complex systems can generate so much data that they may encourage "analysis paralysis."

Labor has always represented the major cost in the laboratory. Historically, the College of American Pathologists (CAP) Workload Recording Method was often used to help identify labor costs and calculate labor productivity. The CAP relied on volunteers to provide the time studies for the different test instruments and methods in use. As many new tests, instruments, and methods were brought on the market, it became increasingly difficult to recruit volunteers to perform the time-consuming studies. Additionally, there were discrepancies among those performing the time studies as to how much labor was actually required for each test. Hospital administration did not always understand the system and its productivity calculations. As hospital affiliations have grown during the last few years, administrators have become interested in comparing how their laboratory's costs and productivity compare with similar size laboratories in their group. The CAP abandoned the Workload Recording Method in 1992. The CAP replaced it with the Laboratory Management Index Program, which is discussed later in this chapter.

Determining Labor Costs

Many laboratories continue to use the CAP Workload Recording Method for determining labor costs. Other laboratories perform their own time studies based on the CAP method. Thus, a basic understanding of the method is required.

Item for count defines for each procedure the entities to be counted.[2] The counting method is standardized to eliminate ambiguity in deciding what constitutes one procedure. Most chemistry and hematology procedures are simply counted by test, such as glucose or hemoglobin. The microbiology procedures are not as easily counted. For example, a request for culture may signify very little work preformed if there is no growth or considerable work if numerous pathogens require identification. In cases such as this, individual test components (for example, plate, tube, specimen, or slide) are counted. *Raw count* is the tally of items for count.

Unit value per procedure represents the mean number of laboratory workload units (WLUs) required to perform the procedure once. Each unit is equivalent to 1 minute of technical, clerical, and aide time involved in directly performing the procedure.

Unit values are based on the preanalytical, analytical, and postanalytical time required. The following is an explanation of those times.

Preanalytical time—initial handling of the specimen—includes receipt of the specimen by the laboratory, sorting specimens, logging the patient's name and other required information on laboratory forms or in the computer, preparing the worksheet, labeling the sample, loading the sample into and unloading the sample from a centrifuge, separating the serum and plasma, and delivering the sample to the work area.[2,3] The time the specimen is spinning in the centrifuge or is being incubated is not included. The specimen collection time is not included, because this procedure has its own unit value. *Daily and periodic activities* include only the steps that are routinely required but not repeated for each sample. This includes time for the preparation of reagents, solutions, controls, standards, and samples. Also include is the glassware wash time, including washing, drying, and sterilization of equipment used in the procedure. When an instrument is used, time required for cleaning, warmup, calibration, and shutdown is included.

Analytical time generally represents the least amount of time in the three major areas studied. Analytical time includes diluting the specimen, adding reagents, adjusting the analytical instrument, introducing the test into the instrument, taking readings, and removing the test from the instrument.

Postanalytic time—recording and reporting time—includes calculation of results, recording of results on report and laboratory record forms or entering them in the computer, checking, sorting, and filing of completed reports. Also included is time for telephone calls (incoming and outgoing) related to the initial report. *Maintenance and repair time* includes scheduled and minor unscheduled maintenance performed by nonlaboratory personnel and is not included. *Direct technical supervision time* includes time for evaluating quality control results and verifying and approving patient results.

In addition to the above activities, a personal fatigue and delay factor should be included in the time estimate to account for the "human factor." An additional 15% is considered reasonable to account for this element.

The time studies do not include the performance of standards or quality controls. These samples are counted separately in the raw count and are given the same unit value as a patient procedure. Serum/reagent blanks are included in the time studies and must not be counted as separate procedures.

When a procedure must be performed a second time to resolve a problem, it is counted as a repeat. A repeat is equivalent to one raw count. Some procedures (for example, radioimmunoassays) require duplicate performance of certain steps. When a procedure requires the multiple analysis of each specimen, it is considered a replicate analysis and part of the procedure. Replicates are not counted individually. Time for replicate analysis is included in the unit value studies.

COST ACCOUNTING

Because the large laboratories already have a cost accounting system in place with which the laboratory manager will be expected to work, this chapter discusses the basics of cost accounting and tries to simplify what can be a complex subject.

Cost Accounting Methods

There are three basic ways of looking at laboratory costs: the macro, micro, and incremental methods. The *macro* method (historical method) looks at the total costs assigned to each of the laboratory's cost centers (sections). This method is useful for preparing budgets and comparing total costs of the different sections. It can also be used to establish "relative values" for estimating average test cost within that section.

The *micro* method (engineering method) defines all of the specific costs related to performing a single test. The micro method is more accurate and more time consuming than the macro method. The micro method is most useful for setting test fees and evaluating different instruments and methods. Because of the difficulty and time required to perform the micro method, it would be impractical to micro cost account every test. Because a small number of tests actually account for the most frequently performed tests, it would be wise to micro analyze these tests first.

The *incremental* method is a modification of the micro method in which the cost of performing additional tests is calculated. This is most useful when the laboratory manager is interested in bidding competitively for additional testing.

The Macro (Historical) Method

Regardless of the type of laboratory situation, the macro method is appropriate. In the hospital laboratory, the manager will not be responsible for determining overhead (hospital-allocated) costs. The hospital controller will provide those data. However, the laboratory manager may be required to help provide information regarding the assignment of direct costs to the proper cost centers in the laboratory. If you are the manager of an independent laboratory, you may have the responsibility for performing many of the duties performed by hospital controllers in determining and apportioning direct and indirect costs.

Direct costs are directly traceable to the performance of a specific test or provision of service. Direct costs include labor to collect, prepare, perform, test, record, and report the test. Direct costs also include supplies, instrument maintenance, repair and depreciation, reagents, standards, controls, proficiency testing, development, and any repeats or duplicate tests required to produce a billable product.

Indirect costs can be attributed to the production of a test or service but are not directly involved in the production. These costs may be called overhead and may be intradepartmental or extradepartmental. Intradepartmental indirect costs may include shared equipment (eg, refrigerators and centrifuges) and shared services (eg, clerical and supervisory personnel). Extradepartmental (institutional or corporate) indirect costs may include space, utilities, billing, administration, and other shared or non–revenue-producing services apportioned to the laboratory.

The following example is a simplified look at the macro method of cost accounting for a hospital laboratory.

Gather the laboratory's cost figures, including all direct and indirect costs the laboratory must recover. It is imperative that all costs be available for the final accounting to be accurate.

Define cost centers. The small laboratory may find it most practical to lump costs into one unit for the entire laboratory. In a larger laboratory with supervisors responsible for their own sections, it may be advantageous to assign costs to those sections. This will allow the laboratory manager to hold each section supervisor responsible for costs in his area. There are two types of cost centers in the laboratory: revenue producing and non-revenue producing. Revenue-producing cost centers perform billable tests or services. The non–revenue-producing cost centers may be sections with their own supervisors. In the example shown in Table 31-1, the major sections of the laboratory, including chemistry, hematology, microbiology, blood bank, histology, and phlebotomy, represent the revenue-producing cost centers. The non–revenue-producing cost centers are laboratory administration and physician remuneration. When preparing a cost report, the laboratory manager may define as many or as few cost centers as needed to provide the necessary information and meet the needs of the employer. The examples given are for illustration purposes only.

Accumulate direct costs. This is a difficult task and represents the bulk of work in performing cost accounting.

Calculate labor costs. Labor costs often represent 60% to 70% of the direct costs in a laboratory. The fringe benefits must also be considered along with the cost of salaries. In some hospital laboratories, the cost of fringe benefits is included in the hospital allocation of overhead costs to the laboratory. The cost of fringe benefits, such as FICA, retirement plan, health insurance, life insurance, disability insurance, and worker's compensation is high (often exceeding 20% of the salary).

Determine equipment costs. Equipment costs include the cost of purchase, lease or rental, depreciation, site preparation, installation, training, computer interface, and maintenance and repair. A common method of estimating annual equipment costs for a purchased instrument is to divide the purchase price by the number of years the instrument is expected to be in use. Some accountants will calculate the cost of capital (the cost of the money tied up in an instrument over its useful life) to determine the value of the money tied up in the instrument purchase as compared with its future worth if invested. With this type of accounting, a cost higher than the purchase price will be used. When projecting the cost of maintaining analytical equipment not covered by a service contract, a rule-of-thumb estimate commonly used is 10% to 15% of the retail price of the instrument per year.

Accumulate supply costs. Supply costs include reagents, standards, controls, cost of proficiency testing programs, pipettes, tubes, slides, laboratory report and request forms, office supplies, and all other consumables used in the laboratory. Other costs include expenses for continuing education, library, or any other

Table 31-1
Example of Laboratory Costs

| | Revenue-Producing Cost Centers | | | | |
	Chemistry	Hematology	Microbiology	Blood Bank	Histology
Salaries	$180,000	$116,000	$86,000	$58,000	$70,000
Equipment	$30,000	$15,000	$8,000	$4,000	$9,000
Supplies	$38,000	$21,000	$18,000	$12,000	$13,000
Other	$6,000	$4,000	$2,000	$2,000	$6,000
Subtotal	$254,000	$156,000	$114,000	$76,000	$98,000

| | Non–revenue-Producing Cost Centers | |
	Laboratory Administration	Physicians
Salaries	$102,000	$220,000
Equipment	$34,000	
Supplies	$25,000	
Other	$6,000	
Subtotal	$167,000	$220,000

items that are directly related to the cost center and not included under salaries, equipment, or supplies.

Determine laboratory administration costs, which include the salaries of the laboratory manager, secretaries, clerks, and other personnel not directly associated with the performance of billable tests or procedures within a specific revenue-producing cost center. The cost of office equipment and the laboratory computer system is included in this section. Glassware wash up and media preparation costs, including salaries, supplies, and equipment costs associated with providing these services, are included in this section. Other costs include expenses for continuing education, library, or any other items that are directly related to the laboratory and not included in one of the above groups.

Include physician remuneration costs. Some laboratories hire the pathologist, others work out contractual agreements, and some pay on a fee-for-service basis.

Apportion nonrevenue costs to the revenue-producing cost centers. Table 31-2 shows laboratory administration and physician costs apportioned to each department based on its percentage of the total costs of the revenue-producing centers. In this example, the nonrevenue costs were distributed according to the percentage of total costs represented by each revenue-producing cost center. These costs could also be allotted according to the total revenue each center produced, or any other equitable way could be used. One should

strive to apportion these costs as fairly as possible to provide a true representation of where costs actually belong. This information becomes vital when trying to establish individual test costs.

Allocate overhead (institution) costs. The costs of housekeeping, maintenance, building depreciation and insurance, utilities, and other overhead costs are commonly allocated to the laboratory on the basis of the amount of square footage the laboratory occupies. Table 31-3 is an example of the allocation of these expenses to each of the revenue centers.

The human resources, payroll, and food services costs are often allocated to the laboratory on the basis of the number of employees in the laboratory. Purchasing department costs may be allocated on the basis of the percentage of the total purchases handled by the purchasing department for the laboratory. The costs of the medical records department, hospital computer service, and other central administration costs may be apportioned according to the percentage of the laboratory direct costs as compared with the total hospital direct costs. Table 31-3 also shows the allocation of overhead costs and the basis of their allocation.

FEE-SETTING BY THE MACRO METHOD

Once the macro method allocation of costs is completed, the patient-charged WLUs can be applied to the costs and used as relative value units (RVUs). Table 31-4

Table 31-2
Example of Laboratory Nonrevenue Cost-Center Apportionment

		Revenue-Producing Cost Centers				
		Chemistry	Hematology	Microbiology	Blood Bank	Histology
Revenue center direct costs		$254,000	$156,000	$114,000	$76,000	$98,000
Nonrevenue center indirect costs						
Laboratory administration	$167,000	$60,000	$37,300	$27,300	$18,200	$23,400
Physicians	$220,000	$80,000	$49,200	$35,900	$24,000	$30,900
Total laboratory costs		$394,800	$242,500	$177,200	$118,200	$152,300

shows an example of the relationship between total costs and patient WLUs. If an automated chemistry procedure has been time studied and found to require 2 WLUs, the cost for performing this would be 2 × $1.23 or $2.46 according to the macro method. By performing the allocation of costs for each revenue-producing center in the laboratory, the laboratory manager has a calculated basis for setting fees by RVU. This approach can be refined by defining more revenue-producing cost centers for the laboratory. There comes a point, however, when the time spent defining and allocating costs to a multitude of laboratory revenue-producing cost centers becomes counterproductive. Thus, one should establish the minimum number of cost centers in the laboratory that is essential. As the following micro approach to cost accounting example demonstrates, there can be significant differences between the cost of a test calculated by the macro method compared with the micro method.

The Micro (Engineering) Method

This method is time consuming and difficult. It is most reasonably performed for the highest volume tests. These are often the tests that a laboratory performing reference testing wants to market at competitive prices. In this scenario, the laboratory manager will need to

Table 31-3
Example of Allocation of Overhead Costs

Indirect Costs	Amount	Allocation Basis	Laboratory Revenue-Producing Centers				
			Chemistry	Hematology	Microbiology	Blood Bank	Histology
Building maintenance, depreciation, housekeeping and utilities	$350,000	Square footage	$120,000	$50,000	$68,000	$34,000	$78,000
Human resources, payroll, food services	$70,000	Personnel	$29,000	$14,500	$10,500	$5,500	$9,500
Purchasing	$50,000	% purchases	$21,000	$12,000	$7,000	$4,000	$6,000
Central Administration	$280,000	% direct costs	$101,900	$62,600	$45,700	$30,500	$39,300
Total allocated institutional overhead Costs			$271,900	$139,100	$131,200	$74,000	$132,800
Total laboratory costs			$386,000	$237,000	$174,000	$116,000	$149,000
Total costs			$657,900	$376,100	$305,200	$190,000	$281,800

Table 31-4
The Relationship Between Total Cost and Patient Workload Units (WLU)

	Revenue-Producing Centers				
	Chemistry	Hematology	Microbiology	Blood Bank	Histology
Total costs	$657,900	$376,100	$305,700	$190,000	$281,800
Charged WLUs	$535,000	$280,000	$170,000	$120,000	$190,000
Cost per relative value unit	$1.23	$1.34	$1.80	$1.58	$1.48

know the cost of performing a test as accurately as possible.

The total cost per test can be determined by adding together the cost per test of direct and indirect labor, direct and indirect materials, equipment costs, and overhead expenses.

Direct labor costs include the costs of technical personnel who actually perform the testing. By dividing the annual cost of technical labor by the annual total of WLUs performed, the direct labor cost per WLU is derived. If a new test is being evaluated, the direct labor cost per test is computed by multiplying the WLUs for the new test by the direct labor cost per WLU.

Indirect labor costs represent the cost of all other laboratory support and supervisory personnel costs. The indirect labor costs are calculated by dividing the total cost of support and supervisory personnel by the total WLUs and then multiplying the result by the number of WLUs for the individual test.

Indirect materials costs encompass the costs of shared equipment and supplies that cannot be directly allocated to individual tests. The costs of the laboratory computer system, centrifuges, refrigerators, and office equipment and supplies are included in this area. The cost per test is calculated by dividing the annual cost of indirect materials by the laboratory's annual WLU volume and then multiplying this by the number of WLUs for the individual test (Box 31-1).

Overhead costs include the hospital's allocation for utilities, housekeeping, administration, and other costs, including profit if it is an investor-owned facility. Some hospitals require that the laboratory multiply the total laboratory-related costs by an overhead factor to calculate the allowance for overhead costs when pricing new tests. Other hospitals will assign a fixed cost to be recovered by the laboratory. In this case, the overhead costs can be allocated by dividing the total overhead costs by the total WLU volume and assigning the cost per WLU.

A simplified example of this micro approach is described in Box 31-2.

Because only 528 (63%) of the total 840 tests in Box 31-2 can be billed to patients, the actual test cost per patient billable test is $10.33. If the hospital had not built its profit or contribution into the overhead allotment of costs, this would have to be added. Before pricing the test, the laboratory manager must also consider fixed third-party reimbursement, bad-debt rate for laboratory fees, competitive pressures, and whether it would be more cost effective to continue sending the test to a reference laboratory.

If the manager had only calculated costs based on the macro approach, 2 RVUs × $1.23, a test cost of only $2.46 would have been established. However, the XYZ test requires dedicated equipment at a higher cost

Box 31•1

Equipment Cost Calculations

Equipment Description	Replacement	Useful Life (b)	Annual PM Contract (c)	Annual Tests (d)	Cost $[a/b) + c]/d$
Analyzer	$11,900	7 y	$1,200	840	$3.45
Pipettor	$950	7 y	—	840	$.16
Total equipment cost					$3.61

PM = preventive maintenance

Box 31·2

Case Example: Test Cost Analysis

A laboratory has been sending the XYZ test to a reference laboratory. The test volume has reached a point where the laboratory manager decides to evaluate the cost effectiveness of performing the test in his own laboratory. The laboratory anticipates performing 258 patient tests and 312 other tests (standards, controls, repeats), for an annual total of 840. The XYZ analyzer has been assigned 2 WLUs per test.

The hospital controller provides the following data:

CHEMISTRY SECTION: ANNUAL COSTS

Direct labor: $0.38/WLU
Indirect labor: $80,000
Indirect materials: $56,000
Annual overhead: $251,000
Annual WLU volume: 480,000

Using the calculations explained above and the equipment costs and materials Costs forms, the laboratory manager is able to derive the costs in the following test cost analysis summary:

Materials Costs

Item Description	Unit Cost (a)	Items/Unit (b)	Items/Test (c)	Cost (a/b) × c
Reagents	$33.67	100	1	
Calibrator	$21.00	1,000	1	$.02
Sample cups	$17.50	1,000	1	$.02
Pipette tips	$31.00	1,000	1	$.03
Disposable cuvettes	$9.75	100	1	$.10
Total materials costs per test				$.51

TEST COST ANALYSIS SUMMARY

Direct labor: $ 0.76
Indirect labor: $ 0.34
Direct materials: $ 0.51
Indirect materials: $ 0.24
Equipment: $ 3.61
Overhead: $ 1.05
Total costs: $ 6.51
Cost/patient test: $10.33

per test than most tests performed in the laboratory. The test volume is rather low, and a high ratio of nonpatient to patient tests exists. Thus, the micro approach is most useful in evaluating new procedure costs prior to committing to performing them in house.

The Incremental Method

The incremental method looks only at the extra costs for performing potentially added testing volume. Incremental costs would not exist if additional testing were not performed. If the additional testing can be performed using existing equipment and testing personnel,

the incremental costs would be consumables and incidental associated costs, such as courier service or teleprinter installation. Equipment service contracts, cost of calibrators, and certain other expenses can be ignored. Testing personnel costs would not be included as long as overtime or additional personnel were not required to perform the extra testing. If extra labor costs were required, those costs would be considered incremental.

As an example of incremental cost accounting, a physician's clinic calls and offers to send a local laboratory a minimum of 500 12-test chemistry profiles per month if the laboratory will accept $7.00 per profile. The laboratory knows it can handle the additional testing on existing equipment without adding personnel costs. The laboratory calculates the cost of reagents and consumables required for the additional testing and determines the incremental cost to be $5.88. Thus, the potential margin (profit) would be $7.00 − $5.88 × 500 $560.00 per month.

The laboratory manager in this example must also consider other variables. Do the additional 500 tests per month put the laboratory near its maximum capacity, and would the additional cost of new instrumentation or extra labor costs allow the laboratory to still come out ahead financially? By offering this special pricing, will the laboratory be forced to give similar pricing to its current customers? If so, the anticipated profit must be compared to the amount of revenue lost with a lowering of price to the current customers. Are there any overlooked costs, such as the need to install a teleprinter in the clinic to meet the reporting demands of the clinic? On the positive side, will the offering of $7.00 chemistry profiles lead to any "pull-through" business, resulting in additional testing in other areas of the laboratory? Will the extra testing volume require more reagents, which will allow the laboratory to receive a discounted price for the reagents? There may be many other factors that must be considered prior to making the decision. If the decision is made to accept the proposal, the laboratory manager should closely examine future cost reports to see if the proposal had the desired effect.

Comparing the Cost Effectiveness of Two Methods

When justifying the acquisition of new equipment to administration, the manager should be aware that the speed, accuracy, and precision of the new equipment does not carry as much weight as the bottom-line figure of how much the new method will cost and how much revenue it will generate.

Automated equipment is able to reduce the cost of labor in the laboratory (Table 31-5). However, before the cost of automated equipment can be justified, one must perform a sufficiently large workload to reach the break-even point and surpass it to show a profit. Naturally, the instrument manufacturer's sales personnel will be eager to share this information with you. Unfortunately, the sales representative's figures often suggest that unreasonably small workloads are adequate to justify the equipment purchase. Thus, the ultimate responsibility for realistically evaluating the cost falls to the laboratory manager.

The following formula is useful when comparing two methods to determine the volume of tests to break even. The break-even point occurs when

$$A_1 (X) + B_1 = A_2 (X) + B_2$$

Table 31-5

Unit Values for 12 Commonly Performed Chemistry Tests With Manual and Semiautomated Equipment

Test	Manual Unit Value	Semiautomated Unit Value
Glucose	8	4
Urea	8	4
Uric acid	10	4
Calcium	14	4
Phosphorus	10	4
Total bilirubin	15	6
Total protein	12	4
Albumin	12	4
Cholesterol	8	6
SGOT	10	4
LDH	10	4
CPK	13	4
Total	130	52

where A_1 variable costs per test of method 1, X break-even volume, B_1 total fixed costs of method 1, A_2 variable costs per test method 2, and B_2 total fixed costs of method 2.

To perform this comparison, you must know the annual fixed and variable costs associated with each method. The institution-allocated indirect costs and the laboratory cost center's indirect costs are fixed. These indirect costs are the same for each method being compared.

The fixed direct costs for each method will not be the same. They include the cost of equipment depreciation and maintenance for that method. The variable costs for each method will depend on the method's direct costs for labor, reagents, and disposable supplies.

As an example of how this cost comparison method can be used, consider a laboratory situation in which 6,300 12-test chemistry profiles are being performed annually. This laboratory wants to purchase a semiautomated analyzer. A cost study and determination of break-even volume are provided in Box 31-3.

The laboratory's institution-allocated costs for this cost center total $22,000, and the laboratory cost center's indirect costs are $6,800. The direct labor cost of each WLU in this laboratory is $0.142. Thus, the direct labor cost for performing a manual profile is $18.46 (130 × $0.142). The direct labor cost for performing the same profile on semiautomated equipment is $7.38 (52 × $0.142). The purchase price of the new semiauto-

Box 31•3

Worksheet for Comparing Cost Effectiveness of Two Methods

Procedure: *Chem. 12-Test Profile*
Method 1: *Manual*

VARIABLE COSTS PER TEST

Direct labor	$18.46	
Reagents and supplies	7.04	
Total variable costs per test		A_1 $25.50

FIXED COSTS

Institution-allocated indirect	$22,000	
Cost center indirect	6,800	
Equipment depreciation	860	
Equipment maintenance	400	
Total fixed costs		B_1 $30,060

Method 2: *Semiautomated*

VARIABLE COST PER TEST

Direct labor	$7.38	
Reagents and supplies	4.55	
Total fixed costs		A_2 $11.93

FIXED COSTS

Institution-allocated indirect	$22,000	
Cost center indirect	6,800	
Equipment depreciation	3,571	
Equipment maintenance	2,500	
Total fixed costs		B_2 $34,871

mated equipment is $25,000, depreciated over 7 years at an annual cost of $3,571. The maintenance cost per year is $2,500. The reagent and disposable supplies cost is $2.55 per profile. Using the break-even formula,

$$A_1 (X) + B_1 = A_2 (X) + B_2$$

we find

$$25.50 (X) + 30,060 = 11.93 (X) + 34,871$$
$$13.57 (X) = 4811$$
$$(X) = 355$$

Thus, 355 profiles must be performed annually to reach the break-even point. Because this laboratory is currently performing 6,300 profiles annually, the semiautomated equipment is justified.

Determining Cost-Effective Instrument Operation

The break-even formula is useful for performing cost studies when the purchase of new equipment is questioned. However, often a laboratory has more than one instrument available for performing the same test. One of the most cost-effective means of controlling costs in the laboratory is using the proper procedures and instruments for testing at the proper times. The cost of performing stat tests will always be unproductive when compared with batching of samples. However, serving the acutely ill patient often requires immediate performance of a test. If one determines the most cost-effective means of performing such a test, it is possible to make the best of a bad economic situation without lowering the quality of patient care or wasting money.

By comparing the variable direct costs of labor, reagents, supplies, and equipment for the different instruments used in the laboratory that are capable of performing the same tests, the manager can determine the most cost-effective use of the alternatives available.

In the following discussion, the labor, reagent, supply, and instrument costs of performing a stat glucose on a semiautomated analyzer are compared with the respective costs on a discrete automated analyzer. Because the instruments are already in the laboratory and being used for many different tests, instrument depreciation and maintenance costs per test are based on current volume. The instrument costs for depreciation and maintenance are calculated per test by dividing the total of these two costs by the number of tests performed on the instrument annually.

Assume the semiautomated equipment requires a minimum of one zero calibrater, one standard, and one control per test run. Thus, if only one stat patient test is performed, an additional three nonpatient tests must also be performed. The discrete analyzer needs to be calibrated only once every 90 days (manufacturer and government approved). In addition, the discrete analyzer requires only two control determinations each 8-hour shift. The WLU value for the semiautomated procedure is 4, and the WLU value for the discrete analyzer is 3. The cost per WLU in this laboratory is $0.142. These data and the reagent and disposable supply costs per test are summarized in Table 31-6.

The summary indicates that the semiautomated instrument is the most cost effective for stat glucose assays. However, this is deceiving. The most cost-effective method is dependent on how many stat glucose tests are performed per 8-hour shift. For instance, if another stat glucose test were performed within the 8-hour shift, the semiautomated cost ($3.37) would remain the same, because all the work would be repeated. With the discrete analyzer, which requires that only the single patient test be performed, the cost is $2.64 for the second stat glucose assay (Table 31-7). Batching of samples

Table 31-6
Cost Comparison of Stat Glucose Assays Done on Semiautomated Equipment and Discrete Analyzer

	Semiautomated	Discrete Analyzer
Workload unit (WLU)	4	3
Workload per run		
Zeroes	1	0
Standard	1	0.1*
Controls	1	2
Patient	1	1
Total	4	3.1
Labor cost ($0.142/WLU)	0.57	$0.43
Reagent and supply cost/test	0.39	0.85
Total reagent and supply cost	1.56	2.64
Instrument cost/test	0.31	1.36
Total instrument cost	1.24	4.22
Cost per stat run	$3.37	$7.29

* Nine standards are used to calibrate every 90 days. $9 \div 90 = 0.1/d$

brings a different conclusion. Table 31-8 shows the cost of performing different volumes of glucose runs with the same data.

Evaluating Productivity

Each laboratory manager must define acceptable productivity. No two laboratories are exactly alike. Thus, it is difficult to state an ideal productivity rate. The laboratory manager must first determine the current produc-

Table 31-7
Cost Comparison of Performing Each Additional Glucose Assay

	Semiautomated	Discrete Analyzer
Labor	$0.57	$0.43
Reagents	$0.39	$0.85
Instrument	$0.31	$1.36
Total	$1.27	$2.64

Table 31-8
Labor, Supply, and Instrument Cost of Glucose Assays

Patient/Run	Semiautomated	Discrete Analyzer
1	$3.37	$7.29
2	$4.64	$9.93
3	$5.91	$12.57
5	$8.45	$17.85

tivity rate for the laboratory. Then this rate must be monitored and action taken to improve productivity or prevent a lowering in productivity. There are three ways to view productivity: (1) as related to paid man-hours, (2) as related to worked man-hours, and (3) as related to specified man-hours.

Paid Productivity

Even though 1 CAP unit is equivalent to 1 minute of time, no person is able to achieve 60 WLUs/h paid (100% productivity). Paid absentee time is usually 10% to 20% of total paid time. This is dependent on the employee's benefits, including paid vacations and holidays, paid sick time, paid time away from the laboratory (eg, continuing education, jury duty, personal leave), and overtime hours actually worked. Each laboratory's benefits and employee use of sick leave will vary. The amount of overtime must be controlled. When overtime is paid at the customary time-and-a-half rate, every paid hour of overtime includes pay for 30 minutes of time not worked.

Paid hours represent the entire personnel burden in the laboratory, excluding only the laboratory physicians, doctoral-level clinical scientists, and students. All paid time, productive or nonproductive, must be included. The institution's payroll clerk can provide the number of paid hours needed for this calculation.

$$\text{Paid productivity} = \frac{\text{Total WLUs}}{\text{Total paid hours}}$$

Paid productivity is the most commonly used measure to determine cost-effective use of personnel. To calculate the paid productivity of each section in the laboratory, the manager needs to apportion the time of department-shared supervisors and clerks by allocating their time to the various departments (similar to the step-down method used for allocating costs). An example of paid-productivity calculation is given in Box 31-4.

At the time of this printing, the CAP reported the median paid productivity ranged from 34 to 36 units per paid hour for community hospitals and from 31 to 35 units per paid hour in university and other teaching hospitals.

Because of the wide discrepancy of laboratory situations, it is often useful for the laboratory supervisor to present productivity to administration as worked, specified, and paid productivity. This will help justify what may at first appear to be an unacceptable paid productivity. On the other hand, the calculation of paid, worked, and specified productivity may objectively show the need to reduce personnel.

Worked Productivity

Total worked hours are the total paid hours minus the total paid hours not worked (eg, paid vacations, holidays, sick leave, continuing education leave). These figures should also be available from the payroll clerk.

$$\text{Worked productivity} = \frac{\text{Total WLUs/year}}{\text{Total worked hr/yr}}$$

Worked productivity will naturally be higher than paid productivity. However, worked productivity will never reach 100%. If it does, either the workload data are incorrect or the staff is overproducing at a rate con-

---

Box 31•5

Worked Productivity Example

If the five FTEs in a laboratory section each annually average 15 days vacation, 10 holidays, and 6 sick-leave days, worked productivity is 83.7%.

Total paid time/FTE/y	2,080 h
Minus nonworked paid h/FTE/y	
Vacation (15 days × 8 h/d)	120 h
Holidays (10 days × 8 h/d)	80 h
Sick leave (6 days × 8 h/d)	48 h
Nonworked paid time/FTE/y	248 h
Total worked h/FTE (2,080 − 248)	

$$\text{Worked productivity} = \frac{\text{Total WLUs}}{\text{Total worked hours}}$$

$$\text{Worked productivity} = \frac{460,000 \text{ WLUs}}{9,160 \text{ h } (1,832 \times 5 \text{ FTEs})}$$

$$\text{Worked productivity} = 50.2 \text{ WLU/h}$$

$$\frac{50.2 \text{ WLU/h}}{60 \text{ min}} \times 100$$

$$= 83.7\%$$

---

sidered hazardous to quality. Many laboratorians set a goal of 50 to 52 units per worked hour. The worked productivity is often the best way for management to evaluate the laboratory's labor productivity (Box 31-5).

Specified Productivity

A list of the items included in the CAP time studies is presented earlier in this chapter. Many other activities are performed by the laboratory personnel that are not part of the CAP workload unit time. These activities include the following:

Laboratory administrative duties, such as compiling workload statistics, budgeting, recruiting, orientation, discipline, performance evaluation, and employee scheduling

Lunch and coffee breaks mandated by law or contract

Education of others in formal programs, such as residency or medical technology schools

Accounting, billing, and related activities

Box 31•4

Paid Productivity Example

If a laboratory section employs five full-time equivalents (FTEs) and produces a total of 460,000 workload units (WLUs) annually, the paid productivity rate is 73.7%.

$$\text{Total paid time} = (8 \text{ h/d} \times 5 \text{ days/wk}) \times 52 \text{ wk/y}$$

$$= 2,080 \text{ h}$$

$$\text{Paid productivity} = \frac{\text{WLUs/y}}{\text{Total paid h/y}}$$

$$\text{Paid productivity} = \frac{460,000 \text{ WLUs}}{2080 \text{ hr/FTE} \times 5 \text{ FTE}}$$

$$= 44.2 \text{ WLUs/paid h}$$

$$\frac{44.2 \text{ WLUs/paid h}}{60 \text{ min/paid h}} \times 100 = 73.7\% \text{ paid productivity}$$

Purchasing and procurement time, including sales visits, demonstrations, and the inventory of supplies

Computer activities

Clerical support, mail handling, photocopying, typing letters, courier activities

Clearly identified research and development

Grouped in-service education, bench training, lecture

Laboratory staff meetings and other meetings, including safety committee, infection control committee, and consultations with pathologists and other specialists

Preparation of reports, such as a tumor registry, transfusion reactions for utilization review, and similar activities

Morgue activities and decedent affairs

Laboratory procedures that do not have a unit value assigned

Any other activities not included in the CAP time studies

The CAP manual includes a "Non-Specified Hours Weekly Worksheet" and a "Laboratory Staffing Analysis Employee Diary," which are valuable in collecting data for studying specified productivity.

Total specified hours are total worked hours less all paid hours for untimed activities.

$$\text{Specified productivity} = \frac{\text{Total WLUs}}{\text{Total specified hours}}$$

If specified productivity is more than 100% and no workload recording errors are evident, more personnel are indicated. Demanding 100% or higher productivity forces employees to take shortcuts, and the quality of patient care will suffer (Box 31-6).

Determining Staffing Needs

One of the most common uses of workload recording is in determining the number of full-time equivalents (FTEs) required to perform the laboratory's workload. The easiest calculation is to use last year's workload figures and change them by the percentage of change forecast. For example, if one anticipates a 5% increase in work, the current total of FTEs is multiplied by 1.05 for determining the FTEs required to undertake the increased workload. This approach is valid only if the workload recording method has been used for several years and the data obtained are acceptable, the laboratory's present rate of productivity is satisfactory, and the forecast change in workload is reasonably accurate.

If one wants to increase paid productivity by 5%, it will be necessary either to reduce paid hours by 5%

Box 31•6

Specified Productivity Example

Assume the five FTEs each average 30 minutes of breaks per day, 30 minutes of staff meeting time per month, and 1 hour of inservice education per month. In addition, the administrative time included in the five FTEs totals 10 hours per week. Purchasing functions require an extra 4 hours per month.

SPECIFIED TIME

Breaks (0.5 h/d × 229 d/y × 5 FTEs)	572.5 h/y
Meetings (0.5 h/d × 12 mo × 5 FTEs)	30 h/y
In-service (1 h/mo × 12 mo × 5 FTEs)	60 h/y
Administrative (10 h/wk × 49 wk)	490 h/y
	1152.5 h/y

TOTAL UNTIMED HOURS

Total worked hours	9,160 h/y
Total untimed hours	152.5 h/y
Total specified hours	8,007.5 h/y

$$\text{Specified productivity} = \frac{\text{Total WLUs/y}}{\text{Total specified h/y}}$$
$$= 57.4 \text{ WLUs/h}$$

$$\text{Specified productivity} = \frac{57.4 \text{ WLU/h}}{60 \text{ min/h}}$$
$$= 95.7\%$$

---

or to increase volume by 5% without allowing a concurrent increase in paid hours beyond the present level. By performing worked- and specified-productivity studies, the laboratory manager can identify areas in the laboratory where change is needed. By studying productivity of various work shifts, he may discover ways to reorganize workload or personnel in such a manner as to allow a reduction in paid hours. The workload recording program and productivity studies provide an objective approach for determining staffing needs. Otherwise, the manager has only a subjective feeling about whether the laboratory is understaffed or overstaffed.

Computing the Labor Component of Test Costs

The cost of labor in the laboratory is often 60% to 70% of total direct costs. Before performing a cost-effectiveness study, the manager must know the labor cost of performing a WLU in the laboratory. Cost accounting by the macro and micro approaches demonstrate how each laboratory procedure is unique. The macro approach compares patient-charged WLUs with total costs. The macro approach does not appreciate the relationship of a procedure's workload time to its individual reagent, instrument, or nonpatient (standard and controls) requirements.

When performing a cost-effectiveness study, it is necessary to know the labor cost of the WLU in the laboratory. If the laboratory participates in the Monitrend service, the cost of salary expense/100 WLUs is supplied. If this figure is $14.20, divide by 100 to obtain the WLU cost of $0.142.

Laboratories that are not using Monitrend can divide the total WLUs for a period into the cost of laboratory technical, clerical, aide, and appropriate laboratory administrative (excluding physicians) pay for the same period. Because of the variation of productivity from month to month in many laboratories, a calculation should usually not be based on less than 3 months' data. If the laboratory performed 412,500 WLUs in 3 months and the cost for laboratory salaries (excluding physicians) for that period was $58,575, the laboratory labor cost per WLU is $58,575 divided by 412,500 WLUs, or $0.142/WLU.

Productivity is the output of the laboratory compared with its resources. In the past, WLUs were used to determine technologist workload. Because the billable test is easily understood, determined, and monitored by most laboratories, it can be used as a universal unit for comparison purposes. Today, more laboratories are looking at measuring total production factors and are using productivity ratios. There are several major programs available for this purpose, including the CAP's Laboratory Management Index Program (CAP-LMIP), the Volunteer Hospitals of America's Data Comparison Reporting System (VHA-DCRS), Health Care Development's Lab Trends, Monitrends, and the Mecon Peer program. The VHA-DCRS program has more than 1,000 hospitals. The CAP-LMIP has more than 1,000 clinic, independent, and hospital laboratories enrolled.[4]

Although each program has its own strengths and weaknesses, a brief description of the CAP-LMIP follows as an example of the type of information the laboratory manager will supply and receive when participating in such a program.

The CAP-LMIP is based on input and output units instead of WLUs.[4–6] Productivity can be assessed using output units, such as total billable tests. Input units (eg, personnel, salary, consumables, equipment) are used to evaluate labor and expense costs. Peer comparison is based on output units, not hospital bed size. This allows laboratories performing similar output (billable tests) to compare productivity based on the cost of their input (resources) independent of hospital bed size or the type of laboratory.

All participants of the CAP-LMIP receive the basic LMIP, which allows evaluation of total laboratory operations and is most applicable for small laboratories. Participants may also subscribe to the comprehensive LMIP, which includes six sectional productivity modules: chemistry, transfusion medicine, immunology, hematology, urinalysis, and microbiology. Specimen procurement and anatomic pathology modules are also available.

CAP-LMIP TERMINOLOGY

Total laboratory FTEs are a measure of labor or personnel time. One FTE is 1 person working 40 hours per week for 52 weeks per year (2,080 paid hours per year). Doctoral-level clinical scientists are included in this figure, but pathologists and other laboratory personnel are not.

Laboratory technical FTE refers to the actual testing personnel. This usually includes technicians, technologists, cytotechnologists, and histotechnologists. Nontechnical FTEs include laboratory secretaries, receptionists, couriers, phlebotomists, morgue attendants, and supervisors (who do not perform testing duties). If a supervisor spends 50% of his time on the bench performing testing, 0.5 FTE would be counted to reflect this technical activity.

Laboratory paid hours encompass all paid time, including vacation time, holiday time, sick time, education time away from the facility, actual overtime hours, and other paid time off (eg, jury duty). Actual overtime hours are counted on a one-for-one basis as the actual number of hours paid during call-back periods, whether the employee is at home or called in. Laboratory paid hours include all personnel on the laboratory payroll, excluding only pathologists, other laboratory physicians, students, and volunteers.

Laboratory worked hours are the total paid hours minus the paid time off (eg, paid vacation time, holiday time, sick time, education time away from the facility, jury duty). The actual number of hours worked overtime is included on a one-for-one basis (excluding pathologists, other laboratory physicians, students, and volunteers). CAP-LMIP participants provide the following information to CAP on a quarterly basis:

1. Billable tests
2. Billable tests performed on site
3. Billable tests referred out
4. Inpatient billable tests
5. Outpatient billable tests
6. Nonpatient billable tests
7. Hospital inpatient days
8. Hospital inpatient discharges

9. Total laboratory FTEs
10. Laboratory technical FTEs
11. Laboratory paid hours
12. Laboratory worked hours
13. Total laboratory labor expenses
14. Laboratory technical labor expense
15. Laboratory consumable expense
16. Laboratory blood and component expense
17. Laboratory equipment and maintenance expense
18. Laboratory equipment depreciation expense
19. Laboratory referred test expense
20. Outpatient visits

The CAP-LMIP reports the following to the participants:

Productivity Comparison Ratios

1. On-site billable tests per total FTE
2. On-site billable tests per technical FTE
3. Percent technical FTEs per total FTEs
4. On-site billable tests per worked hour
5. On-site billable tests per paid hour
6. Percent worked hour per paid hour
7. On-site billable tests per total billable tests

Use Comparison Ratios

1. Inpatient billable tests per day
2. Inpatient billable tests per discharge

Cost-Effectiveness Ratios

1. Consumable expense per on-site billable test
2. Depreciation expense per on-site billable test
3. Direct laboratory expense per on-site billable test
4. Total labor expense per total on-site billable test
5. Technical labor expense per patient day
6. Total laboratory expense per discharge
7. Total laboratory expense per patient day
8. Referred billable test expense per billable tests
9. Total expense per total billable tests
10. Cost of blood as percentage of total expense

Users of programs such as the CAP-LMIP have found the most commonly valued ratios in order of importance to be:[7]

1. Direct costs per test
2. Consumable costs per test
3. Salary costs per test
4. Tests per worked hour
5. Tests per technical FTE
6. Tests per total FTE
7. Tests per paid hour

The CAP-LMIP and programs like it are not only useful for monitoring labor productivity, but also allow the laboratory manager to evaluate the cost effectiveness of supply and equipment use. These programs establish performance benchmarks available only through external peer comparison. The program ratios are useful for monitoring changes made by management. For instance, if a new chemistry analyzer was purchased with the goal of reducing the cost of supplies and labor, after the instrument is in use, the technical labor expense per billable chemistry test and consumables expense per billable chemistry test should reflect this improvement.

Identifying Program Areas

Variance analysis is one of the best means a laboratory manager has of detecting problem areas. Many institutional and laboratory computer programs provide monthly cost reports. By comparing actual expenses to budget expenses, the laboratory manager can detect problem areas and deal with them in a timely manner. Productivity ratios and comparison with peer laboratories through programs such as the CAP-LMIP are extremely valuable. Without these reports, the manager might devote time and effort to areas that seem inefficient but actually are not. Good cost analysis is an essential tool for the laboratory manager.

REFERENCES

1. Diagnostics: Just who is the customer? In Vivo The Business and Medicine Report 12(7):10, 1994
2. Workload Recording Method and Personnel Management Manual, 1992 ed, pp 7–9. Northfield, College of American Pathologists, 1991
3. Cost Accounting in the Clinical Laboratory: Tentative Guideline, pp 10–11. Villanova, National Committee for Clinical Laboratory Standards, 1994
4. Sodeman T, Griffith J: Financial Management in the Clinical Laboratory—American Society for Clinical Pathologists Workshop. Cincinnati, The Christ Hospital, 1994
5. Sodeman TM: Your lab's productivity. CAP Today June, 1993
6. College of American Pathologists: Laboratory Management Index Program. Northfield, College of American Pathologists, 1994
7. Hunter LL, Pomerantz P: Practical tools for evaluation. Clinical Laboratory Management Review 8(5):439, 1994

ANNOTATED BIBLIOGRAPHY

Brase SJ, Matysik MK: How to speak "finance." Clinical Laboratory Management Review 6:2, 1992
    This article provides good explanations and examples of balance sheets and cash flow statements.

Carpenter RB: Laboratory cost analysis: A practical approach. Clinical Laboratory Management Review 4:3, 1990
> A method for performing cost analysis in a smaller laboratory without use of a computer is presented. Useful worksheets and examples are included.

College of American Pathologists: Laboratory Management Index Program. Northfield, College of American Pathologists, 1994
> The program is described with definitions of terms and examples of the output.

Cost Accounting in the Clinical Laboratory: Tentative Guide, pp 10–11. Villanova, National Committee for Clinical Laboratory Standards, 1994
> This guideline should help standardize laboratory cost accounting. It provides an excellent description of the concepts of cost accounting plus techniques for application. Included are many worksheets, formulas, and examples that make this manual essential to the student and manager.

Frangedakis BJ: Cost accounting for the small laboratory. Lab Med September:596–597, 1993
> This is a good source for examples of quality control and proficiency testing cost calculations.

Getzen TE: What is value? Clinical Laboratory Management Review 8:6, 1994
> This article discusses the calculation of actual value, cash flow, rate of return, present value discounting, and risk.

Hunter LL, Pomerantz P: Practical Tools for Evaluation. Clinical Laboratory Management Review 8(5):439, 1994
> This article includes results of a survey that identified and ranked the value of the tools laboratory managers use to evaluate the various aspects of laboratory productivity.

Simmers NR: A tool to evaluate equipment purchases. MLO 25: 37–40, 1993
> Discounted cash flow analysis is presented as a tool to evaluate instrument purchases.

Sodeman T, Griffith J: Financial Management in the Clinical Laboratory—American Society for Clinical Pathologists Workshop. The Christ Hospital, Cincinnati, 1994
> This workshop presents an excellent and comprehensive overview of the subject with examples from the presenters' laboratory.

Sodeman TM: Your lab's productivity. CAP Today June, 1993
> This article discusses why the College of American Pathologists switched from the workload recording method to the LMIP.

Tirabassi CP: Cost accounting in the POL. POL Adviser November, 1994
> This article presents an excellent explanation of cost accounting for the physician's office laboratory and includes useful worksheets and examples.

Workload Recording Method and Personnel Management Manual, 1992 ed, pp 7–9. Northfield, College of American Pathologists, 1991
> This manual describes the WLU system and lists WLU values.

32

Coding, Billing, and Reimbursement Management

Diana Voorhees

For many years, laboratories were accustomed to billing for their services and receiving payment that reflected nearly 100% of the billed amount. As government health-care programs, primarily Medicare and Medicaid, approached a prospective rather than retrospective payment system, laboratory reimbursement changed. In 1984, the prospective payment system was implemented for inpatient reimbursement. This system identified a specified reimbursement per inpatient visit based on patient diagnosis. This was the first sign of "managed care" and "capitated payments." Laboratories would continue to be reimbursed for outpatient services according to the procedures performed. These procedures, however, were to be identified with five-digit numerical numbers or codes from current procedural terminology (CPT). CPT codes would also be linked to a predetermined amount of reimbursement, another sign of emerging capitated payment.

CURRENT PROCEDURAL TERMINOLOGY CODING

These five-digit numerical codes identify specific analytes, methodologies, assays, stains, consultations, interpretations, and so forth. As the acronym implies, these codes identify *procedures* performed for billing purposes. CPT catalogs laboratory services in the 80000 series of codes by discipline (Box 32-1).

How and When to Use CPT Codes

All Medicare, nearly 100% of state Medicaid, and many private or commercial insurance payers require use of CPT to identify services. These payers will deny payment for any service not identified with a CPT code—no code, no payment. It is important to assign accurate and effective CPT codes to services. To be accurate and efficient, one must be familiar with CPT format and use. Many CPT code descriptions contain words or phrases that duplicate words or phrases in codes immediately listed above or below. To conserve space, a coding description that is indented includes all verbiage prior to the semicolon in the preceding description (Table 32-1).

CPT 81000 describes the method and components of a urinalysis prior to the semicolon. Because the following two codes are indented, the portion of the description for CPT 81000 prior to the semicolon applies to CPT 81002 and 81003 as well. The portion of the description following the semicolon differentiates the four codes. CPT 81000 includes a microscopic examination, as does 81001, but the chemical solution is automated. CPT 81002 does not include a microscopy, and the dipstick results are read visually. CPT 81003 includes no microscopic examination, and the results of the dipstick are read by an automated means.

Unlisted Codes

Each of the previously listed CPT sections includes at least one miscellaneous or "unlisted" code, which can be assigned to a procedure when no other code is applicable. For example, the hematology section includes CPT 85999 to identify a miscellaneous hematology or hemostasis procedure. Providers should limit the use of these codes because they produce no reimbursement unless a manual or paper claim is accompanied by documentation explaining the merit for test performance and value of results. Most payers/insurers encourage "electronic" billing. Such claims usually transmit codes and fees in addition to patient demographics. Because

509

Box 32·1

Current Procedural Terminology Laboratory Services Catalog

80002–80019	Automated multichannel chemistry tests
80050–80092	Organ- and disease-oriented panels
80100–80299	Drug testing and therapeutic assays
80400–80440	Evocative/suppression testing
80500–80502	Clinical consultations
81000–81099	Urinalysis
82000–84999	Chemistry and molecular diagnostics
85002–85999	Hematology and hemostasis
86000–86849	Immunology
86850–86999	Transfusion medicine
87001–87999	Microbiology
88000–88299	Anatomic pathology, cytopathology, and cytogenetics
88300–88399	Surgical pathology
89050–89399	Miscellaneous procedures

descriptions are omitted from electronically transmitted claims, the payer cannot decipher the type of procedure being billed when an unlisted code is used. Thus, payment will automatically be denied by government payers. A manual claim provides necessary information for payment. The drawbacks to manual claims include the increased time required to produce a paper document, increased expense for billing personnel to produce paper claims, delayed payment, and possible medical review by the payer to determine medical necessity.

Table 32-1
Coding Descriptions

CPT	Description
81000	Urinalysis; by dip stick or tablet reagent for bilirubin, glucose, hemoglobin, ketones, leukocytes, nitrite, pH, protein, specific gravity, urobilinogen, any number of these constituents; with microscopy
81001	automated, with microscopy
81002	without microscopy, nonautomated
81003	without microscopy, automated

Coding Updates

The CPT changes annually. Changes are categorized as additions, deletions, or description revisions and are summarized in Appendix B of CPT. If a code is added to CPT, it bears a "●" symbol to the left of the code. If a code is deleted from CPT, it is listed in parentheses. There may be a reference to another code that substitutes for the deleted code. The symbol "▲" precedes a code with a change in description (Table 32-2).

During the previous year, CPT 83519 was described as an "Immunoassay, analyte, by radionuclide technique (eg, RIA)." The new description restricts use of this code for a *quantitative* assay. Providers must be timely in recognizing annual coding changes. To continue identifying a *qualitative* analysis with CPT 83519 would be noncompliant with government billing regulations. To bill a hepatitis C antibody with a methodology code would be noncompliant when a specific code has been added. Billing with an obsolete or deleted CPT code leads to payment denial.

Technical Component Versus Professional Component

The Medicare program equates the professional component (PC) of a service with a physician component or physician-rendered service. The technical component (TC) is the service or portion of a service rendered by any other health-care professional. Some codes have both components, few have only a PC, and most have only a TC (Table 32-3).

If a physician bills Medicare for a TC-only service, no payment will be issued. Conversely, if a hospital clinical laboratory bills a PC-only service, payment will be denied.

Modifiers

On occasion, a service may be more extensive than usual, less extensive than usual, bilateral, repeated for second opinion, referred to another laboratory, and so

Table 32-2
Coding Updates

CPT	Description
●86303	Hepatitis C antibody; confirmatory test (e.g., immunoblot)
(86365 has been deleted)	
(86411 has been deleted. To report, see 86971)	
▲83519	Immunoassay, analyte, quantitative; by radiopharmaceutical technique (eg, RIA)

Table 32-3
Examples of Technical Components and Professional Components

CPT	Description	Component(s)
83150	Homovanillic acid	TC only
80500	Clinical pathology consultation; limited, without review of patient's history and medical records	PC only
88302	Level II—surgical pathology, gross and microscopic examination	TC and PC

forth. These exceptions may be reported by adding two-digit numerical modifiers to the end of a code. While there are numerous modifiers, only five are listed in the laboratory and pathology section of CPT (Table 32-4).

If a billing program cannot report an eight-digit code, the modifier may be converted to a five-digit code (eg, 09926 for -26) and reported on the line following the regular CPT code. Multiple modifiers may be indicated with -99 following a code (or 09999 on the following line).

Because most clinical laboratory services are reimbursed on a fee schedule or by a percentage of charge and performed in a routinely similar manner, the -22 and -52 modifiers have little use. Pathologists may find these modifiers helpful. Hospital billings for the technical components of procedures are processed by Medicare intermediaries, which do *not* recognize modifiers.

Modifier -32 is informational and has no impact on reimbursement. In reality, most laboratories are unaware that a procedure may be mandated by a third-party payer.

Table 32-4
Five Modifiers Listed in the Laboratory and Pathology Section of Current Procedural Terminology

Modifier	Circumstance
-22	Unusual procedural services
-26	Professional component
-32	Mandated services
-52	Reduced services
-90	Reference (outside) laboratory

The -90 modifier indicates that a laboratory is billing for an analysis that was performed by another laboratory. Hospital laboratories do not recognize modifiers, and due to more recent billing guidelines, this modifier is infrequently used.

The most applicable modifier is -26, which only requests payment for a physician component of a service. Medicare recognizes the merit of a pathologist's interpretation of certain test results; in these instances, the -26 modifier is appropriately used to bill for the interpretation.

Intermediaries and Carriers

Briefly, a Medicare carrier is an insurance company that bids for and is awarded the contract to process part B claims for Medicare beneficiaries. Part B claims typically include outpatient hospital billings, independent laboratory services, physician office laboratory services, clinic billings, and all physician-rendered services. Part B services are billed to Medicare on an Health Care Financing Administration (HCFA) 1500 form.

A Medicare Intermediary is an insurance company that also is awarded the Medicare contract to mediate the claims process primarily for hospital inpatient services, part A. As hospitals developed outreach programs for rendering outpatient medical services, the hospital billing offices handled outpatient billings as well. Hospital part A and B billings are transmitted using a UB92 claim form.

Because hospital-generated billings are processed by intermediaries, only a TC is reimbursed. Remember, intermediaries do not recognize CPT modifiers; therefore, when a hospital bills with CPT 88302 on a UB92 form, only the TC is reimbursed. If a pathologist provides interpretation of a specimen associated with CPT 88302, the professional component would be billed directly to a Medicare carrier on a HCFA 1500 form with the addition of -26 modifier (88302-26). The carrier would then reimburse only the PC of the procedure.

Because independent laboratories, physician office laboratories, and clinics send all Medicare claims to a carrier, a "global" billing would be appropriate when both TC and PC are provided. The appropriate CPT code (eg, 88302) would be indicated with no modifier. The carrier would reimburse both TC and PC.

OTHER HCPCS CODES

The CPT is actually level I of the HCFA Common Procedural Coding System (HCPCS). CPT is authored by the American Medical Association, and therefore most codes historically identified physician-provided proce-

Table 32-5
Level II HCPCS Codes (Examples)

HCPCS	Description
J7190	Factor VIII, per IU
J7197	Antithrombin III, per IU
P9010	Blood (whole), for transfusion, per unit
P9012	Cryoprecipitate, each unit
P9021	Red blood cells, each unit

dures. To supplement these codes, the HCFA established level II HCPCS codes. Level II codes are alphanumeric, five-digit codes that are nationally recognized. Most level II codes that impact laboratories are found in the J or P series of these alphanumeric codes (Table 32-5).

Level II codes are collectively found in a separate book and are available through HCFA or other coding publishers.

Level III codes are assigned by local carriers to fill voids in CPT and level II coding. These codes are also alphanumeric (W, X, Y, Z), include five digits, and may only be used when billing the carrier that assigned them (Table 32-6).

The status of these level III codes should be verified annually.

FEE SCHEDULES

Clinical laboratory procedures are reimbursed by Medicare according to the clinical laboratory fee schedule. Most CPT codes are recognized on this fee schedule. Medicaid, which varies by state, may frequently exempt recognition for CPT codes that are Medicare recognized. The clinical laboratory fee schedule identifies a predetermined amount of reimbursement for each CPT code by Medicare locale. Payment for a laboratory service is always the lower of the (1) provider charge, (2) local fee schedule amount, or (3) national limitation.

Table 32-6
Level III HCPCS Codes (Examples)

Code	Description
W8012	Chlamydia antibody, serum
Y8257	Cyclosporin level
X8410	LASA
X8414	Spontaneous blastogenesis assay

A local fee schedule may identify an allowable fee for a code that is higher than the provider's charge. In this instance, the charge, which is lower than the Medicare allowable, would be the reimbursed amount.

In recent years, Medicare has targeted high-volume laboratory tests that appear to be generously reimbursed by local carriers and intermediaries and increasingly consuming the program budget. This list of procedures now includes nearly all of laboratory CPT. Thus, a national limitation or "cap" has been superimposed on area fee schedules. Therefore, reimbursement for a CPT code by a local Medicare payer would be superseded by the national limitation if the national limitation were lower than the local allowable.

When Medicare initiated the fee schedule reimbursement, it replaced fee-for-service reimbursement. To wean providers into the fee schedule process, reimbursement was initiated at 115% of the fee schedule amount (at the 60th percentile of the median of all national fee schedules). This 115% was to be annually decreased to 100% of the fee schedule's 60th percentile. Some hospitals may be reimbursed at the 62nd percentile if they meet requirements and are classified as a rural facility. Once the 100% level was attained, however, the caps continued to drop to 96%, 93%, 88%, 84%, 80% (1995), 76% (1996), and now 74% (1998). Economic increases will be curbed by Congress for 5 straight years, and with the caps consistently dropping, chances for future economic increases look bleak.

Exemptions From Fee Schedule Payment

Not all clinical laboratory procedures are reimbursed according to the fee schedule. Certain procedures are exempt (Box 32-2). Therefore, these procedures are generally reimbursed at a percentage of the provider charge. This percentage may vary depending on type

Box 32·2

Procedures Exempt From Fee Schedule Payment

1. Nondiagnostic services (transfusion medicine)
2. Consultations
3. Procedures attached to new current procedural terminology codes
4. Procedures identified with unlisted codes
5. Other physician services
6. Anatomic, surgical, cytopathology services

of laboratory, Medicare contract, and application of Medicare fee schedule (see below).

Medicare Fee Schedule

This fee schedule usually applies to reimbursement of physician services and is the outcome of the research and development of the resource-based relative value scale (RVS). Pathologists were first exposed to fee schedule payment in 1992. When a procedure includes a technical component that is exempt from the clinical laboratory fee schedule, the TC may be reimbursed by the Medicare fee schedule.

An RVS delineates a value for individual medical procedures relative to other procedures. For example, CPT 85060 identifies a physician's written interpretation of a peripheral blood smear. The Medicare fee schedule currently aligns this procedure to a relative value of 0.69 units. This total relative value is further segmented into relative value units (RVUs) as in Table 32-7. This particular CPT code, 85060, relates to a professional component only.

Compare the above procedure, CPT 85060, with another procedure, CPT 88305. This latter code describes a midlevel, gross and microscopic examination of tissue, such as bone marrow biopsies, breast biopsies, cell blocks, and heart valves. This code demonstrates an example of a procedure with both TC and PC. The global or total RVU is 1.86. RVUs are further delineated in Table 32-8.

To convert a relative value of a procedure into a payment amount, a conversion factor is used. The national conversion factor for nonsurgical physician services is approximately $35. Thus, $35 multiplied by 1.32 for CPT 88305, as an example, would produce reimbursement to a physician of $46.20. In actuality, the conversion factor is also adjusted for geographic cost practice variances.

Other Payment Methods

Numerous RVSs exist; thus, not all RVSs align the same value to every procedure. Therefore, conversion factors cannot be substituted from one RVS to another. Many

Table 32-8
Further Delineation of Relative Value Units (RVUs)

Component	RVU
Work—PC	0.75
Work—TC	0.00
Practice expense—PC	0.53
Practice expense—TC	0.50
Malpractice—PC	0.04
Malpractice—TC	0.04
Subtotal—PC	1.32
Subtotal—TC	0.54
Total	1.86

private or commercial payers use these systems for payment purposes. Providers often purchase these scales as a mechanism to evaluate their current fees.

An alternate guideline for governing payment is a usual, customary, and reasonable (UCR) set of data. These data are usually based on tracking provider charges to determine what charge is actually usual, customary, and reasonable by locale. Such databases may also be purchased and are still used by many commercial payers.

Of course, traditional payment methods have included fee for service and percentage of charge. The Medicare fee schedule, RVS, and UCR systems of tracking provider charges and guiding reimbursement of services have provided data sets that encourage and assist in the development of managed care. These data and provider billings and costs will continue to require development and monitoring to evaluate outcomes and areas of change in managed care.

OTHER CODING SYSTEMS

International Classification of Disease-9 Codes

While CPT codes identify *procedures*, International Classification of Disease-9 (ICD-9) codes identify diagnoses. ICD-9 codes provide rationale and justification for procedures being ordered and performed. Without this justification, procedures may be performed, but payment will be denied. Thus, it is important for ICD-9 codes to reflect patient status. Some procedures are considered screening procedures and are not covered by Medicare. The ICD-9 code may indicate whether a procedure should be covered and reimbursed. For ex-

Table 32-7
Relative Value Unit (RVU) Segments

Component	RVU
Work	0.45
Practice expense	0.22
Malpractice liability	0.02
Total	0.69

ample, a prostate-specific antigen determination is only covered for male patients when Medicare providers report diagnosis codes associated with known carcinoma of the prostate to establish a baseline (ICD-9 185), known neoplasms impeding the bladder (ICD-9 188.8), lymph node neoplasms (ICD-9 196.5 and 196.6), prostate carcinoma in situ (ICD-9 233.4), or family history of prostate cancer (ICD-9 V16.5).

Ancillary ICD-9 codes or "V" codes relate to signs, symptoms, and conditions; their use is important in substantiating procedural orders. More than one ICD-9 code may be used when filing a claim to government payers. These codes are required when filing all inpatient and outpatient claims to government payers.

Revenue Codes

Hospital laboratories must use revenue codes for all claims forwarded to government payers. These three-digit codes identify the hospital department where a service was rendered. These codes are required for all hospital billing whether impatient or outpatient. Hospital supplies and other items, which are not procedures, have no CPT code and would be billed under a revenue code. When CPT or other HCPCS codes are used for identifying procedures, it is occasionally important to crosswalk a CPT-coded procedure to a specific revenue code. While most hospital clinical laboratory procedures crosswalk to the general revenue code 300, specific revenue code requirements exist for certain services, such as those related to autologous and directed units. Laboratory revenue codes are listed in Appendix 32-1.

Certification Codes

Certification codes are required for all laboratory billings except those generated in the hospital setting. These codes, also three digits, indicate to government payers whether a laboratory has met requirements for performing a billed procedure. These codes are listed in Appendix 32-2. For example, a laboratory certified to perform general microbiology procedures but not specifically parasitology testing would not be reimbursed for parasitology testing. CPT codes are linked to categories of certification codes for Clinical Laboratory Improvement Act delineation of testing.

Diagnosis-Related Group Codes

Diagnosis-related group (DRG) codes classify inpatient stays into payment groups according to diagnosis(es) indicated on claims. These groups also direct reim-

bursement because each DRG code is aligned to a specific dollar amount. When a hospital files a Medicare claim on a hospital inpatient, an intermediary uses an editing system to examine diagnosis coding and group the visit accordingly into a payment category or DRG. There are approximately 270 DRGs. Reimbursement for a particular DRG will vary from one facility to another within the same geographic area. Thus, negotiations and cost documentation are important factors when establishing payment levels with Medicare. While the payment base is the same for every facility, certain factors provide added dollars. These factors include teaching versus nonteaching status, type of capital equipment, and disproportionate shares of welfare service.

Ambulatory Patient Group Codes

Ambulatory patient groups (APGs) comprise an outpatient prospective payment system that parallels the inpatient DRGs. While other outpatient payment mechanisms have been proposed, APGs were chosen for experimental reimbursement by certain Medicaid agencies. HCFA is also proposing acceptance of APG for Medicare due to the following comparative advantages:

1. Includes complete range of outpatient services
2. Clinically based and reflects costs
3. Flexible in inclusion of varying ancillary services

While this outpatient prospective payment program is mandated by Omnibus Budget Reconciliation Act (OBRA) 90, HCFA projects a "phase-in" approach. Laboratory services are not currently targeted for the initial phase.

REIMBURSEMENT PROCESS

Reimbursement should be considered a cyclic process. The process begins with how a service is ordered and progresses through the initiation of a service (eg, blood drawing), provision of testing and results, identification of service (applicable coding systems), establishment of an appropriate charge, accurate billing and generation of claims, and receipt of fair and appropriate reimbursement. This process should be completely evaluated to ensure a complete cycle that ends with accurate reimbursement. The process should also be evaluated on a periodic basis to detect impedances, correct errors, and verify a continuum. This evaluation is also necessary to maintain compliance with government regulations.

FRAUD AND ABUSE

Noncompliance with government regulations can result in one or two categories of misuse.

Fraud

Fraud may be briefly defined as an intentional deception or misrepresentation that knowingly results in an unauthorized benefit. Fraud is a felony, and if a conviction results, it leads to a maximum penalty of $25,000 per infraction or 5 years of imprisonment. These penalties are projected to be increased.

Abuse

Abuse describes incidents or practices that deter from accepted medical, business, or financial practices and cause unnecessary cost or improper reimbursement by government programs. Abusive practices are considered misdemeanors and may result in fines of up to $10,000 per infraction (plus treble damages) and suspension from the abused programs.

   Practices that lead to fraud and abuse include upcoding, double billing, and unbundling or fragmentation. Upcoding is the practice of attaching a CPT code to a procedure that will be reimbursed more than an appropriate amount. For example, a provider in Florida might perform a cell count on spinal fluid and not accompany the count with a differential. The correct CPT code would be 89050, cell count only, which precipitates a $6.70 reimbursement from Medicare. If the provider billed Medicare using CPT 89051, count *and* differential, $7.80 would be reimbursed. This differential amount, $1.10, would be falsely reimbursed on every billing.

Double billing may occur if a hospital-based pathologist, intending to bill for only an interpretation of a surgical specimen, forwards a CPT-coded claim without the -26 modifier. The hospital would, for example, bill an intermediary for the TC (histologic preparation) surrounding a bone marrow biopsy with CPT 88305. The physician's interpretation should be billed with CPT 88305-26 through the carrier. If the modifier is not used in this instance, the carrier would reimburse globally (both TC and PC); the TC would be reimbursed twice.

   An example of unbundling or fragmentation includes billing component tests of a panel or profile with individual CPT codes rather than one code that reflects the composite testing. Note the scenario in Table 32-9 using allowables from the state of Illinois.

   Fragmentation usually leads to an inappropriately higher level of reimbursement. CPT coding assignments should be as specific as possible. Medicare is currently addressing editing capabilities to prevent payment for unbundled claims.

Specific Coding

As previously indicated, if a specific CPT code exists for a procedure, the procedure should be identified with that code rather than an alternative code. A qualitative or semiqualitative immunoassay for an immunoglobulin M (IgM) *Chlamydia* antibody should be coded with CPT 86632, which specifically identifies an IgM antibody to *Chlamydia*. Occasionally this same procedure is linked to CPT 86317, a quantitative immunoassay for an infectious agent antibody. Also, codes change annually. If CPT 86317 were to reimburse more than 86632, attachment of 86317 could be misconstrued as upcoding as well.

Table 32-9
Abuse Scenarios Using Allowables From the State of Illinois

Incorrect Coding			Correct Coding		
CPT	Test	Allowable	CPT	Panel	Allowable
82465	Cholesterol	$6.15	80061	Lipid	$18.95
83718	High-density lipoprotein	11.58			
84478	Triglycerides	8.10			
	Total	$25.83			$18.95

FUTURE TRENDS AND ISSUES

The topics and information presented in this discussion provide a base for building continued understanding and added knowledge of coding, billing, and reimbursement management in the medical laboratory. To present and thoroughly discuss all related issues would require a separate text.

The last 2 years have been interesting for laboratory reimbursement. We have seen government payers' scrutiny of laboratory operations result in massive paybacks and penalties. Fraud and abuse are constantly on every laboratory administrator's mind. The laboratory continues to be targeted for Medicare and Medicaid reimbursement cuts. As personnel decreases are mandated by certain economic outcomes, it becomes more crucial than ever to implement cost-effective management and ensure *complete* and *appropriate* payment for services. Administrators will potentially be faced with direct billing requirements, coinsurance mandates, ap-

propriateness of discounts, competitive bidding for Medicare contracts, and APGs, the outpatient cap on government payment. What government payers have implemented and mandated is increasingly adopted by private payers. Managed care will continue to evolve.

REFERENCES

1. CPT, 4th ed. Chicago, American Medical Association, 1995
2. Department of Health and Human Services: ICD-9-CM. Salt Lake City, Medicode Publications, 1995
3. Medicare Carriers Manual. Department of Health and Human Services
4. Voorhees DV: Mistakes to avoid in CPT coding and billing. MLO June, 1991
5. Federal Register, U.S. Washington, DC, Government Printing, 59(235), 1994
6. Code It Right. Salt Lake City, Med-Index Publications, 1992
7. Voorhees DV: Pathology and laboratory changes, reimbursement update. Salt Lake City, 8(3), 1993

APPENDIX 32–1 REVENUE CODES

The following groups of revenue codes are appropriate for identifying clinical and other diagnostic laboratory services. Each code is accompanied by a standard abbreviation for billing purposes. Substitute the appropriate number from each subcategory for the "X" in the three-digit heading.

30X: *Laboratory*—Charges for the performance of diagnostic and routine clinical laboratory tests

Subcategory	Standard Abbreviation
0—General classification	LABORATORY or (LAB)
1—Chemistry	LAB/CHEMISTRY
2—Immunology	LAB/IMMUNOLOGY
3—Renal patient (home)	LAB/RENAL HOME
4—Nonroutine dialysis	LAB/NR DIALYSIS
5—Hematology	LAB/HEMATOLOGY
6—Bacteriology and microbiology	LAB/BACT-MICRO
7—Urology	LAB/UROLOGY
9—Other laboratory	LAB/OTHER

31X: Laboratory pathological—Charges for diagnostic and routine laboratory tests on tissues and culture

Subcategory	Standard Abbreviation
0—General classification	PATHOLOGY LAB or (PATH LAB)
1—Cytology	PATHOL/CYTOLOGY
2—Histology	PATHOL/HYSTOL
4—Biopsy	PATHOL/BIOPSY
9—Other	PATHOL/OTHER

38X: Blood—Charges for blood; separately identified for private payer purposes

Subcategory	Standard Abbreviation
0—General classification	BLOOD
1—Packed red cells	BLOOD/PKD RED
2—Whole blood	BLOOD/WHOLE
3—Plasma	BLOOD/PLASMA
4—Platelets	BLOOD/PLATELETS
5—Leukocytes	BLOOD/LEUKOCYTES
6—Other components	BLOOD/COMPONENTS
7—Other derivatives	BLOOD/DERIVATIVES
9—Other blood	BLOOD/OTHER

39X: Blood storage and processing—Charges for the storage and processing of whole blood

Subcategory	Standard Abbreviation
0—General classification	BLOOD/STOR-PROC
1—Blood administration	BLOOD/ADMIN.
9—Other blood storage and processing	BLOOD/OTHER STOR

APPENDIX 32-2 Laboratory Certification Codes

010 Histocompatibility testing (tissue typing)
100 Microbiology
    110 Bacteriology (with antimicrobial susceptibility)
    120 Mycology
    130 Parasitology
    140 Virology
    150 Other
200 Serology
    210 Syphilis
    220 Serology—other
300 Clinical chemistry—routine
    310 Clinical chemistry—routine
    320 Urinalysis—clinical microscopy
    330 Chemistry—other (toxicology)
    330 Chemistry—other (endocrinology)
400 Hematology
500 Immunohematology
    510 Subgrouping
    520 Antibody identification
    530 Compatibility testing—cross-match
    540 Blood typing for paternity tests
600 Pathology
    610 Histopathology
    620 Oral pathology
    630 Exfoliative cytology

33

Financial Ratios for Laboratory Management Decision Making

James W. Sharp

NEW GOALS AND CHALLENGES

The Tax Equity Fiscal Responsibility Act (TEFRA), passed in 1982, ushered in a new operating environment for hospital clinical laboratories. Before TEFRA, the goal of the clinical laboratory was to provide quality laboratory services in a timely fashion. Now the goal is to provide quality, timely laboratory services in a cost-effective manner.[6]

The shift in emphasis has created new challenges, and new challenges require new resources. Today's laboratory decision makers need a thorough understanding of laboratory economics and access to detailed quantitative cost data. The purposes of this chapter are twofold: first, to present an overview of an effective laboratory information management system and second, to demonstrate how this system provides the essential data necessary to make critical operational and functional management decisions.

Most businesses are split into marketing and sales, production and manufacturing, and accounting and finances.[3] The marketing and sales division identifies the need for a product and its likely markets; the manufacturing people are responsible for efficiently producing the product; and the financial division sees that the products are produced, marketed, and sold at a profit.

Similarly, a clinical laboratory has three functional divisions (Fig. 33-1). In the laboratory, the marketing and sales function is called utilization and is controlled by the physicians on the medical staff. By ordering laboratory tests to diagnose disease and monitor therapy, for example, physicians ultimately determine the number and types of tests processed and performed in the laboratory.

The type of clinical tests performed by the laboratory range from the simple, highly automated, routine chemistry tests to the complex, esoteric, labor intensive, low-volume hormone assays. The physician sets the service-level requirements for each test. For example, a test may be ordered in a stat mode with a 2-hour turnaround time requirement, or it may be ordered in a routine mode with a 24-hour turnaround time. Because it is more expensive for the laboratory to provide the rapid service, physicians control, to a large extent, laboratory costs.

The operations, or production, division of the laboratory processes and produces the test results. This division is under the control of the laboratory director or the laboratory manager. These individuals produce the physician-requested output (laboratory tests), using an efficient combination of input factors (labor, materials, and equipment).

The hospital administrator controls the financial side of the laboratory. Decisions about test prices affect laboratory revenues, and decisions about employee pay policies affect laboratory expenses. Therefore, the hospital administrator determines the laboratory's profit or gross margin (excess of revenues over expenses).

Figure 33–1 shows the interrelationships between the three laboratory divisions. Decisions made in one sphere have an impact on the other two. For example, a financial decision to raise test prices made by the administrator might cause a decrease in the number of tests physicians order and lead to an overall decrease,

519

Hospital Clinical Laboratory

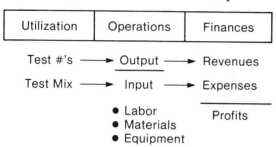

FIGURE 33–1.   Interrelationships among three laboratory division.

rather than an increase, in revenues. In addition, the "productivity" of the laboratory would suffer because it would be doing fewer tests.

THE THREE-STEP PROCESS

Managing a clinical laboratory is a three-step process. The manager first sets appropriate and realistic goals, then develops a system for evaluating and measuring progress toward those goals, and finally takes corrective action when necessary.

Laboratory goals and objectives are determined through a strategic planning process. In strategic planning, certain external, environmental factors and internal, laboratory factors are examined and analyzed.[3] A thorough analysis of the external factors uncovers the opportunities and constraints in the current economic climate. Internal factor analysis identifies the strengths and weaknesses of the laboratory. The strengths and weaknesses are matched with the opportunities and constraints, and appropriate goals and objectives are determined.

Some of the environmental factors examined are the impact of recent legislation on laboratory activities, current economic trends, projected industry growth rates, impact of new technologies, local competition, and community expectations.[2]

For example, an analysis of recent legislative activity might reveal that an increasing number of hospital patients are covered by fixed-rate insurance, such as diagnosis-related groups (DRGs), health maintenance organizations (HMOs), or prospective payment organizations (PPOs). This means that a significant percentage of laboratory tests are reimbursed at a set rate regardless of the laboratory's charges for these services. This severely limits the effectiveness of the strategy of increasing test prices to raise revenues.

An analysis of economic trends and industry growth rates suggests that the population is growing older. Older patients are usually "sicker," and sicker patients require more laboratory tests. This suggests that laboratory test volume should continue to increase. However, the business community complains about the high cost of health insurance premiums it pays for its employees. This is a powerful downward force tending to negate the upward pull of an aging population's use of health-care resources and laboratory test volume.

Another trend is the shift of patient care from the hospital environment to home health-care centers and outpatient surgery units. There is a parallel shift of laboratory testing from the hospital laboratory to physician's offices.[5] What percentage of hospital laboratory tests will eventually be affected by these shifts? What are the long-range effects of these trends on laboratory revenues?

Every day new and less expensive methods of performing laboratory tests are introduced by various manufacturers. Physicians—and even patients—are encouraged by these manufacturers to perform more diagnostic testing themselves. This trend in technology will probably continue and further erode the test bases of the large hospital laboratories.

The large commercial laboratories see much opportunity in the changing times. These giants are actively competing with hospital and physicians' office laboratories for a shrinking number of laboratory tests. This intense competition is causing a downward trend in test prices, further squeezing already tight operating margins. In addition, the commercial laboratories are offering to manage entire laboratories for hospital clients.[4] This raises questions regarding the adequacy of the quality and service of laboratory testing.

The feelings and expectations of the local community also affect laboratory decision making. For example, does the community expect its hospital to provide complete medical coverage because it is the only hospital in town? If this is so, then the laboratory will be forced to provide a wider variety of tests and services than is economically prudent.

Internal factor analysis involves studying the laboratory's management and organizational structure, its type and use of labor, and its financial condition. For example, an analysis of the organizational and management structure may reveal that the laboratory lacks the ability to respond to the demands and provide the levels of service requested by the medical staff. Instead, the analysis might reveal that because there is no method of calculating data on resource use and distributing it to the appropriate section supervisors, labor and supply costs are higher than expected.

It is important to analyze the work force, because labor costs are the largest budget item. An analysis of the work force may reveal that the majority of the technologists are specialized and capable of working only in certain areas of the laboratory. This lack of flexibility means that it takes more full-time equivalents to staff the laboratory adequately. If, because of unions or other outside forces, laboratory salaries are artificially inflated, cost-reduction strategies will be only marginally successful.

The financial condition of the hospital and laboratory is important in formulating short- and long-term goals. Although a particular strategy may make sense, capital is needed for implementation. The options available to a cash-poor laboratory are limited.

After the external and internal analyses are concluded, goals and objectives are set. What are reasonable laboratory goals and objectives? Since TEFRA, the survival strategy of most hospitals is clear—increase revenues or decrease costs. For the laboratory, increasing revenues means marketing laboratory tests to new, previously untapped sources. Decreasing costs involves lowering laboratory operating expenses. The two strategies are mutually incompatible. That is, a hospital or laboratory must choose one or the other—not both.

For example, marketing laboratory tests to physicians' offices, nursing homes, and local HMOs should increase revenues. If successful, this strategy will also increase laboratory costs. Costs rise because new resources are needed to implement the strategy. A marketing and sales person is needed to approach potential customers. Computer equipment is needed to streamline test ordering and billing. Automated analyzers may be required to speed test processing. All these items increase costs. It is hoped that the increase in revenues will outstrip the increase in costs.

It is not possible for the laboratory to compete for the outside business unless it is given the resources to carry out the job. In this case, the laboratory's goals of increasing test volume while lowering costs are clearly incompatible.

It would not be realistic for a laboratory to define as a goal increasing test volume if the external analysis revealed that the surrounding commercial laboratory competition was great, and the internal analysis revealed that the laboratory lacked the equipment to process large volumes of tests efficiently. Similarly, it makes no sense to set as a goal a reduction in the ordering by physicians of esoteric, expensive tests if the hospital is a teaching or research center. In this case, the hospital's mission directly conflicts with the cost-reduction strategy. It is important that all three laboratory divisions communicate clearly and decide on mutually compatible goals and objectives.

Once the laboratory's goals and objectives are defined, a system should be developed that helps the laboratory manager measure and evaluate progress toward the goals. This management system should accomplish several tasks, including tracking the flow of laboratory revenues and expenses, providing useful data to the proper management person in a timely fashion, and comparing the laboratory's performance against some accepted standards of productivity and efficiency.[7]

From an operational viewpoint, the system should be easy to implement, be inexpensive to operate, and have the flexibility of expanding or contracting to meet the needs of a large or small laboratory. The management system presented here provides a series of ratios that measure laboratory performance over time. Charting and watching the ratios enable the laboratory manager to detect trends and potential trouble spots that need correction or improvement.

Calculating the ratios involves cost-accounting the basic units of laboratory output, but what are the basic units of laboratory output? If the function of the laboratory is to provide physicians with medical information concerning their patients, then the output is an intangible measurement of a physiologic or pathologic parameter in a patient's body fluids or tissues. These intangible measurements or units of information are the laboratory "tests." Therefore, the finished product or output is the test result or billable procedure. A billable procedure is a finished test result charged or billed to a patient or third-party payer.

After the output is defined, all laboratory costs and expenses are related to this unit. For example, labor expense is described as labor cost per billable procedure, and supply expenses are described as supply cost per billable procedure. The ratios are charted or graphed on a monthly basis and provide a means of tracking laboratory performance.

Similarly, use data are described in terms of the billable procedure. For example, billable tests per patient day and billable procedure per patient admission are ratios for evaluating the medical staff's laboratory use patterns.

Before we develop the system, we need to collect the appropriate statistics and financial data. All needed data are collected from the hospital admitting office, business office, or laboratory department management reports. Once the data are gathered, the laboratory is "modeled."

Modeling the laboratory means breaking it down into its component parts. Most clinical laboratories can be viewed at the level of the total laboratory, the laboratory subsection, or the individual cost centers within each subsection (Fig. 33-2). The object is to trace all laboratory revenues and expenses through each of the three levels. Ultimately a portion of these expenses is allocated to each unit of laboratory output—the billable procedure.

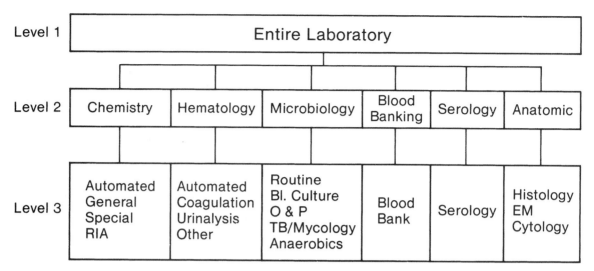

FIGURE 33–2.   Laboratory organization with six major production and cost centers.

This may seem an overwhelming task, but it can be accomplished with a few hours' work with a calculator or computer spreadsheet. Figure 33–2 shows that our sample hospital is organized along traditional lines into six major subsections or production centers. These subsections are chemistry, hematology, microbiology, blood banking, serology, and anatomic. The cost centers within each subsection are also listed.

Tables 33-1, 33-2, and 33-3 are examples of budgets or operating statements for each of the three levels. It is easy to figure the direct labor costs or technical personnel costs for each department. One simply counts the number of technical staff members in each department and lists their total salaries. However, what about the nontechnical salaries or indirect labor, such as those for pathology secretaries, laboratory receptionists, and phlebotomists? They are not usually assigned to a particular area, but their work benefits the entire laboratory. How should their salaries be allocated?

To handle this step, we devise an allocation schedule. This schedule uses a formula for assigning the costs of the nontechnical personnel or indirect labor, the equipment expenses, and professional fees to each subsection and cost center. The formula may differ for each group or item allocated; the only requirement is that it realistically reflects the department's use of that item. Box 33–1 is a description of the budget line items and the formula used to allocate costs for the laboratory subsections and cost centers.

No standard allocation formula applies to all laboratories. Each laboratory manager should be able to cre-

ate accurate formulas for each item and department based on his knowledge of laboratory operations.

Table 33-1
Example of Hospital Laboratory Budget (Level 1)

Revenues	$9,172,526
Expenses	
Salaries	
Technical labor	$1,668,365
Nontechnical labor	
Laboratory receptionists	$197,680
Administrative	$114,525
Nights	$119,873
Phlebotomists	$314,490
Pathology secretaries	$128,804
Professional fees	$1,286,906
Supplies	$1,498,399
Equipment	
Depreciation	$147,506
Service contracts	$105,643
Repairs	$40,842
Other	$115,475
Direct costs	$5,738,508
Indirect costs	$2,215,221
Total costs	$7,953,729
Net income	$1,218,797

Table 33-2
Example of Hospital Laboratory Budget (Level 2)

	Microbiology	Blood Bank	Chemistry	Hematology	Anatomic	Serology
Revenues	$1,006,444	$1,002,114	$4,106,062	$1,457,584	$1,262,867	$337,455
Expenses						
Salaries						
Technical labor	$245,674	$237,429	$557,584	$352,500	$193,455	$81,723
Nontechnical labor						
Laboratory receptionists	$19,217	$13,440	$84,595	$61,845	$8,961	$9,622
Administrative	$11,133	$7,787	$49,011	$35,829	$5,190	$5,575
Nights	$0	$41,955	$35,962	$41,956	$0	$0
Phlebotomists	$46,002	$14,748	$131,439	$98,531	$4,453	$19,317
Pathology secretaries	$12,932	$1,006	$6,333	$4,630	$103,183	$720
Professional fees	$98,215	$98,214	$210,636	$98,214	$683,413	$98,214
Supplies	$144,979	$332,708	$760,486	$140,793	$47,035	$72,398
Equipment						
Depreciation	$13,084	$9,768	$50,804	$45,802	$23,658	$4,390
Service contracts	$9,516	$2,088	$52,313	$32,459	$7,732	$1,535
Repairs	$2,375	$1,661	$10,452	$24,058	$1,107	$1,189
Other	$11,947	$7,796	$49,069	$35,883	$5,198	$5,582
Direct costs	$615,074	$768,600	$1,998,684	$972,500	$1,083,385	$300,265
Indirect costs	$298,183	$312,921	$740,798	$400,102	$340,721	$122,496
Total costs	$913,257	$1,081,521	$2,739,482	$1,372,602	1,424,106	$422,761
Net income	$93,187	($79,407)	$1,366,580	$84,982	($161,239)	($85,306)

O&P, ova and parasites; RIAP, radioimmunoassay procedures; EM, electron microscope

Next, the costs are tracked to the individual cost centers (see Table 33–3). This is important because at this level, the laboratory manager exerts control. That is, even if the manager cannot influence the physicians' patterns of test ordering, he can make sure that the tests, once ordered, are performed as efficiently and economically as possible.

In our sample hospital, the chemistry department is divided into five cost centers. Each cost center performs only certain types of procedures. For example, the automated cost center performs only electrolyte studies and automated chemical tests. When all the costs are allocated, it is possible to calculate the total cost of each type of test.

Operating ratios are tools that help in analyzing laboratory operations. These formulas highlight the relationships among laboratory variables. The ratios provide quantitative information about test ordering patterns, productivity, efficiency, resource use, and financial margins—data that help the manager control costs and improve service.

Figure 33–3 shows how the operating ratios are calculated. Table 33–4 shows how the ratios are applied to the chemistry department cost centers. The same format can be applied to the other laboratory cost centers.

The test use ratios are designed to track physician use of the laboratory. The billable procedures per patient day and billable procedures per patient admission may rise or fall if the physicians alter their test ordering patterns. For example, the ratios increase if the physicians "feel pressure" to diagnose, treat, and discharge patients rapidly and order more laboratory tests.

The resource use ratios monitor the monthly consumption of labor, materials, equipment, and overhead by the cost center. Most of these parameters are under the direct control of the laboratory director and laboratory manager. A rise in the technical labor per procedure, for example, may signal a scheduling problem in a cost center involving the use of expensive overtime labor.

If the supply cost per billable procedure rises at a cost center, the manager should ask why. Are supplies being wasted? Are too many controls or small batches being run? Are ordering patterns resulting in lost dis-

Table 33-3
Example of Hospital Laboratory Budget (Level 3)

	Routine	*Blood Culture*	*O & P*	*TB/Mycology*	*Anaerobic*	*Blood Bank*
Revenues	$500,477	$276,144	$76,837	$53,435	$99,551	$1,002,114
Expenses						
Salaries						
Technical labor	$110,339	$50,571	$53,262	$12,180	$19,322	$237,429
Nontechnical labor						
Laboratory receptionists	$10,956	$3,577	$3,041	$944	$699	$13,440
Administrative	$6,347	$2,072	$1,762	$547	$405	$7,787
Nights	$0	$0	$0	$0	$0	$41,955
Phlebotomists	$23,324	$12,706	$6,481	$2,011	$1,480	$14,748
Pathology secretaries	$7,621	$2,488	$2,115	$656	$52	$1,006
Professional fees	$55,995	$18,281	$15,542	$4,823	$3,574	$98,214
Supplies	$68,836	$54,514	$14,447	$3,887	$3,295	$332,708
Equipment						
Depreciation	$10,152	$1,907	$495	$371	$159	$9,768
Service contracts	$8,152	$556	$512	$187	$109	$2,088
Repairs	$1,354	$442	$376	$117	$86	$1,661
Other	$6,355	$2,075	$1,764	$347	$1,406	$7,796
Direct costs	$309,431	$149,189	$99,797	$26,070	$30,587	$768,600
Indirect costs	$146,707	$50,364	$46,228	$33,339	$21,545	$312,921
Total costs	$456,138	$199,553	$146,025	$59,409	$52,132	$1,081,521
Net income	$44,339	$76,591	($69,188)	($5,974)	$47,419	($79,407)

	Automated-Chem	*General*	*RIAP*	*Special*	*Send Out*
Revenues	$2,208,366	$907,008	$474,800	$237,368	$278,520
Expenses					
Salaries					
Technical labor	$202,072	$178,547	$69,863	$69,853	$37,249
Nontechnical labor					
Laboratory receptionists	$51,387	$18,555	$7,534	$2,495	$4,624
Administrative	$29,771	$10,750	$4,365	$1,446	$2,679
Nights	$35,962	$0	$0	$0	$0
Phlebotomists	$74,655	$29,115	$10,705	$3,620	$13,344
Pathology secretaries	$3,847	$1,389	$564	$187	$346
Professional fees	$127,950	$46,201	$18,760	$6,213	$11,512
Supplies	$207,653	$198,851	$52,707	$24,474	$276,801
Equipment					
Depreciation	$23,144	$17,719	$3,068	$6,404	$469
Service contracts	$20,577	$23,165	$1,171	$6,682	$718
Repairs	$6,350	$2,293	$930	$308	$571
Other	$29,807	$10,763	$4,370	$1,447	$2,682
Direct costs	$813,175	$537,348	$174,037	$123,129	$350,995
Indirect costs	$289,980	$214,749	$80,638	$64,507	$90,924
Total costs	$1,103,155	$752,097	$254,675	$187,636	$441,919
Net income	$1,105,211	$154,911	$220,125	$49,732	($163,399)

Table 33-3
(Continued)

	Automated-Hematology	Coagulation	Urinalysis	Other	Histology	Cytology	EM	Serology
Revenues	$791,497	$282,885	$281,229	$101,973	$1,115,168	$137,739	$30	$337,455
Expenses								
Salaries								
Technical labor	$157,859	$84,531	$87,592	$22,518	$130,589	$52,249	$10,617	$81,723
Nontechnical labor								
Laboratory receptionists	$34,355	$9,113	$14,370	$4,007	$7,117	$1,829	$15	$9,622
Administrative	$19,903	$5,280	$8,325	$2,321	$4,123	$1,059	$8	$5,575
Nights	$24,921	$6,611	$10,424	$0	$0	$0	$0	$0
Phlebotomists	$48,813	$13,242	$30,627	$5,849	$854	$3,547	$52	$19,317
Pathology secretaries	$2,572	$682	$1,076	$300	$103,045	$137	$1	$720
Professional fees	$53,940	$14,308	$22,562	$7,404	$649,239	$34,174	$0	$98,214
Supplies	$62,021	$35,077	$33,815	$9,880	$39,134	$4,759	$3,142	$72,398
Equipment								
Depreciation	$34,267	$9,219	$1,457	$859	$10,254	$1,818	$11,586	$4,390
Service contracts	$23,427	$5,776	$2,233	$1,023	$3,141	$839	$3,752	$1,535
Repairs	$20,661	$1,126	$1,776	$495	$879	$226	$2	$1,189
Other	$19,928	$5,287	$8,344	$2,324	$4,129	$1,060	$9	$5,582
Direct costs	$502,667	$190,252	$222,601	$56,980	$952,504	$101,697	$29,184	$300,265
Indirect costs	$196,910	$76,399	$94,134	$32,659	$267,188	$46,245	$27,288	$122,496
Total costs	$699,577	$266,651	$316,735	$89,639	$1,219,692	$147,942	$56,472	$422,761
Net income	$91,920	$16,234	($35,506)	$12,334	($104,524)	($10,203)	($56,442)	($85,306)

O&P, ova and parasites; RIAP, radioimmunoassay procedures; EM, electron microscope

counts? The ratios pinpoint the troubled cost center and allow for early corrective action.

The most important use ratio is the total cost per billable procedure. In a prospective payment environment, it is vital to determine an accurate total cost per procedure for each hospital product and service. Comprehensive cost data provide valuable ammunition when the hospital competes for patients with HMOs and PPOs. Like DRGs, these prepaid health plans reimburse the hospital on a set fee scale. The hospital that underestimates costs risks bidding too low and locking itself into unfavorable and unprofitable contracts. Accurate cost-per-billable procedure data enable the laboratory manager to put the correct price tag on laboratory services.

The ratios also monitor productivity. Laboratory productivity is measured in many ways, such as the minutes per hour a technologist works on a particular test or procedure or the output of tests from an automated instrument over a period of time. Both of these methods of measuring productivity have a major shortcoming—they fail to define productivity in terms of cost.

In the DRG environment, productivity is defined as output per unit of input. For the laboratory, the output is the billable procedure, and the input is the labor, materials, equipment, and overhead measured in dollars. Productivity is increased by performing more billable procedures or by decreasing input expenses.

The billable procedure per dollar of technical labor ratio measures productivity in terms of labor use. The billable procedure per dollar of equipment cost ratio allows the manager to compare the productivity of two different instruments or analyzers.

The financial ratios allow the hospital administrator to track the laboratory's financial condition over time.[1] A decrease in the margin (profit) per billable procedure may signal a shift in the laboratory's case-mix patterns. That is, a higher percentage of less profitable (lower margin) tests may have been ordered. If the billable procedures per patient admission ratio decreases, the administrator may want to compensate for the de-

Box 33•1

Budget Line Items and the Formula Used to Allocate Costs

Revenues: The revenues are calculated by multiplying the procedure price by the number of procedures. The hospital business office supplies the current price list.

Technical labor: Technical labor includes the salary costs of the technologists and supervisors working in each laboratory department. Data are collected from the department time cards.

Laboratory receptionists: The salary costs for the laboratory receptionists are distributed on the basis of the procedure volume of each cost center. For example, if a cost center performs 6% of the laboratory's billable procedures, then 6% of the laboratory receptionists' salaries are distributed to that cost center.

Administration: This category includes the salaries of the laboratory manager, quality control officer, and research technologist. These costs are allocated in the same fashion as the laboratory receptionists costs.

Nights: This category includes the salaries of the night-time personnel. These costs are allocated on the basis of assignments of the night personnel in the specific cost centers.

Phlebotomists: This category includes the salaries of the individuals responsible for drawing blood and collecting the laboratory specimens. These costs are distributed by multiplying procedure volume by the estimated collection time per procedure in each cost center.

Pathology secretaries: This category includes the salaries of the individuals responsible for typing departmental reports. These costs are allocated on the basis of the percentage of time the secretaries type reports for each cost center.

Equipment depreciation: These costs are distributed on a specific basis for all major equipment items. For example, the depreciation cost of a chemistry analyzer is allocated to the chemistry department. All minor depreciation costs are distributed to the cost centers on the basis of procedure volume. Depreciation is calculated on a 5-year, straight-line basis.

Service contracts: These costs include the maintenance contracts for laboratory instruments. The costs are allocated to the specific cost center on the basis of department records. All general instrument maintenance contracts (eg, centrifuges) are distributed across all cost centers on a procedure volume basis.

Repairs: These are the costs of repairing specific instruments not covered by the maintenance contracts. The costs are allocated into the appropriate departments.

Other: This category includes the costs associated with travel, education, office supplies, dues, and fees. They are distributed on the basis of the procedure volume.

Supplies: These costs are distributed to the cost centers on the basis of data obtained from the laboratory cost ledgers.

Professional fees: This category includes the salaries of the pathologist and the clinical scientists. The costs are allocated to the cost centers on the basis of the amount of time the professionals spent in each center.

Indirect costs: This category includes employee benefits, building depreciation, operation of the plant, administration, and general, housekeeping, cafeteria, and medical records. These costs are allocated on the basis of standard formulas provided by the hospital business office.

creased revenues by increasing the prices of all procedures.

The revenue per billable procedure is the income the laboratory receives from performing and selling one billable procedure. Table 33–3 shows that several of the cost centers operate at a loss. That is, total cost per billable procedure exceeds revenue. This happens because many laboratory managers base prices on estimates of total costs. Unfortunately, these estimates are often low.

If competitive forces allow it, it is better to adopt a pricing policy that yields a constant margin on all tests, for instance, 10% to 15% per procedure. Setting the prices of all tests 10% to 15% above costs protects the laboratory from revenue shortfalls caused by changing test-mix patterns.

This management system is flexible. Many ratios or only a few ratios may be calculated for all or only a few cost centers. Once the laboratory costs are categorized and allocated and the ratios calculated, the only

Utilization Ratios

$$\text{Billable Procedure per Patient Day} = \frac{\text{Billable Procedures}}{\text{Patient Days}}$$

$$\text{Billable Procedure per Patient Admission} = \frac{\text{Billable Procedures}}{\text{\# Patient Admissions}}$$

Resource Utilization Ratios

$$\text{Total Cost per Billable Procedure} = \frac{\text{Total Costs}}{\text{Billable Procedures}}$$

$$\text{Direct Cost per Billable Procedure} = \frac{\text{Direct Costs}}{\text{Billable Procedures}}$$

$$\text{Nontechnical Labor Cost per Billable Procedure} = \frac{\text{Nontechnical Labor}}{\text{Billable Procedures}}$$

$$\text{Technical Labor Cost per Billable Procedure} = \frac{\text{Technical Labor Cost}}{\text{Billable Procedures}}$$

$$\text{Supply Cost per Billable Procedure} = \frac{\text{Supply Costs}}{\text{Billable Procedures}}$$

$$\text{Equipment Cost per Billable Procedure} = \frac{\text{Equipment Costs}}{\text{Billable Procedures}}$$

Productivity Ratios

$$\text{Professional Fee Cost per Billable Procedure} = \frac{\text{Professional Fee Cost}}{\text{Billable Procedures}}$$

$$\text{Billable Procedure per \$ of Labor} = \frac{\text{Billable Procedures}}{\text{\$ Labor}}$$

$$\text{Billable Procedure per \$ of Supply} = \frac{\text{Billable Procedures}}{\text{\$ Supply}}$$

$$\text{Billable Procedure per \$ of Equipment} = \frac{\text{Billable Procedures}}{\text{\$ Equipment}}$$

Financial Ratios

$$\text{Revenue per Billable Procedure} = \frac{\text{Revenue}}{\text{Billable Procedures}}$$

$$\text{Margin per Billable Procedure} = \frac{\text{Margin}}{\text{Billable Procedures}}$$

$$\text{Revenue per Patient Admission} = \frac{\text{Revenue}}{\text{Patient Admission}}$$

FIGURE 33–3. Laboratory ratios.

Table 33-4
Example of Cost Center Operating Ratios

	Automated-Chemistry	General	RIA	Special
Revenues	$2,208,366	$907,008	$474,800	$237,368
Expenses				
Salaries				
Technical labor	$202,072	$178,547	$69,863	$69,853
Nontechnical labor				
Laboratory receptionists	$51,387	$18,555	$7,534	$2,495
Administrative	$29,771	$10,750	$4,365	$1,446
Nights	$35,962	$0	$0	$0
Phlebotomists	$74,655	$29,115	$10,705	$3,620
Pathology secretaries	$3,847	$1,389	$564	$187
Professional fees	$127,950	$46,201	$18,760	$6,213
Supplies	$207,653	$198,851	$52,707	$24,474
Equipment				
Depreciation	$23,144	$17,719	$3,068	$6,404
Service contracts	$20,577	$23,165	$1,171	$6,682
Repairs	$6,350	$2,293	$930	$308
Other	$29,807	$10,763	$4,370	$1,447
Direct costs	$813,175	$537,348	$174,037	$123,129
Indirect costs	$289,980	$214,749	$80,638	$64,507
Total costs	$1,103,155	$752,097	$254,675	$187,636
Net income	$1,105,211	$154,911	$220,125	$49,732
Procedures	105,750	38,185	15,505	5,135
Patient admissions	25,935	25,935	25,935	25,935
Patient days	161,056	161,056	161,056	161,056
Procedure/patient day	0.7	0.2	0.1	0.0
Procedure/patient admission	4.1	1.5	0.6	0.2
Total cost/procedure	$10.43	$19.70	$16.43	$36.54
Direct cost/procedure	$7.69	$14.07	$11.22	$23.98
Nontechnical labor/procedure	$1.85	$1.57	$1.49	$1.51
Technical labor/procedure	$1.91	$4.68	$4.51	$13.60
Supply cost/procedure	$1.96	$5.21	$3.40	$4.77
Equipment cost/procedure	$0.47	$1.13	$0.33	$2.61
Professional fee/procedure	$1.21	$1.21	$1.21	$1.21
Procedure/$ labor	0.5	0.2	0.2	0.1
Procedure/$ supply	0.5	0.2	0.3	0.2
Procedure/$ equipment	2.1	0.9	3.0	0.4
Revenue/procedure	$20.88	$23.75	$30.62	$46.23
Margin/procedure	$10.45	$4.06	$14.20	$9.68
Revenue/patient admission	$85.15	$34.97	$18.31	$9.15

factors that change significantly are the number of billable procedures and the labor and supply use. Most other budget items remain relatively constant from month to month.

This system, which may appear complex, is not difficult to put into practice. Data gathering is the biggest hurdle. It is worthwhile to establish a good relationship with the admissions and business office personnel to obtain better access to the data.

Now that cost efficiency is a watchword in the health-care industry, a comprehensive laboratory management system is a necessity, rather than an option.

Managers who develop a system to set goals, measure progress, and point out trouble spots will use their limited resources more intelligently than managers who do not.

REFERENCES

1. Cleverly WO: Financial ratios: Summary indications for management decision making. Hosp Health Serv Admin 26(3), Special Issue 11:26–47, 1981
2. Greiner LE, Metzger RO: Consulting to Management. Englewood Cliffs, NJ, Prentice-Hall, 1983
3. Kotler P: Marketing Management, 5th ed. Englewood Cliffs, NJ, Prentice-Hall, 1984
4. Sharp JW: The cluster lab: A model for the DRG era? MLO 15(11):40–44, 1983
5. Sharp JW: A DRG survival guide for the laboratory budget. MLO 16(9):38–43, 1984
6. Sharp JW: Directing the post-TEFRA laboratory. Pathologist 39(2), 1985
7. Sharp JW: A cost accounting system targeted to DRGs. MLO 17(9):34–38, 1985

34

Wage and Salary Administration

John R. Snyder

Despite the large expenditures for capital equipment and supplies to operate a clinical laboratory, the wage and salary component of the budget represents approximately 50% to 70% of the department's total operating costs.[19,27] Although many of the functions of compensation management are the responsibility of an institution's fiscal officer for human resources, it is helpful for the laboratory manager to be familiar with the terminology, processes, and procedures used in wage and salary administration.

THE REWARD SYSTEM: COMPENSATION AND NONCOMPENSATION DIMENSIONS

From a department administrator's or supervisor's perspective, it is important to recognize that pay is only one part of the laboratory's reward system. Appropriate financial compensation is necessary to attract and retain personnel who have the necessary knowledge and skills for laboratory operations and are willing to put forth the effort needed to help the laboratory function. However, pay has been identified as a satisfier in some situations, a dissatisfier in other situations, but seldom an effective long-term motivator.

The reward system in the laboratory includes anything that an employer is willing and able to offer and an employee values sufficiently to accept in exchange for performance. The reward process is composed of both compensation components and noncompensation components, as illustrated in Figure 34-1.[17]

Compensation Dimensions

All rewards classified as monetary and in-kind payments constitute the eight compensation dimensions of the reward system.[17] These include the amount of money paid for work and performance in a specified job and money paid for time not worked, for example, holidays, paid vacations, and paid time off for various personal reasons. Other dimensions address continued compensation or job security in the form of loss-of-job income; disability income; spouse or family income continuation after an employee's total and permanent disability or death; and health, accident, and liability protection. Two remaining dimensions include deferred compensation to continue income after retirement and income equivalent payments or perquisites ("perks").

Noncompensation Dimensions

Noncompensation rewards are the work situation factors that relate to the employee's emotional and psychological well-being.[17] Many of these are similar to the motivational factors that behavioral scientists suggest for improving work performance. Henderson[17] identified seven dimensions of the noncompensation reward system: dignity and satisfaction from work performed; physiologic health, psychological well-being, and emotional maturity; constructive social relationships with coworkers; jobs designed to require adequate attention and effort; sufficient resources to perform work assignments; sufficient control over the job to meet personal demands; and supportive leadership and management.

The purpose of this chapter is to introduce the complex area of wage and salary administration as applicable to the clinical laboratory. The chapter begins with a historic perspective of health-care wage determination with citations of significant legislation. Attention is then focused broadly on the accounting of human resources, followed by more specific information about personnel budgeting, financial compensation for laboratory staff and managers, employee incentive systems based on merit, payroll accounting, and benefit plans. The final section addresses arrangements for compensating physician services in the clinical laboratory.

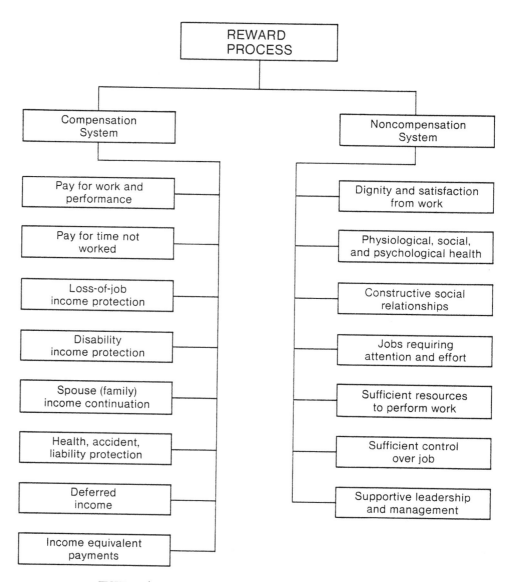

FIGURE 34-1. The reward system: compensation and noncompensation dimensions. (From Henderson RI: Compensation Management: Rewarding Performance, 4th ed, pp xiii, xiv, xx. Reston, VA, Reston Publishing, 1985, adapted with permission)

LEGISLATION GOVERNING COMPENSATION ADMINISTRATION

Wage and salary administration programs in health-care institutions followed a fairly simplistic approach before 1967.[21] The majority of workers were women, and wages were therefore viewed as "supplemental income," because women were viewed as secondary breadwinners. This perception was complicated by a belief that health-care institutions in general, and hospitals in particular, were charitable institutions having limited resources available for improving wages. In hospitals, nurses represented a norm group of "professionals," and wages for allied health professionals, including laboratory workers, tended to fluctuate with nursing salaries.

In the early 1950s, unions entered the health-care fields, which resulted in third-party negotiating through collective bargaining for salary adjustments. The American Nurses Association in 1966 also influenced wage structures in hospitals by establishing a national minimum wage for nurses.

The inclusion of hospitals under the Fair Labor Standards Act in 1967 called attention to the need for an upward adjustment of health-care wages and a study of jobs and job content to guard against problems under the Equal Pay for Equal Work Provisions of the Act. Further modifications resulted from guidelines established in the Economic Stabilization Program under the Johnson administration in 1971. These guidelines determined poverty wage rate levels, and hospitals realized that a large percentage of employees were below or only slightly above the federal guidelines.

Specific legislation influencing compensation practices can be put into four major categories: (1) wage and hour legislation, (2) income protection legislation, (3) antidiscrimination legislation, and (4) wage and price control legislation.[17] The intent of select laws under each of these categories follows.

Wage and Hour Legislation

Laws in this category were established to restrict hours worked and set basic rates of pay.

1935: National Labor Relations Act

This act provided employees the right to bargain collectively for wages and benefits. Nonprofit health-care institutions were excluded from the act until the enactment of Public Law 93-360 in 1974 (see Chapter 16).

1938: Fair Labor Standards Act

After earlier unsuccessful attempts at establishing a regulated minimum wage, the Fair Labor Standards Act (FLSA) established minimum wages for all employees engaged in interstate or foreign commerce or the production of goods for foreign commerce and employees of certain other enterprises. Although specific occupations are exempt, revisions of the act from 1938 have enlarged the number of work groups covered and steadily increased the minimum age. The act also requires employers in covered enterprises to define a fixed workweek and pay time-and-a-half for all hours worked in excess of 40 hours a week. Child labor provisions of the act call for (1) a minimum hiring age of 14 to 16, depending on the kind of work performed and whether the employer is the child's parent, and (2) a minimum age of 18 for work in hazardous occupations.

State Laws on Minimum Wages

Some states have passed their own minimum-wage legislation, and if the state labor laws are more rigorous than federal laws, they supersede the federal statute.

Income Protection Legislation

During the last century, a number of laws have been enacted to provide economic protection for employees who, due to circumstances beyond their control, cannot continue to work.

1911: Workers' Compensation

This enduring piece of legislation is now handled by state compensation laws to (1) provide prompt and reasonable income and medical benefits to victims of work-related accidents or income benefits to their dependents, regardless of fault; (2) provide speedy resolution to disputes arising out of personal injury litigation; (3) relieve public and private charities of financial drains from uncompensated industrial accidents; (4) minimize costs associated with time-consuming trials and appeals; (5) encourage employer involvement in safety and rehabilitation; and (6) promote the study of causes of accidents to prevent future occurrence.[3,17]

1935: The Social Security Act

This law requires employers and employees to contribute equally to guard against loss of income due to termination of employment beyond the employees' control. Although primarily a retirement program, the law also established federal old-age, survivors, disability, and health insurance systems. Amendments to this act established Medicaid and Medicare programs. Significant changes in the act were made in 1983 with the Social Security Reform Bill. Under Title IX of the Social Security Act, unemployment compensation is provided for, but each state establishes amounts of weekly benefits, total number of eligible weeks, the qualifying employer–employee relationship, and waiting time after employment ceases before benefits are received.

Pension Plans

Several pieces of legislation have enacted private retirement protection programs, including the Welfare and Pension Plan Disclosure Act of 1959, the Employee Retirement Income Security Act of 1974, and the Multiemployer Pension Plan Amendment Act of 1980. These acts attempt to improve the operation and financial viability of private pension plans.

1973: The Health Maintenance Organization Act

Most employers provide health and welfare benefits, including life insurance and death benefits, sickness and accident benefits, hospitalization, and medical care. Under the Health Maintenance Organization (HMO) Act, employers covered under FLSA and having 25 or more employees for whom health benefits are provided are required to offer an HMO if available in the area where the employees reside.

Antidiscrimination Legislation

Equal protection under the law is afforded in both the Thirteenth and Fourteenth Amendments to the Constitution of the United States and the Civil Rights Acts of 1866, 1870, and 1871.

1963: Equal Pay Act

This act requires equal pay for equal work for men and women. Equal work is defined as work requiring equal skill, effort, and responsibility under similar working conditions. Similar working conditions are dependent on surroundings and hazards. Under the Equal Pay Act, employers can establish different pay rates based on (1) a seniority system, (2) a merit system, (3) a system that measures earnings by quantity or quality of production, and (4) a differential based on any factor other than sex. Additional protection against discrimination is afforded in Title VII of the Civil Rights Act of 1964. (Other applicable legislation prohibiting discrimination are listed in Chapter 12.)

Tax Investment Legislation

Most tax legislation relates to the deferral or sheltering of income tax payments. Legislation such as the Revenue Act of 1978 and Tax Equity and Fiscal Responsibility Act of 1982 have impacted the take-home pay of employees.

Wage and Price Control Legislation

Wage and price controls attempt to reduce rapid inflation during low levels of unemployment. For example, the Economic Stabilization Act of 1970 allowed identical pay increases to all employees irrespective of high-performing employees.

Although this discussion of the legislation governing compensation is an overview at best, it does lay the groundwork for job analysis and design of a pay structure for clinical laboratory personnel.

HUMAN RESOURCE COST ACCOUNTING

Before beginning a discussion about the mechanics of personnel budgeting, compensation, and payroll accounting, it is helpful to gain a perspective on the costs associated with the human resources entrusted to the laboratory manager's care. This human resource accounting (HRA) process attempts to quantify the value of the "human assets" to the laboratory. Flamholtz[11] states the following:

> A major purpose of human resources accounting is to help managers to use an organization's human resources effectively and efficiently. HRA is intended to provide managers with information needed to acquire, develop, allocate, conserve, utilize, evaluate, and reward human resources.

Human resource costs, like other costs accounted for in the clinical laboratory, have asset and expense components.[9] As an asset, human resources are expected to provide a return on the financial investment in the form of productivity, during future accounting periods. As an expense, human resources will consume some portion of the total financial and physical resources allocated to the laboratory during the current accounting period.

Flamholtz[11] proposed a model for identifying and classifying relevant human resource costs (Fig. 34-2). For an individual already employed in the laboratory, the appropriate categories for historic analysis of human resource costs are acquisition costs and development costs. If employee turnover occurs, separation costs are incurred and added to the acquisition and development costs.

Acquisition Costs

Human resource acquisition costs include recruitment, interview and selection, and hiring costs. Recruitment costs are incurred in advertising, identifying, and attracting a potential employee. Expenditures include personnel department and recruiter salaries, advertising costs, agency fees if used, possible travel and entertainment costs for investigation of leads for possible applicants, and other administrative expenses, such as telephone, postage, and printed recruitment materials. These costs are prorated for the employees netted. If, for example, a single advertisement listing multiple positions, placed in several issues of a professional journal costs $1,200 and nets two employees, the allocated cost would be

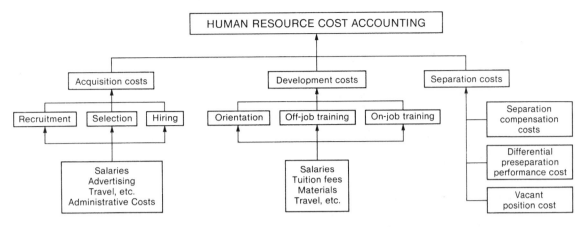

FIGURE 34-2.   Model for measurement of human resource cost accounting. (From Flam-holtz EG: Human resource accounting. InDavidson S, Weil R (eds): Handbook of Cost Accounting, pp 12, 26. New York, McGraw-Hill, 1978, adapted with permission)

$600 per person independent of the number of interviews generated.

Interview selection costs are those incurred in evaluating and selecting the final candidate. These costs include laboratory administration and personnel department salaries for time spent reviewing resumes, checking references, and interviewing. Also, travel and entertainment costs for each candidate become part of the net acquisition cost.

Hiring costs are incurred in bringing the successful candidate into the laboratory and placing the individual in the job. Relocation expenses are an example of actual hiring costs.

Development Costs

Development costs stem from orientation, possible off-the-job training, and on-the-job training until the new employee is prepared to handle a work volume normally expected of an individual in the position. Orientation costs are incurred in lost productive time for the employee and immediate supervisor in ensuring that the new employee is familiar with institutional and laboratory policies and procedures.

Should the new employee need to learn a new skill that cannot be taught in the laboratory by existing technical staff, off-the-job education costs might be incurred. Perhaps the new employee needs to attend a week-long course on how to operate an analyzer in the new employment setting. Costs for this experience would include the employee's salary, course tuition, travel, meals, and lodging.

On-the-job training costs are largely associated with the employee's salary during the period that he is not to a level of expected productivity. This cost obviously is dependent on the breadth and depth of skills of the new employee. For example, an employee with prior experience in general hematology may require a short training period of 1 to 3 weeks in a new hematology laboratory, whereas a general chemistry technologist may require 1 to 3 months to prepare for a position in a special chemistry laboratory.

Separation Costs

If a currently employed laboratorian leaves the institution, additional costs are incurred. Separation costs include separation compensation, differential preseparation performance costs, and vacant position costs. Separation costs may include severance pay for some positions if the separation is at the employer's option. Separation costs probably also include payment for accrued vacation and possibly sick time.

Differential preseparation performance costs reflect a loss in productivity prior to the employee's leaving. Preoccupation with getting ready to leave, or a "short-timer" attitude, tends to diminish the employee's work output despite the fact that there are no changes in the resources consumed.

Vacant position costs may be direct or indirect costs resulting from an unfilled position. If other technical staff are expected to pick up the responsibilities of the vacant position, their own productivity may suffer. This may necessitate overtime and will certainly take its toll on the long-term psychological and perhaps physical well-being of the remaining staff.

To illustrate this model of human resource cost accounting, consider a situation in which a general chemistry technologist is hired to fill a 3 to 11 PM vacancy for a general technologist to work in the chemistry, hematology, and body fluids sections. Assume that acquisition costs, including advertising, travel, appropriately allocated portions of salaries, administrative costs, and relocation, total $3,200. A 3-week orientation on the day shift for the employee to become fully familiar with the procedures used primarily in hematology and body fluids preceded the actual start on the assigned 3 to 11 PM shift. Allocated costs associated with this on-the-job training period are $1,600 (3 weeks of someone else covering the 3 to 11 PM shift at $10.00/h plus the equivalent of 1 additional week's salary of nonproductive work while learning). Also, orientation costs allocated to the preservice experience total $150. Because the new employee will be required to troubleshoot problems in the hematology analyzer, a single-day workshop at a local meeting is planned as off-the-job training. Total costs, including an additional day's salary, are $230. Adding the acquisition costs of $3,200 to the total development costs of $1,980, the total invested "hook value" of the employee is $5,180—and he has not yet begun the shift for which he was hired!

While there are obviously a number of cost estimates included when calculating an employee's human resource value, these costs are often overlooked. The human resource cost accounting model is helpful in gaining a perspective of the monetary investment represented by employees in the laboratory.

PERSONNEL BUDGETING

The personnel budget can be defined as a definite financial plan for personnel expenditures that imposes goals and limitations on staffing in the laboratory. The number of personnel needed for a given laboratory can be determined using workload units and forecast test volume, as was described in Chapter 31. Esmond[10] recommends that line managers be responsible for preparing the personnel budget, because they are ultimately responsible for implementing the plan.

The personnel budget for a laboratory includes the wage and salary calculation for each position and each worker, including anticipated raises and adjustments from a change of employment status.[23] Personnel budgets, prepared by laboratory managers, typically include justification statements regarding overtime pay, vacation relief, and temporary help. Support information may detail calculation of personnel hours required but

General Hospital
Approved Responsibility Center Manpower

Date: _____   Page no.: _____

Responsibility center no.: _____ Responsibility center name: _____

Labor Grade Class	Classification	Approved Full-Time Equivalents	Approved Wage, Salary Range[a]	Additional Data

Wage-earning (hourly) full-time equivalents _____
Administrative (salaried) full-time equivalents _____
Total full-time equivalents _____

FIGURE 34-3. Position control document for a responsibility center.

[a]This column required only if wage or salary ranges are not built into the labor grade classification structure.

Grade Code	Position Title	PT/FT Day Eve	Incumbent	Current Bi-weekly	Projected Annual Base	Anniv. Date	Projected Annual Increase	Projected Total Salary	Hours Per Pay Period Bi-weekly
.01	Dept. Head	FT-D	M. Smith	$1350.77	$35,120	1/2/89	$1756	$36,876	80
.02	Section Supv.	FT-D	J. Wilson	$1200.00	$31,200	3/1/89	$1560	$32,760	80
.03	Technologist	PT-D	F. Bard	$1007.69	$26,200	9/15/89	$1310	$27,510	80
.03	Technologist	FT-N	K. Lewis	$1057.69	$27,500	7/1/89	$1375	$28,875	80
.04	Technician	FT-D	G. Upton	$ 646.14	$16,800	1/2/89	$840	$17,640	80

FIGURE 34-4. Example of laboratory section personnel budget for fiscal year.

not immediately perceptually justified by workload calculations. These may be hours to ensure 24-hour coverage or hours not available to the laboratory if the formula for staffing has not included non–revenue-producing activities or vacation time and holidays. Historic information about turnover rate and absenteeism may also be useful in the budget justification.

Two figures illustrate the categories and detail typically included in a budget. Figure 34-3 is an example of a position control document for a responsibility center.[10] Personnel on this form are expressed in full-time equivalents (FTEs) as defined by personnel policy. Each entry line includes a labor grade classification code and description designating wage and salary ranges matched with skill requirements. The American Hospital Association's Chart of Accounts for Hospitals[1] suggests using a decimal system for coding in which 0.01 represents laboratory supervisors; 0.02, technical specialists; 0.03, technologists; 0.04, technicians; and so forth.

Figure 34-4 displays an example of a laboratory section personnel budget that lists each employee separately.[23] This sample budget worksheet also includes a position or grade code, abbreviated job title or category, number of personnel hours per position, rate of pay, projected annual base salary, and projected annual increase.

FINANCIAL COMPENSATION FOR LABORATORY STAFF

While the process for identifying job content and determining pay structures usually is the responsibility of an institution's fiscal officer, knowledge of the components of the process will help laboratory managers participate in the process, rather than having the result "handed" to them. Figure 34-5 displays the components of the job analysis process, the foundation for a fair and just salary system.

Job Analysis

The first step in designing a compensation system is to define the work content of each job and the worker characteristics (knowledge and skills) required for successful performance of the job. Data for analyzing job activity can be collected by interviews with workers doing the job, observation of the work being done, questionnaires completed by either the person doing the job or his immediate supervisor, or completed journals or logs detailing activities performed.[17] Job analysis is accomplished following the seven steps listed in Box 34-1.[17]

Compensable Factor-Based Job Evaluation

Key to the establishment of a compensation system is identification of compensable factors.[17] These factors distinguish between jobs by establishing degrees of difficulty. The distinction between an entry-level technologist and a senior technologist in a chemistry section might be the ability to solve a problem with a procedure that is out of control due to an interfering substance. Likewise, a distinction may be made between two technical staff members in hematology regarding the judgment used in evaluating an abnormal leukocyte count.

Universal compensable factors as defined by the United States Department of Labor include *skill*—experience, education, and ability; *effort*— physical or mental exertion required; *responsibility*—dependence on the employee to do the job as expected; and *working conditions*—physical surroundings and hazards of a job. These factors are relatively abstract and too general for use in the clinical laboratory.

A more appropriate cost system was developed by the Office of Personnel Management, called the Factor Evaluation System.[17] This method has been used successfully to classify jobs on the basis of the following factors: knowledge required in the position, supervisory controls, guidelines, complexity, scope and effect,

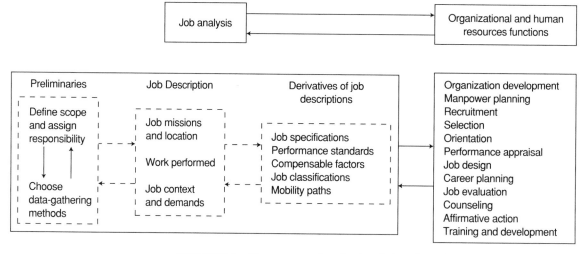

FIGURE 34-5. The process and mechanics of job analysis. (Ghorpade J, Atchison TJ: The concept of job analysis: A review and some suggestions. Public Personnel Management 3:137, 1980)

personal contacts, purpose of contacts, physical demands, and work environment. Each of these factors can be described for a given job and weighted, and the job can then be placed in a continuum of jobs, or a hierarchy.

Designing a Pay Structure

Once a job hierarchy has been established, a pay system needs to be established.[18,22] Heneman and associates[18] define four basic types of conventional pay systems: (1) job-based systems, rewarding the employee for the complexity of task in the job hierarchy; (2) seniority systems, based on length of service; (3) merit systems, which reward performance; and (4) a mixture of the previous three. Heneman and colleagues then define four decision points to consider when pricing (setting wages) within the systematic hierarchy:

(1) whether to establish a single rate or rate range; (2) whether to establish a rate or rage range for each job or for a lesser number of pay grades; (3) what the actual rates, or the minima and maxima of the rate ranges will be; and (4) how to handle current wages or salaries that are out of line.

Consistency is necessary in the pay structure, and pay should reflect the laboratory's goals and competitive levels for comparable jobs in the marketplace.

Principles for a Compensation System

Laliberty and Christopher[21] provide the following principles as guidelines for establishing a compensation system:

- Wages should purchase performance, rather than buy time and talent. Differences in educational degrees and laboratory certifications (generalist versus specialist) reflect talent. Although differential talent should lead to differential tasks, different jobs, and thus a differential wage, many laboratorians are performing similar tasks with the same degree of responsibility despite differential talent.
- A wage should be viewed as an investment; the greater the wage, the greater the rate of performance.
- Wages respond to the supply-and-demand factor. In some instances, this depresses the wage scale; in other instances, it unjustifiably inflates the scale.
- Management essentially controls the work to be performed but does not control the price paid to the worker.
- There is no concept of usage that is absolute. A correct wage justly compensates the employer for the level of performance rendered.
- Wages must be correct in their relationship both within the institution and between the institution and outside sources of competitive employment.
- Fringe benefits are classified as collateral wages

Determining Job Analysis

1. Determine the use of the data and information. This focuses the job analysis questions. Information is useful for developing job descriptions and specifications, compensable factors, job evaluations, and job classifications.
2. Select methods and procedures for securing job data and information. In addition to departmental goals and objectives and existing position descriptions, the organizational chart and a work process chart can be extremely helpful.
3. Schedule the necessary and logical work steps. Use of workload data and the personnel budget are helpful in this step.
4. Identify desired job performance requirements. This step helps focus the analysis on what should happen as opposed to what has happened.
5. Assess the present situation. An assessment must be made of the current job-holder's work performed.
6. Clarify any deviation between identified or observed activities and activities that should be performed.
7. Review the data and the information with the participants. This review offers an opportunity to correct misconceptions, ensure factual information, and ensure that information describing the job is complete.

and must be specifically defined as payment by unit of work.

- Recruitment is based on money; retention is based on fringe benefits.
- Wages have a low priority when the basic wage is adequate.
- The complexity of wage and salary administration requires a formal system.

Compensation Survey

Several of the preceding principles and previous citations note the need for compensation systems to be competitive in the marketplace. Many laboratory managers conduct informal compensation surveys. The key is selecting institutions of approximately the same size,

in a comparable geographic location, with a comparable complexity of laboratory analysis.

A number of professional organizations and other groups conduct periodic national surveys of laboratory personnel salaries. While these data offer a "snapshot" view of salaries, observation of trends is possible. One 1994 national study reported increases ranging from 2% for histology technicians to 7% for histology technologists, for example.[8] Table 34-1 displays median hourly pay rates for seven levels of laboratory personnel subdivided by bed size, type of institution, and geographic location.[8] When comparing laboratory managers' salaries with other managers of patient care services in 1987, Santos found that only pharmacy directors received higher salaries.[26] This study also subdivided respondents by institution size, but used the total number of hospital FTEs. As expected, the larger the institution, the higher the laboratory manager's select salary. At the same service provider level, medical technologists receive less compensation than other allied health professionals who provide primary care.[15]

Equal Pay and Comparable Worth

The difference in pay received by men and women is at the heart of controversy over comparable worth.[31] From a global perspective, it is true that women earn substantially less than men. Some argue that this situation is largely a reflection of wage discrimination. The fundamental problem, as identified by Henderson,[17] is "that when women dominate an occupational field, the rates of pay for jobs within those occupations appear to be unfairly depressed when compared with the pay men receive in jobs where they are the dominant incumbents within the occupational field." The work force in clinical laboratories, composed predominantly of women, is a reasonable example.

The Equal Employment Act cited previously addresses this specific issue by enforcing *equal* (not comparable) pay for comparable *work* (not worth).[17] If charged with wage discrimination under the Act, a defendant must demonstrate that pay differences result from seniority, merit, or quality or quantity of work.

Many studies have attempted to unravel the comparable worth and wage discrimination issues. Muller and colleagues examined the effect of the concentration of female employees within select hospital jobs on wage rates while statistically controlling for differences in the "comparable worth" of various jobs.[25] Medical technologists and laboratory aides were among the 40 hospital positions selected for study. They concluded that hospitals do systematically apply job evaluation criteria when establishing salary levels for job categories and that small but significant pay inequities exist between jobs held predominantly by men and those held

Table 34-1
Median Hourly Salaries in Clinical Laboratories in 1994

	Workplace						Select Regions		
	All Laboratories	Private Clinic/Reference Laboratories	Hospitals	Hospital Bed Size			Northeast	South Central Atlantic	Far West
				<100	100–499	≥500			
Technician (MLT)	$11.80	$11.95	$11.89	$11.00	$11.80–$12.90	$13.00	$13.00	$11.65	$11.94
Technologist (MT)	$14.76	$14.69	$14.95	$13.70	$14.90–$6.50	$16.00	$16.00	$14.45	$17.00
Supervisor (MT)	$17.97	$18.00	$18.00	$15.70	$17.00–$19.80	$20.00	$20.00	$17.00	$20.00
Manager (MT)	$21.00	$21.50	$21.70	$18.20	$22.00–$27.50	$24.30	$23.10	$20.90	$24.00
Cytotechnologist	$17.56	$18.55	$17.50	$17.00	$16.70–$18.10	$18.00	$18.60	$17.10	$19.00
Histologic Technician	$12.56	$11.04	$12.56	$13.10	$11.70–$13.50	$12.80	$14.00	$11.96	$13.47
Phlebotomist	$8.00	$8.00	$8.13	$7.30	$7.90–$9.60	$9.00	$10.00	$7.50	$9.61

From Castleberry, et al: Lab Medicine 26:106–112, 1995; Adapted with permission

predominantly by women. They report that a wage discrimination interpretation is consistent with their findings and encourage continued work with compensation systems to eliminate pay inequities. In a 1992 survey of 619 laboratories, 41% believed women are paid less than men, with the practice occurring more frequently in independent and group practice laboratories.[31]

EMPLOYEE BENEFITS AND SERVICES

In 1982, the Chamber of Commerce of the United States of America calculated that total employee benefits as a percentage of payroll were 36.7%. These benefits are a popular form of compensation because they are for the most part not subject to income tax. Based on the percentage of payroll represented by benefits and the popularity of this portion of the compensation package, laboratory managers are encouraged to study options available in their institution.[24] Many of the benefits are mandated by legislation cited previously. The purpose of this section is to display the range of benefits and services in categories.[17]

Disability Income Protection

Insurance coverage is frequently provided by the employer to ensure continued income in the event of an accident or health-related problem. Major components of this category are included in Box 34-2. Benezra[6] found that 91% of clinical laboratory employers offered paid life insurance, and 99% offered paid sick leave. Pension plans were offered by 89% of laboratory employers.

Loss-of-Job Income Continuation

Benefits in this category are designed to assist employees during short-term periods of unemployment resulting from layoffs or termination (Box 34-3).[17]

Many of the components identified under the disability income protection category have provisions for caring for dependents and survivors of the employee in case of his death.

Box 34•2

Disability Income Protection

Short-term disability or sickness and accident plans
Long-term disability
Workers' compensation in the form of occupational disability insurance
Nonoccupational disability (temporary disability resulting from injury or illness that is not job related)
Social security
Travel accident insurance
Sick leave when an employee is unable to work because of illness
Supplemental disability insurance
Accidental death and dismemberment
Group life insurance with total permanent disability
Disability retirement option

Health and Accident Protection

Health-care insurance benefits cover medical, surgical, and hospital bills resulting from illness or an accident. These benefits are listed in Box 34-4.[17]

For this category of benefits, Benezra found 98% of employers offering paid medical insurance and 71% offering a dental plan.[6]

Property and Liability Protection

Only recently have employers begun to provide employees with personal property and liability protection, including[17] group auto, group home, group legal, employee liability, and fidelity bond insurance.[17] In clinical laboratories, many employers provide group umbrella liability insurance.

Pay for Time not Worked

One of the less recognized benefits is time off with pay. The more common time-off opportunities during which employees continue to receive their daily base rate pay include holidays, vacations, jury duty, maternity leave, witness in court, military duty, funeral leave, time off to vote, and time off for blood donation.[17] Although virtually all laboratories afford full-time, regularly scheduled employees paid holidays and vacation, only 84% in Benezra's survey provided paid maternity leave.[6]

Income Equivalent Payments/Reimbursements for Incurred Expenses

Some employers offer education subsidies, child-care services, subsidized food service, physical awareness and fitness programs, social and recreational opportunities, parking, clothing allowances, emergency loans, and credit unions.[17] Under current cost-containment efforts, education subsidies appear to be declining, although in 1987, employers were still paying 84% of seminar and workshop expenses and 72% of paid employee tuition.[6] Other types of compensation in this category were less frequently paid: parking, 39%; uniforms, 27%; professional membership dues, 26%; child day care, 13%; laundry allowance, 12%; and meal allowance, 10%.[6]

Deferred Compensation

Deferred compensation plans have become increasingly popular in recent years. Such plans allow temporary exclusion of a portion of gross income from taxation until it is paid out in the retirement years. Because not all deferred compensation arrangements are tax exempt, employers and managers must carefully analyze the attributes of qualified, unqualified, and Section 403(b) plans (tax-sheltered annuities).[17]

EMPLOYEE INCENTIVE SYSTEMS BASED ON MERIT

Employee incentive systems are pay plans that reward individuals or work groups for outstanding productivity.[22] Basically, with this approach, technologists or managers are compensated above the normal rate for specific activities, such as cost control, improved output, or creativity in handling a particular situation.[7,35]

Five aspects of incentive programs are essential[14]: (1) incentive plans require a total organization commitment; (2) such plans do not substitute for employee supervision; (3) employees must have faith in their employers; (4) cost-consciousness must be a top priority of the organization; and (5) incentive plans need to be implemented carefully.

For an employee incentive system to be implemented, performance must be based on appraisals with measurable performance standards directly linked to responsibilities in each employee's job description.[5,12] Barros[4] offers the steps outlined in Box 34-5 when developing an employee incentive system based on merit.

Although salary adjustments are calculated at the time of performance appraisal in a merit plan, it is advisable to hold separate meetings between the supervisor and employee to discuss the performance review and the pay adjustment.[33] If a discussion of both of these elements occurs simultaneously, some employees will listen only to the part about their salaries at the expense of the performance review comments; others will tend to become argumentative about the appraisal rating because it is tied to the salary adjustment. In the same situation, managers tend to inflate ratings to avoid a confrontation about why an employee's performance does not warrant a merit adjustment. Also, managers may tend to rush through the process to "get it over with" or focus on employee weaknesses, rather than accomplishments. All of these characteristics negate the goal of employee development in the performance appraisal process.

The literature reports more than a dozen hospitals that have successfully implemented incentive plans.[29] Benefits to these institutions include decreased turnover, increased productivity, decreased overtime, decreased sick time, decreased work hours, increased communication with employees, improved management control systems, increased cash, and above-area average employee compensation.[29] The benefit from incentive plans cannot overcome a basic low salary problem; however, Hamon and colleagues found that a merit pay system led neither to greater satisfaction nor to an increase in average laboratorians' salaries.[16] Other problems have also been reported: Objective performance data are difficult to compile for some positions; aggressive and assertive staff are more likely to be rewarded than more passive coworkers; and evaluators

---

Box 34•5

Developing a Merit-Based Employee Incentive System

1. *Define the system.* The merit system must first be completely conceptualized, published, and then explained to employees, probably in group meetings. The anticipated objectives of the system must be clearly spelled out so that its accomplishments are measurable. Employees will need to understand the benefits of such a system to themselves and management.
2. *Build a foundation.* Because the system relies heavily on job-related responsibilities, it is likely that position descriptions will need careful review and even adjustment. A job analysis or reanalysis may be necessary.
3. *Establish performance standards.* While the position description states what is to be done, the performance standards include criteria for how it is be done.[5,12] Standards should include such terminology as "consistently uses," "not more than two occurrences," or "80% of the time" to specify expectations on such activities as turnaround time and quality and quantity of work.
4. *Be consistent with institution's job classifications.* The revised position descriptions and performance standards must adhere to the job classification system as described in this chapter, and the system must not violate the institution's job classification system.
5. *Set up a scale for performance appraisal.* A scale for evaluation of work needs to differentiate among unacceptable performance, "consistently has not met expectations in all major areas of responsibility"; marginal performance needing significant improvement, "not fully met expectations in areas of responsibility", expected average performance, "has consistently met and occasionally exceeded expectations in all major areas"; above-average performance, "has consistently exceeded expectations in most areas"; and outstanding performance, "has far exceeded expectations in all major areas."
6. *Determine salary increases.* The final step is determining how much merit pay is to be added beyond the usual increase (cost-of-living increases or other adjustments). Barrows suggests using a point system for each of the job responsibilities evaluated in step 5 to provide a quantitative basis for calculating salary increases.

may overrate performance to sidestep an unpleasant confrontation.[34] One final observation by Umiker on the value of seniority raises is worthy of note.[32] When studying the question of when a laboratory employee reaches his peak job performance, he found that job performance usually improved during the first 5 years of employment before reaching a plateau. This plateau often lasted until the 10th year of employment, followed by another gradual upward swing. On further investigation, he found this latter improvement was based on the employee being assigned some additional challenge, promoted, or put in charge of a new procedure. He concludes that raises during the first years of employment based on a seniority system are justified.

PAYROLL ACCOUNTING

The purpose of a payroll accounting system is to document compensation costs incurred in providing laboratory services. Payroll records are also maintained by personnel departments for federal, state, and local tax purposes and to maintain employment history and service files. For the latter, a W-4 form must be filed by all new employees for calculation of income tax withholding exemptions. A payroll accounting system must have a clear-cut procedure for recording and reporting time worked, including attendance, scheduled work hours, and overtime authorization.[28] Managers are typically involved in the time-keeping function of hourly employees; payroll deduction activities for Social Security tax, income tax, and other deductions are handled by the personnel department.

Recording the Payroll

A payroll journal or register maintained by the laboratory manager is a helpful accounting tool.[27] Figure 34-5 illustrates a department payroll journal that documents for each employee the hours worked, salary paid, overtime approved, sick days used, vacation days taken, and holidays and other days used for a given month. The journal shows that for the maximum 171 hours worked in November, all employees were paid a holiday, one employee took 2 days of sick time, one employee took 1 day of vacation, and two employees were paid time and a half (overtime) for working the holiday. This journal helps managers keep abreast of salary expenses incurred.

Payroll-Related Costs

As evident in Figure 34-5, payroll-related cost elements enter into the labor cost calculations beyond the basic earnings of hourly and salaried employees. These include overtime, vacation and sick pay, and holiday pay. Overtime premium pay, as provided for under the Fair Labor Standards Act of 1938, is earned at time and a half for hours worked in a given week in excess of 40 hours. While the figure shows vacation and sick pay as an expense during the actual month it was paid out, Seawell[28] recommends charging the expense over the entire year, the period during which the pay is earned. Not evident in Figure 34-5 are other payroll-related costs that would normally be included in a journal kept in the personnel department, such as payroll taxes, workmen's compensation, life and hospitalization insurance, and pension and retirement plans.[28]

Donated Services

For institutions operated by or affiliated with a religious group, it may be necessary to record donated services.[28] Volunteers who transport laboratory specimens or reports, for example, are providing donated services. These services, work without monetary compensation, are recorded at fair market value if there is an equivalent employer–employee relationship and there is an objective basis for calculating the amount that might otherwise be paid for this service.

ARRANGEMENTS FOR COMPENSATING PHYSICIANS

Recent legislation, written to regulate and monitor the financial activity of the health-care industry, has attempted to influence arrangements for compensating physicians, primarily in hospital settings. The American Hospital Association has determined that hospital-based physician remuneration as a percent of total hospital operating costs ranges from 5.45% in hospitals of less than 50 beds to 9.22% in teaching hospitals of less than 400 beds.

The key factor governing all compensation arrangements with hospital-based physicians is whether the Internal Revenue Service views the arrangement as creating employee status or independent contractor status for the physician. Tax ratings set forth four criteria for determining physicians' employee status[30]: (1) the degree to which the physician is integrated into the operating organization of the hospital for which the services are performed; (2) the substantial nature, regularity, and continuity of the individual's work for such hospital; (3) the authority vested in or reserved by the hospital to require compliance with its general policies; and (4) the degree to which the physician is accorded the rights and privileges the hospital provides its employees. These criteria are met if the physician is on a fixed salary or salary range, and hospital policy prevents the physician from employing associate physicians or substitutes and prevents the physician from engaging in private practice.

Basic Arrangements

While fixed salaries or percentage contracts are the foundation for most physician compensation arrangements, various other components, such as fringe benefits packages and retirement plans, are often included. Remuneration modes are classified in Box 34-6.[20,30]

When reimbursement for different types of services is provided from different sources, accountability becomes a key issue.

Setting Physicians' Fees

While many institutions have historically set fees for services based on a local community average, consideration currently must be given to the demand for services

---

Box 34•7

Setting Physician Fees: Points to Consider

Cost of services rendered
    Expenses incurred (eg, office expense, capital equipment)
    Time involved
Patient demand
    Number of patients
    Each patient's ability to pay
Value of service rendered
    Success or failure
    Severity of disease
    Complexity of treatment
Customary fees in the community

---

and inputs required in providing these sources.[20] Glaser[13] suggests that the areas listed in Box 34-7 should be addressed when setting physicians' fees.

Third-Party Reimbursement Aspects of Physician Compensation

Third-party reimbursement concepts are of significant importance to both the laboratory manager and physician provider. Third parties are agencies such as insurance companies or Medicare that pay for services consumed by their constituents. The current Medicare system has marked similarity to various other cost payers like Blue Cross and Blue Shield plans. Under Medicare, physician compensation arrangements include "fixed" and "variable" types.[20]

Fixed methods: Most fixed methods require that the provider bill for the physician's services. This billing includes both the provider and professional service components.
Variable methods: By this method, the physician may bill through the provider or bill the patient directly.

Compensation components of Medicare are divided into two parts: A, administration and supervision of professional services rendered, and B, direct professional service rendered in patient care.

Physicians' Reasonable and Customary Charges

Provider-based physicians, those whose practice allows for the physician to be compensated for services from billings by the provider, are compensated for reasona-

---

Box 34•6

Physician Compensation Remuneration Modes

1. *Fixed compensation salary.* As described previously, this arrangement treats the physician as an employee, and a physician is compensated for administrative and teaching services for patient-care services.
2. *Percentage of income.* An arrangement may be made that compensates the physician with a predetermined percentage of other gross receipts minus adjustments (eg, uncollectible accounts) or net income (revenue after deductions for direct and indirect expenses). These arrangements typically specify minimum and maximum compensation limits.
3. *Fee for service.* This arrangement compensates the physician for each unit of service rendered. Billing may be either by the institution from which the physician receives a portion or by the physician directly.
4. *Department leasing.* A physician may lease equipment or space from the institution while providing a service. In this case, the patient is billed directly by the physician. Lease fees are then paid from revenues received by the physician.
5. *Combination arrangements.* Other arrangements incorporate a minimum guaranteed income plus some form of incentive compensation.

The Uniform Optional Percentage

1	2	3	4	5	
		Estimated Gross	Uniform	Approved	
	Part B	Department	Optional		
Department	Amount	Charges	Percentage	Carrier	Intermediary
Pathology	$14,800	$200,000	7.5[1]		

Divide Column 2 by Column 3 to obtain the uniform optional percentage. This percentage is applied to all departmental billings and will yield in the aggregate an amount equal to the Part B amount (Column 2).

[1]Rounded to nearest ½ percent.

Source: Medicare Carriers Manual, HIM-14, §8099, Exh. 4; Provider Reimbursement Manual, Part I, HIM-15, §2108.11.

FIGURE 34-6. Optimal method for establishing physicians' charges.

ble and customary charges under part B, professional service. The schedule of charges for part B must approximate the actual net payments to physicians for their professional service. Three possible methods exist for establishing a schedule of charges: optimal, item-by-item, and *per diem.*[20]

Optimal: By this method, the provider determines the professional component for all services rendered to patients. This is accomplished by applying a uniform percentage to the providers' total charges. This method is particularly well suited for clinical laboratories and pathologist remuneration, because most of the pathologist's services cannot be directly traced to specific patients; service is therefore classified as part A. The percentage of gross or net charges constitutes part A remuneration, and part B is calculated separately (Fig. 34-6).

Item-by-item: This method identifies a separate professional charge for each service rendered. Figure 34-7 illustrates how each specific charge relates to the type of procedure. This method obtains a charge rate for part B service similar to that used when a physician charges separately from charges by the provider.

Per diem: This third· method is used when a schedule of charges has all-inclusive rate structures. A fixed compensation arrangement can be made for all inpatient and outpatient services.

Alternate Item-by-Item Method

			Pathology Department				
1	2	3	4	5	6		
	Professional		Estimated	Part B		Approved	
	Component	Part B	Procedures	Component			
Procedure	Percentage	Compensation	(Annual)	Charges		Carrier	Intermediary
M	15%	$2.220	1,100	$ 2.00			
N	10	1,480	200	7.50			
O	5	740	55	13.50			
P	20	2,960	300	10.00			
Q	25	3,700	1,700	2.00			
R	5	740	100	7.50			
S	10	1,480	150	10.00			
T	10	1,480	200	7.50			
	(100%)						
	Total	$14,800					

Column 2: Professional Component Percentage—Show the percentage of time which the physicians collectively spend performing each procedure. (The total time spent should equal 100 percent of the time devoted to direct patient services.)

Column 3: Part B Compensation—Multiply the total amount ($14,800) by each percentage in Column 2.

Column 4: Estimated Annual Procedures—Estimate the number of times each procedure will be performed in the coming year.

Column 5: Part B Component Charges—The physician Part B charge is derived by dividing Column 3 by Column 4 rounded to nearest 50 cents.

Source: Medicare Carriers Manual, HIM-14, §8099, Exh. 6; Provider Reimbursement Manual, Part I, HIM-15, §2108.11.

FIGURE 34-7. Item-by-item method for establishing physicians' charges.

SUMMARY

This chapter has introduced the terminology, processes, and procedures in wage and salary administration of importance to laboratory managers. The reward system was globally described in terms of compensation and noncompensation dimensions. Select legislation governing compensation administration was identified. Costs associated with selecting and developing employees were delineated, as were costs incurred in employee turnover. Two financial strategies, personnel budgeting and payroll accounting, were described as methods for planning for and controlling costs associated with the human resource in the clinical laboratory. The process for developing a financial compensation system was described stepwise from job analysis to design of a pay structure. The range of employee benefits and services, 30% to 40% of payroll costs, was detailed. Managers are challenged to investigate positive outcomes possible by implementing an incentive-based rewards system. Finally, arrangements for compensating physicians were described.

REFERENCES

1. American Hospital Association: Chart of Accounts for Hospitals. Chicago, American Hospital Association, 1976
2. American Hospital Association: Physician remuneration has impact on hospital costs. Hospitals 51, 15:34, 1977
3. Analysis of Workers' Compensation Laws, p vii. Washington, DC, U.S. Chamber of Commerce, January, 1980
4. Barros A: Setting up a system of pay for performance. MLO 18(11):40–45, 1986
5. Berte, LM: Performance standards for the transfusion service. MLO 19(11):33–39, 1987
6. Benezra N: Lab salaries and benefits: Are they keeping pace? MLO 19(1):30–34, 1987
7. Browdy JD: Performance appraisal and pay-for-performance start at the top. Health Care Supervisor 7(3):31–41, 1989
8. Castleberry BM, Yablonsky T, Wargelin L: 1994 Wage and vacancy survey of medical laboratories. Lab Medicine 26:196–112, 1995
9. Dillard JF: Human resource accounting. In Cleverly WO (ed): Handbook of Health Care Accounting and Finance, pp. 223–236. Rockville, Aspen Systems Corporation, 1982
10. Esmond TH: Budgeting Procedures for Hospitals, pp 55–65. Chicago, American Hospital Association, 1982
11. Flamholtz EG: Human Resource Accounting, p 21. Encino, CA, Dickensen, 1974
12. Garcia LS: Creating job standards for a merit pay plan. MLO 18(10):30–36, 1986
13. Glaser WA: Paying the Doctor, p 7. Baltimore, Johns Hopkins Press, 1970
14. Groner DN: Employee incentives. Topics in Health Care Finance 3:63–86, 1977
15. Guiles HJ, Lunz ME: A comparison of medical technologist salaries with other job catergories and professions. Lab medicine 26:20–22, 1995
16. Hamon CM, Snyder JR, Wilson SL, Speicher CE: Job satisfaction of clinical laboratory personnel under two performance-reward systems. Clin lab Sci 4:311–315, 1991
17. Henderson RI: Compensation Management: Rewarding Performance, 4th ed. Reston, Reston Publishing Company, 1985
18. Heneman HG, Schwab DP, Fossum JA, et al: Managing Personnel and Human Resources: Strategies and Programs, pp 280–282. Homewood, Dow-Jones-Irwin, 1981
19. Herkimer AG: Understanding Hospital Financial Management, Germantown, Aspen Systems Corporation, 1978
20. Kaskiw EA, King PH, Morell JC, et al: Physician compensation. In Cleverly WO: Handbook of Health Care Accounting and Finance, pp 757–792. Rockville, Aspen Systems Corporation, 1982
21. Laliberty R, Christopher WI: Enhancing Productivity in Health Care Facilities, pp 109–121. Owing Mills, National Health Publishing, 1984
22. Levey S, Loomba NP: Health Care Administration: A Managerial Perspective, 2nd ed, pp 448–451. Philadelphia, J.B. Lippincott, 1984
23. Liebler JG, Levine RE, Hyman HL: Management Principles for Health Professionals, pp 234–238. Rockville, Aspen Systems Corporation, 1984
24. Lunz ME, Morris MW, Castleberry BM: Medical technologist career commitment and satisfaction with job benefits. CLMR 10:613–615, 1996
25. Muller A, Vitali JJ, Brannon D: Wage difference and the concentration of women in hospital occupations. Health Care Management Review 12(1):61–70, 1987
26. Santos A: Annual salaries of top managers to rise 4.7% in 1987. Hospitals 61(9):52–57, 1987
27. Sattler J: A Practical Guide to Financial Management of the Clinical Laboratory, pp 30–35. Oradell, Medical Economics Company, 1980
28. Seawell LV: Hospital Financial Accounting: Theory and practice, 2nd ed, pp 193–202. Dubuque, Kendall/Hunt Publishing Company, 1987
29. Shyavitz L, Rosenbloom D, Conover L: Financial incentives for middle manager: Pilot program in an inner city, municipal teaching hospital. Health Care Management Review 10(3): 37–44, 1985
30. Stevenson DK: Compensation of hospital-based physicians and key administrative employees. In Cleverly WO: Handbook of Health Care Accounting and Finance, pp 577–591. Rockville, Aspen Systems Corporation, 1982
31. Trotto NE: Job satisfaction in the field: Woman speak out. MLO 24(6):22–28, 1992
32. Umiker WO: Pay raises: Merit or seniority? MLO 15(9): 63–68, 1983
33. Umiker WO: Salary talk: When and how? MLO 18(4): 43–44, 1986
34. Umiker WO, Yohe SM: How to make certain you get merit increase. MLO 17(1):77–80, 1985
35. Williams F: Employee incentive systems. In Cleverly WO (ed): Handbook of Health Care Accounting and Finance, pp 395–412. Rockville, Aspen Systems Corporation, 1982

ANNOTATED BIBLIOGRAPHY

Famularo JJ (ed): Handbook of Human Resources Administration, 2nd ed. New York, McGraw-Hill Book Company, 1986

This handbook contains eight chapters addressing wage and salary administration, covering topics related to job evaluation and pay plans, compensation plans for executives, and establishing and maintaining a wage and salary program. An additional five chapters describe employee benefits.

Henderson RI: Compensation Management: Rewarding Performance, 4th ed. Reston, Reston Publishing Company, 1985

This resource provides a comprehensive discussion of work and rewards, identifying job content and determining pay, the compensation package, and managerial and professional compensation. Readers will find the following chapters useful: Chapter 3, "Government Influences"; Chapter 5, "Job Analysis"; Chapter 7, "Job Evaluation"; Chapter 8, "Compensable Factor Based Job Evaluation Methods"; Chapter 10, "Designing a Pay Structure"; and Chapter 11, "Employee Benefits and Services."

Metzger N: Personnel Administration in the Health Services Industry, 2nd ed. New York, Spectrum Publications, 1979

In this resource, Chapter 3, entitled "Job Evaluation and Wage and Salary Administration," offers a step-by-step approach to job evaluation using ranking, classification, and point methods. Guidance is provided for determining relative value of job factors and degrees.

Sattler J: A Practical Guide to Financial Management of the Clinical Laboratory, 2nd ed. Oradell, Medical Economics, 1986

Using a common sense approach to financial management of the clinical laboratory, this resource provides practical guidance for setting up a system of accounting and record keeping of personnel hours worked and salary. The author describes the application of basic accounting principles to the CAP workload units system.

Seawell LV: Hospital Financial Accounting: Theory and Practice, 2nd ed. Dubuque, Kendall/Hunt Publishing Company, 1987

Written under the auspices of the Health Care Financial Management Association, this comprehensive text provides in-depth coverage of financial accounting and related management considerations. Chapter 8, "Accounting for Hospital Expenses," includes valuable information regarding compilation of gross payrolls, payroll deduction, denoted services, payroll-related costs, and internal control documents.

Williams F: Employee incentive systems. In Cleverly WO (ed): Handbook of Health Care Accounting and Finance, pp 395–412. Rockville, Aspen Systems Corporation, 1982

This handbook is a classic tome, rich in information regarding financial management in health-care institutions. Four specific chapters offer valuable insight regarding wage and salary administration, including Chapter 12, "Human Resource Accounting"; Chapter 20, "Employee Incentive Systems"; Chapter 28, "Compensation of Hospital-Based Physicians and Key Administrative Employees"; and Chapter 36, "Physician Compensation."

35

Inventory Management and Cost Containment

John R. Snyder

The concept of matériel, or inventory, management is not new. It was first recognized in industry around the turn of the century. It took an external force, World War II, to initiate matériel management as a practical entity in industry. Another external force, cost containment, has brought inventory management to the health-care industry. Health care has come to the forefront of public scrutiny within the last 2 decades. The rising costs of quality health care have brought pressures to bear on health-care institutions from the public and the government. Inventory management is viewed as an opportunity to reduce what seem to be spiraling cost increases.

As is demonstrated later, the matériel management department is responsible for approximately 30% to 40% of the total operating budget of a hospital. Matériel management is directly responsible for all supplies—the unit cost of the supplies themselves and the logistical support costs necessary to order, receive, inventory, distribute, and dispose of or reprocess them. It seems only natural that pressure for reducing costs would come to bear ultimately on matériel management.

SCIENTIFIC INVENTORY MANAGEMENT

Today many inventory management and control systems are computerized, but the same basic principles apply to a sophisticated computer system or to an effective manual system that uses ordering charts, economic order quantity (EOQ) wheels, or other devices. There are some advantages to computer systems, because manual systems require the interpretation and implementation of inventory directives by numerous individuals involved in the inventory replenishment cycle. This situation perpetuates inconsistencies between stocking

units: Several items may be seriously overstocked, while many other items are in short supply. Manual systems hinder the reaction to shifts in the management of inventory conflict and permit poor decisions by some individuals involved in inventory replenishment to go undetected. As a result, investment in inventories is often greater than required to produce a desired supply service objective. This excess investment in inventory generally represents potential savings that could be realized from the use of computerized inventory systems.

This does not mean that manual inventory management systems cannot work efficiently. Given trained individuals with sufficient time to consider relevant variables, there is little doubt that manual systems are superior. Unfortunately, time is a luxury that health-care institutions with broad supply lines can rarely afford.

When to Order—Replenishment

The most important operating consideration of an inventory management system is *when* to reorder a particular item. This decision (the reorder point [ROP]) will determine the supply service attained for a given item. The order quantity is of secondary importance in the determination of supply service.

The relationship between the ROP and supply service stresses the importance of promptly issuing purchase orders for stock that has fallen below the ROP. Using valid data to arrive at the ROP is crucial. If purchase orders are not issued at the appropriate time, supply service will suffer adversely. Furthermore, if the data used in arriving at the ROP are not accurate, the computation of the ROP becomes a futile exercise in mathematics. The lead time, the expected demand, and the errors in forecasting expected demand are important elements in determining the ROP. These elements and their roles are discussed in greater detail later in this chapter.

How Much to Order—Order Quantity

Once a decision has been made to replenish a stock-keeping unit, order quantity is the most important operating consideration in realizing inventory investment objectives. The greater the order quantity, the higher the amount of investment required to finance inventories. Once supply service objectives have been established, the ROP becomes secondary in the determination of inventory investment. However, in establishing supply service objectives, management has its greatest impact on the amount of investment to be devoted to maintaining inventory.

The order quantity is set at a level that minimizes the total annual variable cost associated with ordering and holding an item in stock. While a small order quantity will result in a low investment inventory (ie, a low holding cost), the cost of frequently ordering and receiving the item will be greater. When determining order quantity, the total of these costs—ordering and holding—should be held to a minimum. The elements that make up these costs and their role in influencing the order quantity are discussed later. For the most part, minor errors in estimating these costs will have little effect on the computation of the order quantity.

Forecasting—Estimate of Expected Usage

The forecast of demand can affect both the ROP and the order quantity. The forecast is important in determining the ROP because it is necessary to anticipate demand from the time a purchase order is placed to the time it is physically received and available for use by the laboratory. The forecast is also important in determining how much to purchase.

In a computerized inventory management system, one of the most important uses of the forecast of supply demand is the measurement of inability to forecast. The forecast error, or the difference between the forecast and the actual laboratory demand, determines the buffer or *safety stock* requirement that makes up the ROP.

Purchasing

Purchasing systems translate ROP and order quantities for stock-keeping units into acceptable purchase orders and thus are concerned with the practical, everyday problems of purchasing. The system is not concerned directly with supply service, inventory investment, or order requests.

A purchasing system will modify, within defined bounds, order quantities, ROPs, and other inventory management considerations to meet supplier purchase-order minimums, supplier item minimums, order items in standard multiples, and other defined policies.

TECHNICAL DESCRIPTION OF INVENTORY REPLENISHMENT SYSTEMS

Three basic types of systems are used to replenish items normally inventoried: the fixed-quantity, or trigger, replenishment system; the fixed-period, or tickler, replenishment system; and a mixed approach using aspects common to both systems.

Fixed-Quantity System

The fixed-quantity, or trigger, system initiates (triggers) an order at the instant the balance of available stock reaches a predetermined ROP. This approach is sound in concept, but in practice, it ignores the fact that it might be desirable to consolidate all purchase requirements for a given supplier into one purchase order for a given period of time. In addition, whether on a computer or manual system, it is highly unlikely that a purchase order would be automatically created at an instant in time.

Figure 35-1 illustrates the fixed-quantity system for known consumer demand. The graph is commonly referred to as "saw tooth." With known demand, the ROP equals the expected demand during the lead-time period (in this case with known demand of 40 units or 30 days' supply). The dotted line in the chart represents an on-order quantity. Thus, when the available stock reaches 40 units, an order is automatically placed.

Figure 35-2 illustrates the fixed-quantity system for unknown demand. The element of uncertainty introduces a second component in the determination of the ROP. Rather than having a known demand of 40 units per month, the demand is now expressed as an average, assuming that the supply service objective for the item illustrated requires that during the lead-time period, demand of 60 units is reasonable. Thus, if the maximum demand materialized during the lead-time period, the item would be out of stock. To prepare for this contingency, the ROP should be increased to 60 units, 40 units of which represent an average lead-time supply and 20 units, the difference between the maximum reasonable demand and the average. The 20 units designated for contingencies are usually called *safety stock*. Figure 35-

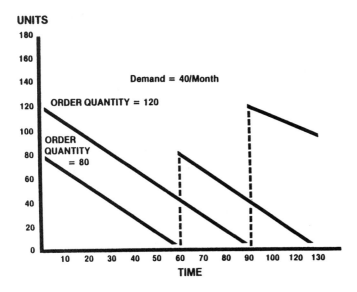

FIGURE 35-1. Fixed quantity replenishment system for known consumer demand.

3 illustrates the fixed quantity system for unknown demand after the introduction of the safety stock.

Fixed-Period System

The fixed-period, or tickler, system initiates a purchase order at the review time regardless of the balance of available stock. The review time is usually established on the basis of the period over which the order quantity is expected to satisfy normal demand. Thus, in the example being discussed, if the order quantity is determined to be 80 units, and the average demand is 40 units per month, the review time will usually be set at 2 months or 60 days.

The parameters for replenishment, order quantity, lead time, average demand, and safety stock are the same generally for both the fixed-quantity and fixed-period replenishment systems. What differs in the two approaches is the action required to initiate a purchase order. In the fixed-quantity system, the quantity ordered remains constant, and the time interval between purchases, *review time*, varies with customer demand. In the fixed-period system, the review time remains constant, and the quantity ordered varies with customer demand.

The fixed-period approach is also sound in concept. However, in practice, it ignores the fact that when dealing with multiple-item suppliers, varying the review time of the various items making up the vendor's line

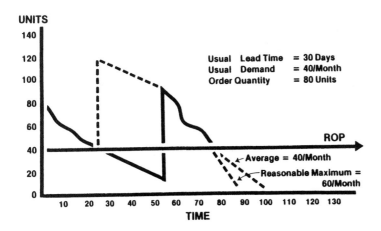

FIGURE 35-2. Fixed quantity replenishment system for unknown demand.

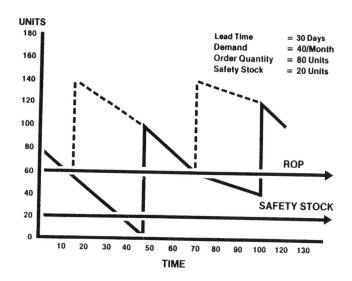

FIGURE 35-3. Fixed quantity replenishment system, unknown demand and safety stock.

can be desirable; this approach probably comes closer to reality than the fixed-quantity system previously discussed.

Figure 35-4 illustrates the fixed-period system for unknown demand. The item illustrated is the same item previously discussed. The dotted line in the chart represents an on-order quantity. Thus, at the review time (regardless of the level of available stock), an order is placed immediately. The quantity ordered is the maximum less the amount of available stock. This maximum quantity is the total of the ROP and order quantity previously determined for the fixed quantity system.

Mixed Replenishment System

The mixed replenishment system uses aspects common to two other systems in an attempt to overcome the impractical aspects attributed to these systems when used alone. Thus, this approach will vary, depending on specific applications. Figure 35-5 illustrates the mixed replenishment system. This mixed approach uses the safety stock and ROP common to the fixed-quantity approach and a maximum and fixed review time common to the fixed-period approach. A purchase order for the item is initiated at the review time only if the amount

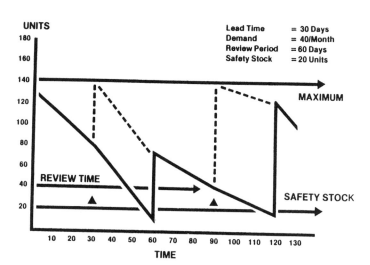

FIGURE 35-4. Fixed period replenishment system, unknown demand and order quantity.

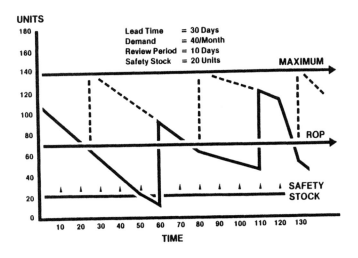

UNITS

Lead Time = 30 Days
Demand = 40/Month
Review Period = 10 Days
Safety Stock = 20 Units

MAXIMUM

ROP

SAFETY STOCK

TIME

FIGURE 35-5. Mixed replenishment system when demand is unknown. Arrowheads denote maximum and fixed review time.

of available inventory is less than the ROP. If a purchase is warranted, the purchase quantity becomes the maximum quantity less the amount of available inventory. Thus, the mixed replenishment approach results in the purchase of an item at irregular intervals in varying quantities.

This method more closely resembles the fixed-period approach than the fixed-quantity approach. Setting a common review period for all items in a supplier's line means that the total requirements at a review period for a particular supplier can be readily consolidated into one purchase order. Setting a frequent review period for the supplier means that the order quantities for the supplier's various items can be established independent of the period review while remaining consistent with the economics of holding and ordering costs. Ordering items from a supplier only when available inventory balances are below the ROP means that frequent purchases of small quantities, with their related ordering costs, can be minimized.

Economic Order Quantity

The initial effort of purchasing and inventory management to control costs was to attack the unit price paid for a given item. Far-reaching tactics were used to achieve this goal. For example, the concept of group purchasing was given a great boost by purchasing agents or matériel managers. Activities such as these are understandable, because the unit price paid for any given item is the easiest factor to measure. Additionally, department heads, encouraged to reduce their spending, typically have only the unit price of supplies in their budget and not a fee for the logistical support

services, such as inventory holding costs and purchasing expense.

A true understanding of matériel management, however, shows that the unit cost is not the only or ultimate answer to reducing the overall costs. EOQ is determined to minimize the total annual variable cost associated with ordering and holding an item in stock. The three relevant cost elements are (1) holding costs, (2) ordering costs, and (3) purchase price of an item, the least important consideration.

Carrying Costs

The total annual variable cost of holding or carrying inventory includes costs incurred from the time an item is purchased and put on the shelf until that item is sold. The components of holding costs can include those listed in Box 35-1.

Box 35·1

Components of Holding Costs

Personal property taxes related to inventory
Rental or depreciation of space and fixtures devoted to inventory
Maintenance of storage space (security and janitorial costs)
Real estate taxes and insurance attributed to storage space
Shrinkage and obsolescence (nonmovement and excess)
Interest costs of money tied up in inventories

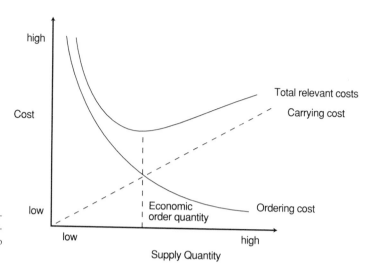

FIGURE 35-6. Opposing cost pressures in inventory management. (Noel, SA, Snyder, JR. Forecast comparisons in inventory management. Lab Medicine 21:91–96, 1990).

Sometimes storage cost is not considered a variable cost, but a fixed or shrunken cost. However, when space is near capacity, this view is unrealistic and can lead to overcrowding. Also, the cost of money tied up on maintaining inventories is sometimes viewed not as the interest cost of money, but as the potential return on investment (ROI) derived from alternative uses of the money.

Ordering Costs

The total annual cost of ordering an item for inventory includes costs incurred from the time the item is identified as being in short supply and ordered until the time an item is received and put on the shelf. The compo-

Box 35·2

Components of Ordering Costs

Stock purchase order forms, envelopes, and postage
Expediting forms, postage, telephone expense
Time related to review, purchasing, expediting, receiving, and payables
Payroll costs related to review, purchasing, expediting, receiving, inspection, warehousing, material movement, and payables
Fringe benefits associated with payroll costs

nents of ordering costs can include those listed in Box 35-2.

From Figure 35-6, it is evident that ordering costs per unit decrease as the size of the order in number of units increases. It is also evident that carrying costs per unit increase as the size of the order increases. To minimize ordering costs, the manager must place fewer orders; to minimize carrying costs, the manager must keep inventory as low as possible. The challenge then is to find a balance between ordering cost pressures for large inventories and carrying cost pressures for small inventories, a balance resulting in the lowest order cost and carrying cost.

Many laboratories today are negotiating with vendors for *just-in-time delivery* of supplies. This purchasing–delivery strategy requires a communications link to the vendor for rapid notification of orders and a sensitive inventory system to trigger the order process. By mechanizing the ordering process, the cost of ordering is diminished; by receiving supplies just when they are needed, the holding costs are diminished.

Purchase Price

The total annual purchase price will not usually be affected by the amount purchased or the frequency of purchase. The only major exception to this is the situation in which the vendor offers item quantity discounts. Once holding costs, ordering costs, and purchase price have been determined, EOQ can be derived through trial and error. (For the purposes of our calculation, we are ignoring for the moment the possibility of item quantity discounts.) Normally the cost of holding inventory is stated as a percentage, such as 20%. This percentage is related to the unit cost of each stock-keeping unit and the annual carrying cost for that item. The cost of ordering inventory is stated as a dollar amount for each line item. This dollar amount carries the assumption that on average, a certain number of line items will be purchased on a single purchase order and accordingly includes costs associated with ordering a line item and issuance and processing of a purchase order.

Figure 35-7 illustrates an item having a known demand of 40 units per month. In previous illustrations, the item was shown as having an order quantity of 80 units. For the purpose of determining EOQ, ROP and safety stock are ignored. Accordingly, using a known demand without consideration of the real uncertainty involved does not change the determination of EOQ. Furthermore, with a known demand, it is also possible to conclude that if an order quantity is set at 80 units, then the average amount of available inventory on hand will be half that quantity (or 40 units). With this background, the EOQ can be found through trial and error. First, if we start with an order quantity of 80 units and assume a purchase price of $1.50, annual variable ordering cost will be $12.00 (six purchases a year at $2.00 each). Thus, the total variable costs equal $24.00. If we use 120 units as the order quantity, total annual variable holding costs will be $26.00. If we try an order quantity of 60 units, total annual variable holding and ordering

costs will be $25.00. Any order quantity other than 80 units will result in a total annual expense greater than $24.00. Thus, 80 units is the EOQ.

Accuracy of Economic Order Quantity

When determining the variable holding and ordering costs, it is possible to make an error in estimating. Furthermore, holding and ordering costs are averages and are not necessarily accurate for one item. For instance, the holding cost of an item that is bulky or must be refrigerated is greater than that of a small item kept in normal bin storage. Also, the annual usage of an item is not always known and may be subject to change as the year progresses. Fortunately, the total variable costs associated with ordering and holding inventory are not very sensitive in the range of the EOQ.

Order Quantity Sensitivity

The example in Box 35-3 illustrates the total annual variable costs of different order quantities. As the order quantity is varied from 60 to 120 units, the total variable cost does not differ by more than $2.00. Accordingly, the necessity of estimating does not negate the EOQ concept, but rather encourages its use.

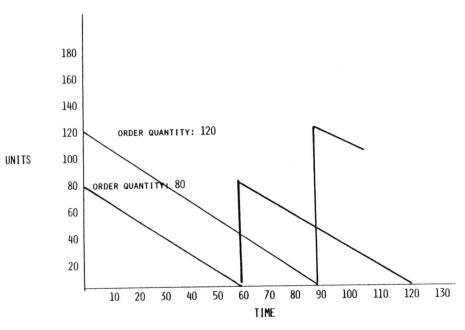

FIGURE 35-7.   Economic order quantity (EOQ).

Box 35·3

Order Quantity Sensitivity

FACTORS

Holding cost
Ordering cost
Purchasing price

EXAMPLES

Purchase price = $1.50

I. Order quantity 80 units
   Annual ordering cost $12.00 (6 orders per year at $2.00)
   Annual holding cost $12.00 (4 units at $1.50 at 20%)
      Total $24.00
II. Order quantity 120 units
   Annual ordering cost $ 8.00 (4 orders per year at $2.00)
   Annual holding cost $18.00 (60 units at $1.50 at 20%)
      Total $26.00
III. Order quantity 60 units
   Annual ordering cost $16.00 (8 orders per year at $2.00)
   Annual holding cost $ 9.00 (30 units at $1.50 at 20%)
      Total $25.00

Item Quantity Discounts

If a vendor offers an item quantity discount, sometimes called a break-point algorithm, the EOQ may require adjustment. The example in Box 35-4 illustrates the required analysis of the item previously discussed. With a purchase price of only $1.50 per unit, the EOQ was 80 units, resulting in a total annual variable cost of $24.00. If the supplier offers a 5% discount for a purchase of 160 units or more, the order cost will decrease $6.00 (three less purchases at $2.00 each), the holding cost will increase $12.00 (40 units more in inventory at $.0142 at 20%), but the annual purchase price will decrease by $36.00 (480-unit annual usage at $0.75 cost reduction per unit). The net change is a savings of $30.00; therefore, the order quantity should be equal to the item break point of 160 units.

Forecasting

The approach for forecasting supply demand or usage that is common to most inventory management systems involves the projecting of the past into the future. This approach differs from prediction, and introducing and anticipating changes in new circumstances still remain

---

Box 35·4

Item Quantity Discount

PRICE-BREAK FACTORS

Holding cost
Ordering cost
Purchase price

EXAMPLE

Normal order quantity	80 units
Normal purchase price	$ 1.50
Normal ordering cost	$12.00
Normal holding cost	$12.00

AT 5% DISCOUNT FOR 160 UNITS

Order quantity	160
Order cost change	$(12)
Holding cost change	$ 12
Purchase price change	$(12)
Net change	$(12)

Box 35·5

Calculating Economic Order Quantity (EOQ) and Changing Variables

Annual units	600
Ordering cost	$8.00
Inventory carrying cost	20%
Cost per unit	$30

The formula used to arrive at the EOQ is as follows:

$$EOQ = \sqrt{\frac{2AS}{1C}}$$

$$EOQ = \sqrt{\frac{2(600)(8)}{(.20)(30)}} = \sqrt{\frac{9600}{.06}} = \sqrt{160,000} = 400$$

$$\sqrt{\frac{2(\text{annual units})(\text{ordering cost})}{(\text{carrying cost \%})(\text{cost per unit})}}$$

$$\sqrt{\frac{2(600)(8)}{(.20)(300)}} = 13 \text{ High cost}$$
↑

$$\sqrt{\frac{2(600)(8)}{(.10)(30)}} = 565 \text{ Low carrying cost}$$
↑ ↓

$$\sqrt{\frac{2(600)(80)}{(20)(30)}} = 1265 \text{ High ordering cost}$$

$$\sqrt{\frac{2(12,000)(8)}{(20)(30)}} = 1789 \text{ High usage}$$

the functions of the inventory manager (Box 35-5). To function effectively, an inventory management system must have the benefit of both forecast and prediction.

Techniques

Several techniques can be used to project the future on the basis of past experience. Generally, these techniques all use the statistical concept of an average.

The Moving Average

The simplest of these approaches is the *moving average,* which produces a forecast for the future that represents the simple average of the periods encompassed by this moving or sliding approach. Each historical period is generally given equal weight. In a 5-month average, each of the 5 months contributes 20% to the forecast of the next period. When the actual experience becomes available for the next period, the oldest experience is dropped, and the most current set of five experiences is again averaged. This approach is good for stable items but generally not for items with upward and downward trends.

Regression Analysis

Regression analysis produces a forecast by fitting a line or curve to a series of experiences. This line is commonly called the "line of best fit." Regression, unlike the moving average, assigns a weight to each experience that varies with the amount of deviation from the average. The greater the deviation, the greater the weight assigned. Unlike the moving average, the regression approach may not be responsive to upward or downward trends.

Exponential Smoothing

Exponential smoothing is a moving average that assigns unique weights to a historical experience. the greatest weight is assigned to the most current experience. For this reason, the smoothing approach is more responsive to upward or downward trends than the moving average. However, the adjustment will always lag behind the trends; the lag will determine the number of periods being used. To compensate for this lag, second-order, or double, smoothing can be used. With double smoothing, forecasting can be highly responsive to trend.

Figure 35-8 illustrates the weights associated with different alpha factors that are used in exponential smoothing. As the illustration shows, an alpha factor of

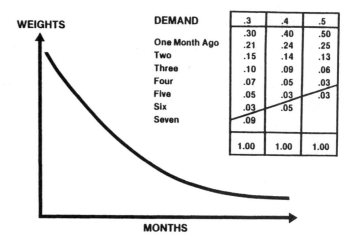

WEIGHTS

DEMAND	.3	.4	.5
	.30	.40	.50
One Month Ago	.21	.24	.25
Two	.15	.14	.13
Three	.10	.09	.06
Four	.07	.05	.03
Five	.05	.03	.03
Six	.03	.05	
Seven	.09		
	1.00	1.00	1.00

MONTHS

FIGURE 35-8. Exponential smoothing in forecasting.

0.3 is equivalent to a 5- to 7-month moving average using unequal weights, while an alpha factor of 0.5 is equivalent to a 3- to 5-month moving average.

Exponential smoothing also has several computational advantages, making it desirable for use in computer applications. These advantages center around the fact that only the old forecast is required for determining the new forecast, with a simple moving average of all historical data retained.

New forecast = Alpha × Demand + (1 − Alpha) × Old forecast

The example in Box 35-6 illustrates how a single smooth forecast is computed with an alpha of 0.3 (a 5- to 7-month moving average). With the current demand of 80 units for the first month, the new forecast becomes 66 units. For the next month only, this figure is used in

determining the new forecast of 67 units. (For illustrative purposes, the calculation is also shown with additional historical data.)

Base Index

The *base index* approach is used most often in conjunction with an averaging technique to compensate for items with seasonal demands. While averaging will smooth out seasonal patterns, the base index approach attempts to reinstate these regular patterns. This approach requires substantial demand history and works by averaging the same month of the year over several years. For example, if traditionally the seasonal peak for an item is July, the July average will be greater than the smoothing or simple average, and this relationship

---

Box 35•6

Exponential Smoothing

EXAMPLE

Old forecast	60
Demand	80
Alpha	0.3
New forecast	0.3(80) + 0.7(60)
	24 + 42 = 66

NEXT MONTH

Old forecast	66
Demand	70
Alpha	0.3
New forecast	0.3(70) + 0.7(66)
	21 + 46 = 67

or

0.3(70) + 0.7(24 + 42)
21   17   29 = 67

will be used to correct the smoothed or simple average when forecasting July.

Adaptive Smoothing

An averaging approach that assigns unequal weight to past experiences, *adaptive smoothing* uses sine and cosine functions, adjusting for trends and seasonal demands while averaging. Accordingly, the weights assigned to past experiences vary considerably, depending on the number of terms used in the calculation. This approach can be responsive and effective but is highly sophisticated and difficult to start up or adjust once in use.

Responsiveness

Throughout the discussion of various forecasting approaches, responsiveness has been emphasized. *Responsiveness* means an ability to react to an indication of a shift in demand. This characteristic is desirable for forecasting. However, because trends or shifts in demands are not always readily discernible, responsiveness must be dampened so as not to cause an overreaction.

It is not uncommon for a trend to be accompanied by sporadic demands on both the high and low sides of the trend. When too few experiences are considered, the magnitude and even the direction of the trend may be misread. Likewise, the forecast approach may react to too few experiences. This applies to forecasting trends where they do exist and, just as importantly, to not forecasting trends where they do not exist. A shift in demand based on a few unusual experiences does not make a trend.

Forecasting Error

An integral part of forecasting is measuring the forecast error. The forecast error is the difference between actual demand and forecast demand. Accordingly, the better the forecasting approach selected, the smaller the forecast error. On the other hand, a realistic understanding of the forecast error enables the inventory management system to establish a sufficient buffer or safety stock to compensate for the inability to forecast accurately. Therefore, regardless of the ability to forecast, adequate safety stock should be available to ensure satisfying

supply service objectives. Obviously, it is desirable to forecast as accurately as possible, because it reduces the need for safety stock, thus minimizing inventory investment. However, because safety stock is dependent on the forecast error, the existence of the forecast error should not necessarily affect supply service. For this reason, the measure of the forecast error is often considered more important than the forecast itself.

Forecasting Illustrated

To gain a better understanding of how forecasting is done and how responsiveness and forecasting errors are handled, let us now examine single exponential smoothing in more detail. This method is probably the one most commonly used in the health-care industry today.

The issue of responsiveness is normally handled through a method called *demand screening*. The current demand used to update the forecast is screened to minimize the effect of the new forecast on any unusual situation manifesting itself in the current demand amount. One should attempt to keep the new forecast from being too responsive to a chance event. On the other hand, if this unusual demand is the beginning of a drastic change, the screening process will retard the adjustment of the forecast to the drastic change. It is more desirable not to overreact to a chance event than it is to respond too slowly to a drastic change in an item's demand. Because the latter should be recognized by the people dealing with distribution and inventory, a manual adjustment can be made.

The screening process works by computing demand limits that range from plus four times the mean absolute deviation (MAD) to minus four times MAD. If the actual demand is outside this range, the demand limit is used instead of the actual demand in updating the forecast. The real demand should be maintained and used when it becomes necessary to reanalyze the item being forecast.

Figure 35-9 illustrates a normal distribution curve, which represents demand in relationship to the forecast. There is a 50% probability that demand will not exceed the current forecast at each level of MAD. The measure of the forecast error commonly associated with this forecasting approach is MAD. This method of error or standard deviation can be associated with any forecasting approach using statistical averages.

Figure 35-10 illustrates that MAD is the average of the absolute forecast error. This average is commonly calculated by exponential smoothing in the same manner as the forecast. In addition to the MAD established in this illustration, there is one other factor used in measuring forecast error—the sum of errors. It is computed

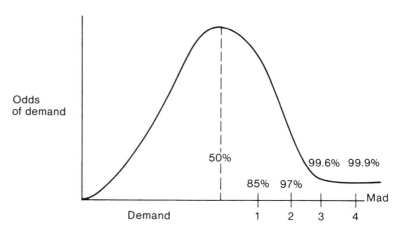

Odds
of demand

FIGURE 35-9. Demand in relation to forecast (MAD, mean absolute deviation).

as MAD is, except that the signed (plus or minus) difference is used.

Reorder Point

Inventory systems should recalculate ROP and safety stocks on a periodic basis, probably once a month. As indicated below, the ROP is composed of the average lead-time supply plus safety stock.

$$ROP = F(LT + RT) + SS$$

where

$$F = \text{Forecast} \qquad RT = \text{Review time}$$
$$LT = \text{Lead time} \qquad SS = \text{Safety stock}$$

$$ROP = (\text{Lead time}) (\text{Demand}) + \text{Safety stock}$$
$$= \text{Reasonable maximum}$$

$$30 \text{ days} + 40/\text{mo}$$
$$40 \qquad + 20 = 60 \; ROP$$

Safety stock has been previously described as the amount needed to increase the average lead-time supply to the reasonable maximum demand for the lead-time period. This reasonable maximum demand is determined by considering supply service objectives for this item. Safety stock is commonly calculated with the statistical approach that is shown in Box 35-7.

Cost Containment

If we view the total cost of purchasing as an iceberg, we see that the unit price paid for an item is only the tip of the iceberg. Because the unit price is the most visible component, it is only logical that it would be likened to the tip or most visible part of the iceberg. However, somewhat out of sight of the users of supplies are two other costs. The middle portion of the iceberg is the cost of acquisition, the cost necessary for purchasing supplies. It is the cost of personnel involved in the paper-flow process of purchasing. Buried deeper in the iceberg is the cost of inventory. The cost of putting an item on the shelf and anticipating its use is composed of such things as shrinkage, obsolescence, depreciation, the cost of personnel to distribute or redistribute the product, and the cost of capital.

To understand more clearly the relationship between the unit price of an item and the costs of logistical support, consider the following information gathered by the American Hospital Association concerning an average 250-bed hospital in the United States. An average hospital has an operating budget of approximately $50,000 per bed per year. Of that, $10,000 per bed per year pays for the unit price of supplies, while another $10,000 per bed per year pays for the logistical support system. Clearly, there is a dollar-for-dollar relationship between the cost of supplies and the total cost of acquisition and inventory. It is also apparent that the matériel management department is clearly responsible for approximately 40% of the total operating budget of the average hospital.

With the understanding that the average healthcare institution is a large business and that the matériel management department is responsible for 40% of the cost of operation of this large business, it is only proper that we view the matériel management function from one of industry's measures of efficiency—return or investment. The matériel management department is definitely a business operation. The process of ordering, receiving, inventory, distributing, and reprocessing (manufacturing) is nothing more than the process of manufacturing and distribution.

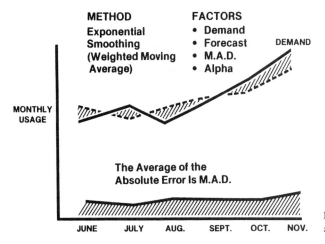

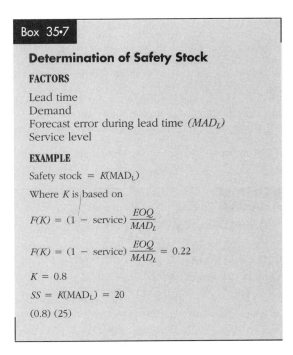

FIGURE 35-10. Mean absolute deviation (MAD) as the average of the absolute forecast error.

For our purposes, ROI is defined as earnings divided by assets. To increase ROI from the vantage point of matériel management, it is necessary either to reduce operating expenses, and thereby increase earnings, or reduce assets. To reduce operating expenses and increase earnings, matériel management has the opportunity to decrease the cost of acquisition, especially with regard to personnel productivity. Additionally, reduced expenses can originate from the reduction of inventory and thereby the reduction of inventory-holding costs. The matériel management department may also decrease assets by reducing inventory. The combination of reduced inventory and increased productivity within the cost of the acquisition process will yield a twofold impact on the increasing ROI.

Cost of Acquisition

The cost of an average purchase order in a health-care institution can range from $25 to $50. Reported actual stated costs have ranged from $60 to $108. Whatever the cost of the purchase order process, it is necessary to understand that approximately 75% of cost is directly attributable to personnel, and only 25%, or even less, is attributable to the cost of supplies for the purchase-order process. Any significant impact on reducing the costs of acquisition will result directly from increasing the productivity of the people involved in the process.

For purposes of illustration, the following case study discusses a cost of acquisition and inventory analysis. In this case study, General Medical Center has invited a consulting team to analyze its matériel manage-

ment program with specific emphasis placed on the impact of this function on the laboratory environment.

Case Study: Cost of Acquisition Analysis

Interviews in purchasing, matériel management, the clinical laboratory, and accounting revealed the purchasing paper flow and accountability system to be

---

Box 35·7

Determination of Safety Stock

FACTORS

Lead time
Demand
Forecast error during lead time (MAD_L)
Service level

EXAMPLE

Safety stock $= K(MAD_L)$

Where K is based on

$$F(K) = (1 - \text{service}) \frac{EOQ}{MAD_L}$$

$$F(K) = (1 - \text{service}) \frac{EOQ}{MAD_L} = 0.22$$

$K = 0.8$

$SS = K(MAD_L) = 20$

$(0.8) (25)$

comprehensive but overly burdened in two particular areas: (1) the requisition process and (2) documentation and accountability files.

The paper-flow process was studied in detail. It should be understood that this study depicts the flow of documentation for a "clean" order, receiving, and accounting process. Various errors, either user or vendor induced, can cause any or all of the system to be "turned" one or more additional times.

It was found that at least two requisitions are prepared before the purchase order is actually typed. Both requisitions were also typed. From the standpoint of productivity, time is wasted in typing each order *three times* at General Medical Center. The first requisition prepared by departmental personnel is a composite for that department for all vendors. The laboratory coordinator's office then prepares from those documents individual requisitions for each department by vendor.

With respect to document files, closed-order files, which are maintained for 7 years, were discovered within the medical center in purchasing, accounting, and receiving. Audit accountability was the only reason given for the need for closed-order files; therefore, the file in accounting was the only file necessary.

The general accountability of the system for audit purposes was found to be excellent. In fact, the mechanism established for accountability was found to be too exhaustive and produced severe limitations to purchase-order productivity. Those limitations are imposed by the following criteria established for purchase orders (Box 35-8).

These restrictions result in significantly reduced purchase order productivity. For example, if two departments within the clinical laboratory order the same item from the same vendor, there will be two distinct purchase orders, receivings, invoices, and so forth. Thus, the purchasing paper-flow system will turn twice. In reality, all that is required is that each expenditure, regardless of vendor and item, be accounted for by department account number.

The paper-flow system was found also to contribute to lead-time-induced inventory. The total time from recognition of a need by the user to vendor action (eg, shipment, back-order) was found to be approximately 9 working days.

One particular area inducing as much as a 2-day delay was the budget control process. While the function and purpose of this were clearly understood, in practice it was not realistic for the clinical laboratory for routine supply items. The budget-control process for such items was probably best performed "after the fact." Critical products for patient diagnosis would not, it seems, be rejected for order because of budget overrun. The budget accountability process should be managed on a periodic basis by exception.

The cost of a purchase order was calculated to be $39.84. The details of how this was calculated are found in Figures 35-11, 35-12, and 35-13.

Recommendations (General/All-Vendor Interface)

The recommendations that follow are suggested areas for consideration. Although potential procedural guidelines are provided, they are not totally comprehensive. They are offered within the confines of the research and thus limited to the clinical laboratory's current procedures and perceived needs. Many recommendations may apply to other departmental areas or be limited because of restrictions imposed by other departmental purchasing areas. Figures 35-14, 35-15, 35-16, and 35-17 demonstrate graphically the specific changes in the cost of acquisition process and the related financial impacts of those changes.

With regard the clinical laboratory and purchasing for routine consumables (value per unit less than $300), eliminate the budget-control process prior to the complete purchasing process. In theory, the budget-control process step within the purchasing process is sound, but in practice, it loses merit and is a greater limitation than its merit warrants.

Eliminate two of the three closed-order files. Three such existing files are not deemed necessary and are potentially counterproductive. Entries to a file after the fact for information relative to a specific order in a given file may not carry through all three files, thus creating discrepancies. The single file necessary should be associated with the accounting department because the control/accountability of that file rests within the accounting department.

Increase the number of pages per purchase order. Productivity within the purchasing process is severely limited owing to the restrictions on the

---

Box 35•8

Criteria Established for Purchase Orders

Only one account number (department) per purchase order
Only one vendor per purchase order
Only one page per purchase order with space for only four items with two-line descriptions or eight items with one-line descriptions

Contribution	Annual Costs	Suggested Factor	Factor	Contribution Cost
All labor costs in purchasing including fringes (excludes department managers)	167,700	100%	100%	167,700
Purchasing department— Manager's salary/ fringes		25%		
All labor costs in accounts payable attributable to payment of invoices generated through purchasing	71,510	Variable	85%	60,784
Labor for receiving and stores	247,946	25%	90%	223,151
Telephone costs for:				
—Purchasing	2,100	50%	40%	840
—Receiving	900	50%	50%	450
—Stores	—	50%	—	—
—Accounts Payable	900	50%	50%	450
Office supplies for:				
—Purchasing	—	75%	—	—
—Accounts Payable	1,416	75%	75%	1,062
—Receiving	—	75%	—	—

Total annual contribution costs (excludes end-user contribution)	$454,437.
Total number of purchase orders annually (includes end-user POs)	19,500
Departmental purchase order cost	$23.30
Average lines per order	3.4

FIGURE 35-11.   Cost of acquisition. Departmental contribution—preanalysis.

number of items on a given purchase order document (four to eight items). This increases "turns" in the paper-flow process, receiving, deliveries to the user departments, and the number of invoices to be processed through accounts payable. Second and third pages of the original purchase order document could have the purchase order number, page number, and so forth recorded on them.

Consolidate orders to vendors across departmental lines and account numbers. All that is required is that a given item on a given purchase order have the account number for the user department associated with it. This would significantly increase the purchase system productivity but is predicated on implementation of the preceding recommendation.

Reduce or eliminate typed requisition process at the user department and laboratory coordinator level. A "card system" for requisitioning is in place for some items in the clinical laboratory. This should be expanded to include all the laboratory items purchased (at least on a routine basis). Each department would submit cards to

Contribution	Annual Costs (Salary/Fringes)	% of Time Involvement* (Factor)	Contribution Cost
Laboratory director	38,000	2	$ 760
Laboratory manager			
Laboratory secretary			
Laboratory purch. clerk	12,500	70	8750
Departmental supervisors (combine all if more than one)	256,485 (12 supervisors)	3	7695
Medical technologists (combine all if more than one			
Others _____			
_____			
_____			

Total annual contribution costs	$17,205
Total number of laboratory purchase orders annually	1,040
End-user purchase order cost	$16.54

FIGURE 35-12. Cost of acquisition. End-user contribution—preanalysis.

Contribution	Total Contribution Cost	Total Orders	Cost Per Order
All departments except requisitioning department	454,437	19,500	$ 23.30 /Purchase order (A)
Requisitioning department (end-user)	17,205	1,040	$ 16.54 /Purchase order (B)

Cost per order for orders from end-user (A + B) = $ 39.84 /Purchase order

$$\text{Cost per order line} = \frac{\text{Cost per order}}{(A + B)} \div \frac{\text{Average lines}}{\text{per order}} = \$ 11.72 / \text{line}$$

FIGURE 35-13. Cost of acquisition. Total contribution cost—preanalysis.

Contribution	Annual Costs	Suggested Factor	Factor	Contribution Cost
All labor costs in purchasing including fringes (excludes department managers)	167,700	100%	80%	134,160
Purchasing department— manager's salary/ fringes		25%		
All labor costs in accounts payable attributable to payment of invoices generated through purchasing	71,510	Variable	85%	60,784
Labor for receiving and stores	247,946	25%	75%	185,960
Telephone costs for				
—Purchasing	2100	50%	40%	840
—Receiving	900	50%	50%	450
—Stores	—	50%	—	—
—Accounts payable	900	50%	50%	450
Office supplies for				
—Purchasing	—	75%	—	—
—Accounts payable	1416	75%	75%	1062
—Receiving	—	75%	—	—

Total annual contribution costs (excludes end-user contribution)	$383,706.
Total number of purchase orders annually (includes end-user POs)	19,360
Departmental purchase order cost	$ 19.82
Average lines per order	4.0

FIGURE 35-14.   Cost of acquisition. Department contribution—postanalysis.

the laboratory coordinator's office on a routine basis. These cards would be compiled by vendor within the laboratory coordinator's office (see the previous recommendation) and forwarded to purchasing for purchase order preparation. Each group of cards would indicate a specific vendor and thereby constitute a single purchase order. The user portion of the purchase order could be returned to the laboratory coordinator's office with the cards to verify the order. Alternatively, the laboratory secretary could be charged with the responsibility of typing the actual purchase order documents and forwarding these to the purchasing department for approval and vendor submission. This would decentralize the work effort of the purchase order preparation but retain centralized purchasing control.

Reduce the total number of copies of the purchase order document. An inordinate amount of paper flows through the system for the relatively small order dollar volume. Eliminating receiving's and purchasing's closed-order file as previously recommended does away with the need for two of the copies. Receiving can function properly with only one copy of the original document. Photocopies (which exist in the system now) can

Contribution	Annual Costs (Salary/Fringes)	% of Time Involvement* (Factor)	Contribution Cost
Laboratory director	38,000	0	0
Laboratory manager			
Laboratory secretary			
Laboratory purch. clerk	12,500	70	$8750
Departmental supervisors (combine all if more than one)	256,485 (12 supervisors)	1.5	$3847
Medical technologists (combine all if more than one			
Others _____ _____ _____			

Total annual contribution costs	$12,597
Total number of laboratory purchase orders annually	900
End-user purchase order cost	$14

* Percent of time involvement is percent of employees' time directly related to the functions of analyzing need for products to be ordered, requisitioning, purchasing, expediting, receiving merchandise, correcting errors, and so forth.

FIGURE 35-15.   Cost of acquisition. End-user contribution—postanalysis.

be used effectively. Receiving's single master copy would be retained until all shipments against the purchase order were complete, with photocopies flowing through the system for partial shipments. With completion of the order, receiving's master would flow through the system. The ultimate effect here is that receiving would have no remaining paperwork on the order—no closed-order file. Because purchasing would not keep a closed-order file, it is not necessary to have a receiving copy for purchasing notification.

Purchasing will now handle errors and expedite on a by-exception basis. The single copy file in purchasing can be updated periodically or on an ongoing basis. For example, the final copy from receiving indicating order completion could be routed through the purchasing department, signaling that the order is complete. At that point, it would no longer be necessary for purchasing to retain its copy of the original purchase document.

In practice, unless accounting is encumbering funds, it is not necessary for Accounting to receive an additional copy of the purchase order. The accounting function is to process invoices for payment based on verification from receiving and the user department that shipment is accurate and complete. Accounting is notified of accuracy and completeness of shipment by receiving's copy of the original purchase document. The lack of an original purchase order copy to accounting controls potential prepayment of the invoice.

If these processes are used, the original purchase order would be reduced from six to four copies: (1)

Contribution	Total Contribution Cost	Total Orders	Cost Per Order
All departments except requisitioning department	383,706	19,360	$ 19.82 /Purchase order (A)
Requisitioning department (end-user)	12,597	900	$ 14.00 /Purchase order (B)

Cost per order for orders from end-user   (A + B) = $ 33.82 /Purchase order

Cost per order line = Cost per order (A + B) ÷ Average lines per order = $ 8.46 /line

FIGURE 35-16. Cost of acquisition. Total cost contribution—postanalysis.

Category	Existing System	Revised System	% Improvement	Dollar Impact
Paper flow process steps	14	10	—	—
Departmental contribution cost	$454,437	$383,706	15.6	$70,731
End-user contribution cost	$ 17,205	$ 12,597	26.8	$ 4,608
Total contribution cost	$471,642	$396,303	16.0	$75,339
Cost per purchase order	$39.84	$33.82	15.1	$6.02
Cost per order line	$11.72	$8.46	27.8	$3.26
Number of end-user purchase orders	1,040	900	—	—
Total number of purchase orders (all departments)	19,500	19,360	—	—

FIGURE 35-17. Comparative financial analysis—cost of acquisition.

vendor, (2) purchasing, (3) receiving, and (4) accounts payable.

The paper-flow process can be significantly reduced. Not only are there fewer pieces of paper flowing through the system, but there are fewer people and less time involved in the process. These two reductions can only result in increased productivity. Through a complete and thorough review and a systems approach to the acquisition process, the matériel management department can significantly affect the process and reduce the cost.

Cost of Inventory

Inventory is like a gas: It will expand to fill the container to which it is allotted. Historically, users of a given supply item will base judgment on the quantity of inventory on the space available for storing an item.

Especially in health-care institutions, which deal with human lives, the technical users of various items would view the ideal inventory as an almost limitless supply available at any given time. However, the product laboratory manager would argue, conversely, that the smallest possible inventory or no inventory would be ideal, because inventory is expensive. Obviously, there must be some median whereby the service level to the user is in harmony with the cost of maintaining the inventory. There must be trade-offs.

The laboratory manager has obviously based his desires on the fact that inventory investment significantly affects many areas within the financial system. Inventory basically is a large nonspendable asset and as such, can severely affect the cash flow system. Inventory requires handling for storage and redistribution, and it requires space for storage. Therefore, inventory affects operating revenues. Also, the monetary assets bound up in inventory represent an opportunity for investment income. To a cash-rich institution, this income opportunity could be realized in the form of high-interest certificates of deposit. At a minimum, the cash-poor institution could use freed working capital to reduce debt. The financial implications of inventory investment clearly state that inventory is an asset worthy of strict management principles.

The following case study analyzes the inventory control mechanisms in the clinical laboratory at the mythical General Medical Center. The financial impact of the recommendations made after the analysis is shown in Figure 35-18.

Case Study: Inventory Analysis

All inventory in the clinical laboratory is classified as "unofficial," because it has been expensed to a user department instead of being maintained as an asset. As is common among clinical laboratories, there exists no inventory control system except the perpetual-card system. The user ultimately controls the inventory. The only control perceived outside the stockroom is the routine schedule for the ordering process. Historically, this has little or no influence on the actual controlling of inventory.

The laboratory stockroom was defined as containing items common to all user departments within the clinical laboratory. A visit to this stockroom verified that the items located there were, in part, common to more than one user department. However, much of that inventory appeared to have been there for quite some time. Some of the items could be better classified as those originally purchased in a large volume and stored there for convenience. Other items stored represent a very small dollar volume and are not worth controlling.

The perpetual card system in place for this laboratory exists in practice but is not properly controlled. For example, EOQs were historically established and did not appear to have been periodically reviewed or changed. Each department had instances where quantity on hand far exceeded monthly usage.

In summary, the inventory control process in the clinical laboratory is determined by the user—not matériel management.

Recommendations

Perform ABC inventory analysis to determine how best to handle the inventory control process of various products or product groups. Analysis of order history for various items is a relatively time-consuming process and may require research of documentation from vendors but will be a significant savings opportunity. ABC analysis is merely a method of determining which items require what type of inventory control. It is not in and of itself an inventory control system.

Establish an effective inventory control program for the clinical laboratory (for at least class A items as defined in the preceding recommendation). Inventory control is best defined here as determining proper EOQs and ROPs for items. Calculations of these parameters for each item would be time consuming and an ongoing process but can be performed with a programmable calculator. (Normally attempts to institute such a system are computer based or assisted.) Effective adherence to calculated EOQs and ROPs based on inventory reduction goals set by General Medical Center would continue inventory control at the user level without the

Department or Class	Existing System				Revised System				% Improvement	Dollar Impact
	DIOH Turn	Total Inv. Value	Holding Costs	Total Inv. Investment	DIOH Turn	Total Inv. Value	Holding Costs	Total Inv. Investment		
Chemistry	51/ 7.2	$42,006	$12,602	$54,608	30/ 12	$25,353	$7606	$32,959	39.6	$21,649
Blood bank	91/4	14,380	4314	18,694	61/6	9591	2877	12,468	33.3	6226
Cytology	65/ 5.0	4820	1446	6266	30/ 12	2256	677	2933	53.2	3333
Histology	228/ 1.6	1263	379	1642	15/ 24	35	26	111	932.0	1531
Immunology	66/ 5.5	15,919	4776	20,695	30/ 12	7301	2190	9491	54.1	11,204
Hematology Coag.	111/ 3.3	28,300	8490	36,3790	37/ 10	9334	2800	12,134	67.0	24,656
Microbiology	64/ 5.7	17,286	5165	22,471	30/ 12	8138	2441	10,579	53.0	11,892
Phlebotomy	94/ 3.9	19,273	5782	25,054	15/ 24	3139	942	4031	83.7	20,973
Urinalysis	182/ 2.0	22,400	6720	29,120	30/ 12	3798	1139	4937	83.0	24,183
Totals	76/ 4.8	165,646	49,694	215,340	32/ 11.5	68,995	20,698	89,693	58.3	125,647

Total holding cost savings $28,996

Total reduced working capital requirement $96,651

[Total inv. value (existing) − total inv. value (revised)]

FIGURE 35-18. Comparative financial analysis—inventory.

necessity of carrying the entire inventory in a stockroom environment and subjecting it to routine physical inventories. As such, this system would control unofficial inventory efficiently.

Use the existing stockroom space in the clinical laboratory for controlling only class A inventory items common to more than one department. To the extent that inventories become more visible, they are more readily controllable and accountable. Although it is apparent that the concepts of keeping an inventory and controlling certain items exist within the current stockroom environment, in essence the wrong items are being inventoried. ABC analysis would identify items that should be maintained within this stockroom environment. Class A inventory should turn so rapidly that creating it as an asset would be of little significance.

In summary, effective inventory management is a strategy for containing costs. If we worked in a perfect world in which a back door to the laboratory led to a supply house containing any and all supply items used by the laboratory, this chapter would not be necessary. However, we do not work in a perfect world, so attention to the inherent costs associated with inventory management and strategies for reducing these costs are essential.

ANNOTATED BIBLIOGRAPHY

Astor SD: Loss Prevention: Controls and Concepts. Los Angeles, Security World Publishing, 1978
> This text covers basic principles of loss prevention, including employee involvement and methods of distribution center security.

Baer DM, Hawkins B, Tymoshuk P, Washington R: Inventory control and purchasing at reduced cost. MLO 26(11):42–46, 1994
> This reference article describes a comprehensive program of inventory control, storage supervision, and purchasing. An inventory management specialist and a supply technician are assigned to the laboratory. Using a bar code inventory system and a computer, inventory data are maintained, and a list of orders to be placed is generated. Monthly reports showing turnover of items, dollar value of inventory, and the delay time in filling orders are provided to laboratory managers.

Bickford GR: The vendor/laboratory manager relationship: Some practical negotiation tips. Clin Lab Mgmt Rev 7:328–334, 1993
> This article encourages laboratory managers to negotiate with vendors on more than just the purchase price of supplies and equipment. Suggestions include free financing, on-site training, and off-site educational opportunities.

Compton HK: Supplies and Materials Management, 2nd ed. Estover, England, MacDonald & Evans, 1979
> A complete discussion of the maintenance of inventory and supplies is covered in this basic reference. Of particular interest are Chapters 5, 7, 9, and 10, addressing the ABC classification, storage cycle, supply flow patterns, and economic order quantity, respectively.

Larson SE: Inventory Systems and Controls Handbook. Englewood Cliffs, Prentice-Hall, 1976
> While written primarily for industry, this text has many ideas and solutions with regard to inventory maintenance that can be used in the clinical laboratory. Chapter 9 covers aspects of "what" and "when" to order. Chapter 12 describes methods for reducing the costs of material receiving, handling, and stocking.

Spechler JW: Administering the Company Warehouse and Inventory Function. Englewood Cliffs, Prentice-Hall, 1975
> This is a practical "how to" book written with a building-block approach to the study of inventory control and cost containment. Chapter 11 deals with inventory control planning, providing examples and discussion of many of the concepts covered in laboratory inventory control.

Stafford AC: Inventory control through focus forecasting. MLO 17(10):49–53, 1985
> This reference article describes four different strategies for inventory management based on the prior-use data: A—the same volume is anticipated as in prior 3 months; B—the same volume is anticipated as in the same 3 months last year; C—a 10% increase in volume is predicted for the next 3 months; and D—a 50% increase in volume is forecast for the next 3 months.

Index

Note: Page numbers followed by f indicate figures; those followed by t indicate tables.